"Long after we're gone, this information will still
be here for those who come next. In that sense,
it is timeless. This planet will continue to present challenges,
often in the form of pathogens and other toxic troublemakers,
to the people living on it. The human body will continue
to hold the capacity for healing—if the coming generations
know how to tap into its cleansing rhythms."

— Anthony William, Medical Medium

"*Anthony's books are revolutionary yet practical. For anybody frustrated by the current limits of Western medicine, this is definitely worth your time and consideration.*"

— James Van Der Beek, creator, executive producer, and star of *What Would Diplo Do?* and star of *Pose* and *Dawson's Creek*, and Kimberly Van Der Beek, public speaker and activist

"*Anthony is a great man. His knowledge is fascinating and has been very helpful for me. The celery juice alone is a game changer!*"

— Calvin Harris, producer, DJ, and Grammy-winning artist

"*I am so grateful to Anthony. After introducing his celery juice protocol into my daily routine, I have seen a marked improvement in every aspect of my health.*"

— Debra Messing, Emmy-winning star of *Will & Grace*

"*My family and friends have been the recipients of Anthony's inspired gift of healing, and we've benefited more than I can express with rejuvenated physical and mental health.*"

— Scott Bakula, producer and star of *NCIS: New Orleans*; Golden Globe–winning star of *Quantum Leap* and *Star Trek: Enterprise*

"*Anthony has dedicated his life to helping others find the answers that we need to live our healthiest lives. And celery juice is the most accessible way to start!*"

— Courteney Cox, star of *Cougar Town* and *Friends*

"*Anthony is not only a warm, compassionate healer, he is also authentic and accurate, with God-given skills. He has been a total blessing in my life.*"

— Naomi Campbell, model, actress, activist

"*Anthony's extensive knowledge and deep intuition have demystified even the most confounding health issues. He has provided a clear path for me to feel my very best— I find his guidance indispensable.*"

— Taylor Schilling, star of *Orange Is the New Black*

"*We are incredibly grateful for Anthony and his passionate dedication to spreading the word about healing through food. Anthony has a truly special gift. His practices have entirely reshaped our perspectives about food and ultimately our lifestyle. Celery juice alone has completely transformed the way we feel and it will always be a part of our morning routine.*"

— Hunter Mahan, 6-time PGA Tour–winning golfer

"Anthony William is changing and saving the lives of people all over the world with his one-of-a-kind gift. His constant dedication and vast amount of highly advanced information have broken the barriers that block so many in the world from receiving desperately needed truths that science and research have not yet discovered. On a personal level, he has helped both my daughters and me, giving us tools to support our health that actually work. Celery juice is now a part of our regular routine!"

— Lisa Rinna, star of *The Real Housewives of Beverly Hills* and *Days of Our Lives*, *New York Times* best-selling author, designer of the Lisa Rinna Collection

"Anthony is a truly generous person with keen intuition and knowledge about health. I have seen firsthand the transformation he's made in people's quality of life."

— Carla Gugino, star of *Jett, The Haunting of Hill House, Watchmen, Entourage, Spy Kids*

"I've been following Anthony for a while now and am always floored (but not surprised) at the success stories from people following his protocols . . . I have been on my own path of healing for many years, jumping from doctor to doctor and specialist to specialist. He's the real deal and I trust him and his vast knowledge of how the thyroid works and the true effects food has on our body. I have directed countless friends, family, and followers to Anthony because I truly believe he possesses knowledge that no doctor out there has. I am a believer and on a true path to healing now and am honored to know him and blessed to know his work. Every endocrinologist needs to read his book on the thyroid!"

— Marcela Valladolid, chef, author, television host

"What if someone could simply touch you and tell you what it is that ails you? Welcome to the healing hands of Anthony William—a modern-day alchemist who very well may hold the key to longevity. His lifesaving advice blew into my world like a healing hurricane, and he has left a path of love and light in his wake. He is hands down the ninth wonder of the world."

— Lisa Gregorisch-Dempsey, *Extra* Senior Executive Producer

"Anthony William's God-given gift for healing is nothing short of miraculous."

— David James Elliott, *Spinning Out, Trumbo, Mad Men, CSI: NY*; star for ten years of *JAG*

"I am a doctor's daughter who has always relied on Western medicine to ameliorate even the smallest of woes. Anthony's insights opened my eyes to the healing benefits of food and how a more holistic approach to health can change your life."

— Jenny Mollen, actress and *New York Times* best-selling author of *I Like You Just the Way I Am*

"Anthony William is a gift to humanity. His incredible work has helped millions of people heal when conventional medicine had no answers for them. His genuine passion and commitment for helping people is unsurpassed, and I am grateful to have been able to share a small part of his powerful message in *Heal*."

— Kelly Noonan Gores, writer, director, and producer of the *Heal* documentary

"Anthony William is one of those rare individuals who uses his gifts to help people rise up to meet their full potential by becoming their own best health advocates . . . I witnessed Anthony's greatness in action firsthand when I attended one of his thrilling live events. I equate how spot-on his readings were with a singer hitting all the high notes. But beyond the high notes, Anthony's truly compassionate soul is what left the audience captivated. Anthony William is someone I am now proud to call a friend, and I can tell you that the person you hear on the podcasts and whose words fill the pages of best-selling books is the same person who reaches out to loved ones simply to lend support. This is not an act! Anthony William is the real deal, and the gravity of the information he shares through Spirit is priceless and empowering and much needed in this day and age!"

— Debbie Gibson, Broadway star, iconic singer-songwriter

"I had the pleasure of working with Anthony William when he came to Los Angeles and shared his story on Extra. What a fascinating interview as he left the audience wanting to hear more . . . people went crazy for him! His warm personality and big heart are obvious. Anthony has dedicated his life to helping people through the knowledge he receives from Spirit, and he shares all of that information through his Medical Medium books, which are life changing. Anthony William is one of a kind!"

— Sharon Levin, *Extra* Senior Producer

"Anthony William has a remarkable gift! I will always be grateful to him for discovering an underlying cause of several health issues that had bothered me for years. With his kind support, I see improvements every day. I think he is a fabulous resource!"

— Morgan Fairchild, actress, author, speaker

"Within the first three minutes of speaking with me, Anthony precisely identified my medical issue! This healer really knows what he's talking about. Anthony's abilities as the Medical Medium are unique and fascinating."

— Alejandro Junger, M.D., *New York Times* best-selling author of *Clean*, *Clean Eats*, *Clean Gut*, and *Clean 7* and founder of the acclaimed Clean Program

"Anthony's gift has made him a conduit for information that is light-years ahead of where science is today."

— Christiane Northrup, M.D., *New York Times* best-selling author of *Goddesses Never Age*, *The Wisdom of Menopause*, and *Women's Bodies, Women's Wisdom*

"Since reading Medical Medium Thyroid Healing, I have expanded my approach and treatments of thyroid disease and am seeing enormous value for patients. The results are rewarding and gratifying."

— Prudence Hall, M.D., founder and medical director of The Hall Center

"How very much we have been moved and benefited from the discovery of Anthony and the Compassion Spirit, who can reach us with healing wisdom through Anthony's sensitive genius and caring mediumship. His book is truly 'wisdom of the future,' so already now, miraculously, we have the clear, accurate explanation of the many mysterious illnesses that the ancient Buddhist medical texts predicted would afflict us in this era when over-clever people have tampered with the elements of life in the pursuit of profit."

— Robert Thurman, Jey Tsong Khapa Professor of Indo-Tibetan Buddhist Studies, Columbia University; President, Tibet House US; best-selling author of *Love Your Enemies* and *Inner Revolution*; host of *Bob Thurman Podcast*

"Anthony William is the gifted Medical Medium who has very real and not-so-radical solutions to the mysterious conditions that affect us all in our modern world. I am beyond thrilled to know him personally and count him as a most valuable resource for my health protocols and those for my entire family."

— Annabeth Gish, *The Haunting of Hill House*, *The X-Files*, *The West Wing*, *Mystic Pizza*

"Anthony William has devoted his life to helping people with information that has truly made a substantial difference in the lives of many."

— Amanda de Cadenet, founder and CEO of The Conversation and the Girlgaze Project; author of *It's Messy* and *#girlgaze*

"I love Anthony William! My daughters Sophia and Laura gave me his book for my birthday, and I couldn't put it down. The Medical Medium has helped me connect all the dots on my quest to achieve optimal health. Through Anthony's work, I realized the residual Epstein-Barr left over from a childhood illness was sabotaging my health years later. Medical Medium has transformed my life."

— Catherine Bach, *The Young and the Restless*, *The Dukes of Hazzard*

"My recovery from a traumatic spinal crisis several years ago had been steady, but I was still experiencing muscle weakness, a tapped-out nervous system, as well as extra weight. A dear friend called me one evening and strongly recommended I read the book *Medical Medium* by Anthony William. So much of the information in the book resonated with me that I began incorporating some of the ideas, then I sought and was lucky enough to get a consultation. The reading was so spot-on, it has taken my healing to an unimagined, deeper, and richer level of health. My weight has dropped healthily, I can enjoy bike riding and yoga, I'm back in the gym, I have steady energy, and I sleep deeply. Every morning when following my protocols, I smile and say, 'Whoa, Anthony William! I thank you for your restorative gift . . . Yes!'"

— Robert Wisdom, *Ballers*, *The Alienist*, *Rosewood*, *Nashville*, *The Wire*, *Ray*

"In this world of confusion, with constant noise in the health and wellness field, I rely on Anthony's profound authenticity. His miraculous, true gift rises above it all to a place of clarity."

— Patti Stanger, host of *Million Dollar Matchmaker*

"I rely on Anthony William for my and my family's health. Even when doctors are stumped, Anthony always knows what the problem is and the pathway for healing."

— Chelsea Field, *NCIS: New Orleans, Secrets and Lies, Without a Trace, The Last Boy Scout*

"Anthony William brings a dimension to medicine that deeply expands our understanding of the body and of ourselves. His work is part of a new frontier in healing, delivered with compassion and with love."

— Marianne Williamson, #1 *New York Times* best-selling author of *Healing the Soul of America*, *The Age of Miracles*, and *A Return to Love*

"Anthony William is a generous and compassionate guide. He has devoted his life to supporting people on their healing path."

— Gabrielle Bernstein, #1 *New York Times* best-selling author of *The Universe Has Your Back, Judgment Detox*, and *Miracles Now*

"Information that WORKS. That's what I think of when I think of Anthony William and his profound contributions to the world. Nothing made this fact so clear to me as seeing him work with an old friend who had been struggling for years with illness, brain fog, and fatigue. She had been to countless doctors and healers and had gone through multiple protocols. Nothing worked. Until Anthony talked to her, that is . . . from there, the results were astounding. I highly recommend his books, lectures, and consultations. Don't miss this healing opportunity!"

— Nick Ortner, *New York Times* best-selling author of *The Tapping Solution for Manifesting Your Greatest Self* and *The Tapping Solution*

"Esoteric talent is only a complete gift when it's shared with moral integrity and love. Anthony William is a divine combination of healing, giftedness, and ethics. He's a real-deal healer who does his homework and shares it in true service to the world."

— Danielle LaPorte, best-selling author of *White Hot Truth* and *The Desire Map*

"Anthony is a seer and a wellness sage. His gift is remarkable. With his guidance I've been able to pinpoint and address a health issue that's been plaguing me for years."

— Kris Carr, *New York Times* best-selling author of *Crazy Sexy Juice*, *Crazy Sexy Kitchen*, and *Crazy Sexy Diet*

"Twelve hours after receiving a heaping dose of self-confidence masterfully administered by Anthony, the persistent ringing in my ears of the last year . . . began to falter. I am astounded, grateful, and happy for the insights offered on moving forward."

— Mike Dooley, *New York Times* best-selling author of *Infinite Possibilities* and scribe of *Notes from the Universe*

"Whenever Anthony William recommends a natural way of improving your health, it works. I've seen this with my daughter, and the improvement was impressive. His approach of using natural ingredients is a more effective way of healing."

— Martin D. Shafiroff, financial advisor, past recipient of #1 Broker in America ranking by WealthManagement.com and #1 Wealth Advisor ranking by Barron's

"Anthony William's invaluable advice on preventing and combating disease is years ahead of what's available anywhere else."

— Richard Sollazzo, M.D., New York board-certified oncologist, hematologist, nutritionist, and anti-aging expert and author of *Balance Your Health*

"Anthony William is the Edgar Cayce of our time, reading the body with outstanding precision and insight. Anthony identifies the underlying causes of diseases that often baffle the most astute conventional and alternative health-care practitioners. Anthony's practical and profound advice makes him one of the most powerfully effective healers of the 21st century."

— Ann Louise Gittleman, *New York Times* best-selling author of over 30 books on health and healing and creator of the highly popular Fat Flush detox and diet plan

"As a Hollywood businesswoman, I know value. Some of Anthony's clients spent over $1 million seeking help for their 'mystery illness' until they finally discovered him."

— Nanci Chambers, co-star of *JAG*; Hollywood producer and entrepreneur

"I had a health reading from Anthony, and he accurately told me things about my body only known to me. This kind, sweet, hilarious, self-effacing, and generous man— also so 'otherworldly' and so extraordinarily gifted, with an ability that defies how we see the world—has shocked even me, a medium! He is truly our modern-day Edgar Cayce, and we are immensely blessed that he is with us. Anthony William proves that we are more than we know."

— Colette Baron-Reid, best-selling author of *Uncharted* and TV host of *Messages from Spirit*

"Any quantum physicist will tell you there are things at play in the universe we can't yet understand. I truly believe Anthony has a handle on them. He has an amazing gift for intuitively tapping into the most effective methods for healing."

— Caroline Leavitt, *New York Times* best-selling author of *With or Without You*, *Is This Tomorrow*, and *Pictures of You*

MEDICAL MEDIUM

CLEANSE
TO HEAL

ALSO BY ANTHONY WILLIAM

*Medical Medium: Secrets Behind Chronic and Mystery Illness
and How to Finally Heal*

*Medical Medium Life-Changing Foods: Save Yourself and the Ones You Love
with the Hidden Healing Powers of Fruits & Vegetables*

*Medical Medium Thyroid Healing: The Truth behind Hashimoto's, Graves',
Insomnia, Hypothyroidism, Thyroid Nodules & Epstein-Barr*

*Medical Medium Liver Rescue: Answers to Eczema, Psoriasis, Diabetes,
Strep, Acne, Gout, Bloating, Gallstones, Adrenal Stress, Fatigue,
Fatty Liver, Weight Issues, SIBO & Autoimmune Disease*

*Medical Medium Celery Juice: The Most Powerful Medicine of
Our Time Healing Millions Worldwide*

All of the above are available at your local bookstore, or may be ordered by visiting:

Hay House USA: www.hayhouse.com®

Hay House Australia: www.hayhouse.com.au

Hay House UK: www.hayhouse.co.uk

Hay House India: www.hayhouse.co.in

MEDICAL MEDIUM

CLEANSE TO HEAL

HEALING PLANS FOR SUFFERERS OF ANXIETY, DEPRESSION, ACNE, ECZEMA, LYME, GUT PROBLEMS, BRAIN FOG, WEIGHT ISSUES, MIGRAINES, BLOATING, VERTIGO, PSORIASIS, CYSTS, FATIGUE, PCOS, FIBROIDS, UTI, ENDOMETRIOSIS & AUTOIMMUNE

ANTHONY WILLIAM

Published in the United States by: Hay House, Inc.: www.hayhouse.com®
Published in Australia by: Hay House Australia Pty. Ltd.: www.hayhouse.com.au
Published in the United Kingdom by: Hay House UK, Ltd.: www.hayhouse.co.uk
Published in India by: Hay House Publishers India: www.hayhouse.co.in

Cover and interior illustration design: Vibodha Clark
Interior design: Charles McStravick
Indexer: Jay Kreider

Cataloging-in-Publication Data is on file at the Library of Congress

Hardcover ISBN: 978-1-4019-5845-9
E-book ISBN: 978-1-4019-5846-6
Audiobook ISBN: 978-1-4019-6160-2

10 9 8 7 6 5 4 3 2 1
1st edition, May 2020

Printed in the United States of America

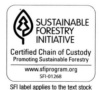

SUSTAINABLE FORESTRY INITIATIVE
Certified Chain of Custody
Promoting Sustainable Forestry
www.sfiprogram.org
SFI-01268

SFI label applies to the text stock

For the underdogs.

This is a message for the people
who are struggling and trying to heal.
My job is to look out for the underdogs
who have been through hell and back.
Think of the living words here as your refuge.

As someone who has suffered or been close
to someone suffering, you hold true clarity.
You deserve to trust yourself again.
You deserve to respect yourself again. It's time.

— Anthony William, Medical Medium

CONTENTS

"Be proud of using your free will to make your own choice to work on your healing. Have compassion for yourself and know that your suffering is not your fault. Your struggles are not your fault. You're accomplishing great things every single hour and day as you work on your healing process with the powerful tools in this book. I believe you can heal. More than believe—I know."

— Anthony William, Medical Medium

FOREWORD

"Have you got any more wild blueberries?" That's what I heard behind me in an aisle of a Whole Foods store. Having just put several packs into my own cart, I was curious about who else might be a fan, so I turned around— just in time to hear the clerk say, "No, I don't think so" to a very disappointed woman. I let the woman know that there were, in fact, still more and offered to show her where they were. As we walked, I asked if she was looking for them because she was following the Medical Medium. Her face excitedly lit up. "Yes! I'm visiting for a few days and can't be without my Heavy Metal Detox Smoothie!"

My encounters with people whose lives have benefited from the Medical Medium's information are becoming more and more frequent, and each one continues to make me smile. Several times a week, I hear from patients, colleagues, friends, and neighbors about the hope, knowledge, and healing tools that Anthony William has given them through his books and online presence. One of my favorite examples is a sign I recently saw in the local health food store: "Due to the high demand for celery, the price has gone up." Why the high demand? Simply put, it's because more and more people are going beyond just talking about improving their health and are actually taking steps to do so.

As a physician, I've always been driven by the idea of proactive prevention, and I encourage my patients, as I do with my own family, to learn as much as they can about their own health, become their own advocates, and be open to both traditional and nontraditional approaches. This means not giving up or waiting around for a condition to get worse. It means looking beyond a medication-only treatment, with the goal of understanding and addressing the root causes of a health concern. It means incorporating impactful, natural healing options with fewer potential side effects. And it means learning about therapies that may not be mainstream or well documented by researchers yet, but that are still benefiting people on a widespread level. A preventative mind-set takes action early.

Anthony's approach has resonated with me from the moment I was introduced to his work, first from his books and then as we collaborated on several treatment plans. I initially wondered if I was drawn to his advice because of my love for fruit, which, rather than vilifying, Anthony values highly and encourages people to consume. But it goes much further than our shared admiration for apples. To me, his insight makes sense. If you've been following him, you know he has been prolific in bringing to light the health burden from chronic infections (such as viruses) and chemical exposures (such as heavy metals). His tools to address these concerns have been a game changer in what I've been able to offer to my patients as part of a treatment plan.

As a specialist in the field of Physiatry (Physical Medicine and Rehabilitation) and Functional Medicine, for more than 25 years I have focused on improving the lives of people who have lost their optimal function due to injury, illness, or trauma. It starts by understanding each person's own unique and often complex story of how they got to their current state of health. Then it's recognizing, within those complexities, what kinds of root causes may be contributing to their story. There are essentially four major root cause categories that contribute to the majority of health conditions, and most of them are well within our power to address. They are: infections, toxic exposures, stress/ trauma (both physical and psychological), and severe deficiencies (malnutrition, dehydration, sleep deprivation, isolation from nature or from others, immobility). And when the body is constantly on guard trying to repair and protect itself from these factors, it goes on high alert, and we feel it. The result could be pain, inflammation, fatigue, or any of the many symptoms that leave us feeling that something's wrong.

Looking at a problem from this perspective explains why many chronic illnesses don't get better, even when patients have tried a variety of medications or surgeries.

Having a plan that includes removing or reducing the root causes and risk factors,

along with strategies to help the body heal and increase resilience, is when people start to reclaim their health. Self-care approaches play a big part in this kind of plan.

Now, here's where the dilemma lies. A self-care plan is often the part of the medical prescription that gets forgotten. And even if it is addressed, questions often arise. Where do you start? What's important? How extensive an approach or how radical a change is needed to make a strong impact? How do you implement it so it fits into your daily life? That's where *Cleanse to Heal* comes in.

As you read through *Cleanse to Heal*, you'll be amazed by the amount of information Anthony William shares. He starts with a detailed explanation about toxins, what they are, where we're exposed to them, how they affect us, how our body is designed to effectively deal with them, and why it often fails to do so. He then delves into what it means to cleanse, which is like a chance to hit a reset button and start at a fresh, new physiological baseline. He also discusses other popular philosophies and how they compare and contrast with his.

Then come his cleanses! The 3:6:9 Cleanse that has been changing lives worldwide is deconstructed in depth and reconstructed into three different versions, including simplified and advanced ones. Even more cleanse options, all true to his principles, focus on more targeted strategies. Down to their core, the cleanses illuminate the power of the food we choose to eat: not only the *kinds* of foods, but the ways we combine them and when we eat them. And just when you think you couldn't possibly learn any more, Anthony gives you a giant toolbox with suggestions for condition-specific supplements (herbs, vitamins, minerals).

The food-based strategies (including recipes), the supplement options, the spiritual wisdom, the empowering advocacy, the whys, the dos and don'ts, the troubleshooting advice, and the deeply compassionate soul that this information comes from make *Cleanse to Heal* the Medical Medium's ultimate resource.

I am honored to write this foreword for Anthony William. I do so in reverence to my father, whose devastating battle with lung cancer, just over two decades ago, awakened me to the realities and limitations of the traditional medical model. My brother and I had spent countless hours in a frantic search for lifesaving information, and I was astounded to learn that holistic approaches and alternative therapies were helping people around the world, yet were never mentioned to my father as options. This also made me realize that his "preventive care" (which consisted of diagnostic screenings and medications to treat symptoms) hadn't actually addressed his root-cause risks. Those insights, along with seeing this resilient, strong man feeling helpless, completely shifted the way I thought about medicine and what medical care needs to include to help keep chronic illnesses from destroying lives.

We can't control what kind of toxins or stressors we were exposed to in the past and we may not always be able to control the kinds of environments we are currently or will be in, but taking actions to minimize their impact is very much within our control. Giving us powerful tools to do so is the gift that Anthony William has been sharing with the world!

— Ilana Zablozki-Amir, M.D., dipABPMR, IFMCP

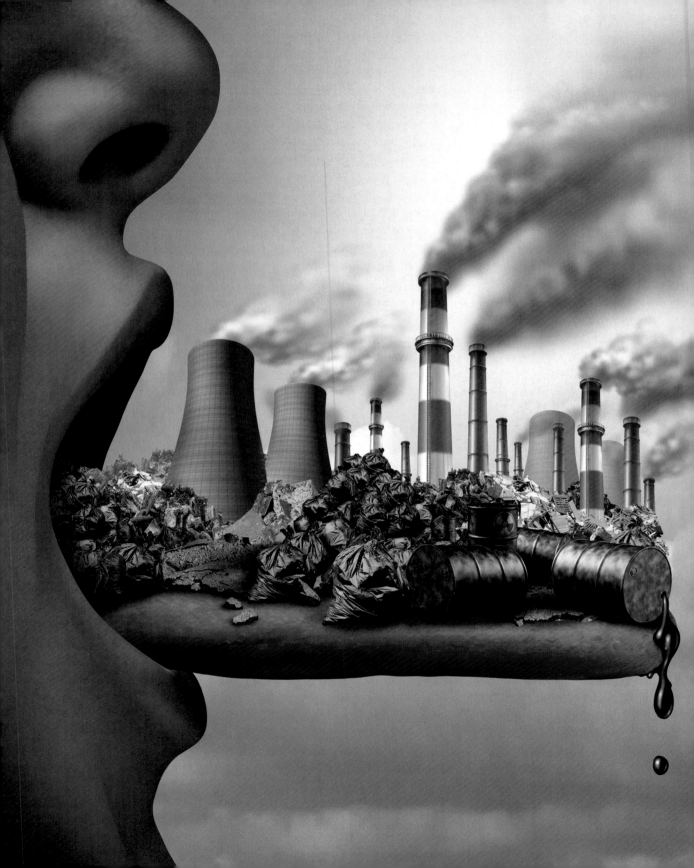

PART I

WE NEED TO CLEANSE

"Chronic illness is growing at an alarming rate.
Even with the massive amounts of organic food being
cultivated now, even with the awareness about removing processed
foods from our diets, even with the newest healing modalities,
sickness is present like never before. No one is escaping illness,
not unless they have the right information to
stop the ticking clock."

"This is not a lifestyle book. It's a lifetime book.
In a sea of false truths, this is about saving lives."

— Anthony William, Medical Medium

CHAPTER 1

Cleanses from Above

The cleanses in this book come from above. They are not man-made. They are from a higher source.

Cleansing is truth, a truth you're about to embark on as you read further. Whatever you believe in, whether God, the Universe, the Light, or the Creator—or if you believe in nothing at all, that we're just floating through space together on this rock—know that the information about cleansing in this book is separate from all the other noise out there. It comes from a different place. It's not jumbled misinformation or gathered bits and pieces of gimmicky confusion. This is real and it works.

It's also needed with urgency on this earth. Chronic illness is growing at an alarming rate. Even with the massive amounts of organic food being cultivated now, even with the awareness about removing processed foods from our diets, even with the newest healing modalities, sickness is present like never before. No one is escaping illness, not unless they have the right information to stop the ticking clock.

It takes a force greater than us, a helping hand from above.

AN ARMY IN HIDING

What if I told you that there are thousands of people hiding away from the world? What if I told you that it's really hundreds of thousands? What if I told you that it's really millions? People who use what little life force they have left to pick up what they need from the store on off hours, when they know it won't be crowded. People who don't go out for a lighthearted dinner and a movie because they don't feel well enough. People who miss their best friend's birthday party, engagement party, bachelor or bachelorette party, wedding, and baby shower—they miss it all—because they aren't up to it. They don't even have enough energy to shop for a card. Do you think there's just a handful of these people? There's a whole army of them.

Many of them have found the advanced healing information in this book series and begun their healing process, and are recovering enough to reenter the world. Many more have not yet found this information. I call the chronically ill the forgotten souls. It's one thing to ignore them. It's another to forget they exist. Because they have to live their lives in a

3

way that doesn't draw attention—sometimes they don't even have the energy to converse if given the opportunity—we're not reminded of them as we go about our days.

Or they're just barely able to function in the world, sitting in the cubicle next to us at work or showing up at school drop-off and pickup, prompting us to believe everything is fine. When we see them, it can look like nothing's wrong. "Well, you look good," we may say to a friend who's struggling, thinking we're being helpful. What we can't see are the pain, dizziness, body temperature fluctuations, burning sensations, anxiety, depression, troubling thoughts, fears, brain fog, and fatigue with no answers in sight. We can't see our friend's mind taken over by doctors' appointments and worries about how she's going to find the resources to sustain herself. We can't see her need to be validated and accepted right where she is in this moment, while being encouraged that someday it will get better.

Whether we offer them witness or not, the army is out there. Whether we respect them, ignore them, or forget them, there are far more people physically and mentally suffering today than there were 30 years ago, 10 years ago, or even 5 years ago.

ACTUAL AWARENESS

No one is safe from becoming ill. With what we're up against in today's world and what that's doing to our bodies, nobody is guaranteed that one day down the road, they won't develop their first set of symptoms when they least expect it. This knowledge is not about living in fear. It's about not living in denial.

How many people do you know who struggle with their health? Chances are, whether they show it or not, most of the people in your life do. And chances are, you're one of them—whether you're dealing with acid reflux, high blood pressure, anxiety, eczema, psoriasis, brain fog, depression, or fatigue. You're far from alone. Living with symptoms has become the new normal.

Much of the time, people coexist with their ailments, accepting them and never questioning why science hasn't offered answers, as suffering has become the status quo. Sometimes, though—an increasing amount of the time now—people's symptoms start to impede their quality of life. They start to lose joys and privileges. They join the hidden army of those stuck at home or even in the hospital with mystery health issues. As they consult doctor after doctor and expert after expert and have trouble functioning on a day-to-day basis, their spark starts to go. They lose hope.

Awareness is a term we all use now. It's supposed to mean a lot. Heralded and exalted as a powerful and empowering word, it's supposed to attune us to our feet on the ground and the people we spend our time with and to help us through our days. What's awareness, though, if we're not becoming aware of what's really happening inside of us? If we're not becoming aware of the truth that we're more and more challenged by symptoms, conditions, and illness as we go through our lives?

It can seem as though everyone is a health expert these days, sharing their opinions of what works for them or what hasn't worked for them. That's easy to do when we're not chronically ill and remain unaware of what can go wrong. When we're 20 years old and making our shakes with protein powder or almond butter, or eating high protein and cutting out grains, and we're sharing on social media about how we're feeling pretty good, that represents one moment in time. Even as we're feeling indestructible, sharing about the energetic shifts we've felt with our trendy diet and exercise routine, we don't realize what could be developing within—going awry along the way—and what we could be facing in the future. New exposures or existing ones that have been causing problems out of sight could, down the road, lead to myalgic encephalomyelitis/chronic fatigue syndrome (ME/CFS), or any of a host of other symptoms and conditions—if we don't have true awareness of what creates these problems.

IS CLEANSING A MYTH?

A rising belief in the health world is that we don't need to take special detox measures because the body does so naturally. Some health professionals even go further, saying that cleanses don't actually cleanse us. This is just backlash from the cleanses of the past (and present) that weren't good for us—the reckless cleansing business of powders, books, and programs that weren't built around how the body works or what the body needs. And so dieticians, nutritionists, and other practitioners try to safeguard their patients' health by teaching them that the body's natural cleansing processes are enough, not realizing that they're not fully informed in their advice; they haven't received complete training in how the body works when it comes to detox.

What the experts don't understand is that we're not only up against daily toxins. We're up against pathogens: viruses and bacteria that are rapidly moving through the population, causing autoimmune diagnoses and more in people all the way from children to the elderly. We're up against toxic heavy metals, pesticides, herbicides, solvents, petroleum-based products, and other modern-day chemical warfare that's subliminally part of our everyday lives.

The experts who claim we don't need to detox also don't understand that the high-fat diets most everyone eats—in whatever shape those diets come, whether no-rules standard eating; "balanced" diets of moderation; intuitive eating; trendy paleo or keto; or plant-based approaches that emphasize nut butters, oils, and soy—don't allow for the natural processes of detox that professionals say happen on their own. Fat thickens the blood, and that inhibits the body's day-to-day cleansing ability. Many influencers, dieticians, nutritionists, health coaches, doctors, and other health professionals even recommend high-protein diets, not realizing that high protein automatically means high fat because peanut butter, nuts, salmon, eggs, and chicken contain ample amounts of fat, and that with this advice, they are inhibiting the very detox processes they say should be enough to get us by in life.

We can't have it both ways. We can't tell people to fill the bloodstream with fat, creating an inability for the liver to naturally release poisons on a daily basis, and also say that we don't need to embark on cleanses and detoxes. As healthy as a recommended diet may seem because it cuts out fast foods, fried foods, and processed foods, if it emphasizes fat and protein—no matter if it's animal protein based or plant based, whether it's called keto, paleo, vegan, or some new term—it is going to make the liver sluggish with its overload of fat.

In all this confusion, people need at least the sound information that keeping the blood thinner with more fruits, vegetables, and leafy greens and lower fat is the only way to stand a chance of detoxing the toxins our bodies create as natural byproduct and waste from their internal processes, never mind detoxing the outside toxins we're exposed to on a daily basis.

When the liver is sluggish from fat, the heart must pump harder. A fat-filled bloodstream also minimizes oxygen, allowing pathogens to thrive. Plus toxins enter the excess fat cells, which then accumulate around organs once someone reaches the age when they can't spend two hours a day exercising like they used to—and when keeping processed foods out isn't enough to keep a spare tire from developing around the waist. Health experts don't realize this epidemic of sluggish livers is happening, so "slow metabolism" and hormones take the blame instead of a high-fat diet over too many years.

What's worse is this: too often, influencers and health professionals who make pronouncements that try to debunk the "myth" of cleansing don't understand the struggle of someone who has been chronically ill. They don't get what it is to go from doctor to doctor and receive diagnosis after diagnosis—or non-diagnosis after non-diagnosis—and still have no answers about how to feel better. These are people who truly need to detox. They need to know the truth about pathogens and toxic heavy metals and how to eliminate them from the body in order to recover from their chronic symptoms and suffering.

Imagine what it is to be someone with a chronic illness—or maybe you already know all too well. What is that like to see on your social media stream someone who can work out for an hour or two a day and has no visible body fat? What is it like to be told you can attain the very same thing if you get up off the couch, go to the gym, and start making protein shakes like they do? What is it like to be told that if you don't feel well enough to do that, then you must be creating your roadblock with emotional issues and negative thoughts? That you must not be thinking positively enough or engaging with the universe the way you need to be? This is what people are being told. They're being told that they don't need to cleanse; they need to get with the program of mastering their mind. They're being told that they're creating their problems and their illnesses, and that it's their fault. It's making an entire segment of the population—those who are dealing with the reality of chronic symptoms—question their very sanity.

Is cleansing a myth? No. It's a vital tool for anyone concerned about their health. It's a very real technique to fight against the burdens of our modern world, as long as you go about it the right way.

LIFESTYLES OR LIFESAVERS

When cleansing is regarded with a touch more respect, it's still not given its proper due. The trend today is to think of cleansing as short term and therefore less worthy and to think of "lifestyles" as potent somehow, longer term than they really are. "You should be taking on a whole lifestyle," people are told, "in order to make your life better." Lifestyles tend to be image-focused, with the buy-in fairly pain free (if you can afford it). Traditionally, they were material—carry a certain handbag, dress a certain way, drive a certain car—and sometimes centered around a certain hobby or sport. Over time, many lifestyles have shifted toward wellness. Exercise classes such as aerobics were an early trend. Then yoga, Pilates, and spinning, with flashy, healthy-seeming foods or supplements, were incorporated into these lifestyles.

Paradoxically, lifestyles tend to be about quick changes in looks and attitude. They're about building a brand and then calling a brand a lifestyle . . . even though it's inevitable that when people get sick and develop symptoms and conditions that confuse multiple doctors, they'll realize whatever lifestyle they've adopted isn't making the problem go away and didn't prevent it in the first place. Lifestyles are not so much about putting in the work, as far as the true nitty-gritty of cleaning up the body's toxins and pathogens goes. They're more about putting in the work to build a platform and sales to the point that someone's own take on a lifestyle may even become a full-time job. That's a different form of work than digging out the poisons, viruses, and bacteria from the body that will ultimately get you sick years down the road, if they haven't already.

When we're watching a lifestyle in the short term, we can be easily deceived, thinking and trusting that what we're seeing in the moment is truth and not what someone needs to show to protect their brand. If we follow people on social media long term, we will see how things can start to go wrong and opinions can change. If we watch them over the course of 5 or 10 years or even longer, we will see problems develop. Looking back, we could ask, "Why didn't that protein shake with almond butter or gluten-free avocado toast save them from their symptoms?"

The answer: because the lifestyles that people are adopting do not look at the true causes of what's behind chronic illness. Without addressing what's really happening inside our bodies, it's just a game that people are playing, one they've gotten wrapped up in purposely or sucked into innocently. Lifestyles are guessing games—they guess with our health using the massive amount of misinformation that's circulating.

The cleanses in this book, and the cleanses throughout the Medical Medium series, speak to what's truly going wrong inside of our bodies that no trendy lifestyle approach can ever address—because that truth of what's going on inside of us is unknown to the lifestyle creators. In today's world, no matter what lifestyle a person subscribes to, they are still falling ill. People are—forgive the expression—dropping like flies. Symptoms are stopping them in their tracks, bringing them to their knees, and forcing them to redesign their lives around feeling unwell. Even if they subscribe to the best-seeming diet trends and they're making photo-worthy smoothies and meals at home and keeping processed foods out of their diets, they're still coming down with chronic symptoms and disease at a faster rate than ever before in history.

People's lifestyles aren't saving them. Lifestyles don't get to the guts of what's keeping somebody ill. They don't draw from knowledge, insight, and wisdom about what's truly plaguing someone, hindering them from living the life they deserve to be living. They don't look out for the person who has pesticides or toxic heavy metals deep inside their organs or viruses active inside their body or a broken immune system or emotional injury. They don't solve the mystery of why someone is sick at all.

Maybe we're in our mid-30s, sharing photos of our adrenaline highs taken in front of the mirrored walls of the gym or the grassy hills of a running trail. It doesn't mean it's going to stay like this. It doesn't mean that two years later, Hashimoto's thyroiditis isn't going to develop and force us into bed, as it does for thousands of women and men, when everything had seemed like it was going okay. Sharing beautiful images of plates stacked with "balanced" foods doesn't mean that ME/CFS isn't suddenly going to appear.

And if we do go down, forced to second-guess everything we've ever heard, the people who haven't fallen yet will continue to spread misinformation. Rather than doubt their own messages, they'll believe that the predecessor who became ill simply did something wrong or that their body was faulty. The person with Hashimoto's or ME/CFS will all too often be made to feel like a loser or a failure. Maybe they got the diet wrong, the thinking will go. Maybe they have emotional problems and are making up the symptoms or created them by not thinking positively. Maybe it's just who they are.

There's a mentality out there of "the strong will survive," and it can create a feeding frenzy in the healing arts world, with social media fueling it further. The sharks survive, and everybody else becomes bait for the sharks. We forget we're all in this together. We forget we're all potential victims of chronic illness, whether Hashimoto's, ME/CFS, or any of hundreds of other afflictions. Especially when we're younger and haven't experienced health challenges yet, we think we've found the Holy Grail with each newly named trend and lifestyle. We don't realize we're repeating the same mistakes of previous generations over and over, whether we're trying a high-fat, high-protein diet, staying away from fruit, or

exercising fanatically. It doesn't matter what we call it—plant based, paleo, the "new" keto, or high fat. It's so easy to think we know better than the people who've been there, done that, and are suffering.

All of this is nothing compared to where it's headed in a couple of years. It's only going to become a bigger mess. The images we see of what people are doing for their health will only become more alluring and misleading to those who are at the start of their healing journeys, searching for answers to their symptoms and conditions. The promise of a youthful vibrancy will send us to videos and podcasts for all our answers. The potential for misinformation is huge as the people who make the videos and podcasts repeat what their nutritionists or trainers or friends told them, or the theories they read about in articles, and the garbled messages are celebrated as gospel.

People who've been through chronic health problems for months or even years possess a real knowing. Especially those who've tried everything to get better and who've kept on struggling with their symptoms—they are aware that we are each vulnerable, much as the healthy ones may want to believe otherwise. As distancing as it can be for those in pain to watch others seem to live their best lives, that vantage point gives them perspective to understand the tender balance of life. Even if they doubt themselves in the face of so much messaging that they are somehow weak or faulty, they possess a deeper wisdom that can enlighten us all if we listen: nobody who gets sick deserves it; there has to be more to the story.

And there is more to the story. There is so much more to safeguarding your health and healing than we know. There is so much more simplicity to it than we dare to believe.

It takes a measure above a lifestyle in order to solve and remedy these problems. It takes a book with truths and answers and direction to bring us out of the depths of struggle and into the light of healing. So this is not a lifestyle book. It's a lifetime book. This is not about building a brand. It's about building your recovery. This is not about selling you a cleansing product, with clothing to match to create your lifestyle. In a sea of false truths, this is about saving lives.

While each cleanse may seem like a short-term measure, the hard work involved in even the nine-day 3:6:9 Cleanse—the cornerstone of this book—has long-term payoffs. These cleanses are ones you can turn to throughout your life. They are about holding the keys to bring yourself back into health, about rising out of the ashes of suffering no matter what comes your way, about true well-being and real answers for survival here on a planet that can too often be unforgiving. Even 50 years from now, wherever you find yourself, they will be here for you as lifesavers.

SURVIVAL OF THE LESS TOXIC

Here's some perspective for you: whoever is luckiest to be born with the least amount of toxins, and to have the stronger constitution because of that, subsequently does not contract as many viruses along the way in life as others do. Maybe fortunate circumstances mean they have fewer toxic heavy metals in their system than someone else. Maybe the people they come into contact with in relationships have fewer pathogens to share and

pass along. Maybe their family lineage is slightly less toxic because their forebears were raised on farms rather than in cities during the Industrial Revolution, so there were fewer toxins to pass down from generation to generation. Maybe they grew up with substantially reduced stress because they had all the resources they needed and tremendous emotional support from family.

It's not survival of the fittest. It's survival of the ones who come into this world less toxic, with lots of love, support, and resources (it all counts) at the same time—and then happen to stay that way while here on earth. It's the chance of what resources their ancestors had before them, how minimal their ancestors' exposures were, and what privileges they've experienced themselves: love and support to protect their adrenals, less contact with the poisonous matter in our everyday world, and fewer viruses and bacteria in their path. These are the lucky ones who dominate the health movement and social media. Often, they were raised with an abundance of confidence and perhaps even some entitlement, giving advice as though their protein shakes or workout routines are what have protected them and made them money.

Those in this position often say that they work for humanity, for the universe, for the light. They package up their good health and the profits they make with their platforms and try to claim that it's all positivity coming back to them for the good they're doing for humankind. This new technique has the unfortunate effect of making you feel that if you're sick, or not making money, or not able to take care of yourself or rise above your symptoms, then you are not working for good and not useful. An elitist class of the healthy is developing, with the influencers saying they're being rewarded tenfold for their gift to humanity of spreading the word about keto or an exercise regimen as the great epiphany. Again, the millions dealing with very real problems that have not been properly diagnosed, treated, or understood are left to feel that they're not being positive enough or taking the right actions for the universe to reward them. They think less of themselves because what they're being told to do isn't helping at all, which leads them to believe the messages that say they're attracting negativity and creating their own problems. They aren't being told the truth, which is that real physiological causes—viruses and other pathogens, plus toxins and poisons that are stealthily abundant in our world and in our bloodlines—are behind the epidemic of chronic and mystery symptoms.

Only luck has prevented the influencers from struggling in this way. I keep stressing this point because the pernicious assumption that people who haven't been trapped by chronic symptoms simply understand the secrets of life better than those who get sick is so ingrained in our culture that the truth bears repeating (again and again!). If you have ever found yourself lying in bed, scrolling through somebody's feed of waterfalls, beaches, and smoothie bowls with peanut butter, wondering where you went wrong to land yourself on your little mattress island apart from the world, know this: you didn't go wrong. You are not faulty or less-than. The reality is that outside circumstances and inherited poisons and pathogens, not internal weaknesses, determine the challenges we face. There's a generations-long backstory to the health that each of us experiences. The fortunate ones are born with fewer toxins, experience less pharmaceutical injury as young ones, and continue

through life dodging bullets by happenstance. We can't help it if we come into this world with struggling livers or toxic heavy metals from those before us in the bloodline (who couldn't help it either) or if we end up with viral exposures to which we're more vulnerable because a lack of support or financial stability has done a number on our immune system.

Not that our health is a fixed state—not by any means. Just as someone who's been lucky for decades can come up against an exposure that leads to a health challenge at any time, so too can someone who has suffered health challenges change their fate. The key is to know how prevention and healing really work. Before we can grasp whether cleansing is needed or beneficial, or what the right kind of cleansing is, we must recognize this. Otherwise, we're swimming through a sea of confusion, all of it unsubstantiated by medical research and science, and it's virtually impossible to discover the truth.

There's no reason to blame anyone in all of this. We shouldn't begrudge anyone their good health. The influencers are just as scared as the rest of the world, and most of the time, they really do think they're doing good. They don't want to believe that there are as many health threats in our midst as there are, because that kind of hypervigilance is unsettling. And then there are the influencers with health problems who tell everyone what they're doing to manage their symptoms and conditions by shifting foods and exercise routines. While it may give them temporary relief and allow their health issues to ebb and flow or come and go, it may not work for many other people, because it's still a guessing game process that never uncovers the real cause. Only with that true knowledge of the cause can they heal for good and teach others how to rid themselves of symptoms.

What's worse than knowing about the health threats in our world is suffering and not knowing why. It's exhausting trying to discover what works and what doesn't. It's exhausting trying to get results and not seeing them—or getting some results and then losing them. It's exhausting spending exorbitant amounts of money on hope after hope. It can break you down and bewilder you, even if you're on the right track, because there is always another competing claim out there to cast doubt on what you're doing. The chronic fatigue you're trying to alleviate gets compounded by the fatigue of trying to find answers.

When you finally find salvation in information that works, when you finally learn how to use it to move forward and heal, it's a feeling like no other. It's a feeling that does exist and is achievable. You don't even have to have a positive attitude in order to achieve it. You could be cranky, miserable, negative, disheartened, bitter, and even angry and you can still experience it, because when you take the right steps, the body strengthens quickly and helps get you to the finish line of healing.

FOOD WARS

When it comes to information about food, there's a lot of fluff out there. We could even call it smog. That smog is designed to keep people occupied and to obscure the truth—and the food wars are part of that smog.

By "food wars" I mean arguments between opposed food belief systems. You know the type I mean: the claims that this way of eating is better or even morally superior, while that way of eating is silly or ignorant, all of it rooted in guesswork and ideology, not truth. These battles often get in the way of conversations about cleansing. If we're kept busy with resentment toward another group, if we're distracted standing up for our own philosophy while trying to discredit the other side, we'll miss out on what's really happening inside the body, and we'll never take the time to seek out answers.

The most vocal in the food wars are the people who feel the least sick. They're the ones who have the stamina to fight about plant versus animal protein and whole grain versus grain free and removing fruit or allowing only low-glycemic fruit—and have the stamina to attack anyone who doesn't fall into their own belief system. In support of their claims, they tend to spout scientific research studies paid for by sources with vested interests in the outcomes, because they are out of touch with the person who's been to 20 doctors and is still lying in bed with no answers about why they're sick. Perhaps they've experienced small inconsistencies with their health—they've had a little less energy here or there, faced mild acne or eczema, dealt with drawn-out rebound times from workouts, maybe had a cold or cough that stuck around a little too long, or dealt with bloating or a minor digestive issue, so they had to go on a round of antibiotics, any of which can get someone thinking about eating better. Somewhere along the way in their diet research process, they became staunch supporters of a belief system, enough to take up the cause and attack the other side.

Meanwhile, all sides in the food wars are still sick. What the arguments ignore is that millions are still struggling, whether from thyroid disorders, ME/CFS, fibromyalgia, Lyme disease, multiple sclerosis (MS), eczema, psoriasis, acne, endometriosis, polycystic ovary syndrome (PCOS), fibroids, crippling anxiety or depression, or any of hundreds of other diagnoses or non-diagnoses. Just like in any war on this planet, the smog of battle distracts from the suffering of those who don't have the strength to fight.

Balanced Diet, Moderation, and Intuitive Eating

Balanced diet—you'll hear the term everywhere as a guiding principle about how to eat. That's supposed to be the great wisdom about food. Funny thing is, every single person has a different definition of what a balanced diet is, because no one eats exactly the same way.

A "balanced" diet sounds like one that's regulated in some form or fashion to properly care for humans. Think about it, though: What authority actually determines what makes a diet balanced? Is a balanced diet a colorful array of foods? Is it a mix of vegetables, fruits, proteins, and fats? Everyone has a different interpretation. What none of it considers is this: How can we determine if a diet is balanced when we don't know the true cause of autoimmune disease and the hundreds of labels that are given to symptoms and conditions under the autoimmune umbrella? What person, health professional or otherwise, has the right to claim that you're not on a balanced diet, or to offer a balanced diet, when they're in the dark along with the rest of medical research and science as to why someone is sick and how they can recover? It's merely a guessing game of removing processed foods and bringing in vegetables, nuts, and seeds, and that's not an answer. Before anyone can

weigh in with authority on a balanced diet, they need to understand chronic illness.

Everyone has a different emotional connection or disconnection to their food. They eat what they *think* is a healthy diet, not realizing that the "everything in moderation" advice they grew up with has made their food choices *too* varied, making too much room for troublemaker foods on their plate and not leaving enough room for nutrient-dense options. Or they make a point on social media of shunning a certain food in the name of a more balanced diet, not mentioning to their crowd that the real reason they avoid, say, fruit or potatoes is because someone they knew used to say (mistakenly) that "sugar is sugar" whenever they reached for any form of carbohydrate—and so they've felt guilty about even healthy carbs ever since. People are constantly changing their approaches to food, sometimes on a monthly basis, because they're constantly in search of the right way to eat. Those who claim, "I intuitively eat; that's how I stay healthy" eventually get sick all the same. "My body feels like it really needs these eggs," for example, falls under the category of justifying cravings without knowing how those foods affect your health. Eating "intuitively" doesn't mean that you know what causes your symptoms or conditions. We were all exposed to confusing food messaging in our formative years and difficult circumstances around food, whether it was not enough food on the table, a lack of resources to buy fresh fruits and vegetables, putdowns from family members, illnesses that affected what we could stomach, or societal values and images. Somewhere along the way for each of us, that particular combination gelled and created the foundation of how we think about food. And then we kept being exposed to new headlines and trends and opinions and beliefs and theories and life circumstances that built on that.

It's a natural, animal instinct to have hang-ups around food, because our survival revolves around it. We are not alone. Hyperawareness about what we eat is built into who we are as human beings, and we don't need to be ashamed about that. We don't need to punish ourselves about what we eat, nor do we need to punish ourselves for worrying about what we eat. What we need is to be mindful that amidst all the influences that have informed our relationship with food is very little actual truth—because we're not taught the truth about how to feed ourselves for lasting health, or what a healthy cleanse looks like. (Hint: it's not starvation or torture.) It's all still guessing games out there, with the very same experts who are saying that people should find a balanced diet not sure what a balanced diet even looks like for themselves.

Animal Versus Plant Protein

In all the noise and misinformation out there about protein, you can usually hear a distinction between two camps: animal protein versus plant protein. The plant protein camp is much smaller. It's minute, really, when compared to the size of the animal-protein camp. Plant protein proponents are fighters, though, with strong conviction—until they start to experience a few symptoms and feel the world blaming their symptoms on their plant-based diets. Overwhelmed, they surrender at rapid rates to the other side.

Meanwhile, those in the animal-protein camp are just as sick, with just as many symptoms. The difference is that animal protein doesn't come under the same scrutiny; no one in the mainstream is tearing down their diet and blaming it as the cause. They get a free pass from having the food they eat considered to be related to their health struggles. Plant-based folks don't get this immunity. The minute they start to deal with fatigue or brain fog or pain or any other symptom, it's blamed on their diet. The sad part is, not only do the meat eaters blame the plant-based person's sickness on their diet; the plant-based person herself quickly loses all loyalty to fruits and vegetables and easily believes the animal protein eater's claims.

Both camps are at least considered to be healthier than standard diets. Both avoid processed foods, fried foods, and most grains. Both tend to believe in the ketogenic philosophy—the theory that high fat is good and carbohydrates should be limited if not eliminated altogether. And neither camp is taking the right measures to cleanse and detox.

Neither those who promote animal protein nor those who promote plant protein know the true causes of today's symptoms, conditions, illnesses, and diseases. Neither camp realizes that lack of protein has nothing to do with why someone is not getting better or why they're sick to begin with. Neither camp even has real science to back up their beliefs. Conventional medical science doesn't believe in the plant-based movement or in a healthy high-fat diet or healthy high-protein diet; conventional medical science has never believed food is behind illness at all. While, yes, you'll find studies about food playing a significant role in instances such as type 2 diabetes, conventional medical universities are still not focused on teaching that food is behind conditions and illnesses, even if the students who attend these medical universities are.

So it makes sense that everyone is confused about cleansing and detoxing. It makes sense that health professionals are spreading the mistaken belief that your body does enough daily detoxing on its own if you eat a "balanced" diet. Misinformation about why health issues exist in the first place is rampant—how would anyone know the truth about how to address the underlying causes through specialized cleansing if they hadn't experienced it or seen it for themselves?

RESPECT

All of this food confusion means that when family, friends, or even strangers see you cleansing, they may question and discourage you. In certain situations, with certain cleanses that get attention, that can be sage advice. There are harsh cleanses out there.

You may still encounter doubt, though, when you're doing precisely the right cleanse from this book, or simply bringing some Medical Medium information into your life. Because there's a history of cleansing the wrong way, it's understandable that fear will linger around the words cleanse and detox, that people you know will try to protect you—because they haven't been given an understanding of what our bodies are up against and what causes illness.

So many people who develop symptoms or get diagnosed with a condition or disease experience a lot of peer pressure to keep on going to doctor after doctor and to stick with the status quo of what life looks like for a sick person. That pressure can be to eat a certain way: for example, to rely on mainstream comfort foods or to get "enough" fat or protein in your diet, whether plant based or animal. That peer pressure can feel disheartening and can even be misleading, as peer pressure so often is. When you find an opportunity to heal, people will keep on making judgments. You may hear, "You're trying another cleanse?" They may be skeptical, just as you may be, that after everything you've tried, this is finally the answer.

Or maybe they had a bad experience themselves with a cleanse or diet that was gimmicky and man-made and didn't have a foundation in the truth of how to get out certain toxins and bugs that make us sick. Maybe it gave them a (figurative) bad taste in their mouth that led them to worse eating habits in rebellion. They don't realize that the Medical Medium cleanses come from a source above and that they address the real reasons why people are sick. When we have our guard up from being let down time after time, sometimes we're not prepared to see when the truth has finally come to visit us.

Those who are nervous for you when you start one of the cleanses in this book don't know that this is specific cleansing for specific problems. They're still susceptible to trendy misinformation and even the old-fashioned "everything in moderation" advice that's still circulating. They don't know what you're going through in this moment with your health. They don't understand the beating heart of desire you have within yourself to heal.

When you're feeling good or ignoring your own symptoms, it's easy to misunderstand those who aren't feeling well and what they go through. That is, unless you're the family member or other loved one paying witness to the daily battles of someone in your life. Sitting beside them in waiting room after waiting room, trying to keep them mentally refreshed and stable even as they spend another day unable to move from the couch, supporting them in any way possible, sometimes even entering the depths with them or literally holding them up—you know the struggle is real. Your heart aches when you see the worry and fatigue in their eyes as they search and search for answers to chronic illness. You live their story with them.

Everyone has a different threshold for health problems. One person may become frantic upon developing a symptom such as acne that's painful or makes them embarrassed to go out. For another person, it may be brain fog that rattles them to their core when it prevents them from accomplishing focused tasks like schoolwork or a to-do list. Some people carry on with their aches and pains or fatigue, not getting upset because they consider it normal or part of getting older. Then there are those who experience several if not dozens of symptoms at once. They might have reached a state of what looks like calm on the outside—as a coping mechanism for the overwhelm of bearing it all. Everyone handles health disruptions in their own unique way, and it's all valid and legitimate.

We must hold respect for those suffering from any kind of health impediment whatsoever. Years ago, the world had to be educated about cerebral palsy, strokes, muscular dystrophy, stutters, speech disorders, Down syndrome, and other pronounced difficulties so that we could be taught to show respect. It's a new world now, and we need to bring education to a whole new level—because nearly everyone is dealing with a symptom or condition of some kind, whether mild or severe. In addition to understanding and honoring those with the disabilities and disorders we've come to recognize, we need to honor those who struggle to get through the day with other chronic symptoms and no answers about why.

When someone starts to feel unwell, the respect they receive from those around them tends to drop, unless they're an elder (in which case they're expected to have problems) or a child. For the people in between, it's almost like a class system, with the class of the sick and the class of the not-so-sick. We're being divided: the chronically ill are swept under the carpet, treated with disregard, or ignored, while those who can hide their symptoms do, pretending they're okay and keeping their struggles private so classmates don't get suspicious or coworkers don't tell the boss. We're living in a time where we're practically punished for symptoms, taught that we shouldn't hold self-worth if we're not optimizing and performing at the top of our game.

And yet medical science and research never get the blame for not having the answers about why so many people are chronically suffering. Instead, it's the person who gets the blame for being sick, the person who's either told or made to feel that it's their fault one way or another. Because science hasn't yet discovered the physiological reasons for the epidemic of chronic and mystery illness, people are left to search for cosmic explanations.

That's why the trend of believing that health is a manifestation of who you are as a person has been able to take hold. In the absence of information, in the age of "cause unknown" and the autoimmune theory, it becomes permissible to blame the person who is suffering for their own suffering. This is how someone starts to believe that it's who they are as a person that attracted their symptoms, that they brought it upon themselves by being lazy or not creating the right energy or not thinking positively enough, or that at some fundamental level they made the choice to stay sick. Or they come to believe that their body is letting them down or turning on them, which robs countless people of their self-trust. Eventually, in the future, everyone will have a symptom or condition they can use to relate, which will make it feel safer to reveal one's own health struggle. In reality, those who haven't struggled or suffered—yet—or who haven't been the support system for someone who has, those who haven't yet had to scratch and claw for answers, don't have the life experience to hold true clarity. As someone who has suffered or been close to someone suffering, you do. And you deserve to trust yourself again. You deserve to respect yourself again. It's time. With the healing steps in this book, you can tap into your body's gifts of renewal and learn to do just that.

HOW THIS BOOK WORKS

In the rest of Part I, "We Need to Cleanse," you'll find insights into where we find ourselves today with our health and how to make sense of the cleansing theories out there. In the next chapter, you'll discover the true reasons for today's epidemic of burnout. Following that, you'll find Chapter 3's wake-up call to the poisons and pathogens that threaten our health, starting before we're even born—and that continue to hold us back in life as we encounter them in our everyday. If you think you couldn't possibly harbor any toxins, this chapter will open your eyes to the countless hidden

exposures in our way. Along with advice on avoiding common daily toxins, it will illuminate the toxins we can't help encountering and get to the heart of why it's critical to know the right way to cleanse.

Continuing on in Part I, you'll find the chapters "What about the Microbiome?," "Intermittent Fasting Revealed," and "The Juicing versus Fiber Debate" for answers about these trendy topics. It's critical that you don't get derailed from cleansing by misled theories, and these chapters will offer precisely the knowledge you need to save yourself from misinformation and stay on track. It's also critical to read Chapter 7, "Troublemaker Foods," for answers about foods that can work against your healing.

And in Chapter 8, to wrap up Part I, you'll find a guide to choosing a cleanse, whether from Part II, which provides Original, Simplified, and Advanced versions of the 3:6:9 Cleanse, or Part III, "Other Life-Saving Medical Medium Cleanses." You'll even come away from Chapter 8 with an understanding of how these cleanses fit with the other cleanses from the Medical Medium series. Don't despair if cleansing seems too involved, complicated, or out of reach. There's an option for you.

No matter which cleanse you decide is right for you to start with, you'll find it useful to read through all of Parts II and III, since understanding how the other life-saving cleanses work helps illuminate how the 3:6:9 Cleanse works, and understanding how the 3:6:9 Cleanse works will help you see how this most efficient cleanse may be useful for you someday, even if you're not quite ready to try it—yet.

Part IV, "The Insider Cleanse Guide," starts with "Critical Cleanse Dos and Don'ts" such as why lemon water is on our side (so it's a "do" while cleansing), how to handle cleanse interruptions, and even how to make sense of water fasting and juice fasting. In Chapter 20, "Your Body's Healing Power," you come to understand your body's healing process as it detoxes and what to expect in terms of bowel movements and weight loss. Chapter 21, "Cleanse Adaptations and Substitutions," offers modifications and alternatives to the most common cleanse foods and drinks from Parts II and III. And then Part IV wraps up with sample menus for Original, Simplified, and Advanced versions of the 3:6:9 Cleanse and recipes to get you through your Medical Medium cleanse.

Part V, "More Spiritual and Soul-Healing Support," will provide precisely what it sounds like. Offering an anti-bullying tool kit, revelations about the physical reasons why cleansing can get emotional and how to weather those feelings that arise, and a message of spiritual support to remind you that healing is possible, this section of the book is here to be your anchor. No matter what new heights your healing brings you to, these living words will be available to offer grounding whenever you need it.

At the end of this book, you'll find Part VI, "Knowing the Cause and the Protocol," with extensive lists of supplements for your specific symptoms and conditions—and insights into what causes each health issue. Here, you'll find guidance on whether to incorporate supplementation into a Medical Medium cleanse and which supplements to avoid and why, as well as how to bring herbs and supplements into your everyday life. Keep it nearby to use as a reference tool in your day-to-day.

AN ARMY OF COMPASSION

You just found something different. You found an escape hatch. And you found it for a reason. Maybe it's for you. Maybe it's for someone else in your life too. Maybe it's for health trouble you're dealing with now. Maybe it's to head off trouble that would otherwise be headed your way.

This book that you've brought into your life is timeless. The ultimate resource for getting your health back, it stands apart from the noise because its information comes from above—it comes from God. Bigger than any of us, it is meant to be a resource for the ages, one that anyone can turn back to whenever they or a loved one is in need.

You don't have to hide anymore. I believe in you and all that you're going through, all that you're struggling with. I understand if you're battling symptoms that are confusing and feel like they're holding you back, getting in the way of expressing yourself or becoming your true self. You're accomplishing more than you know through the process of struggling with your symptoms or illness—and there are answers about why we get sick. They do exist. You don't have to be without the knowledge of how to heal anymore.

Be proud of using your free will to make your own choice to work on your healing. Have compassion for yourself and know that your suffering is not your fault. Your struggles are not your fault. You're accomplishing great things every single hour and day as you work on your healing process with the powerful tools in this book. I believe you can heal.

CHAPTER 2

What's Causing Burnout

It's human nature to push our bodies past the limits they offer us. We like to push ourselves to the max. We don't know when to back down, when to stop, when to take breaks, when to put on the brakes. If we can, we will try to get away with anything, from multiple jobs to multitasking to overthinking in all different realms, whether because we're forced to take on a certain amount of work to survive or because we're blessed with the luxury of pushing our creativity as far as we can. We often need to teach ourselves to back off, learn balance, and manage our output. If we're not careful, we can burn out.

Every single person has a different scale of limitations and a different burnout level. One person can push themselves in one way while a friend would burn out long before. We always look to each other's level of work and accomplishments, whatever others may be doing in whatever field, and compare ourselves. Whether careers, hobbies, athletics, academics, social media, or any number of other areas of life, our burnout point may be shorter or longer than theirs. We can't judge anybody for that, and we can't judge or shame ourselves on any level.

There are different reasons for everybody's different cases of burnout. Toxic heavy metals are a factor, and that's one reason why it's important to consider the Heavy Metal Detox Cleanse you'll find in Chapter 17. Varying degrees of toxic heavy metals in various regions of the brain can quicken somebody's burnout—because when metals are saturating neurons, electrical impulses burn hotter and more inconsistently, neurotransmitters become weakened and diminished, and electrical activity in the brain can be strained, making it harder for one person to complete a task in the time frame another person may be able to do it. This doesn't mean one person is smarter and the other less smart. It means that when we talk about preventing and understanding burnout, we need to consider that toxic heavy metals are a leading cause. It's what I call *toxic heavy metal burnout*.

Then there are chronic illnesses and chronic symptoms. Underlying, low-grade viral infections are more common than anyone realizes. Often, someone is unaware that one or more of the over 60 varieties of Epstein-Barr virus (EBV) and/or one or more of the over 30 varieties of shingles virus and/or cytomegalovirus or other viral strains are lying deep inside their liver, creating neurotoxins as waste and releasing them into the bloodstream, and from there inflaming nerves and creating mild neurological fatigue. This can quicken somebody's fatigue response when they're doing a lot of work or even a lot of play. They may tire faster than someone else, "short circuit" faster, or perhaps they can't handle as much emotional stress, and what no one can tell them is that it's a form of viral burnout.

And then there's someone who's emotionally injured. They've been hurt by betrayal, a broken heart, a breakup, divorce, broken trust, or loss, or maybe they've lost their job or community. When someone has gone through tremendous stress in life, burnout can happen a lot faster. This often goes hand in hand with posttraumatic stress symptoms (PTSS) and obsessive-compulsive disorder (OCD), with memories and experiences deep in the brain that may emerge easily from day-to-day triggers. Living with this can make it harder to sustain oneself and keep from burning out.

Someone can also have multiple burnout factors contributing at once. For example, they could have some low-grade viral activity brewing that's creating a hypothyroid issue at the same time they have low adrenals at the same time they have a sluggish, stagnant liver that's led to a diagnosis anywhere from small intestinal bacterial overgrowth (SIBO) all the way to Lyme disease and beyond. And then on top of it all, someone could have some toxic heavy metals such as mercury, aluminum, and copper inside their liver and brain while they're going through a lot emotionally and also working very hard to sustain themselves financially and provide the resources they and their loved ones need. Or maybe you're living with someone who's under constant stress and duress, creating a situation that's weakening your energy reserves as it takes up what we call "brain space." This alone can create a case of burnout.

Some people have just one factor, some people have many, and then there are people who seem healthy overall—who don't have a lot of heavy metals (at least not yet), who don't have a lot of viral inflammation (at least not yet), who somehow haven't hit too many emotional pockets with family or relationship trauma. Burnout can still occur if they put in too many hours, whether on a creative job they feel passionate about or a job that may not be as fulfilling and yet pays the bills. When we haven't learned where our boundary lines are, we can hit a wall. Even when we learn to read our burnout signs and signals, sometimes there's not a lot of choice. People have it hard; there are a lot of situations where we're forced to get up in the morning and push ourselves to do what we have to do, whether burnout comes or not.

Whatever cause or causes we can put our finger on for our burnout, it's critical that we don't go to a place of self-blame. All too often, *burnout* is used as a label—just like blaming genes, or metabolism, or the autoimmune theory that the body attacks itself—a label that excuses authorities from looking harder for underlying answers and a label that makes someone feel that they're the problem. You're not burnt out because there's something wrong with who you are and you simply haven't worked hard enough at creating balance in your life. Remember, it's human nature to push ourselves as hard as we can. We are up against substantial challenges on this planet, and it's not your fault if you're battling toxic heavy metals or a viral load on top of adrenal compromise or emotional challenges.

You *can* help yourself find relief by addressing the hidden contributors to burnout and using the tools in this book series to sustain yourself. Are you eating well? After reading the chapters to come, you're sure to have a whole new definition of "eating well." Are you getting enough sleep and allowing enough time to recoup amid all the hard work? Are you taking the right supplementation? See Part VI, "Knowing the Cause and the Protocol," for detailed supplement support. And, of course, are you cleansing to rid yourself of toxins and pathogens? We are up against more than we know in this world. With the Medical Medium cleanses in this book, we can provide ourselves and our families with critical protection.

"One of the most important foundations to hold on to is that no matter what, in the end, it's not your fault. Once you take the blame off your own soul and realize your symptom, condition, illness, or disease is not your fault— and not your body's fault—you can become truly empowered."

— Anthony William, Medical Medium

CHAPTER 3

A Wake-Up Call to What's Inside Us

We can choose not to see everything we're exposed to and how that threatens our health. We can know it exists and ignore it, pretending it doesn't exist or living in denial. We can even not know it exists, because we haven't learned. These would all probably be good approaches if we didn't have the option to fix it, a viable way of cleansing and detoxing and ridding the troublemakers that we inherit and continually encounter and that are stored inside us. Maybe it would be positive not to know or to pretend they're not there. Maybe it would help ease us emotionally as we started getting sick down the road—if we didn't have a way to get ourselves better.

The path of not knowing is not your path. You do know now, because you're holding this book. You know there's a way to clean up and heal from the troublemakers that create the epidemic of chronic suffering, so you know not to be afraid in the face of information about our exposures. You can see with clear eyes that it is best to know, to become an expert, so you can share this information with others in your life and protect them at the same time you protect yourself.

Don't we all want to have choices? Or do you want everything decided for you, even decisions that could be to your detriment? Wouldn't you prefer to be able to stand up for yourself, to know what is truly going wrong, and to be able to defend yourself? Everybody should be able to defend themselves, their family, and other loved ones from harm—and yet that's not always how the world works. We're not always allowed to defend ourselves from certain angles. Many of us get cheated out of being able to protect ourselves by rules and systems created by industries and hierarchy, by whatever institutional environments we operate within in this governing world.

Against sickness and disease, we often feel most powerless. Many of the poisonous chemicals and toxins we inherit or are exposed to and re-exposed to throughout our lives are propelled and governed by industries and money rather than our best interest. We're being sickened by sources and substances we never got a chance to have a say in—because we were supposed to be kept in the dark. At the same time darkness is what's affecting us, it's what's infecting us too. Spiritually speaking, darkness wants us to be in the dark.

A lesser quality of life, a shortened life span, or a lesser quality of life *during* a shortened life span: Why should we accept this as the new normal? That's what's happening in today's society. It's the new normal to have reproductive system conditions, autoimmune diseases, emotional and mental challenges, and other health problems—at the same time it's the new normal to disrespect people for their challenges, illnesses, and diseases. We're still in an age where we treat the chronically ill like lepers. And we were never supposed to treat people with leprosy like lepers in the first place! We're still in an age of the old normal, hiding away people who suffer, sweeping them under the carpet. This is a repeated strategy of the industries because it controls you while allowing for profit and gain—and not profit that goes in your pocket. The difference now is that because of social media, the chronically ill can have a voice, give themselves some visibility, and connect with each other. They still deserve more respect than they receive throughout their struggles.

They even deserve more respect when they find healing through avenues such as the books in this series. Constantly, people young, old, and in between are ridiculed for the mere fact that they are healing. They're doubted, too, by skeptics questioning whether they were sick to begin with. It's tough enough to put in the work to overcome your chronic symptoms. To get flak for it at the same time makes the climb to healing even harder. This is another tactic that condones hate speech against the chronically ill, attempting to break their spirits to keep them down. It's often employed by those who haven't struggled enough with symptoms or illnesses yet to understand. It's easy for people who haven't been there to purposely demean individuals who are fighting for their freedom, health, and right to heal. If you never acknowledged how down-and-out someone was, it's easy to brush aside their wins along the way. If you never paid witness to their fade from daily living, it's easy not to appreciate how momentous it is when they come back to life.

Troublemakers. I give that name to toxins, poisons, and pathogens because it's what they do: make trouble in our bodies, our brains, our lives. No matter how much you may want to believe that you haven't encountered viruses, bacteria, and toxic heavy metals (to name a few) and that they haven't had any effect on you, nor will they ever hurt you, the truth is that any symptoms you experience are physical proof of the fact that something is going on inside your body. No one is spared from exposure in this day and age.

Troublemakers are inside us all, and they're not helping any of us. Some of these troublemakers were inside our ancestors too. When we inherit troublemakers from the generations before us, it's no one's fault. We can't blame our parents or their parents or their parents for what the world exposed them to, and we can't blame ourselves for our children's struggles. What we can do is wake up, open our eyes, and turn on the light. Only then, with all the information clearly in front of us, can we defend ourselves and the ones we love from sickness and disease.

This is your chance. Take it.

WHAT'S INSIDE US

Even with symptoms from mild to severe creeping up on so much of the population, people often don't want to know that they have toxic heavy metals or any kind of pathogen inside their bodies. This occurs mostly with younger people. Any kind of bug living inside them seems like an impossibility. Individuals in their late teens, 20s, and even early 30s would often rather think that the reason they're dealing with a symptom or condition is a lack of protein or good fat in their diet, some kind of imbalance in their digestive tract, too many carbs, or even fruit creating a problem. Only when they've exhausted all those options, found they weren't the answers, and become wiser from the experience are they ready to realize and accept that toxins, viruses, or other pathogens inside of them could be making them sick.

Everybody has a different set of poisons and toxins within their bodies. While similar, the exact mix is unique for everyone. Someone might have worked in an office with plug-in air fresheners where their lungs were saturated with toxic oil for years, while someone else might have worked in an office filled with mold. Someone might have worked in landscaping and dealt with constant gasoline exposure from equipment. Maybe someone worked outside near heavy traffic and a tremendous amount of exhaust, so they were regularly breathing in carbon monoxide, lead, petroleum byproducts, and nitrogen dioxide. At the same time, to get ready for those jobs, they were all relying on different conventional body products and laundry products such as makeup, hair dyes, deodorants, perfumes, colognes, and dryer sheets, meaning that they breathed in and even swallowed problematic ingredients, or that those ingredients soaked into their pores. That buildup is inside the body now too—not to mention the toxic heavy metals such as mercury, aluminum, lead, and copper that we're exposed to from various sources and that we enter into this world with at birth.

And then there are pharmaceuticals. We all have pharmaceuticals inside us; no one is pharmaceutical-free. You may argue and say that there are people who have never taken a drug, whether prescription or over-the-counter. Well, we come into this world with drugs already in us because our parents or their parents took them. And if you're someone who comes from a line of ancestry where no one ever took a single medication going back through all past generations, what about food raised with antibiotics? Did you or an ancestor ever eat an animal product that wasn't organic or wild? If you can answer "no" to that too, then you were *still* exposed to antibiotics because pharmaceuticals are in our water systems. And if you can guarantee that you've never consumed tap water from a public water supply in a restaurant, coffee shop, hotel, or home; you've never bathed in or brushed your teeth with tap water; and you've never eaten food cooked in tap water—not ever—then that would be a miracle. We all have drugs in our bodies.

Planet Earth is not a pure place. It isn't easy to live here or thrive here. Maybe there are other planets where there are no toxins, no exposure to anything harmful, where people's cells have never experienced poisons from the Industrial Revolution. Not this planet. We all have pharmaceutical-raised pathogens and bits and pieces of industrial waste inside us, some of us more than others, with poisons and toxins residing in our cells and never leaving until we do something about it. We can't assume we don't need to cleanse. We can't assume our bodies just take care of everything naturally if we eat what seems like the best trending diet or what's considered "right." We're grossly mistaken if we accept that eating any given version of "healthy" and "balanced" and "intuitive" cancels out the need to cleanse.

As we've covered, there are people in the health profession who believe otherwise—and believe otherwise with conviction. They're anti-cleanse and anti-detox, and they believe that with moderation and exercise, your body cleanses and detoxes naturally. We already examined the myth of "moderation," so you're aware by now that however well-meaning, these professionals are misguided and misdirected. Their education doesn't teach them the true causes of chronic illness, because medical science and research don't have the answers about what's causing hundreds of symptoms and conditions. So how would health professionals know? They're in the dark about what we're exposed to every day, how very unnatural those troublemakers often are and what they do to us.

Our bodies need to be assisted with cleansing and detoxing because we're up against too much for it all to come out on its own. Instead of letting it out naturally on a daily basis, we gather more. We're constantly up against the poisons, toxins, and pathogens buried in our cells and tissue, such as mercury deep in the brain leading to depression, anxiety, or even Alzheimer's and viruses deep in the liver leading to Lyme disease, lupus, and other autoimmune conditions, as well as new troublemakers we collect in the present. If we cook on a gas stove, those carcinogenic gas fumes are entering through our airways and being stored deep in our bodies as we fry up our eggs.

The solution isn't to stop living our lives. The solution is to assist our bodies with the right cleansing and detoxing techniques so that our inevitable exposures don't hold us back. It's to make medicinals such as celery juice and the Heavy Metal Detox Smoothie a more regular part of our routines between cleanses. It's to become more aware of the toxic exposures we do encounter and to limit them when we can, which is exactly what the next section of this chapter is geared to help you do. Otherwise, the troublemakers build up more and more, making us more and more likely to develop viral- and bacterial-caused symptoms because those exposures have not only fed the bugs; they've weakened our immune system against the pathogens. That's not what any of us wants, is it?

HIDDEN EXPOSURES

It's one thing to talk about toxic troublemakers. It's another to understand how they work inside our bodies and how bad they really are. Our natural human instinct is to believe only what we can see and ignore what we don't see, resorting to denial as we look toward the noise and stay focused on distractions. Toxic substances and pathogens can mean nothing to someone if they don't see them in front of their eyes. Rarely do we witness a direct exposure and its effects—for example, someone being sprayed by pesticides and instantly falling ill. By far the more common example is when small accumulations of pesticides that no one ever saw build up inside someone's liver, brain, and even breast tissue and reproductive tissue over time, setting the stage for symptoms to occur many years later.

None of this is our fault. Industries keep us in the dark and even keep themselves in the dark. If they knew this was happening, that people were getting sick from exposures, they would likely stay in denial that it was even occurring. Our choice, then, is to see it for ourselves—it's the only way to protect ourselves and our families.

In the coming pages, we'll look at some of the most common, surprising, invisible (or near invisible) troublemaker exposures and what they do to us if we aren't aware.

Mercury

So many of us hear "mercury" as an empty word, believing it has nothing to do with our lives on any level. Truth is, there are endless ways to get mercury exposure, and it has a very real effect on our lives. Even if you weren't exposed to mercury recently, it doesn't mean you weren't exposed at one point in your life. Almost without a doubt, you were exposed at conception. We all were. Our ancestors were inundated with mercury toxicity, and they've passed that mercury along from generation to generation through contaminated sperm and egg.

Mercury has been in our world for thousands of years, and not naturally. Sure, it's a natural element. We've mined it from the earth, though, and brought this toxic substance up into our lives throughout the ages. It's still in industrial use today. Perhaps you've heard that it's used in certain types of lightbulbs. At one time in your life, you might have broken one of these bulbs and inhaled the microscopic vapor

particles of mercury. You might have had a pharmaceutical of some kind that could have contained traces of mercury. Our water supply has mercury in it, both the ocean and freshwater sources. Restaurant food prepared with tap water that's not filtered, in some cities, can contain mercury. You may be from a generation that still has mercury fillings. Maybe you or your family members have worked in factories over the years that exposed you to mercury. The car industry, for example, uses mercury in many different auto parts. Today's technology still uses mercury in its manufacture, and mercury is still used in many batteries. We often think of mercury as inside these products, not realizing that the manufacturing process can actually leave residue on the outsides of batteries, certain lightbulbs, and the like, residue that can contain minute levels of mercury.

If you think it's impossible that you've gotten exposure from any of the above mercury sources, well, we're all still exposed, because it falls out of the sky. It's not because the universe drops mercury pellets on us. It's not the god Mercury shedding tears from above. Mercury doesn't exist only in the shiny silver globule form we may picture sliding out of a broken thermometer of the past. It can also exist in minute, particulate form. The mercury we breathe in comes from vaporized solutions being emitted by airplanes and jets that eventually reach us through the air.

Mercury is not tolerant or kind when it resides inside of us. It weakens our immune system, causes emotional struggles and mental struggles, and feeds viruses aggressively, allowing them to prosper, become more toxic, and create more viral toxins in the body. This can lead to a myriad of neurological problems and diagnoses, including neurological Lyme disease, MS, fibromyalgia, ME/CFS, bipolar disorder, schizo-phrenia, attention-deficit/hyperactivity disorder (ADHD), and autism, to name only a few. When mercury feeds a pathogen such as the Epstein-Barr virus, it leads to the virus releasing a heavy metal–based neurotoxin—that is, a poison even stronger than the poison it consumed. Mercury-based neurotoxins are highly toxic to nerves throughout the body. They can create symptoms such as fatigue, tingles, numbness, tics, spasms, anxiety, depression, emotional disturbances, migraines, headaches, ringing in the ears, weakness in the limbs, and difficulty sleeping.

You don't need a lot of mercury saturation to experience a health problem. It could be the most minute exposure from the most obscure area of your life that wreaks havoc later. That's why we can't afford to think of mercury as distant. Only with vigilance can we avoid and shield our families from new exposures whenever possible while actively working to remove what's already in us.

Air Fresheners, Scented Candles, Conventional Laundry Detergent, Fabric Softener, Perfume, Cologne, and Aftershave

We all walk around as if it's normal and actually good to be surrounded by synthetic chemical products meant to create pleasing smells. Who are they actually pleasing? If no one really likes the smell of cologne, neither the people who wear it nor those who interact with them, why are so many people using it? All it takes is five people wearing cologne in a room of a hundred to overpower the air.

Don't underestimate the toxic levels of this category. Just because these products have fragrances we've been taught to identify as

pleasing, whether inside our home or on our body, it doesn't mean they're safe. These are some of the most hazardous chemicals to be concerned about, creating a future of health deprivation.

We think, for example, that by using an air freshener, we're creating a more pleasing environment. Once we unleash that plug-in air freshener, though, our sense of smell instantly becomes disabled. When you're living in a home or working in an office or other environment with a plug-in air freshener spewing chemical-laden oil into the air, you may not smell it anymore. After plugging them into the wall, many people forget air fresheners are there and don't notice when they've run out because the walls, bedding, pillows, furniture, air vents, and window shades have become so saturated. And while we become desensitized to that scent, it's nearly impossible to smell anything else.

These chemically scented, vaporized poisons hurt the lungs—their waxy, oily residue builds up in the lung sacs. If you're someone who doesn't smoke and yet you love plug-in air fresheners, you're better off removing your plug-in air freshener and starting to smoke. That's right; you actually have a better chance of longer-lasting health and vitality without complicated diseases if you smoke cigarettes than if you breathe plug-in air fresheners day in and day out. Does that put it in perspective?

The oily film from air freshener doesn't only affect the lungs. It also ends up in the liver when it enters the bloodstream from the lungs. Plus we swallow air freshener when we breathe it in through our mouth, and that brings it to the intestinal tract, from which it enters the bloodstream and heads to the liver as well. Air freshener residue in that organ can reduce liver function. If a really inquisitive surgeon opened up the body of a patient who had lived for years in a space highly saturated with air freshener, that surgeon would smell the air freshener scent seeping out of the patient's blood and cells.

The chemicals in synthetic scents can lower the immune system rapidly. What does that mean? It means that when the chemicals enter our bloodstream, our natural killer cells, lymphocytes, and other white blood cells absorb them, and that instantly weakens our immune cells and even kills some off. Our white blood cells need clean, fresh, oxygenated blood; with chemical scents, our white count becomes hindered. Exposure to a heavy dosage of air freshener, scented candle, cologne, perfume, or similar scent could mean three to four days of a weakened and lowered immune system. Pathogens can take advantage with an uprising—especially because the synthetic scent chemicals can, at the same time, feed viruses and bacteria, allowing them to prosper and reproduce, leading to further illness. Someone who's prone to urinary tract infections (UTIs), sinus infections, or flare-ups of fibromyalgia, ME/CFS, lupus, MS, eczema, psoriasis, or Hashimoto's may experience a new flare-up following exposure.

It seems like a really neat idea to plug in a device that releases a scent that makes you think of wildflowers. In the end, they're not real fragrances. They're synthetic and man-made in a factory, formulated by a group of people testing scents around a laboratory table and picking the one they like best. Air fresheners sprayed from a bottle or can and scented candles are just as bad. Even if they're called "natural fragrances," don't be fooled. This is the same tactic as listing "natural flavors" in a food's ingredient list as a secret label for MSG. It's difficult to find an enclosed space these days that's free of chemical scent. When we move to a different home, it's tough to find an apartment or house that doesn't have a lingering scent in the walls. Out in the world, we're exposed in stores, malls, hotels, restaurants, offices, friends' and families' homes, and public restrooms more than ever before in history. Hop in a taxi or ride service car, and you're likely to find air freshener coming through the vents. We inhale it just from being near people who have the scent on their clothes from air fresheners at home—on top of whatever scented laundry detergent, dryer sheets, deodorant, shampoo, hair product, lotion, aftershave, cologne, or perfume they use.

We live in a world where chemical sensitivities are becoming much more prevalent. That means that these chemical exposures are not only a nightmare for the individuals already suffering with sensitivities; they're creating new cases of chemical sensitivities for people who didn't previously have them. Years ago, it was older people who would complain about smells, saying, "I need fresh air," "Can you put out that fire?", "Please shut the window," "Close the front door; you're letting dust in," or "I don't like the smell of that cologne." They were the ones who had lived long enough to become sensitive. Now it's not like that anymore. Younger people are developing actual chemical sensitivities at rapid rates due to all they're exposed to, and the complaints of older generations are nothing in comparison to what the younger generations are up against.

Now, don't let this all put you into fear and chaos. While out and about, we can do our best to take measures to avoid these scents. For example, we can choose not to walk by the perfume counter at the department store; to purchase bath, body, and laundry products that are unscented or only scented with pure essential oils; and to find an alternative to the café around the corner that burns scented candles. Because we can't always avoid them, though—we can't ask the person standing next to us on the train to go home, shower, and wash their clothes in unscented detergent—we at least need to make our own homes, cars, and wherever else we spend extended periods of time into oases from these scents. If we have any say at our workplaces, it's ideal to establish scent-free policies. And of course, because we can't dodge every exposure, cleansing is critical so that we can continually release and rebuild.

Fungicides

There was a day when cash money smelled like cash money. You can probably still remember from childhood the distinctive paper smell of a five-dollar bill—the smell of green. In the U.S. at least, that smell has been taken over by fungicides. We're not supposed to realize this. No one's supposed to know anything about it. And you'd never know, because no one talks or writes about it. If you noticed that your cash from the ATM smelled different, you'd only think that the bank started adding a scent or perfume. That scent is the scent of fungicide, and if you pay attention, you'll find it gives your nose a little sizzle. When it's particularly strong, it can even make your chest tight.

Chemical companies are somehow indoctrinating institutions and corporations into using fungicides on products of all kinds, even government products such as paper money. Clothing is a huge industry and another example of fungicide use. Most clothing today is

laced with fungicides—again, no one would know. You wouldn't know that's what you're smelling, you wouldn't know that you'd been exposed, and you wouldn't know how it could affect your health. You'd just think some sort of scent got into your new sweater from the store or warehouse, if you even noticed it, and you'd go about your day.

Fungicides have a perfume-like scent. It may not have registered if you wear perfume, cologne, or scented body spray; if you wear clothes laundered with scented products; if air fresheners are present in your home, car, or place of work; or if you otherwise live surrounded by synthetic scents. These scents can sabotage your defense mechanism: your sense of smell. If you're shopping with a friend, say, and that friend is wearing perfume or cologne, you're not going to be able to smell the fungicides on the jacket you're trying on. It's when you eliminate the smells around you that are toxic—the conventional detergents and fabric softeners and the air fresheners, scented candles, perfumes, and colognes—that you start to notice the fragrances around you. Your sense of smell becomes sharp, and you register that the money that just came out of the ATM or the shirt inside the package that just arrived is laced with fungicides.

Life choice is taken away from the human race when it comes to this sort of chemical warfare. Chemical giants have learned how to sell their chemicals and keep it quiet, how to get their products into mainstream society without us questioning it, leaving us to be poisoned without our knowledge. Freedom of choice is gone—at the same time we're repeatedly told that we have control over our choices. In this area, it isn't always true.

Are fungicides one of the worst exposures we're up against? Yes, they actually are. Fungicides contain a tremendous amount of copper, a toxic heavy metal partially responsible for everybody's eczema and psoriasis. Have you noticed the explosion of eczema and psoriasis nowadays? Most everyone is developing it at some point in their life. And fungicides can be so strong on manufactured clothing that they send a child or adult to the doctor with complaints of headaches for weeks, with no one able to trace the problem back to that source. Fungicides make life more difficult when life is already tough enough. They get inside our brains and bodies, mostly inside our livers, and denature cells, which weakens them. They break down the body's immune system defenses and serve as food for pathogens such as the over 60 varieties of Epstein-Barr and other viruses, even bringing us closer to a possible cancer diagnosis in the future because certain aggressive strains of certain viruses are partly responsible for cancer.

Chemical companies have slid fungicides into so many different industries and products without telling the wider world. They make decisions, and we don't get a say. Instead, we can try to avoid fungicides with all our might, and it's very helpful to do so. The only way to do that is to become aware. It's hard to avoid them if we don't start to pay attention to that perfume-y scent, and if we don't know where fungicides can appear.

Where do you need to watch out? Well, we know it's on paper money, so apparently it was sold to the government. We know it's often on clothing, so apparently it's been sold to material and garment manufacturers. Sporting goods can be laced with fungicides, brand-new furniture can be laced with them, cardboard boxes can now be coated with them, paper goods can smell of them, they can be applied to car interiors, they can be on the outsides of water bottles, and now dry cleaning can even be fungicide-based. We end up eating them in our food too, since fungicides are used on some crops.

Plug-in air fresheners are also filled with fungicides. One reason why is that the moist, oily nature of chemically scented plug-in air fresheners means their mist coats every item in a home, including the walls and ceiling. They're so strong that they can even get inside walls and saturate them, sometimes seeping all the way through perimeter walls so that you can smell the air freshener from outside the house. This coating can trap moisture and breed mold. Fungicides are meant to help prevent mold and other fungus from growing in people's houses as a result, which would seem like a worthy use of fungicides. Quite the contrary. Fungicides can create *stronger* molds, ones that mutate and can become immune to fungicides, making the mold impossible to stop. It's yet one more reason of many why use of air fresheners should be terminated.

The fungicide applications we've covered are not exhaustive, because the list is growing every day. You may start to notice the noxious perfume and nose sizzle of fungicides from other sources in your daily life. Sometimes we can avoid them, sometimes we can keep those items out of our lives entirely, and sometimes we can't help that a fungicide-coated package was delivered or that we're staying overnight in a scented hotel room.

That's why we cleanse—because we don't have full control over every exposure and every way that industries pollute us. Do control what you can. If you have plug-in air fresheners, pull them out of the wall. Wash new clothes before wearing them. When you buy a new piece of furniture, put a blanket on it for a few weeks to absorb the worst of the fungicides, and then remove and wash the blanket several times. Small, thoughtful steps like these are part of your new survival system.

Gasoline

We act as if gasoline is safe, as if breathing it in is completely harmless, with no effects on our body or health whatsoever. We act almost as cavalierly with gas at the pump as if it were water. Once in a while over the years, I've heard old stories of people siphoning gasoline with a rubber hose using their mouth and then spitting it out, as if this practice can't be that bad for you.

Gasoline has been through a lot of phases of toxicity. It used to have lead in it. How dangerous was that? When the world realized the lead levels were too toxic for human safety, unleaded gasoline was introduced—as though lead had been the only thing harmful about it. Around the same time of the switch from leaded to unleaded gasoline, many gas stations also started switching over from full service to self-serve. That means that in the time of leaded gasoline, the people exposed directly to the gas were mostly limited to gas station attendants, farmers who worked with tractors, and folks who worked in lawn mowing and landscaping. If you were the person sitting in your car getting full service, you only really got exposed to the fumes when you opened your window to speak to the attendant and pay. Those days are over in most places now, and the number of people directly exposed to gasoline has increased exponentially due to pump-your-own stations.

And again, just because lead isn't being added to gas anymore doesn't mean gas doesn't have other components that are just as dangerous, some even more dangerous than lead. Methyl tertiary butyl ether (MTBE) isn't the only additive of concern either; its removal doesn't solve the problem. As a solvent, gasoline has ghost-like qualities, with a highly rapid rate of saturation of cell tissue, even when all we've done is inhaled its fumes into our lungs. And when gasoline does land on skin, it travels through skin tissue as if you have no skin on your body. Your skin is meant to be your body's first line of defense; having your largest organ covering you is meant to protect your blood, immune system, and the rest of your organs. Solvents such as gasoline that are created to run industries bypass this protection mechanism. One drop of gasoline on your skin will drive through layers instantly and enter the bloodstream immediately as if there were no barrier. That's the potency of solvents. From the bloodstream, they can go to your brain, although your liver will try to stop gasoline—absorb it, contain it—as much as it can, and so your liver is where much of your gasoline gets stored in the end. It's kind of like your uncle storing a whole bunch of gas cans in a barn over the years. The gas may be stale, only he knows discarding it takes special care, and he's too flat out with other farm chores to handle it properly, so it stays stored away, just as gasoline sits in your overloaded liver.

We breathe in gas fumes while filling our cars—fumes from our own pumps, fumes from people filling their tanks at neighboring pumps, and exhaust fumes from cars starting up all around us. Many gas stations don't have clips on the nozzle handles, so we have to hold the handle in place the whole time, with our faces only a couple of feet from the gas pouring into our tanks. Plus droplets occasionally splatter onto our hands when we're not using gloves at the gas pump. These are real exposures. People who've had increased exposure because they pumped gas for a living, and those who still do today, have for the most part not enjoyed a high quality of life. Gasoline can be a life shortener—and yet our teenagers are at the gas station every week pumping their own gas into their first cars. There are no signs at the gas pumps saying, CHILDREN AND YOUNG ADULTS SHOULD NOT PUMP GAS. There are no signs saying, TRY NOT TO BREATHE IN GAS FUMES or WEAR RUBBER GLOVES WHEN OPERATING GAS PUMP or STAY AWAY IF YOU HAVE LUNG PROBLEMS or KEEP YOUR DISTANCE IF YOU HAVE A CHRONIC ILLNESS.

It wouldn't take anything for the petroleum industry to create a disposable mask that blocks solvent fumes that you could easily grab from a dispenser at the station. It's a prime example of how the world doesn't always look out for our best interests. That's why the information in this chapter and the rest of this book is here: to look out for you. As worrisome as it may sound that gasoline breaks down the immune system and weakens nerve cells, making us more susceptible to viruses and bacteria and speeding their growth so that we're more vulnerable to neurological illness, it's worse not to know. It's worse to never get a shot at protecting yourself and your family.

Instead of living in fear, you can call around and seek out full-service gas stations or, if you can't find any, gas stations that have a clip on the nozzle so you can at least keep a little distance. You can purchase a box of disposable nitrile gloves to keep in the car for pumping gas. If you're chronically ill and you have a relative who doesn't have the same susceptibility and doesn't mind pumping gas, you can enlist their help. If you must pump your own gas and hold the nozzle in place, you can be cautious about the wind direction and stand upwind so the fumes aren't blowing directly toward you. And to address the exposures from our past and the new ones we can't avoid, we can take the powerful step of cleansing.

Pesticides, Insecticides, Herbicides, Chemical Fertilizers, and Lawn Treatments

Nowadays we focus more on organic food than ever before—it's the number-one focus for many who are health minded. Not everybody eats organic, though, and even the committed have a hard time eating *all* organic, so we do still end up eating foods that were treated with pesticides. And yet ironically enough, food is the least of our worries when it comes to pesticide exposure.

Pesticide drift is virtually everywhere. People are continually getting insecticide and other pesticide lawn treatments at their houses, condominiums, and apartment buildings across the country and around the world to treat certain worms, aphids, mosquitos, and other bugs. Even worse, herbicide treatments are popular for parks and lawns too. This is really damaging: insecticides, other pesticides, and herbicides denature and damage our cells in critical places such as our brain. No one has been spared from inhaling herbicides, because they drift and travel far and wide. Herbicides are used in little backpacks by landscapers in every neighborhood across this country to spray for weeds in lawns and garden beds. One person's herbicide application on a lawn travels miles and miles, thinned out enough that we can't smell it, yet it's present enough that it ends up in somebody's lungs. Herbicides are also used in agricultural destinations around the globe. Farmlands spray heavy, heavy applications of pesticides too, which drift for hundreds of miles. I'm sorry to say that even if you've been spared herbicide and pesticide exposure for years by living in a little oasis, it doesn't mean you're not going to travel in the future, perhaps enrolling in school in a different location, and move to a place where you encounter your first exposure.

It doesn't take a lot of pesticide, insecticide, herbicide, or chemical fertilizer to be detrimental. All you need is a little, and you likely won't even know it happened. Meanwhile, it can be an instant cell killer. That's why you'll see red DANGER and CAUTION warnings and skull and crossbones images on many of these labels: to signal that if you ingest them or they come into contact with your skin, you'll be in grave danger. In truth, the majority of us are exposed on at least a weekly basis from breathing them in from the air around us, if not from sitting in the grass at the local park or walking barefoot across a treated lawn. Indoor pesticide treatments for pests such as bedbugs, fleas, and ants are another source of exposure.

Need any more convincing that this is serious? Herbicides, insecticides, and other pesticides can speed up the advance of every single degenerative disease. Chemical fertilizers that are used to green up and speed up the growth of grass, shrubs, and hedges are in the same classification, affecting the body in similar ways. They can all end up stored in our deep tissue areas. Herbicides and many insecticides can get stored deep within our bones too, causing bone marrow and white blood cell conditions.

If you still think you haven't been exposed, think again. Mosquito treatments (and sometimes other pest treatments) occur in every state in this country throughout the spring, summer, and fall—and mosquito treatments are some of the most dangerous insecticides. That's why spraying happens at nighttime. Authorities are worried about an epidemic of neurological issues if the mosquito spray is used when people are out and about during the day—they know that too many health problems could develop in the population too rapidly if they spray during the day, that within minutes and hours, people could start exhibiting tics and spasms, severe aches and pains, dizziness, ischemic attacks, strokes, weakness in the limbs, motor skill issues, confusion, severe brain fog, and migraines. So they spray at night. Maybe you've even come home late from a party when the spray was floating in the air. Nighttime spraying isn't great for the jogger who likes to run at night or in the predawn morning either—and that exposure is tough to track because the spraying is so discreet. The local emergency room could get a few more cases overnight of tightness of the chest. They'll send patients home with anti-anxiety pills, and no one will be aware of the fact that inhaling mosquito spray was what landed those patients in the hospital. By morning, the insecticide has settled into the grass and plants of our yards and parks, which means we can still get exposure, though on a smaller scale.

These chemical formulations stay deeply embedded in our organs and continue to wreak havoc for years to come. It's not as though one exposure from last year stopped causing trouble—and yet instead of blaming these very real toxic exposures, we blame our bodies or even our thoughts for creating our illnesses. These products have an extremely long shelf life inside our body. They're "gifts" that keep on giving, and the only way to change that is to rid them from our organs through cleansing.

Radiation

Here's an unknown source of radiation: luggage that's been through airport security. When your bags go through the scanners that allow agents to analyze their contents, the bags collect radiation that stays on them for years—centuries, even. The next time your knapsack or tote or briefcase goes through the scanner, it collects more radiation, and that accrues and accrues and accrues with every trip. Airport security is using more radiation than ever before right now. Every year, it increases. As a result, we should be discarding our carry-on bags every three trips. The checked bag scanning process tends to emit less radiation, so you can discard checked bags less often, more like every six trips. (And those are one-way trips, by the way. Round trips count as two trips.)

Now, I know this isn't welcome information. I know it sounds drastic and jarring, especially with the popularity of expensive luggage and in this age of reuse. *Can I afford to buy a new bag every few trips? Isn't it wasteful?* you may be asking yourself, and rightfully so. The bigger question is, can you afford not to? Especially if you have babies or children who spend any time near your luggage that's been on multiple flights, can you afford to expose them? (More on protecting little ones in a moment.)

No one wants to age quickly—to get gray hair faster or wrinkled skin or degenerative bone diseases. No one wants to shrink and lose their height. No one wants their fingernails and toenails to lose their vitality and color. No one wants their teeth to discolor and decay or their eyes to glaze over with cataracts or degenerative retina disease to develop. We simply don't want to age; we're always talking about anti-aging and never talking about the radiation exposure that contributes to it. Radiation speeds up the aging process rapidly. It causes much faster deterioration of cell tissue; vitality gets sucked out of every cell exposed to radiation. While the body's cells are always renewing, radiation doesn't just disappear. We need to work on actively ridding it with the 3:6:9 Cleanse and the Heavy Metal Detox. (The Heavy Metal Detox addresses radiation at the same time as toxic heavy metals.) Otherwise, radiation within us has a shelf life that outlasts our body. When we're in our grave, hundreds and hundreds of years after we've died, we're still radiating.

Radiation also lowers the immune system. It's critical to keep our immune system strong so we can fight the pathogens and battle the toxins that we come up against every day. When we fly, we already get a tremendous amount of radiation exposure. There's still nuclear fallout floating in the sky, for one, from tragedies such as Fukushima, Hiroshima, and Chernobyl, and there's more of it up high. For another, everybody on the plane has just been through scanners and placed their scanned luggage in the overhead bins, concentrating all that radiation directly over our heads, which gives us extra radiation exposure. With all of this—on top of the radiation exposure we get from sources other than flying, such as X-rays, CT scans, MRIs, devices such as cell phones, and even food and water—if we can take a step to protect our health, well-being, and vitality, it's worth taking.

We also need to think about where we're storing our luggage between trips, especially if we have little ones. When there are children in the house or we're chronically ill, we need to be most mindful about not keeping well-traveled bags nearby. What if you're using your child's bedroom closet to store the family carry-ons that have been on five, six, or seven trips? What if you sleep four feet away from the backpack you've taken on 10 flights and it's radiating there, right next to you, every night? These are questions to consider. If you have kids, do whatever you can to change luggage regularly. Be particularly careful about letting babies near bags that have been on a flight with you. If you don't have children in the home and you can't afford new bags, stow them as far from where you spend time in the home as possible.

What about the items that were *in* the luggage when it went through airport security? It's really the largest item that collects the most radiation, and that item is the piece of baggage itself. Computers, phones, and clothing are smaller, and we store them separately and spread out when we're not flying. That is, we don't usually keep an exact set of shirts, pants, and sweaters from a trip shut together in one drawer, where all the radiation it picked up will be concentrated. These smaller items tend to be replaced more often than luggage too; we cycle through them, so this doesn't need to be a big source of worry. Same with snacks you might have packed in your carry-on to eat while traveling. When we eat food that's been through the scanner, yes, we'll get a small dose of radiation. Food sold at the airport has been scanned too, though. You may need to

eat while traveling, and you especially need to drink liquids, so go ahead and pack your snacks, drink your water, and plan to take care of yourself with cleansing steps such as the Heavy Metal Detox Smoothie afterward.

This is what I mean about living our lives. Some exposures we can't avoid. Some, like luggage, we can limit. Either way, it helps to be aware. Then we can make smart choices, such as choosing a more economical bag next time you purchase luggage so you won't mind letting it go before long, and sparing your kids from sleeping next to radiating carry-ons. If you're concerned about the waste aspect of discarding your travel bags over time, think about the waste aspect of becoming ill and hospitalized—and the costs that occur on all levels of life when that happens.

Now, it's possible that someday, radiation at airport security will get more attention. If it does, be prepared to hear experts say that the radiation levels that luggage picks up, if detectable, are safe for the body. That won't mean the radiation really is safe—it's like telling us mercury fillings are safe. Sometimes tools and knowledge are behind the times. Hold on to what you've discovered about the truth here.

Plastics

Plastic is getting more and more attention lately, particularly when it comes to the environment. As we become more and more aware of how much of it is around us, the reality that plastic exposure isn't good for us either is also starting to sink in. There are plastics in pharmaceuticals and PVC pipes. So many items, such as meats, are wrapped in plastic. The list goes on. Because plastics are everywhere, and because there's already a lot of fear and chaos surrounding plastic bottles, bags, packaging, and straws, my goal is not to make you more afraid. Rather, it's to get you thinking about trying to remove years of accumulated plastics from your body.

What does it mean that plastic isn't good for us? Well, plastic is a petroleum-based byproduct. It's a concoction of various chemicals, toxic to the human body, added together to create polymers. Formulations come in different ratios to create different degrees of hardening, with some plastics stronger for industrial use and others flexible, like a plastic bag. Problematic as plastic is, it's a useful resource for many applications. We can't run away from it and hide from it and rid it from our lives entirely. Sometimes we rely on plastic in the kitchen to make our healing recipes. High-quality blenders, juicers, and food processors are worth using and don't pose the risks that cheap, disposable plastics do. While we can limit plastic straws and stop using plastic bags, the next thing you know, you'll be using water that was pumped through your house in PVC pipes (which, while a safer route than metal pipes, will still lead to plastic exposure). What about the plastic hair clip you touch, the computer keyboard, or the shoe made from faux vegan leather? Plastic is everywhere. Even if you think that you've made choices to keep plastic out of every area of your life, be aware that in every state in this country, you're still breathing it in through the air due to burning plastics from agriculture. Certain times of year, in hot weather, are difficult for sensitive people due to accumulated toxins in the air; burning plastic is one of those toxins.

So we inhale plastic, we eat it, we drink it. We're all exposed—we can't run, we can't hide. Plastic items have a runoff we can't see.

When saliva touches it or water touches it or any kind of oil, including the natural oil from the skin on your hand, touches plastic, it takes a little plastic along with it. This is on a minute scale, barely detectable. It's still enough that it adds up. When this plastic runoff enters the body, it doesn't leave, because our diets and lifestyles today don't allow it to leave. With the other poisons and contaminants we're exposed to daily that are also entering our body, plus the way we eat, we're not able to detoxify properly. It's not like plastic is the only thing we have to worry about. As you can see from this chapter, so much is coming into our body all at once.

Plastic tends to stay active in the body, reacting to other poisons and toxins. If you have troublemakers such as insecticides, other pesticides, fungicides, or solvent-based conventional cleaners inside your body, they're interacting with the nano-sized plastic film that's coming off the plastic you're touching, eating, and drinking that's entering your body. When the other chemicals in your body interact with that plastic petrochemical film, its composition changes, making it even more toxic than it would be otherwise.

Plastic ends up in organs all through the body. No organ is safe from it or devoid of plastic exposure. In the summertime, we sit on plastic lawn furniture heated by the sun. We sit on plastic beach chairs while we put on suntan lotion, and when that sunscreen on our arms or legs or back gets sandwiched between our skin and the plastic chair, a reaction occurs that makes the plastic leach more. That's only one prime example. Suntan lotion on our skin against plastic pool toys has the same effect. And do you ever go camping with a tent made from nylon, polyester, and other forms of plastic? What about plastic clothing and plastic shoes, which are getting quite popular? Stand next to a home with vinyl siding as the wind is blowing? Sit inside a home with open vinyl windows as a breeze comes in? Vinyl flooring is big now too. What about your driver's license and credit cards—do you ever handle those? That's why we can't run and we can't hide from plastic.

Again, my goal is not to make you afraid. I know plenty of you are wary of plastics as it is. Others, though, will be skeptical that it could possibly affect them, and so I need to make it clear that we're all exposed from multiple angles. While any steps you take to be mindful about your plastic use certainly do help, even if you use zero disposable plastic in a day, you're going to get exposure elsewhere, and plenty of it. We need to actively cleanse the plastics that have been in our body all these years, before we were wise to them. Otherwise, plastics become part of our organs, including our liver and even our skin.

Plastics don't just become part of our organs; they infiltrate them and oversaturate them. When the liver gets tired, stagnant, and sluggish from various factors in our lives, including high-fat diets (whether "healthy" or obviously unhealthy ones), it has trouble filtering additional plastic coming into our body. As the main filter of our body, our liver can only hold on to so much. And so when plastics slip out of our liver, they end up getting to cells in other parts of the body, creating a film-like coating between cells in connective tissue, muscle tissue, and nerve tissue. The film can become like a barrier that doesn't allow cells to breathe, potentially starving cells of oxygen and causing cell death to increase in certain areas of the body. This is, on an individual cell level, like the concern we have about children and plastic bags and the reason they're printed with warnings about the danger of suffocation. As a result of plastic exposure, cells adapt and mutate, with new cells that are produced becoming infused with plastic residue.

We want to be proactive about ridding plastics from the body. When we're young, it's easy to feel indestructible, and yet all of us are going to get older someday. As plastic film and residue build up inside us, we may not feel it in the present—we may not feel if it coats the cells inside our lungs, for example. That doesn't mean that down the road, it won't affect us. We need to be concerned now about what we're putting in and on our bodies so that we're not paying the price dearly later. Cleansing is a critical way of ridding plastics from organs such as the liver—getting plastics away from critical life-supporting cells and helping prevent illness.

THE TROUBLEMAKERS LIST

The examples I just shared are, I'm sorry to say, only some of the exposures we encounter day-to-day. What follows is a list of some of the most common troublemakers in our world that can pose problems with our health if we don't actively cleanse them. If you want to know more about how we encounter these and how they affect us, as well as how long it can take for the body to let go of each, you'll find further information in *Liver Rescue*. As you scan these lists, remember: The goal here is not overwhelm and fear. The goal is knowledge and power. Becoming enlightened to what can harm us is our only chance of protection.

Viruses and Viral Waste Matter

- Cytomegalovirus (CMV)
- Multiple varieties of herpes simplex virus (HSV) 1 and 2
- Multiple varieties of human herpesvirus (HHV)-6, HHV-7, HHV-8
- Multiple varieties of the undiscovered HHV-9, HHV-10, HHV-11, HHV-12, HHV-13, HHV-14, HHV-15, HHV-16
- Over 30 varieties (all but one undiscovered) of shingles
- Over 60 varieties (most of them undiscovered) of Epstein-Barr virus (EBV)
- Viral waste matter (byproduct, neurotoxins, dermatoxins, and viral corpses) from these herpes-family viruses

Toxic Heavy Metals

- Aluminum
- Arsenic
- Barium
- Cadmium
- Copper
- Lead
- Mercury
- Nickel
- Toxic calcium

Pharmaceuticals

Some medications for certain circumstances can be life-saving. There are times when they are truly necessary. The opposite occurs with many medications as well, with life-threatening situations that can arise. What we need to be is aware: aware that excessive use can burden the liver, aware that different prescriptions provided by different doctors who aren't all on the same page (or different self-prescribed over-the-counter medications) can create a cocktail your liver and other organs don't like, and aware that even without taking a single medication in your life, you can end up with them in your system due to our food and water supply. With cleansing, old pharmaceuticals can start to come out of the liver immediately. If your doctor feels you need to be on medication in the present, by all means follow their instruction. At least you can focus on clearing out old pharmaceuticals you ingested in the past that have stuck around in your system.

- Alcohol
- Antibiotics
- Antidepressants
- Anti-inflammatories
- Biologics
- Blood pressure medications
- Hormone medications
- Opioids
- Prescription amphetamines
- Recreational drug abuse
- Regular immunosuppressants
- Sleeping pills
- Statins
- Steroids
- The Pill
- Thyroid medications

Chemical Industry Domestic Invaders

- Aerosol can air fresheners
- Cologne and aftershave
- Conventional cleaning products
- Conventional hair dye
- Conventional laundry detergent, fabric softener, and dryer sheets
- Conventional makeup
- Conventionally scented body lotions, creams, sprays, washes, and deodorants
- Conventionally scented shampoos, conditioners, gels, and other hair products
- Dry cleaning chemicals
- Hairspray
- Nail chemicals (such as polish, remover, adhesive)
- Perfume
- Plug-in air fresheners
- Scented candles
- Spray tan
- Spray-bottle air fresheners and mists
- Talcum powder

Bacteria and Other Microbes

- *C. difficile*
- *E. coli*
- Food-borne toxins (Includes many uncataloged microorganisms. Even when killed off through cooking, the microbe bodies remain toxic and can build up in the system.)
- Methicillin-resistant *Staphylococcus aureus* (MRSA)
- Mold
- Over 50 groups of *Streptococcus* strains
- Parasites
- *Salmonella*
- *Staphylococcus*

Chemical Neuroantagonists

- Chemical fertilizers
- Chlorine
- DDT
- Fluoride
- Fungicides
- Herbicides
- Insecticides
- Larvicides
- Other pesticides
- Smoke exposure of any kind

Petrochemicals

- Carpet chemicals
- Chemical solvents, solutions, and agents
- Diesel fuel
- Dioxins
- Engine oil and grease
- Exhaust fumes

- Gas grills, stoves, and ovens
- Gasoline
- Kerosene
- Lacquer
- Lighter fluid
- Paint
- Paint thinner
- Plastics

Troublemaker Foods

For a full list of foods that can interfere with our health, including explanations of how they affect us, see Chapter 7, "Troublemaker Foods."

Toxic Adrenaline from Emotional Traumas

Emotions are never the cause of illness. They can merely be triggers that put great stress upon the adrenals, in turn leading the glands to release corrosive adrenaline that lowers our immune system. When this occurs on a regular basis, it can set the stage for health struggles if we have underlying susceptibilities from the other troublemakers in this chapter. Because of this immune system factor, repeated or prolonged instances of excess adrenaline can particularly affect you if you're dealing with a viral condition. Again, though, these emotional experiences are not the reason you become sick. While sometimes we're forced into difficult situations or forced to make decisions that don't help us due to a lack of support or resources, and we often can't guard against these traumas, they don't ultimately need to disempower us. We can turn it around by taking care of our health and

empower ourselves by cleansing. For further insight into emotions and healing, see Chapter 25, "The Emotional Side of Cleansing," and Chapter 26, "Empowered Souls."

- Abuse
- Being ignored
- Betrayal
- Broken trust
- Constant letdown
- Extreme adrenaline-based sports and activities
- Family stress
- Fear
- Financial stress
- Having the (figurative) rug pulled out from under you
- Heartbreak
- Mistreatment
- Not being heard
- Not being understood
- Prolonged overabundance of adrenal stress
- Unfulfilled promises

Radiation

- Airplane travel
- Cell phones and other technological devices
- Continual atmospheric fallout from past nuclear disasters
- CT scans
- Food and water supply

- MRIs
- PET scans
- X-rays

Troublemaker Food Chemicals

- Aspartame and other artificial sweeteners
- Citric acid
- Formaldehyde
- Monosodium glutamate (MSG)
- Natural and artificial flavors
- Nutritional yeast
- Preservatives
- Alcohol

Rainfall Exposure

- Precipitation contaminated with chem trails (not just contrails)

TIME TO GET YOUR LIFE BACK

Now that you know what's inside your body, do you want to know how to let it go? The rest of this book is here for you. In Chapter 8, "Your Guide to Choosing a Cleanse," you'll discover many options available to you for wherever you may be with your health.

We're each in a different place in life, and we deserve individual approaches.

Our body cannot rid these toxins we've accumulated without our active help. Even with all this new knowledge, if you don't want to cleanse, or if your circumstances don't allow any change in your diet, you still hold new power: the power to minimize any new troublemakers entering your body. While there's so much we can't control, such as outdoor air quality, there are basics within our reach. Find the items in this chapter that you feel you can control—for example, use nitrile gloves at the gas pump, avoid sharing drinks or bites of food with friends, pull your air fresheners out of the wall, throw away scented candles, stop wearing perfume or cologne, switch to natural detergents—and take it from there. Maybe your job right now requires an exposure you'd rather avoid. You don't need to panic—that adrenaline rush wouldn't serve you anyway. Instead, limit what other trouble-makers you can and start to think about whether you can ask for a change in working conditions or find another career path for yourself in the future. Take one step at a time.

When you're ready, the cleanse options in this book are here for you, and Chapter 8 will guide you in how to choose the right one. Taking a few days or mornings to switch up your food routine is worth it. Cleansing gives us back years of our life—years we don't even know we've already lost and don't realize we can gain back.

CHAPTER 4

What about the Microbiome?

The term *microbiome* has exploded in popularity. Because it sounds like an advanced word and because it's everywhere, people tend to think the concept must be wholly understood. The way conversations are framed now, it's "If you don't know anything about the microbiome, then you don't know anything about health." That means that you may find yourself wondering why the 3:6:9 Cleanse and other Medical Medium cleanses aren't entirely centered on microbiota, or gut flora.

Here's the truth: the microbiome-explains-everything trend is an indication of the growing awareness that chronic symptoms and illness are taking over the population. That awareness is good. It's better than the days when people had such a hard time being believed that their trouble getting out of bed wasn't laziness, that their brain fog or bloating or stomach cramping or poor digestion wasn't their fault, and that their pain wasn't in their head. The microbiome trend is not ultimately moving us forward, though, because its fundamental premise—that an imbalance of fungi and *Candida* and a lack of beneficial bacteria and unproductive microorganisms in the gut are responsible for the health complaints of our modern world—is

inaccurate. Much as this goes against new popular thinking, the truth is that our health does not all come down to the complex world of healthy microorganisms in our gut. Any disruption there is merely a sign of a deeper problem.

So many people walk around with guts filled with unproductive fungus, yeast, mold, acid, low levels of beneficial bacteria, and rotting, putrefied fats and proteins stuck to the linings of their intestinal walls, yet they have no complaints about their overall health. They function perfectly fine in everyday life. Compare that to someone whose gut isn't dealing with all of these factors and yet can barely function enough to get out of bed or someone who is dealing with mystery pain or high anxiety. You can add all of the beneficial microorganisms you want to your gut, choose the best probiotics, focus on improving your microbiome, and in the end, if you're walking around with a low-grade viral infection for years, or *Streptococcus* bacteria inside your organs or even intestinal tract, this focus on good bacteria is not going to take you to a secure place with your health, healing, and recovery. Killing off pathogens and removing their fuel sources from the body is the only way to address the real issues behind mystery illness—which includes chronic illnesses that may be labeled with names and yet aren't understood by medical research and science. You can't kill unproductive bacteria or viruses with probiotics. The cold, hard truth is that the microbiome trend is not the panacea we're seeking to address chronic illness.

ANOTHER WAY TO BLAME OURSELVES

Is it true that we *have* a complex world of microorganisms in our guts? Absolutely. Is this the answer to everyone's suffering? No. That's only another theory as the health world scrambles to understand why everybody is sick. It's not even a new theory. It's back to the old territory of *Candida* blame and telling us our guts are where all our problems are. It's another way to blame ourselves for illness—which doesn't get us anywhere, because it's not our fault.

Anybody who's spent enough years in the health realm knows that it's the same old, same old. The reason the microbiome is taking off as a concept is that there's a younger crowd coming up who didn't experience the last three to four decades of *Candida* blame. These 20-somethings and even 30-somethings were still growing up and weren't a part of the wellness world yet, so now they're fresh blood, primed to fall prey to the misdirection and scams that claim "It's all in your gut" and "It's all about yeast, mold, and a balance of good bacteria," and that push probiotics. Older people have been through all that already, only it's the younger generations who have the big presence on social media. They're the ones it's easy to influence and sell to there. They haven't been through 30 years of "Your gut is why you're sick"; they haven't followed all the gut guidance there is and stayed sick.

The older generations have been there, done that. When they find Medical Medium information, they're learning and accepting the truth that they actually have pathogens that have been creating and sustaining their chronic illness symptoms. They're wise enough to know that *microbiome* is just another term for "It's all in your gut. Eat 'better,' and here, take some beneficial microorganisms." That never works for long-term healing and never did—and yet the 22-year-old who has a social media presence and is experiencing their first signs of bloating doesn't know that. They're easily swayed by the microbiome theory, which is more convincing than ever because it has funding behind it now. It's a financial endeavor outpacing the *Candida* scare tactics of the past, a new push repackaged with a new name to create a new distraction to keep everybody from the truth of why sickness is growing exponentially. It's a prime example of how the alternative health market can be just as confusing and corrupt as the conventional health market.

This is a classic equation. It takes a little-understood problem (that more and more people are suffering from chronic health complaints) and combines it with a little-understood aspect of our health (the mysteries of digestion) to create the appearance of a sound solution—rather than admit, "We don't have the answers yet."

And here's what makes it especially sneaky: the microbiome trend is not wholly bad. Writing it off entirely doesn't serve us, because of course it makes sense to take care of our gut. We need to know the *right* way to do that, though. And more importantly, the gut doesn't happen to be the source of all our problems. If we stay focused there, we'll lose sight of the answers that could save us.

THE REAL SOURCE

Before we go any further, let's establish that it's impossible to create a healthy microbiome when we're not educated about troublemaker food. Inside of our body is a complicated warehouse of millions of items jostled about, and it's trying to create balance constantly. Twenty-four hours a day, seven days a week, there is never a moment when our body is *not* trying to harness balance within us. We can call that what we want; if you want to call that "microbiome," then by all means, do that.

The main concern as our body tries to maintain balance is keeping the immune system strong against pathogens. How many destructive, problematic, disease-causing viruses and bacteria are active inside us, and how robust is our immune system in the face of them? That's the real foundation, where the truth lies about what's been happening to people's health over the past decades. You could have all the beneficial bacteria you want in your gut, and even all the undiscovered productive microorganisms that medical research and science don't yet know about, and you're still not going to get anywhere until you know how to address the pathogens in your body—pathogens such as the aggressive EBV strains that can cause breast cancer when the right toxins are in the body to feed them, or the strep that causes intestinal inflammation, or the shingles strains that cause ulcerative colitis. Only when medical research and science understand what truly causes the epidemic of chronic and mystery illness will they get past merely managing symptoms and feeling helpless as patients get sicker and sicker. Meanwhile, medical communities play all the guessing games they want: removing gluten from the diet; playing other elimination and food combining games; being concerned about something called lectins; encouraging the masses to swallow probiotics, collagen, and fish oil in high quantities; and getting patients on hormones, high-fat keto diets, or high-protein diets at the functional medicine doctor's office. Until medical communities are past guessing, they won't break the barrier of healing. People's symptoms will keep getting worse and worse.

(By the way, high-fat and high-protein diets are the same thing. Eggs, nut butters, chicken, and fish—some of the standbys of each—are high in both fat and protein. And food combining is another example of rehashing a practice that's been around for decades; it's another technique that's being sold to the younger crowd right now. It hasn't offered answers to anyone with chronic illness for the past 30-plus years, and yet it's taking on a whole new life because there's a whole new audience for it.)

One of the confusing parts of this is that when people start to be concerned about their microbiome, they tend to make several changes at once. They remove some processed foods from the diet, get on supplements, start exercising a little. You can start to notice yourself getting better that way as you recalibrate your health. If someone tags your improvement with "microbiome," it's easy to think your gut was the foundation of your health—without realizing that no one actually knows what happened.

Here's the truth. When we're eating troublemaker foods, we're feeding the dangerous pathogens—the viruses and unproductive bacteria—that cause some of the biggest health problems. And pathogens such as *Streptococcus*, *E. coli*, *Staphylococcus*, HHV-6, CMV, human papillomavirus (HPV), EBV, and shingles don't care about how much good bacteria you have in your gut. Good bacteria in your gut do not stop bad bacteria (or viruses) from causing harm or damage throughout the organs and body; healthy microorganisms do not kill, stop, or even thwart dangerous bacteria and aggressive viruses. Instead, those viruses and unproductive bacteria look for food they like, ignore productive microorganisms, and go about their business of wreaking havoc and creating inflammation.

People who have real problems such as severe ME/CFS, advanced fibromyalgia, or debilitating rheumatoid arthritis (RA), Hashimoto's thyroiditis, MS, lupus, connective tissue disease, eczema, psoriasis, or other autoimmune diseases have often been from doctor to doctor, told to swallow all kinds of fish oil and probiotics, even removed many gut-disruptive foods such as gluten, and still they suffer with their neurological symptoms. That's because the gut is not the answer to why we're sick. Instead, the gut is a pathway for us to deliver chemical compounds from food and supplementation as well as fuel sources such as carbohydrates that convert into blood glucose. Viruses and unproductive bacteria get into the bloodstream and take up residence deep in organs and other parts of the body before they make trouble for our gut. Even if our gut gets sick because it becomes inhabited by viruses or unproductive bacteria, that happens regardless of how many beneficial microorganisms we have or don't have.

Even if a probiotic product could kill off pathogens in the gut (and it can't), that wouldn't take care of the pathogens in our liver and other organs, where illness first begins and where illness continues to advance. Also be mindful that fish oil supplements contain traces of mercury. There is no fish oil in production that is exempt from containing trace mercury, which ends up feeding viruses in your body. (For more on fish oil, refer to Chapter 27, "What You Need to Know about Supplements.")

Viruses and unproductive bacteria are responsible for chronic illness, along with toxins such as toxic heavy metals and whatever stressors may be weighing on us that weaken our immune systems, whether a lack of resources or emotional struggles. This combination of toxic troublemakers is why we're sick. And to be clear, emotional hardships are not the root cause of illness. They simply act as triggers that, when we already have a lowered immune system, can make us more susceptible to the pathogens and toxins that really cause illness. We can focus on the microbiome all we want. That's not going to minimize our toxic heavy metal levels or stop the mercury in our system from feeding EBV and creating lupus.

Meanwhile, the world's current focus on the microbiome is at least helpful because it's encouraging people to think about what they put in themselves. So if someone told you to think about your microbiome, you might have taken a food out of your diet that no one realized was feeding EBV in your body and in turn creating your lupus symptoms. It takes more than removing that one food to heal the underlying problem and get better. If you have mercury and other toxic heavy metals in your system, which are more common than anyone realizes, you want to actively cleanse those out because it's impossible to remove toxins just by trying to create a healthy microbiome. Your immune system is still going to be weakened if you have toxic heavy metals inside of you, and a healthy microbiome is not going to fix that either. Creating a healthy microbiome is simply not the answer for chronic and mystery illness, neurological problems, and widespread issues such as fatigue that so many theorize it to be.

Is a healthy microbiome helpful? Of course. If your gut is in balance, that can help if, for example, you develop a case of food poisoning; you'll be less likely to be injured by the food-borne toxins or microorganisms. A healthy microbiome helps with absorption of nutrients too. With all that said, do medical communities actually know how to create a thriving microbiome? And who's to say, with all this talk of microbiome, that we have it right about what's "healthy"? It's solely a guessing game at this point by both the alternative and conventional industries to sell products and make money. The truth is that *Candida* is part of how we absorb nutrients, and yet so many professionals will advise you on how to get *rid* of it. They don't realize what a beneficial fungus it is and how without it we can't thrive—because nutrient absorption depends on *Candida* breaking down food. If we're trying to help the microbiome while killing off beneficial fungus, then we're already off the mark.

Even if we're talking about a truly healthy environment in the digestive tract, one that allows *Candida* to do its work without overgrowing, one that is less acidic and fosters a proper pH and has an abundance of good bacteria inside it, the gut is not the answer to chronic illness. The health world has been focused on the gut for years as the source of all our problems, and the theories just keep cycling through with new names. Sure, an imbalance in gut flora can be an indication of a disruption somewhere in the body—just that, though: an indication, not a cause. For the true causes of chronic suffering, we need to look to what this world does to the liver, as in my book *Liver Rescue*. The liver is where problems take root as unproductive bacteria, viruses, mold, and toxins move in—and getting our liver healthier by cleansing it in the right way is how we get a healthy microbiome in the end anyway. Liver care is the real key to creating health in the rest of your body, and cleansing is the ultimate liver care.

When your liver is stagnant and sluggish from harboring a toxic and pathogenic load, it produces less bile to digest high-fat, high-protein foods. Low bile production ultimately leads to low hydrochloric acid in the stomach, so those foods rot and putrefy in the intestinal tract, not allowing for proper nutrient absorption. This is just one example of how the liver is responsible for gut health. When you're eating what professionals believe is healthy for your gut, the truth can be that it's unhealthy for your liver, and anything that's unhealthy for your liver defeats the purpose of what you're trying to accomplish: healing your gut. Remember, your intestinal tract is merely a pathway for fluids, nutrients, phytochemical compounds, and fuel to enter your bloodstream, move on to your liver, and be delivered to the rest of your body. Only with this awareness of the complex interplay can we wake up to what we really need to feel better.

CLEANSING FOR TRUE BALANCE

This is all to say that there's a reason this is not a book about balancing your microbiome. There's a reason it's not all about fermented foods—there's a reason it doesn't hold up probiotics, kombucha, yogurt, kefir, sauerkraut, and apple cider vinegar as the answer. They never were the answer, and they haven't suddenly become the answer as their popularity cycles around again, this time on social media. They were and are a distraction as the search for the Holy Grail of understanding chronic illness continues. The 3:6:9 Cleanse and the other life-saving cleanses from Part III focus on restoring balance in the ways that can truly move you forward.

Again, toxic heavy metals do not care about healthy microorganisms. Viruses do not care about healthy microorganisms. They don't battle each other. They don't have confrontations. They don't even fight for the same food; problematic, aggressive microorganisms such as viruses and unproductive bacteria do not seek out the same fuel that healthy bacteria do. Healthy bacteria look for nutrients that can be found in fruits, vegetables, leafy greens, herbs, and juices made from these ingredients. Celery juice is one of the most powerful tools to supply these nutrients; it feeds all beneficial microorganisms in our gut while destroying unproductive bacteria and viruses there and is the most powerful nutrient delivery system to our microbiome.

Our healthy bacteria do not look for gluten, eggs, milk, cheese, butter, or other animal products. Healthy bacteria do not even look for yogurt, kefir, apple cider vinegar, or fermented foods. Not even *Candida* looks for these foods, not unless it's trying to save your life and gobble up troublemaker foods in order to stop bacteria such as strep or *E. coli* in your gut from having a feeding frenzy on them. Our healthy bacteria look for antioxidants and life-giving phytochemical compounds so they can withstand the constant onslaught of poisons and toxins that we ingest, environmental troublemakers that we're exposed to, and even our own excess adrenaline production when we're living with an overabundance of stress. Pathogens such as *E. coli*, strep, EBV,

shingles, and HHV-6 love gluten. They love the proteins and hormones from eggs. They love the lactose and fats from milk, cheese, and butter. Unproductive viruses and bacteria thrive on these food sources, consuming them rapidly and building up their strength in numbers regardless of how much good bacteria you have residing inside your intestinal tract, bloodstream, or body. Viruses and bacteria don't care what else is happening; if they have these food sources, it will allow them to thrive. Pathogens thrive on these food sources because they are mucus-producing foods, and pathogens tend to hide within the mucus, using it as a shield. While feeding on these foods, pathogens also release toxins that stimulate the body to produce more mucus, further protecting the pathogens. Meanwhile—I'll say it again, so it sinks in—your beneficial microorganisms just want clean, healthy foods: fruits, vegetables, leafy greens, herbs, and fresh juices such as celery juice. Feeding the beneficial microorganisms won't help balance out the pathogens. Only removing the foods that pathogens like, and using anti-pathogen measures such as celery juice, can send pathogens on their way.

So the next time you see a headline about the microbiome as some new health answer, remind yourself that no matter the updated take on the term, it's yet another indication of a misguided focus. Remember this: you can never get a healthy microbiome if you don't know what you're really going after—if you don't know how to target certain viruses and bacteria, if you don't know to go after toxins, if you don't know how to remove mercury and aluminum, or if you don't know that toxic heavy metals are oxidizing and causing sickness and hardship in the first place. Only when we get these real instigators out of our body are we going to take ourselves to better health. Any of the measures in this book will help you in that quest. To start with, consider cutting out the troublemaker foods from your diet with Chapter 15's Anti-Bug Cleanse and bringing in the Heavy Metal Detox Smoothie (recipe in Chapter 23). In the process, you'll set the stage for bringing order back to your gut. For extra gut support, try Chapter 18's Mono Eating Cleanse.

"People who have real problems such as severe ME/CFS, advanced fibromyalgia, or debilitating RA, Hashimoto's thyroiditis, MS, lupus, connective tissue disease, eczema, psoriasis, or other autoimmune diseases have often been from doctor to doctor, told to swallow all kinds of fish oil and probiotics, even removed many gut-disruptive foods such as gluten, and still they suffer with their neurological symptoms. That's because the gut is not the answer to why we're sick."

— Anthony William, Medical Medium

CHAPTER 5

Intermittent Fasting Revealed

Intermittent fasting is a temporary Band-Aid that can support someone short term if they're not sick. We shouldn't see it as anything beyond short-term support for not-so-sick people, though—and even for those people, to get any of the positives, it needs to be done correctly. If you're an intermittent faster and you've come across this chapter, I'm going to offer you tips so that you can still do your intermittent fasting with the least consequences down the road for your body. It's best to eventually graduate out of intermittent fasting into one of the cleanses inside this book.

When you're sick and trying to recover from a chronic illness or symptom that's impeding your life, intermittent fasting will not give you the long-term relief you need; it can only hinder you, possibly even worsening your illness or condition. While I know so many people are into intermittent fasting, you shouldn't incorporate it into the 3:6:9 Cleanse, which is specifically geared to cleanse the body. Intermittent fasting does not translate to cleansing. What is someone eating on the other side of an intermittent fast? What's going on with their health? There are complexities here that make it unwise to combine intermittent fasting with the 3:6:9 Cleanse or any other cleanse in this book.

If you're still looking for an intermittent fasting option, you'll find a technique at the end of Chapter 16, "Morning Cleanse," that you can try separately from the 3:6:9 Cleanse. Keep in mind that when you're intermittent "fasting," you're never truly fasting. Not until you go 24 hours without food or beverages other than water can you call anything a fast. The body doesn't start its fasting process until the sun has risen twice. So if you're withholding foods in the morning or for most of the day and you eat a meal before 24 hours have passed, or you drink black coffee or even squeeze lemon into your water within those 24 hours, you stop the process of fasting from beginning. (That's not to say you *should* be fasting instead. While water fasting has its time and place, it should be done only with great care and in special circumstances.) Point is, the name of this technique is flawed to begin with, which showcases that the "experts" in intermittent fasting are unaware of how the body's processes really work.

WHY PEOPLE LIKE INTERMITTENT FASTING

Let's talk about the short-term positives of intermittent fasting. Not-so-sick people who like intermittent fasting say that they feel clearer and have more energy and better focus. The reason this occurs is that when they remove food for more than two to three hours, the body starts to run on adrenaline (also called epinephrine), which works as a natural amphetamine. That adrenaline races to the brain and ignites electricity there. So if you're someone who's not so sick and not so compromised—meaning that you still have adrenaline reserves—and you withhold food for long enough, you'll start running on those reserves of adrenaline. That's what brings the clarity, focus, and temporary energy.

Another reason some people report feeling better when they start intermittent fasting is that they're removing one to two of their fat-based meals for the day. When you give your body a break from a fat-based breakfast (and possibly lunch) that would have included radical fats such as avocado, peanut butter, almond butter, milk, cheese, bone broth, eggs, or other animal proteins (because animal proteins are always intertwined with fats), you automatically start to feel better because you're allowing your body to do a bit of cleansing. The right way to give your body this break would be to follow the Morning Cleanse that you'll read about in Chapter 16. It's the healthier option to protect you. And if you're still really attached to intermittent fasting, then the intermittent fasting option in that chapter is the way to go. Giving your body a break from meals really gives your liver, pancreas, and other organs a break from high-fat foods. (More in a moment.)

THE CAFFEINE MISTAKE

A huge mistake with intermittent fasting is that people are running on caffeine all day, slowly trashing their adrenal glands. Their caffeine addiction is forcing their adrenals to pump a harsh blend of adrenaline through their body for hours and hours. It's a truly unhealthy practice, and down the road, it's going to lead to aging, damaged skin, brain fog, severe focus and concentration problems, fatigue, hair loss, and weight gain. These symptoms may not show themselves in someone's 20s. They tend to surface later in the 30s and 40s. Even if someone is experiencing weight loss or stable weight right now, they can still gain weight from it later, once the adrenals have been trashed enough or the liver has become stagnant and sluggish enough from excess adrenaline caused by caffeine use. This comes back to the reality that intermittent fasting experimental practices are Band-Aids that don't address what people or their bodies truly need.

(For more on caffeine, see Chapter 7, "Troublemaker Foods.")

MORNING RELIEF FROM FATS

The popular trend in intermittent fasting is to consume nothing with sugar in the morning. The method of choice for many people is coffee, water, and no calories. I recommend not running yourself on only coffee and water. I recommend at least bringing in celery juice, coconut water, lemon water, and raw honey while, if possible, leaving out caffeine, which you'll see in the intermittent fasting option in Chapter 16, "Morning Cleanse." Professional hobbyists in the field of intermittent fasting think that the avoidance of sugar is why they're thinking more clearly and feeling better at certain parts of the day. They don't realize it's not the sugar; again, it's because they stopped eating fat.

When you're eating fats in the morning, you're burdening your liver, forcing it to produce bile, which stops the cleansing process that your liver was trying to accomplish throughout the night as you were sleeping. All those poisons are supposed to be flushed out in the morning and leave your body. Instead, people normally eat high fat–based foods in the morning—for example, peanut butter on their oatmeal, avocado toast, or eggs. This stops the poisons that the liver was gathering overnight from leaving the body. Instead, the poisons get trapped in the bloodstream and enter organs such as the brain.

Intermittent fasting eliminates fats by accident, with no one realizing it's the *fats'* absence, not the removal of sugar, that has people feeling better in the morning. Not realizing that fats were the real culprit is a great compromising mistake that will set you up for failure long term. Inevitably, people don't know that if they're losing weight or maintaining their weight through intermittent fasting, especially if they're able to exercise, it's because they're eating less fat in a day. They're keeping dietary fat from entering the bloodstream for long enough—often 16 to 18 hours—that they can maintain or even lose body fat. It gives the body a chance to rid itself of old fat that it's stored in organs and body tissue. Experts of the intermittent fasting theory and experiment don't realize this is the "why" of any results people get. They also don't realize that when withholding food throughout the morning and most of the day, they only appear leaner because they didn't fill their intestinal tract with food, which normally causes a natural expansion that widens the abdominal region. The temporary difference between eating and not eating is especially apparent for people who tend to experience bloating from meals. We need to factor in dehydration too: when intermittent fasting, many people are on caffeine drinks of various kinds, which causes a diuretic effect, or they don't drink enough water in the morning or the rest of the day. All of this can create the *illusion* that someone is leaning out and developing extra muscle definition on an intermittent fast. They don't realize that intermittent fasting is an unbalanced way to do this, and that there are much more balanced solutions.

The improvements people see with intermittent fasting can include a reduction of high blood pressure and improvement of A1C levels, blood sugar, and cholesterol levels. It's all because the liver is catching a break for a moment, with no fat or protein consumed for many hours. People don't realize that they would see these same benefits from lowering fat in their diet overall without needing to go hours without food. When fats are removed from a diet for long enough, it thins the blood enough to help reverse all kinds of symptoms and conditions.

This is one of the key reasons why historically, when someone went on a whole-food, plant-based diet, many symptoms could improve: because they were naturally consuming less fat than normal. When the current plant-based movement was in its early days, plant-based diets were very much low-fat—less fat and more carbohydrates were recommended. I've been teaching this for over 30 years. Nowadays, due to diet trends, plant-based diets are getting fewer results because they've become ketogenic plant-based diets, which is to say, high fat. Even the paleo diets of years ago had lower fats in them than they do now.

Because people are hitting plateaus with these diets and not getting the results they desire anymore, they're leaving, altering, or combining paleo, keto, and high-protein, plant-based diets with intermittent fasting—with no one teaching them (because no one knows) that the reason intermittent fasting can get results is because it halts the consumption of fats for part of the day. Instead, people are hearing that maybe sugar is the problem, and so avoiding sugar for part of the day must be the Holy Grail. Or they believe that an intermittent fast helps by giving your digestion a break and allowing that energy to go to fat loss, cell regeneration, and body repair, which can actually happen when the liver is not contending with a lot of fat in the bloodstream. Again, though, no one realizes it's the break from fats that allows your body to repair and let go of body fat. These diets and intermittent fasting are all part of a guessing game. The simple truth is that lower fat improves your health. There are better ways to lower fat in your diet—namely, the 3:6:9 Cleanse and other cleanse options in these pages.

A RECIPE FOR BURNOUT

People also adopt an intermittent fasting approach because they notice that if they withhold eating for long enough, they can get through a larger part of the day without eating foods they regret or eating too much. When you eat the "wrong" breakfast in the morning, it can set the stage for eating "off" all day long. Intermittent fasters get around this by withholding food as long as they can and using caffeine as a stimulant to get by. If enough hours

pass this way, then when you do start eating, you're already at the end of the day and don't have to make so many food choices, or there's not a chance to eat as many calories before bedtime. There are so many more reasons why someone chooses intermittent fasting as they try to "hack" their health and miss the truth in the process. A better approach would be to drink coconut water all day long, because the downside of withholding food and critically needed glucose and mineral salts while running on adrenaline all day is that you're eventually going to come to a point when it's time to eat, or you even reach a point of breakdown, and then it's going to be hard to *stop* eating because you've gone into glucose, carbohydrate, and mineral salt deficit. Intermittent fasters often find themselves bingeing on troublemaker foods, even if it's just on their "cheat day," when they give themselves permission to indulge once a week. Then there are those who find themselves bingeing on troublemaker foods without making it public. Those in either crew never learn how to truly heal or take care of themselves with food.

Even if they choose what seem to be healthier food options at first, after too many weeks of starving themselves of carbs—and carbs translate to glucose that's critically needed for brain function—plus too many weeks of using caffeine to stimulate adrenaline to replace that glucose for the brain, intermittent fasters can reach a point of burnout. This can mean more focus and concentration problems than you ever had before you started, even if it seemed like focus and concentration improved at first. It's a slippery slope and a rabbit hole you have to try to avoid. If you're living with any neurological symptoms (such as anxiety, tremors, tics, spasms, shakes, dizziness, vertigo, balance issues, eye floaters, migraines, trigeminal neuralgia, nerve pain, tingles, or numbness, to name a few), keep in mind that even if they improve with intermittent fasting, it's temporary, and they most often come back and eventually worsen—because intermittent fasting does not remove toxic heavy metals or kill off viruses and bacteria that are at the root of these symptoms and conditions. When the nervous system is sensitive, it's critical to keep a consistent balance of glucose and mineral salts so that nerves don't weaken and your health doesn't decline.

SAVE YOURSELF FROM UNNECESSARY HARDSHIP

Intermittent fasting experts are trying to teach people to hack their health by not eating. It's another man-made self-plan. Intermittent fasting originated from people who were under a lot of stress, experiencing hardship,

loss, or struggle of some kind. These are the sorts of emotional challenges that can make eating very hard, or make somebody sick to their stomach, or make it hard to enjoy food and therefore prompt them to withhold food, perhaps only sipping tea throughout the day or eating very little because they're so unsettled and uneasy about what's happening in their life in that moment. This is how the idea of intermittent fasting came about.

I'll say it one more time: it's a Band-Aid, a temporary Band-Aid to get us through hardship before everything goes wrong with the intermittent fasting practice.

We don't need to make life any harder on ourselves. If you're into intermittent fasting, I recommend instead that you stick to the cleanses in this book. Learn how your body works so that you don't prematurely age, weaken your liver, set yourself up for chronic illness, blow out your adrenals too early in life, and end up lost and sick.

"You are far from alone. You are part of an empowering movement. By standing up for yourself, you are standing up for the crowd of people with hopes and dreams for their lives who do not deserve to be held back by chronic suffering."

— Anthony William, Medical Medium

CHAPTER 6

The Juicing versus Fiber Debate

Here's a surprisingly hot-button topic that gets in the way of people trying and committing to celery juice and other fresh, healing, cleansing juices: pulp. Certain health professionals share concern that when you juice anything, you're getting rid of what they believe to be the most important part: fiber. They believe that by extracting the fiber, you're extracting all the nutrients and throwing away the very component that's supposed to keep the small intestinal tract and colon healthy, care for the microbiome to feed good bacteria and lower bad bacteria, and allow for regular bowel movements. They believe that juicing denatures food, that it takes a whole food in its natural state and practically destroys it, minimizing what it has left to offer the body. This sounds like a great argument, a noble cause to fight for. It's quite the opposite. Let's look at the real deal.

A MISLED QUEST FOR FIBER

The only people who are lacking fiber in their diet are those who eat mostly processed food. If you've been convinced that fruit is bad and you've taken it out of your diet (which I don't recommend), you're still getting enough fiber. Even people who eat predominantly fast food tend to get enough fiber. A standard American diet with the worst varieties of gas station burritos, drive-through burgers, sausages, pancakes, waffles, and deep-fried and greasy abominations still gives someone enough fiber.

The reason health professionals think we need more fiber is that, "healthy" diet or not, people are experiencing constipation. That sluggish peristaltic action that slows down bowel movements doesn't come from a lack of fiber, though. It comes from inflammation. And that inflammation comes from pathogens feeding on both high-quality and low-quality sources of food, including cheese, gluten, and much-revered eggs. Consider whole-wheat bread. That's packed with fiber, and in many circles, it's thought to be a healthy source of it. Trouble is, it's also packed with gluten, and gluten feeds the viruses and unproductive bacteria that create intestinal inflammation, which can in turn make it difficult to go to the bathroom. That leads someone to seek out more fiber in hopes of moving along intestinal tract blockages.

It's not a matter of getting enough fiber. We get enough fiber. It's a matter of getting the right varieties of food that don't feed unproductive bugs in the gut that lead to more damage to the intestinal tract linings. If you're someone who gravitates to a healthier diet, staying away from fast food and other processed foods and incorporating more fruits, vegetables, healthier whole grains, nuts, seeds, and even avocado, you're supplying yourself with ample fiber, and that fiber is helpful in some ways. The even more helpful aspect? Eating higher quantities of healthy foods leaves less room for foods that feed unproductive bacteria and viruses, which can create intestinal disorders. Leaving out those troublemaker foods, not adding in more fiber, is the real key to gut health.

Let's break down what troublemaker foods can do to the gut. Take white bread, considered unhealthy in part because of its lack of fiber. Even people with white bread in their diet get enough fiber from other sources, though, unless they're living solely on white bread. The real issue, just as with the whole-wheat bread, is gluten. It's gluten feeding *Streptococcus*, *E. coli*, *Staphylococcus*, and hundreds of other varieties of unproductive bacteria—with strep's many strains leading the way as they create issues such as celiac disease and SIBO. It's gluten feeding viruses such as shingles, which lies inside the intestinal tract and creates colitis, or the Epstein-Barr virus, which along with strep is responsible for celiac. It's gluten feeding the various pathogens that inflame the linings of the colon and cause irritable bowel syndrome (IBS). These causes of chronic gut problems all remain mysteries to medical research and science.

Nerve damage around the digestive tract lining is another factor here. Millions of nerve cells line your stomach, small intestinal tract, colon, and surrounding areas. These nerves can become inflamed too, creating a host of different symptoms including varieties of gastroparesis and cramping, discomfort, bloating, and slowdown or stoppage of peristaltic action. That inflammation isn't happening due to a lack of fiber. Fiber is not the issue.

And where does fiber fit when it comes to hydrochloric acid? It doesn't. Nearly everyone is walking around with low hydrochloric acid and digestive problems because of it—they're not breaking down their proteins. Fiber isn't a solution here, because fiber doesn't make you break down proteins.

Fiber also doesn't break down fat. We rely on bile for that, and nearly everyone's bile reserves are low too. That's due to the weakened, stagnant, sluggish livers people walk around with, and that's in turn due to diets too high in fat and troublemaker foods feeding pathogens that live inside the liver, intestinal tract, and even stomach. As a result, pathogens can create ulcers in the gut: *E. coli*–based ulcers, strep-based ulcers, and even herpes-based ulcers caused by viruses such as herpes simplex 2. The ulcers don't form from a lack of fiber in the diet. They form because poor foods in the diet feed pathogens.

Where does peristaltic action originate? Does it come from fiber? Not necessarily. Your central nervous system creates peristalsis. Signals that come from your brain down to your small intestinal tract move food through you. Some people have a robust connection between their brain and intestinal tract. It almost doesn't matter what you put in them; their digestive tract will peristaltically move that food along regardless of how fibrous it is. Someone can live off white, processed food—they can fill their stomach up with lots of white bread, white rice pudding made with processed sugar, and the like—and it will move through perfectly.

If, on the other hand, you have trouble going to the bathroom, with less peristaltic action, that's not the fault of a lack of fiber. While you may use fiber as a tool to help you manage your constipation, your intestinal tract didn't become dysfunctional in the first place from not getting enough fiber.

Troublemaker foods such as gluten and eggs are the real problem here, along with other troublemakers we're exposed to, such as toxic heavy metals—because troublemaker foods and toxic troublemakers (1) weaken the central nervous system's ability to communicate with the intestinal tract and (2) feed pathogens such as strep, shingles, *E. coli*, and various unproductive fungi that can reside inside the intestinal tract. A high level of fat in the diet overall, whether from healthy or unhealthy fats, is also significant, because a steady diet of high fat slowly injures the liver over time, making it stagnant and sluggish, which means it creates less bile, and that low bile can be the true issue—meaning that a weak liver is one real reason why you end up relying on more fiber to move food through the gut.

Instead of focusing on cleaning up pathogens in the intestinal tract and colon to reduce inflammation, raising hydrochloric acid production to break down proteins, and rejuvenating the liver so we can break down both fats we're consuming in the present and old, rancid fats caked on our intestinal wall linings, we're told to worry about fiber. We treat fiber as wisdom for the ages, the answer to everything, when really, making fiber your dietary focus is like doing a forceful broom sweep of the intestinal tract without fixing the floorboards—that

is, without addressing any of the underlying problems. It's why people tend to get sicker and sicker with their gut issues, relying on more and more fiber laxatives that only act as Band-Aids while the digestion issues continue.

How *do* we address the underlying problems? Fiber isn't the answer, because a lack of fiber didn't start the issues. Instead, we fix gut issues and get your body working again with the very technique that's so often written off: juicing as medicine.

THE REAL WASTE

Let's consider the arguments of anti-juicing enthusiasts. A big part of the reasoning is that making a vegetable or herb into juice wastes the most important part of it: the fiber. Well, now you know that you get plenty of fiber from the rest of your diet, so adding a juice or two to your day won't deprive you. Besides which, fiber isn't the most important part of a vegetable, fruit, or herb—and we'll cover even more about this in a moment.

The next part of the rhetoric that juicing is bad is that throwing out all that fiber is wasteful. Interesting. So if instead of making juice from a serving of vegetables, you were to eat them whole, would you save your poop? Because whenever we eat vegetables (or anything else), our body is processing out that fiber, and we're flushing it down the toilet. That's how fiber is supposed to work; fiber doesn't stay in the body. We excrete it, and then we send it away to the septic tank or sewer system and don't think about it.

When we juice, though, we see the fiber pile up and that makes us worry that it's wasteful. The waste that comes from juicing fruits and vegetables does not hurt our planet. We can even compost it and turn it into garden soil. You can't turn your poop into garden soil safely.

Again, the real issue is that most food waste in our lives is "out of sight, out of mind." When we do more of our own food prep and start feeding ourselves at home, we see the rinds, peels, seeds, and scraps of fruits and vegetables pile up. It's an illusion to think that this means we're producing more garbage in general, though. What about all the waste we never see that goes into making the bags and boxes of processed foods we buy? What about all the waste from eating out? Dinners, lunches, snacks, even coffee purchased when we're away from home—they all produce piles of waste behind the scenes. Everything produces waste. Whether or not we see that waste determines whether we feel guilty of a crime.

There is no crime in juicing, even though people get picked on when they do it. All that fiber and pulp they throw away that's supposedly the healthiest part and really isn't—again, that isn't waste that hurts the planet. It only helps; it's a harmless byproduct of a process that creates medicinal extracts that people are using to heal themselves so they can save the world.

Meanwhile, coffee drinkers don't get picked on in the same way. Think of the massive piles of coffee grounds that get dumped into the garbage every day. Not only that; think about the sugar so many people stir into their coffee. How much land was mauled and rainforest destroyed so that sugar cane could be grown? No matter how healthy you think you are, the foods you choose lead to waste. The foods you put in your body create waste. That's how the cycle works. We can't pretend that the person who decides to juice some

fresh produce is the perpetrator of a food crime of which everyone else is innocent.

Rather, we need to respect the person who brings juicing into their life. We need to honor that individual who fills up their fridge with vegetables and herbs and piles up their counter with fruit. This is about the body getting exactly what it needs for survival. It's about preventing illness so that they're not a draw on the medical system. The person who eats what they think is healthy—whether keto, paleo, vegan, or any other popular diet—and yet isn't juicing and giving their body everything it needs will rely more on the medical system later, and that creates waste long term. The person who's generating juice pulp and fiber now will rely less on the medical system and create far less waste in their lifetime. What's a true waste is if we don't try fresh, healing juices because we've gotten caught up in a philosophy, theory, or agenda.

FIBER SKELETONS

Fiber itself: Does it contain nutrients we need? Are we missing out on those nutrients with juicing?

Fiber only contains nutrients that can be separated from it, which means that no, we're not missing out. Quite the opposite: if those nutrients were inseparable from the fiber, we'd never be able to absorb them; only when nutrients get released from fiber (whether through chewing, digestion, blending, cooking, or especially juicing) can we access and benefit from them.

Say a lab analyzes what nutrients a plant food contains. That doesn't mean our body benefits from all of them; those nutrients are useless if the body can't extract them easily and they stay locked inside the fiber and we eliminate them—that is, if we poop them out. As much research as you may find about what's inside a certain food, that nutrition is only useful to us if we can access it. Some nutrients really hide inside fiber; much of the time, our body can't extract the nutrients hiding inside a plant food's fiber so easily. A lab may be able to extract them and put their medicinal properties to use, whereas the body can't on its own.

When you eat a piece of lettuce or a celery stick, for example, or a piece of raw cauliflower or cucumber or tomato, you'll get a lot of nutrients—those nutrients that the body can easily separate from the fiber. Your body can't access, absorb, and assimilate *all* the nutrients, though, because as you can read throughout this book, our bodies are weakened. Fiber gets in the way. We need help—help from a machine in extracting those precious minerals, enzymes, trace minerals, antivirals, antibacterials, antioxidants, and healing phytochemical compounds that we can't get any other way. I'm talking specifically about juice extracts here, not blended drinks. Our bogged-down, broken-down digestive tracts can struggle to get a fraction of the nutrients even in blended smoothies, because the fiber is still there. Many health professionals believe that throwing whole foods in a blender is the answer to so much, and while that's a great concept—and you'll see in some of the cleanses in this book that blended foods hold an important place in healing—it's not going to cut it as the sole approach. We also need to extract juices to create separate medicines.

Remember, you are most likely getting more than enough fiber in your diet. Even if you need to keep using fiber as a tool to help move your bowels, don't let that eclipse juicing. Fresh juice extracts are key to repairing the digestive tract, among other aspects of our health.

My gut is fine, you may be thinking. *It's strong. I don't need help.* The truth is, even the healthiest people can't extract every nutrient hidden inside fiber with their digestive strength alone. It's not possible. You could have the strongest digestive tract with strong enough bile and hydrochloric acid reserves (everyone's reserves are at least somewhat weakened at this point) and you could exercise regularly, and you're still not going to get everything you need from fruits, vegetables, herbs, and healthy grains as they are. Not to mention that your digestive system will weaken over time if juicing isn't a part of your life. Your body shouldn't have to process mega amounts of fiber, not with everything we're up against in this world—more than ever before in history. Juicing is a critical way to be proactive. It saves our body from extra work and helps protect our digestive system from losing strength. Juicing provides respite.

Fiber is essentially present in a plant food to hold the fruit or herb or vegetable together. That's its purpose. Health professionals are not yet aware of the reality that fiber is there to give a food a skeleton so it can stand up or hold its shape to receive sun in the field or grove as it's growing. It's there as a structure to hold the plant cells together: the juicy plant cells that hold the real nutrients. Fiber isn't there to help you go to the bathroom. Rather, that happens to be a benefit of fiber for people with mild to severe gut injuries from real issues that are being ignored.

The best dietician will recommend fiber for many digestive problems without knowing what's really causing those problems.

That's no disrespect to dieticians. There are some amazing ones out there. The answers they need simply aren't in the literature yet. Fiber has never fixed an illness or disease. When you stop eating fiber, your problem comes back. Fiber doesn't kill off the *E. coli* or *Streptococcus* bacteria that injure the intestine with divots, creating diverticulitis and diverticulosis. It simply moves food through when peristaltic action is weakened. Bowel movements are about so much more than fiber; digestion is so much bigger than fiber. It's all part of a symbiotic process that involves the liver, stomach and rest of the gut, and nervous system—and real healing is about taking care of all these in ways we were never taught. So if you fear a lack of fiber if you drink a daily juice, don't worry anymore. You're going to get more than enough fiber in any one of these cleanses. Much more critically, you're going to benefit from the cleanses' diverse healing components to address what's going on in your body at a much deeper level.

THE DANGER OF BEING MISLED

Why do people turn to juicing in the first place? Because they've been sick with chronic symptom or illness and they see juicing for what it is: life-saving medicine. They rely on it to bring them back to life. Why take that away with misinformation?

When a professional who's vocal in the health arena advises against juicing, and particularly advises against juicing celery because they say we're better off getting the fiber, it shortchanges people of their health and their family's health. That's what happens when we put blind faith in belief systems and letters behind a name, and it's dangerous. If we see a quote that juicing is bad, silly, or wasteful and we see "Ph.D." or "M.D." to go with it, and we follow that professional's words because of these markers we're supposed to trust at face value, we get derailed. We shorten our life pan. And we never realize that we put our lives and our families' lives in the hands of a mere theory that a misled, fallible human being had along the way.

What about me? If you find yourself wondering why trust me and why follow my belief system, know that I don't offer beliefs, a belief system, or theories. If you've read my other books, and if you read Chapter 24, "Living Words for Underdogs and a Note for Critics," at the beginning of Part V, you'll know that the information I share does not come from me. It comes from above, from the highest, nonbiased source so you can heal.

CHAPTER 7

Troublemaker Foods

Chances are, you're reading this book or sifting through its pages because you've experienced a symptom. Maybe it interfered with the quality of your life or your performance or how you feel emotionally. Maybe it was a perplexing symptom or set of symptoms that sent you to one doctor, two, or more. Maybe you received a diagnosis, whether of an autoimmune condition or not, and maybe it was passed off as hormones or stress. And if that isn't your story, then chances are it's the story of a loved one, close acquaintance, or friend. You find yourself now in this chapter, about to look over foods that you feel have been good to you in your life. You've enjoyed them and even been told some of these foods are healthy.

I wouldn't tell you that a food is bad for you because I'm guessing. I wouldn't insult who you are as a person. I don't play games. You didn't come across a book that's all "pro" this and "anti" that. The only "antis" here are *antiviral* and *antibacterial*—in the name of your healing. I'm all about the truth of what's occurring inside your body and how you can finally heal.

When you wake up each day and instantly come to the realization that the symptom you're battling is still there, or that your next doctor's appointment for your chronic condition is still on the horizon, and part of every day is absorbed by the fact that you're not feeling well, it matters to me. I believe that you have the right to heal and be symptom free. More than believe—I know. I understand what you're going through every hour as you emotionally, mentally, and physically struggle with a symptom that's most likely mysterious in nature to doctors and other health professionals; even if they've given you a diagnosis or they have a name for your symptom when you describe it to them, if it hasn't gone away, it's still a mystery to them. I know that it's hard and there's nothing easy about any of it.

It's not just that the foods you'll read about here aren't good for you. It's about something that's happening inside of you that's a mystery to your family, friends, doctors, and medical research and science. People are sick from two presences inside their bodies: toxins and pathogens. That's critical to know when you think about food. If you understand how certain foods play a role in continuing to keep you sick, you can see the light and gain clarity—and get to a place of healing.

THE TROUBLEMAKER FOODS LIST

Here's an overview of the foods covered in this chapter. For an easy one-page table, turn to Chapter 15, "Anti-Bug Cleanse."

Level 1

- Eggs
- Dairy
- Gluten
- Soft drinks
- Be mindful of salt consumption

Level 2

All of the above PLUS:

- Pork
- Tuna
- Corn

Level 3

All of the above PLUS:

- Industrial food oils (vegetable oil, palm oil, canola oil, corn oil, safflower oil, soybean oil)
- Soy
- Lamb
- Fish and seafood (other than salmon, trout, and sardines)

Level 4

All of the above PLUS:

- Vinegar (including apple cider vinegar, or ACV)
- Fermented foods (including kombucha, sauerkraut, and coconut aminos)
- Caffeine (including coffee, matcha, and chocolate)

Level 5

All of the above PLUS:

- Grains (other than millet and oats)
- All oils (including healthier ones such as olive, walnut, sunflower, coconut, sesame, avocado, grapeseed, almond, macadamia, peanut, flaxseed)

Bonus

For even better, faster results:

- Cut out salt and seasonings entirely (pure spices are okay)
- Avoid radical fats entirely for a period

And also limit or remove:

- Alcohol
- Natural/artificial flavors
- Nutritional yeast
- Citric acid
- Aspartame
- Other artificial sweeteners
- Monosodium glutamate (MSG)
- Formaldehyde
- Preservatives

WHY TO AVOID THE TROUBLEMAKER FOODS

It helps to think of the troublemaker foods in levels, with Level 1 the most important to remove from your diet if you want to protect your health. When you're working hard to heal, it's best to avoid all of these foods through Level 5 and even "Bonus." Understanding the "why" behind each food that we'll explore will give you all the incentive you need to hold off on them. For physical support as you let foods

go, turn to Chapter 20, "Your Body's Healing Power," and for emotional support and
insights into cravings, turn to Chapter 25, "The
Emotional Side of Cleansing."

Level 1

Eggs

I understand that we all have a deep
emotional connection to eggs. While maybe
not *everybody*, the majority of the population does. Many of us grew up eating eggs
prepared by our mothers, fathers, grandparents, uncles, and aunts, so they have a special
place in our hearts. Eggs at brunches, holi-
day breakfasts, or diners with friends after a
night out—eggs are fun. We bond over them,
whether sunny-side up, poached, scrambled,
hard-boiled, or in French toast, egg sandwiches, or simple eggs and cheese. So when
you tell people to stop eating eggs, a reaction occurs that's distinct from when you tell
people to stop eating other foods, a jolt that's
more intense than hearing "You need to go
gluten-free." Letting eggs go is an emotional
occurrence all on its own. Some people may
feel it's like losing a part of themselves to give
up eggs—that's how attached they are. Some
people may dream about them.

The messages out there about eggs can
get confusing. We often hear that they're a
healthy food—a perfect food, even—and a
well-balanced source of protein. The truth is
that long before pathogens such as unproductive viruses, bacteria, and even funguses
invaded our bodies and created our current
culture of chronic illness as the new normal,
eggs were a survival food. While they weren't
good for us, they at least weren't detrimental

to our health—before the explosion of viruses
and other bugs.

If you haven't discovered that little spark of
doubt inside of you yet telling you that eating
eggs may not be that good for you, consider
the saying "eggs in moderation." That came
about because of (valid) concerns about egg
consumption and heart disease.

And if you're someone who's going to read
this with ruffled feathers because you don't
want to give up your eggs, you may decide to
run and quickly look up scientific research and
studies to support your comfort food. Know
that all egg studies that are positive are paid
for. To put it simply, people are paying science
to do studies on eggs so that you keep eating
them. You couldn't get a study funded these
days to follow through on why eggs really are
bad for us. It would never stick. Everybody
involved would be at high risk of never being
employed again.

A couple of critical mistakes along the way
changed eggs' role from quick and easy survival food in a pinch to a food that lessens our
ability to survive. Without your permission and
without anyone telling you they were going to
do this, the medical industry and Big Pharma
made a decision for you. There was no town
hall meeting; you had no say in the matter and
no way to vote on the issue. They took a common survival food that so many have leaned on
over the centuries and used it to experiment in
a negligent manner. Now, these may be strong
words. When you consider the degree of suffering in adults and children and especially womankind with chronic illness, and the rise of that
suffering in recent years, these words may not
be strong enough to describe the coldhearted
malice and deceit behind what they have done
with your eggs. They took an important survival

food, and without your consent and without being held responsible, they raised pathogens with it. Chronic illness is at an all-time high because of it, and people are still in the dark about the truth of what's happening.

Here's the story: Decades ago, before your time for most of you reading this, eggs were used in scientific research laboratories as food for microorganisms. Unproductive bacteria and viruses—such as *Streptococcus*, *Staphylococcus*, the Epstein-Barr virus, HHV-6, herpes simplex 1 and 2, shingles, cytomegalovirus, even HPV and retroviruses such as human immunodeficiency virus (HIV)—were all toyed with, manipulated, and raised in labs using eggs as the pathogens' food source. That is, eggs were used to keep aggressive bugs alive: the same bugs that today give us endometriosis, fibroids, PCOS, cervical and ovarian cancers, breast cancer, MS, fibromyalgia, rheumatoid arthritis, lupus, Hashimoto's thyroiditis, and ME/CFS in record numbers. If those don't raise an eyebrow for you, then consider eczema, psoriasis, acne, vertigo, balance issues, dizziness, tinnitus (ringing/buzzing in the ears), tingles, numbness, mystery aches and pains, ongoing fatigue, unexplained blurry vision, eye floaters, white or dark spots in the vision, brain fog, crippling anxiety, and depression.

Many of the pathogens that were raised on eggs in labs in the early 1900s through 1930s were privately categorized, patented, and censored from the outside medical system. That is, the viruses were not made publicly known to medical schools and doctors. It took virologists stumbling upon the viral strains in people's bodies years later for these viruses such as Epstein-Barr virus and HHV-6 to be discovered. In private circles, EBV was a

well-kept secret for decades before the virus was identified by heroic virologists.

Pathogens such as these viruses cause a staggering majority of today's ailments—and in addition to eggs, toxins that take up residence in our bodies feed the pathogens. Eggs, then, are at the top of the list of foods you want to avoid while cleansing, because they too are fuel for the bugs that cause us pain and suffering and lower quality of life as the years go by. Eggs even feed the viruses that are responsible for almost all cancers. It's fine and dandy to call eggs a perfect food and hang your hat on that because of what you've been taught, plus the fact that they taste so delicious and are hard to resist in so many ways. Once you start to learn the truth, though, that eggs could contribute to someone developing reproductive cancer (or another type of cancer) over time, they hardly seem worth eating anymore if you have health concerns. Egg whites don't get around this issue. Whether you're eating the whites or the yolk or both together, they feed pathogens all the same.

Many of us have learned that food is medicine. Well, not all food is medicine, even if it has something good in it, and even if it has something *seemingly* good for us in it. Just because a food contains a nutrient doesn't mean there's not another component of that food that we're not being told about that's bad for us—and cancels out any benefits from the nutrient. Spinach is real medicine. Wild blueberries are medicine. Celery juice is medicine. Even potatoes (without butter, cheese, cream, oil, and milk) are medicine, because potatoes carry lysine, which helps the body knock down the very viruses that eggs feed. Meanwhile, food diet programs out there will often exclude potato. It's a prime example of how everyone is guessing.

I'm not going to sugarcoat this and say you might have an egg allergy. Yes, people can have egg allergies, including mild versions that go undetected and yet can cause some trouble. Blanketing the general issue with eggs as "egg allergies," though, would take away from the valuable information that there's a larger reason why eggs don't serve us when we're worried about our health.

We think eggs are a great protein source. Eggs have been married to the word *protein* on purpose, as a marketing strategy. Truth is, the proteins in eggs feed viruses, unproductive bacteria, and fungus—because that egg protein was used in labs long ago as a food that viruses and other pathogens were trained to consume. When we think egg protein is good for us, we have to realize that we cook our eggs, destroying and denaturing the protein so our bodies can't utilize it anyway. We often hear that the omega-3 in eggs is good for us. That gets destroyed once an egg is cooked, too. And while we can use raw egg protein, it still feeds the pathogens that keep us sick, so that cancels out the benefits.

Consider the hormones in eggs. We're not talking about added hormones here; we're talking about the naturally occurring hormones in even free-range, organic, backyard eggs. If you raise your own chickens, realize that even your own chicken eggs will still feed pathogens. An egg is a ball of hormones to grow a baby chicken, and those hormones feed viruses and bacteria as well—bacteria such as *Streptococcus*, which causes acne, bladder infections and other UTIs, chronic sinusitis, lung infections, sties, and even most ear infections. Eggs' naturally occurring hormones disrupt our endocrine glands, causing our own hormones to become imbalanced. The hormones in eggs also feed cysts in the reproductive system—cysts that were created by viruses when women with reproductive conditions were told to eat more eggs. It's like somebody playing a bad joke on these women who have suffered.

Eggs are not blood sugar balancers. Everyone thinks they keep us stable and that they're perfect for diabetes. In truth, eggs are not the perfect food for blood sugar disorders or diabetes. Eggs cause insulin resistance and put us in a constant vicious cycle because inside an egg are both sugar and fat together. When you combine sugars and fats, that's how you get insulin resistance, which can lead to diabetes in the first place. Why is there sugar in eggs? It's the critical carbohydrate needed for the developing chicken's muscle growth—it's the only way for it to get the strength to break out of the shell. Eggs are a high caloric source, which is why people feel that eggs stabilize them. Some people think they've found the Holy Grail when they're frying up their eggs in coconut oil. It's as if they've outsmarted the egg monster that's trying to get them sick without them even realizing it. I'm sorry to say they haven't.

Realize that people with a lower pathgenic load—that is, fewer viruses and bacteria—can get away with eating a lot that people who have ME/CFS or Hashimoto's thyroiditis can't get away with. The fewer pathogens you have, the more you can get away with eating some eggs . . . for now. We're in a new age, where younger people are dealing with a lot of viral mutations that are spurring an epidemic of chronic illness like never before seen in our history. Many older people have fewer pathogens and can get away with eating a few eggs here and there. Our younger generation, especially young womankind with all the reproductive system disorders they're facing, plus eczema, psoriasis, and fatigue, are not getting away with eating eggs today and are suffering as a result. Meanwhile, they're told eggs are a superfood, or the most important protein source they can get.

When you get a symptom or condition or disease or diagnosis, you won't blame the eggs. No one does. Eggs are so coveted that they have immunity. You'll blame another source long before you blame an egg for your symptom, condition, or sickness. You'll blame mold or a piece of fruit you ate a week ago, or you'll blame your body (like medical research and science do), or you'll blame the universe or you'll think you created it. You won't blame eggs. No one will.

I'm the messenger. I'm not the one who ruined your eggs. Big Pharma and the medical industry ruined your eggs. Not the amazing professionals who work for them. The industries did it, by decades ago using eggs to raise the pathogens that plague us today. How come you don't know about pathogens causing all of your chronic conditions and suffering? Why are you told instead that your body's attacking you and that it's your genes? Because if the truth were out there about these pathogens and how they're keeping us sick today, the leaders of the industries would be in a lot of trouble. There would be hell to pay, especially from the moms whose babies have suffered. The truth would cause a revolt and an uprising.

You will find that almost everyone diagnosed with autoimmune disease eats eggs. The same goes for most anyone diagnosed with breast cancer—they're told to eat eggs every morning. Even if someone is getting a

little better because they're removing other foods you'll explore in this chapter, it doesn't mean they're out of the woods. Think of how much further they would go in their healing process if they removed eggs.

Eggs are detrimental, even if they have some good qualities. It's like knowing someone who's likely to harm you physically or emotionally and yet still has one or two really good qualities in them. You know better than to be in denial about the hurt a bully like this could create. As much compassion as you may feel for them, you know to stay away because they'll cause more harm than good. That's how you have to think about eggs.

Dairy

Maybe you've heard that dairy is mucus-forming. Sometimes it feels like you hear it everywhere. When we're consuming dairy products such as milk, cheese, butter, and more, we don't realize just how mucus-forming they really are. And *why* is it mucus-forming? The irony is, nobody knows why. Here's an answer: every time dairy is consumed, it clogs up the liver in an acute manner. That's one cause of mucus production.

Dairy doesn't just get broken down, digested, and sent on its way through the digestive tract in a timely fashion, as many other foods do. Instead, dairy sticks around. First, it slows down the absorption and assimilation of other foods that may be in the gut at the same time, ones critical for sustaining life because of their advanced nutrition: fruits, vegetables, leafy greens, and herbs. These hold minerals, vitamins, undiscovered antivirals and antibacterials, and other nutrients and healing phytochemicals that get caught up in dairy's film and lose their vitality and value before they can be drawn into the bloodstream through the walls of the intestinal tract, brought to the liver through the hepatic portal vein, and converted into more useful, methylated nutrient forms for the body. Once we've consumed a food and the digestion process has started to draw out its nutrients, those nutrients only have a certain amount of time before they're not useful anymore. The nutrients need to reach the liver in a timely fashion because the liver practically ordains them so they don't die or become ineffective as they travel through the body. That is, as one of its over 2,000 undiscovered functions, the liver offers a chemical compound that brings longer-lasting life to the nutrient and keeps it from oxidizing. In our blood are electricity and conductivity that interfere with these nutrients unless the liver's special chemical compound is bonded to them for protection.

Dairy clogs up the digestive freeway, allowing pathogens to thrive in our small intestinal tract and colon that shouldn't, ones such as unproductive funguses, molds, bacteria, and viruses. Because dairy doesn't break down, digest, or leave the system easily, it smothers critical oxygen. When dairy finally does get broken down and drawn through the intestinal tract walls into the liver via the hepatic portal vein, it slows down liver function, making the organ stagnant and sluggish in an immediate, acute manner. This leads mucus to form. When your body's filter—your liver—becomes clogged, all of the toxins that escape your liver as a result and enter your body increase histamine compounds, which feed and form more mucus.

(This is why an increasing number of babies and small children are exhibiting allergic reactions, digestive disturbances, or constipation when consuming dairy products. These little ones' livers are struggling from dairy. Don't be concerned about human breast milk, though. It's in a completely different category than animal dairy.)

Lymphatic vessels also become clogged with dairy byproduct. It's the job of the lymphatic highway to control pathogens. Our lymphocytes (white blood cells) are in our lymphatic system for a reason: to seek out and destroy invaders. Dairy products get in the way of natural killer cells, allowing invaders to thrive. A thriving invader (that is, pathogen) is highly toxic to our lymphatic highway. The poisons it produces stimulate blood vessels and tissue to produce fluid that becomes mucus-y, which is another reason why dairy is so mucus-forming.

For example, when someone gets the flu virus, it goes on a feeding frenzy inside their body, gobbling up foods it likes to eat such as the residue from eggs, dairy, and gluten. In this process, the flu virus eliminates a poison, and that poison stimulates the formation of mucus. (If you're not actively eating those foods, the flu virus finds old "storage bins" of egg, dairy, and gluten residue inside your liver, from when you consumed the foods months or even years ago. The fewer storage bins you have in your body, the less mucus-y you get when you get the flu—another reason to cleanse with the tools in this book.) The mucus that results when the flu virus excretes its poison after consuming egg, dairy, and gluten residues is the mucus that causes cough and sinus congestion when we have the flu. Our body forms the mucus to slow down the virus and trap it.

Now, what about when we don't have the flu? Most individuals have pathogens inside of them—other viruses such as Epstein-Barr and bacteria such as *Streptococcus* that feed on the natural hormones and protein in dairy and release their own toxins that cause a mucus response. If we have a pathogen load in us, such as an elevated level of strep—which many children and adults do without knowing it—then these dairy reactions can all be heightened, taking the form of a dairy allergy. Someone doesn't have to be diagnosed with a dairy sensitivity to be sensitive to dairy, though. Similar to the situation with eggs, anyone can start to develop symptoms as a result of milk, cheese, butter, cream, whey or whey protein powder, kefir, yogurt, sheep's milk, goat cheese, or other dairy in their life, and those symptoms go far beyond those we associate with dairy allergies. When you want your body in a state of healing, it's best to avoid dairy.

One of the reasons it can be hard to cut dairy out of your diet is that the unproductive viruses and bacteria that feed on dairy get hungry and ornery when you take dairy away. The bugs realize they're starting to starve. As some of these bugs slowly die, they release a toxin, and in response your adrenal glands produce an adrenaline blend to act as a natural steroid to protect your immune system from overreacting. With all this going on, we can feel emotionally unstable without knowing why, and that can cause us to feel a need for comfort food. If we go ahead and reach for that ice cream, pizza, cheesy pasta, or cheeseburger—some of the foods these bugs like—then the bugs' fuel starts to get replenished. This is what gives dairy its addictive quality: the bugs in our system thrive on it and practically beg for it. (For more on pathogenic die-off and cravings, see Chapter 25, "The Emotional Side of Cleansing.") When you realize this is what's going on behind the scenes in those moments when you're tempted to reach for a piece of cheese, it gives you a lot more power to say no.

Gluten

To this day, medical research and science still don't understand why gluten is so disruptive. We're told it's because people have gluten allergies or conditions such as celiac disease. That doesn't explain *why* so many people are sensitive to gluten, though. Are we even as sensitive to gluten as we hear? Yes, we are. What you won't hear is the true reason why we react to wheat and other sources of gluten.

Think about this. Do you know any 80-year-olds who've eaten gluten their entire life and never exhibited a single gluten sensitivity symptom? We can probably all think of folks of that generation who feel fine when they eat wheat. Now think about how many people you know, whether children, teens, or people in their 20s, 30s, 40s, 50s, or 60s, who stay away from gluten at all costs because of celiac or other problems with this protein substance.

One of the most common reasons people avoid gluten is because doctors and health professionals of today have told them that gluten causes inflammation or even autoimmune disease. This is not a practice of yesterday. It is a recent theory put out there into the world without any actual understanding of how gluten could cause inflammation or why gluten sensitivities often coincide with autoimmune conditions.

Here's the truth: gluten feeds pathogens. The very viruses that create autoimmune conditions thrive on gluten. *That's* what causes inflammation. It's not the other way around, with gluten triggering inflammation that triggers an autoimmune response in the body. It's gluten feeding bugs that lead to inflammation in the body as the immune system tries to eradicate them. Keep in mind that medical research and science still don't know this.

There are only two causes of inflammation: (1) physical injury, by force or toxic exposure and (2) pathogenic activity in the body. Pathogens can cause inflammation either by entering organs or tissue, which can cause its own kind of cell injury, or by feeding on certain troublemakers and troublemaker foods in the system and eliminating inflammatory poisons and byproduct. A food such as gluten cannot itself cause inflammation. Instead, it feeds the pathogens that can cause inflammation. This is why so many people, especially from older generations, can eat gluten and not get inflamed. In order for inflammation to occur, they need certain pathogens present in the body to feed on the food. It's pathogens such as viruses, not gluten, that are the true cause of celiac disease.

This reality behind autoimmune diagnoses remains a mystery to medical research and science. Even our best doctors and practitioners get confused here, explaining countless symptoms and conditions as the body's own immune system attacking itself. When you hear this, know that it really means medical research hasn't gotten to the root of an illness yet, so their best explanation is that it's the body's fault. In truth, your body's immune system would never destroy your thyroid (which is the theory behind Hashimoto's thyroiditis, with no proof at all). Your body's immune system would never destroy your skin (which is the mistaken theory behind eczema and psoriasis, with no proof at all). And it's not possible for gluten to cause your immune system to react in a way where it attacks your intestinal linings, causing damage, which is a mistaken theory behind celiac disease. It's a pathogen such as a virus that eats gluten and causes the intestinal damage.

What your immune system does is go after the pathogens that create autoimmune conditions. The reason gluten comes into play is because it's fuel for pathogens. Gluten feeds the viruses such as the over 60 varieties of EBV that create, for example, fibromyalgia, Hashimoto's, eczema, psoriasis, multiple sclerosis, Lyme disease, PCOS, endometriosis, psoriatic arthritis, lupus, ME/CFS, ALS, and more—which are all classified these days as autoimmune. Well-meaning practitioners go along with the outdated theory that came out of the 1950s of the body attacking itself as an explanation for chronic conditions that science doesn't yet understand. Today, it has this new twist, where the idea is that gluten causes inflammation that confuses the body, spurring a self-attack. This is not advanced information. It's misleading, even if there is no ill will behind it.

I've talked before about how gluten feeds the bugs that create symptoms and conditions, and health professionals have already started using this Medical Medium information in their practices. They're getting results for patients by helping them understand the source of their suffering: that gluten is fuel for pathogens, so when it's in the diet, those viruses and even unproductive bacteria in their system can embed themselves more deeply into organs, damaging cells and advancing autoimmune and other chronic illnesses. When you have any sort of health concern, whether autoimmune or not, removing gluten is one step. The next step is understanding why it's disruptive in your body and plays a role in your condition so you can protect yourself and heal.

You may not have pathogens in your body that are readily feeding off gluten right now. You may be able to eat wheat and other sources of gluten and feel okay. That doesn't mean you won't experience symptoms down the road. Everybody carries bugs, and they're in different strains and varieties that take different amounts of time to proliferate. You could have a mild pathogenic environment brewing in your body that's creating the mildest of symptoms you don't even realize are a problem. Many people go on a cleanse with no particular health desire besides cleaning house—and only as they're going through it and evaluating afterward do they realize they're feeling better now and were living with more limitations before than they knew.

After removing gluten, they find they have more energy, which they didn't expect because they never thought of themselves as being sensitive to it. They find they can think better, with less brain fog. They find they require less sleep and are free of achiness they had learned to ignore. They find that mild swelling or water retention they didn't even realize they had is surprisingly reduced—all because a mild, systemic inflammation that had been going undetected as they were living their busy lives is now absent with gluten out of the diet. They were so used to their symptoms that they didn't even realize they were issues, let alone that those issues could have been working their way into something bigger if they hadn't given their bodies a break from gluten.

Soft Drinks

Whether you call it soda, soft drinks, or pop, it's not good for any kind of cleanse. Many soft drinks and flavored carbonated waters come in aluminum cans—and aluminum is something you're trying to *detoxify* during a cleanse, not something you want to add to your body at the same time. Soft drinks also frequently contain aspartame, high fructose corn syrup, flavoring, and carbonation, which, even if you're not drinking out of a can, still cause problems.

Advising you that it's fine enough to consume natural-seeming soft drinks and seltzers from the health food store while trying to cleanse would be reckless and unsupportive to you. It's almost always going to lead us into trouble to reach for a soft drink; we're going to grab one with "natural" flavors (which are MSG-based) or GMO beet sugar. The healthiest soft drinks are still man-made. They're not whole foods. Even if they contain an herb, they're basically concoctions—albeit creative, imaginative ones—that still contain manufactured ingredients and are created only to please the palate.

Soft drinks can also throw us out of whack by throwing off blood sugar and making us hungrier for the wrong things. They often contain caffeine too, which revs up our adrenals and can cause several types of imbalances that work against us when we're trying to detoxify. (More on caffeine soon.)

Bottom line: soft drinks don't promote cleansing and healing.

Excessive Salt

We're often told that salt is healthy to have in our diet, as long as it's in high-quality forms such as sea salt or Himalayan salt; therefore, we should be fine to use as much as we'd like because they're nutritious, high-mineral salts. While it's true that these are nutritious salts that are higher in minerals, these stand-alone salts still prevent the body from cleansing. They don't contain the life force that, for example, the mineral salt in celery juice does. The salt that's in celery juice is a subgroup of sodium (called sodium cluster salts) that's suspended in hydrobioactive water. One of the sodium cluster salts' many jobs is to bind onto toxins and draw them out of the body. Another is to destroy pathogens. This special sodium, which you can read more about in my book *Celery Juice*, is part of why millions around the world are healing with celery juice.

Regular salts—including sea salt and Himalayan salt and any other salts considered nutritious—are not detoxifiers. When we consume them, they dehydrate us by moving water away from the places where we need it in our body and redirecting that water to areas in our body where we don't need it. This can slowly pickle our organs in just the way salt is used to preserve foods. It can also cause swelling, and people already have enough inflammation, swelling, water retention, and unwanted weight gain. Salt only makes these symptoms worse. Fluid retention is the last thing you want when detoxing and cleansing.

Now, a small pinch of high-quality sea salt or Himalayan rock salt added to a recipe you made at home is not the most concerning factor. It's the sodium in restaurant meals, prepared foods, packaged foods, and maybe even in our friends' and families' home cooking that we need to watch. Even high-end packaged snacks like dehydrated crackers made by a very well-meaning, sustainable company and advertised with a long list of bullet points describing how good they are for you can be too high in salt.

"Salt to taste" is a phrase that's thrown around a lot. Everyone has free will to toss as much salt as they want into a dish—often reaching for the salt shaker to sprinkle more salt on top of food that was already made with salt, perhaps from packaged ingredients such as sauce that already contained salt too. It means that most of us have acclimated to high levels of salt, more than the body can handle healthily, especially during a cleanse.

In the amounts we're subjected to in everyday life—at the levels used to make consumers happy—salt dehydrates us. Again, the last thing you want while trying to cleanse is to retain fluid at the same time you're chronically dehydrated. Salt preserves toxins and poisons inside the body; it holds on to them and concentrates them in our organ tissue, pushing critically needed water away from organs and making us more dehydrated at the same time that water pools and gets retained in areas that aren't helpful. When we're dehydrated, it's nearly impossible to cleanse. And as it is, most people have already been chronically dehydrated on a daily basis for years. Further, salt disrupts the body's immune system by removing water from our natural killer cells, interfering with their ability to seek out and destroy pathogens.

Again, we're talking about salt that we add to food here. That's different from the sodium subgroup in celery juice that helps us cleanse and detox and fight pathogens. It's also different from the salt found in Atlantic sea vegetables— that is, edible seaweed such as dulse and kelp. A sea vegetable is different from dehydrated ocean water (sea salt) because the sea vegetable contains a naturally controlled amount of salt from the ocean that's both inside the vegetal material and also, when dry, on its surface. Sea vegetables benefit us because they grab on to and eliminate toxic heavy metals and radiation from our bodies, and because of their salt limit, they don't contain enough sea salt to interfere with this process. So there's a distinction between table salt—even the highest-end table salt—and the naturally occurring sodium found in healing foods. Sprinkling dulse on a salad is so much different from having salt in your food multiple times every single day. A piece of seaweed cannot be compared to how much salt is on one slice of pizza alone. Between the salted cheese, the sauce, and the crust, not to mention toppings, pizza is a salt bonanza—and that's not salt that's doing any healing work, the way the sodium in celery juice or sea vegetables is.

That's why it's a good idea to take a break from added salt use when you're trying to cleanse. Look out for salt in seasonings and be cautious in restaurants, asking for food prepared without salt. When you're taking such care to heal, there's no reason to undermine it by continuing to pile on the salt.

Level 2

Pork Products

Pork puts a heavy load on the pancreas, heart, and liver. If someone is eating pork—whether in the form of bacon, sausage, ham, pork chops, barbecue ribs, pulled pork, canned pork product, pork rinds, or lard—their blood becomes very thick. This is a different level of blood thickness than if someone were eating an avocado or a handful of nuts or a piece of salmon. The variety of fat in pork products, the consistency and heavy nature of it, saturates the blood like nothing else. Even if you think most of the fat in the pork you're eating is gone—for example, if you cut the fatty part off a pork chop—you're still getting a large amount of fat, more than the body can handle, because there's fat intertwined throughout the meat. Blood thickened by pork fat is so hard on the pancreas, pushing the gland to labor so much by spilling many months' worth of its reserves of insulin and enzymes to prevent calamity. Why? Because most everyone ends

up eating a sugar pretty close on the timeline to eating pork, if not right alongside it, whether that sugar comes in the form of barbecue sauce, bread, or dessert. So while the high level of fat from the pork is still in our bloodstream, the pancreas is releasing insulin to handle the high level of sugar—and it's that fat getting in the way of the sugar that puts the pancreas on overload to save us with months' worth of insulin and enzyme reserves in one day. The pancreas can finally reach a point of exhaustion in this process. It has often landed people in the hospital overnight with cases of pancreatitis without anyone knowing that's the real cause.

Then there's the part where pork fat gets in the way of detoxing and cleansing. When blood is this thick with fat, it can't remove pathogens and toxins from certain organs such as the liver. The liver exhausts itself producing large quantities of bile to try to break down the fat in order to keep the blood thin enough that the heart doesn't have to labor so much in the process of pumping blood through veins that are crowded with fat. When the bloodstream is this laden, it means virtually no cleansing whatsoever in the brain. We frequently talk about purifying the mind. When we're eating pork, we work against that because we're not cleansing the brain. Blood vessels filled with higher levels of fat because you've consumed any variety of pork means less oxygen getting to brain cells. It means fewer healing phytochemical compounds from the nutritious foods you're eating (including celery juice) getting to brain cells too. Thick blood causes the heart to pump harder, and that means increased pressure in the blood vessels when blood finally enters the brain. While that pressure is in the mildest form, it's pressure nonetheless—which ends up putting pressure on brain tissue. It's pressure that pushes toxins deeper into brain cells rather than letting them leave, so that toxins end up accumulating in the brain.

As I mentioned earlier in the book, you'll find that any cleanse in this book focuses on lowering fats. One reason is to thin out the blood. When you thin the blood, poisons readily surface in cells and tissue and enter the bloodstream freely so they can finally exit your body. Avoiding pork products is a big part of giving yourself the chance to let go of toxins so your body and mind can heal.

Tuna

It's no secret that tuna is high in mercury. So is a lot of fish from our oceans, lakes, and rivers. Tuna stands out because it's such a popular fish eaten on a regular basis, with canned tuna a family staple going back decades.

Maybe you don't eat a lot of tuna fish sandwiches or tuna sushi rolls yourself. It's possible that generations before you in your family line, someone did, and unfortunately, we inherit poisons and toxic heavy metals from our ancestors' contaminated sperm and egg. We've come to a point in human history where we don't have the luxury to eat tuna ourselves anymore if we're concerned about our health. The days of blithely enjoying some tuna fish salad are long gone. We're at a point where mercury is one of our greatest enemies. It's building rapidly in cell tissue as it gets passed from generation to generation. Mercury is responsible for many symptoms and conditions that people struggle with on a daily basis, such as autism, ADHD, brain fog, Parkinson's, memory loss, bipolar disorder, and Alzheimer's. It also feeds pathogens such as the

over 60 varieties of EBV, which create illnesses from thyroid disorders, ME/CFS, Lyme disease, and autoimmune disease to skin rashes, PCOS, and endometriosis. Mercury is behind so much suffering—so we want to rid our bodies of it, not put more mercury into ourselves.

One problem that amplifies tuna's mercury issue is when it's packaged in an aluminum can or packet. When the traces of mercury in tuna touch the traces of aluminum in a can or foil packet, a destructive interaction occurs that instantly creates a dangerous byproduct. This crusty neuroantagonistic toxin oxidizes and grows rapidly and breaks apart in a shedding process. It's an aluminum-mercury neuroantagonistic byproduct that's worse than the mercury or aluminum itself, which on their own can already be highly toxic for the liver and brain. Again, we're talking about traces here, so you won't notice yourself falling ill immediately after eating a can of tuna. In the long run, though, it can add up and lead to some serious brain diseases years and years down the road.

Maybe it's not your style to slop tuna out of a can, drop mayonnaise on it, and throw it between a couple slices of bread. Maybe you're into the more hip, sophisticated way of eating tuna: at sushi bars. While I know that seems elevated, we can't get away from the truth that if we're cleansing, we don't have room for tuna in any form. Consider keeping tuna out of your life entirely while you're trying to heal. If you love seafood, if that's where your heart is, maybe rely on some other fishes that are lower in mercury—while keeping in mind that all fish has some level of toxic heavy metals. Try to keep away from tuna.

Corn

One important reason to stay away from corn is that it's so rare that the corn we have access to is organic. When someone feels license to eat corn, they're eating nachos, corn chips, corn tortillas, corn dogs, canned corn, popcorn, corn cereal, corn flour, corn meal, corn oil, high fructose corn syrup, and more—all of it made from conventional corn. And when we're eating conventional corn, which too often means an aggressive form of GMO corn, that can get us into trouble.

Genetically modified corn harbors toxins that humankind has never been exposed to—until now. These are toxins foreign to the human body that we're exposed to through genetic alteration of food. That poses a risk when you're trying to cleanse and detox. It also poses a risk if you're pathogenic; that is, if viruses and bacteria in your body are creating symptoms and conditions. Corn has the potential to feed these bugs, allowing them to proliferate, and that can lead to more pronounced health issues.

It's not always easy to stay on the organic corn train, making sure that any corn you consume was grown organically with non-GMO seed. Even if corn was grown without synthetic pesticides, herbicides, or fungicides sprayed on it, it doesn't ensure it's not genetically modified, or GMO-contaminated. That's the reality we're living with today.

Another reality is that the pathogens that reside inside our bodies are so used to feeding on sources of conventional GMO corn from different times and occasions in our lives (because GMO corn was used to raise pathogens in labs over the more recent decades) that these pathogens can develop an appetite for corn. Bugs such as EBV and shingles, because they've been trained to feed on unproductive conventional corn from our previous corn meals and snacks, will readily attempt to fuel themselves from organic corn too.

Corn was an amazing, healing, nutritious food in its day. While it still holds some good nutrition, corn has been too tampered with and altered for us to benefit from what it has to offer—the bad outweighs the good, because of the toxic nature of GMO corn feeding pathogens. If you're still going to eat corn after reading this, select some fresh, organic corn once in a while outside of cleansing. It's best to keep corn out of your diet altogether when you're working on detoxing and healing.

Level 3

Industrial Food Oils
(including vegetable oil, palm oil, canola oil, corn oil, safflower oil, soybean oil)

These types of oil are extremely unproductive in any kind of detox because not only are they a source of fat that thickens the blood, blocking toxins and poisons from leaving the body in a cleanse and burdening the vascular system; some of these oils are also astringent and acidic, irritating the linings of the digestive tract. Further, industrial food oils create inflammation because they have the potential to feed pathogens such as the many strains and mutations of strep, E. coli, staph, and hundreds of other unproductive bacteria inside the small intestine and colon, as well as viruses in the liver such as the many strains and mutations of EBV, shingles, CMV, HHV-6, and herpes simplex 1 and 2. As you read earlier, pathogen activity creates inflammation. These oils also put unnecessary stress upon the pancreas and liver, resulting in weak digestion and insulin resistance, which inhibits healing foods from doing their job of cleansing and healing the body and stops critically needed carbohydrates from entering into cells throughout the body. Keep these oils out of any cleanse.

Soy

It's always best to stay away from soy while trying to heal for the simple reason that soy is very rich in fat. Even though soy's natural oil is distributed in its whole-food form, which is different from straight soybean oil, soy is still high in fat, which has the potential to thicken the blood and prevent the body from cleansing.

The other risk that soy products of any kind pose is the GMO factor. GMO foods are toxic to our body systems and lower our immune system. The nutrients in GMO foods are not the same nutrients your immune system feeds on to gain strength. Our liver cannot convert or transform GMO nutrients to make them usable, because they are foreign to our planet and our body. When you're cleansing toxins and poisons, your immune system needs to be sharp, strong, and productive in every way—especially because our immune systems are already burdened with the viruses and unproductive bacteria that everyone is walking around with, in particular when struggling with symptoms or conditions. Using any possible GMO source such as soy when your immune system needs the most powerful healing phytochemical compounds, trace minerals, antioxidants, antivirals, antibacterials, and natural sugars to help it guide toxins out of the body while cleansing can be contradictory.

Just because you're consuming organic soy doesn't mean it's guaranteed not to be GMO. That's because GMO contamination has been part of the organic soy supply for many years now. Gambling with whether your soy is GMO or not may be something you don't mind at other times in your life. Let's try not to gamble while you're in the middle of a cleanse, when your immune system needs to be strong and productive and on the ready. GMO food is foreign to the human body. Even if you can't feel a sensitivity, histamines can rise when we eat GMO sources such as soy, with overall inflammation in the body elevating in reaction, because anything GMO is a foreign substance to our body, just like when chemical companies create dangerous toxic chemicals that our body can react to as well, since toxic chemicals can injure tissue. We're trying to lower inflammation during a cleanse, not instigate it, so it's best to stay away from soy when you want your body in detox mode.

Lamb

The reasoning behind keeping lamb out of a cleanse is similar to why you want to keep pork out of a cleanse: like pork, lamb is high in fat. Too much fat in the bloodstream slows down a cleanse or detox. Lamb isn't generally quite as high in fat as pork is; that's why it's lower on my list of foods to avoid. It's still higher in fat than most other animal proteins, though, and the goal in a cleanse is to make sure you're not consuming too many varieties of fat, lamb being one of them.

Part of why a cleanse needs to be low-fat to no-fat is because when we're detoxing, the heart has enough to keep up with as poisons exit the organs. As poisons and toxins leave our organs and enter the bloodstream, the goal is to keep our blood as thin as possible so these toxins can leave the bloodstream as quickly as possible through elimination such as perspiration from the armpits, bowel movements, and urination. Those poisons and toxins moving through the system already increase our heart rate mildly because nerve cell receptors in the brain detect that the blood is becoming toxic. This signals the brain to then send a direct message to the heart to accelerate its rate of pumping to flush toxins out of the bloodstream more quickly. That doesn't have a negative effect on the heart if we keep the blood thin.

If the blood becomes too thick from someone eating lamb (or pork, soy, or industrial food oils) while trying to cleanse, it's like sucking jelly through a straw, and that becomes a burden on the heart. Now the heart must pump harder because the blood has become thick; it's difficult to draw blood through the veins when it's filled with fat. When you keep foods such as lamb out while cleansing, the blood can remain thin and more toxins and poisons can freely leave through the bloodstream. Heart rate can elevate slightly and safely as those troublemakers exit quickly, with no stress on the body.

All Fish and Seafood
(except for salmon, trout, and sardines)

As I mentioned under "Tuna," there are varieties of fish that contain lower levels of toxic heavy metals such as mercury. Even though that's the case, there are other toxins in seafood that should concern us, that we don't want to accumulate in our systems, especially during a cleanse. We don't want to battle our detox with additional toxins.

What are those other toxins? At the top of the list are dioxins: a historic industrial waste product. Dioxins are in everything already, with traces of them (sometimes at the mildest, mildest levels) in all foods. In fish, we're looking at larger amounts of dioxins. The reason

that should concern us is that dioxins lower our immune system, because a large part of our immune system is inside our lymphatic system, and that's where dioxins accumulate and pool when they first enter our body. Dioxins there end up hampering our lymphocytes; dioxins act like a smokescreen or snowstorm that slows down and weakens the lymphocytes inside our lymphatic system. They're also an aggressive variety of free radicals, basically toxins that are destructive to the cells in our body.

Fish happens to be high in dioxins because the ocean and freshwater sources are where the majority of dioxins float. We don't want to be adding this variety of toxins to our bodies while cleansing. As you know by now, the immune system needs to be strong and reliable during a cleanse, not weakened.

Dioxins can create cancer, in that they feed the aggressive viruses that can turn into and create cancer cells—dioxins are a food that these pathogens like. That's one more reason to avoid most fish and other seafood when you're trying to cleanse and heal.

Salmon, trout, and sardines are different in part because they are higher in trace minerals than other fish. That doesn't mean you should be eating salmon, trout, or sardines every single day, unless you are really into fish. If you rely on it, these three are best. If, on the other hand, you eat fish only because you're looking for beneficial omegas, you can obtain those omegas by consuming sea vegetables.

Another reason to choose salmon, trout, and sardines over other fish and seafood is that they're lower in mercury, especially sardines. That's not to say they're mercury-free—when you hear that salmon is farm-raised, for example, don't let that mislead you into thinking it doesn't contain mercury, dioxins, or radiation from the ocean. Farm-raised has additional concerns, such as antibiotics and antifungals used to keep the fish from developing fungus and bacterial infections, so it's not a safer bet. You want to go with wild-caught salmon, trout, and sardines, if you can, due to the fact that you won't be dealing with those antibiotics and antifungals, both of which can contain toxic heavy metals too.

Lastly, nuclear fallout and nuclear power plants discharging runoff have contaminated our oceans and waterways for decades. Sardines, salmon, and trout are better options than other fish and seafood because they're lower in radiation—sardines especially, due to their size.

That doesn't automatically mean that all fish on the small side are lower in contamination. Some small fish such as mackerel are oilier and can contain more mercury. Why do oily fish and mercury go together? For the same reason that the fat cells in our body become intoxicated and loaded with heavy metals such as mercury: unknown to medical research and science, toxic heavy metals such as mercury dissolve and disperse within fats. This happens because the acids in fats cause a rapid oxidation process in mercury, and in turn, the metal expands and saturates the entire fat cell, making it even more toxic. While salmon may be oily and on the larger side, it's not the oiliest, and it's one of the healthiest the ocean has to offer due to its trace minerals. If you want to eat some fish while trying to cleanse, make it wild-caught salmon, sardines, or freshwater trout.

When it comes to fish oil supplements, don't get sold by advertising that says "mercury-free." This is a false claim. There is no technology that can completely free fish oil from mercury residue. The essence of mercury is still left behind in so-called clean fish oil, and it can be even more toxic than eating a can of tuna because of the engineering involved. The removal process creates a powerful homeopathic charge within the essence of mercury that's left behind in the fish oil. It's now in a much more methylated state, and that methylmercury can travel deeper into cell tissue throughout the body. As an alternative, look for a fish-free EPA/DHA supplement in my supplement directory.

Level 4

Vinegar
(including apple cider vinegar)

Vinegar dehydrates the body on a deep, deep organ level, and when you're cleansing, you don't want to dehydrate the body. Vinegar preserves poisons, trapping them in your organs—and not so that it can then drive them out of your body. Toxins dehydrate us, as they require an abundance of water to dilute them and eventually flush them out of our cells so they can safely leave our organs without hurting us. Rather than help flush out these toxins, vinegar allows toxins to penetrate our cells and organs because it sucks the water out of cells, and that even drives poisons and toxins deeper into organ tissue.

Picture this: a jar of pickles, with cucumbers sitting in a bath of water and vinegar. If the water in that jar had traces of fluoride, lead, arsenic, pesticides, or any other variety of chemical poison, the vinegar would bind onto those toxins, pushing them deep into the pickles, possibly all the way to the core. That's how vinegar works. Well, we have water in our blood too. Toxins also float in it, and it's a good thing that the water is present, because normally, it's supposed to carry toxins along and flush them out. When we consume vinegar, though, suddenly we're the jar of pickles, and our organs are the cucumbers getting pickled. The vinegar begins by separating the toxins in our blood from the water clinging to them. This allows the toxins to burrow into organs, glands, and connective tissue—which works precisely against what you're trying to accomplish on a cleanse. Vinegar also sucks water out of our cells, robbing us of deep hydration reserves in organs such as the liver.

If you're thinking that apple cider vinegar is exempt from all this vinegar talk, think again. Yes, ACV is more nutritious than other vinegars, because it's made from apples, which are nutrient-rich. It's not that much more nutritious than red wine or grape vinegar; grapes hold nutrition just as apples do. All of these fruits are in fermented form, though, and we can't get away from the truth that no matter the source, vinegar dehydrates the body on a deep, systemic level, causing trouble by keeping poisons inside the body when we're trying to get rid of them.

Fermented Foods (including kombucha, sauerkraut, and coconut aminos)

Based on the popularity of fermented foods, you would think that anything fermented is good for us. That's not the case. Fermentation is not a healing technique. It's a survival technique that was developed back in the day to preserve food. Consider yogurt. Most yogurt is a dairy product, and all dairy feeds viruses and unproductive bacteria, the very source behind so much chronic illness. Keep in mind that it's only a theory that the microorganisms in yogurt are beneficial. The damage done by the dairy itself, even if it's raw, unpasteurized yogurt, outweighs any theoretical benefits: the dairy protein and lactose feed the bugs causing your symptoms. Just because you don't have symptoms right now doesn't mean you won't develop them down the road, with yogurt feeding the sleeping giants such as Epstein-Barr virus or unproductive bacteria that you don't realize are inside your body. (Nondairy yogurts such as coconut yogurt and oat milk yogurt don't solve the issue. Again, fermentation itself is not a healing technique. More in a moment.)

Any kind of fermented meat or fermented animal flesh product should be avoided at all costs. The microorganisms on animal flesh are the microorganisms of death. They're part of the decaying process when an animal dies—they develop or arrive on the scene to break down the carcass, and they thrive on rotting flesh. These are not healthy microorganisms for a healthy gut.

Out of all the fermented foods, fermented vegetables and herbs such as kimchi and sauerkraut are the most beneficial—in the sense that they don't harbor the same microorganisms that reside on decaying flesh. These microorganisms from decaying plant matter are more agreeable and healthier and not as offensive to our bodies. They're still not the right kind of microorganisms for cleansing and healing.

What type of microorganisms we take into our body makes a big difference. There are millions of beneficial microorganisms inside each one of us. None of them are the ones sitting on a fermented vegetable. So while at least we could receive a benefit from the nutrients in the vegetable that's been fermented, it's not enough benefit to warrant filling every meal with fermented vegetables. We only get so many meals in our lifetime, and each one is critically important to our health. You'll be much better off eating some raw basil, spinach, or mâche than you will filling your plate with fermented cabbage or other fermented vegetables. That's because the good microorganisms inside you feed and thrive on herbs such as basil and celery juice. They thrive on leafy greens such as arugula, lettuces, kale, and spinach. And they thrive on fresh, raw vegetables such as cauliflower and fruits such as apples. Those are the beneficial microorganisms we're *supposedly* trying to replace when we eat fermented foods. In reality, fermented foods aren't doing the job we believe they are. They're not choice foods for the healthy microorganisms that reside in our body. The true goal is to feed the healthy microorganisms inside of our gut with the foods our body really wants, and you just saw a partial list of what those foods are.

This is why people have remarkable, life-changing results from drinking celery juice versus kombucha tea. There are millions of people globally drinking celery juice and receiving benefits they've never experienced from other modalities they've tried. They can drink kombucha tea for a month straight and never receive any benefits to relieve their chronic illness. Meanwhile, you can drink celery juice for a month straight and see the healing difference. Celery juice not only addresses the pathogens such as the over 60 varieties of Epstein-Barr virus and over 50 groups of *Streptococcus* bacteria behind chronic illness; it also feeds good bacteria, creating your healthiest intestinal environment as a perk.

The only reason that some people who are sick with chronic illness seem to benefit from eating fermented foods is because they've gotten rid of troublemaker foods from their diet at the same time. People tend to make choices for their health all at once, so while they're bringing in fermented foods because they heard that would help their microbiome, they're cutting out gluten and limiting cheese too—and it was the removal of gluten and lowering of dairy that helped them feel better. The minute you stop eating greasy fast foods, you're going to see benefits. Adding fermented foods and even other similar changes at the same time are not going to be enough to heal, though. As you discovered in Chapter 4, "What about the Microbiome?", when someone is sick, the microbiome is not the real problem. Eating fermented foods to fix your microbiome will neither fix your microbiome—for all the reasons you just read about—nor fix your health. The real problems are much deeper, and that's what the cleanses in this book are here to address.

Fermented foods have been around for centuries. We've had fermented foods within the healing community for years, and they became particularly popular in Western culture in the 1960s and '70s. They've never fixed our health. Chronic illness has exploded worldwide in past decades. Fermented foods have not been an answer. No one has had a chronic illness alleviated because of them. It's like we're backtracking when we bring fermented foods and the microbiome into the health conversation. All it does is support old theories that never got anyone better in the first place. It's a constant reignition of an old theory with a new name, convincing people to try an approach that was never the answer. Fermented foods don't address the toxic heavy metals behind chronic illnesses or the viruses behind health struggles such as lupus and fatigue.

It's like the world of chronic illness is a swampy pond of misinformation. Whenever you try to escape the swamp and start to find the truth and the real answers—for example, that pathogens are behind chronic illness—a ghoul jumps out of the pond, grabs your ankle, and tries to pull you back in, telling you that the real reason you're sick is that you're eating lectins, or you're missing collagen, or your microbiome is off and you need fermented foods, or it's all in your head, or you created your illness through bad thoughts, or your body is attacking itself with an autoimmune response. If you don't grab on to the answers in this and every other Medical Medium book, if you don't fight for the truth, the ghoul will constantly try to pull you back through the mud and into the haunted swamp of misinformation, where you'll be forced to swim with everyone else, along with the ghouls and pond monsters.

Caffeine
(including coffee, matcha, and chocolate)

Caffeine has two effects that you don't want during a cleanse. One, it dehydrates the body, which is a theme of the foods in this chapter. Two, it prompts the adrenal glands to pump unnecessary levels of adrenaline into your bloodstream, causing a variety of compromises to your brain, liver, and kidneys.

Caffeine gives the adrenals a sense of fight or flight without our actual life circumstances being fight or flight. Now, fight or flight is a privilege we hold, an option for when we're dealing with stress, loss, or confrontation. Fight or flight is the release of complex blends of life-saving hormones from the adrenals, blends that medical research and science don't yet even comprehend. It's for when we're in a time of need and require the ability to think or act fast for survival.

When we consume caffeine, it creates a boy-who-cried-wolf situation. It's a kid pulling the fire alarm at school when there's no fire. If

you're consuming caffeine all day long, you're continually telling your body that there's a crisis, prompting your adrenals to respond all day long. That can create a numbness. When a real crisis comes, we may not respond appropriately because we're basically immune to the experience of adrenaline hitting the central nervous system. And the specific blend of adrenaline that fight or flight triggers can be highly toxic to the body because it's highly acidic and corrosive to the nervous system and organs. This kind of adrenaline release is not meant to be used every day, let alone multiple times a day. It's meant to be used sparingly. Over time, this adrenaline blend can slowly scorch the liver as the organ sponges up the adrenaline to protect you.

Caffeine feels good. It gets us to get up and go. It gets our adrenals to kick in, gives us that boost, gets us up and dancing to the music, ready and pumped up to move, start the day, and get to work. We pay a price for relying on caffeine to do that. All of that squeezing of the adrenals is supposed to be preserved for special situations that warrant it. When an event that's truly stress-inducing—that needs an immediate reaction—occurs, there may be a delay, a disconnect, a time lapse. A true crisis message can be drowned out by all the hits of adrenaline our brain has become used to from our caffeine habit, and it may be harder to process news and make a decision or offer guidance to a loved one in the face of it. The brain may not respond fast enough.

When we do make a decision in the grip of a caffeine addiction, we can make a mistake, one that can make life harder than it would have been naturally. To make ourselves feel better when we don't like the outcome of that mistake, we may tell ourselves, "It was meant to happen" or "It's a lesson you needed to experience" or "You can grow from this." We lean on these trendy spiritual sayings instead of waking up to the reality that caffeine addiction was throwing off our game. How do you learn the real lesson if you don't see that a situation didn't turn out the best way because you stopped everything you were doing and said, "I have to go get my coffee"? Or because at a crucial moment, you said, "I can't start this until I have my matcha tea" and as a result, lost an opportunity? When something has that much control over your life, it's not about giving you pleasure anymore. It's about taking something away that you weren't even aware was being taken away.

That's the long-term reason to consider cutting back on caffeine. In the shorter term, during a cleanse, you'll benefit from avoiding caffeine altogether to give your adrenal glands and liver a much-needed break from all the false alarms.

Experiencing life without reliance on a stimulant is a positive direction to take for physical and spiritual elevation. In recent years, we've been told that consuming matcha tea and high-quality chocolate every day is healthy. In reality, daily consumption of these forms of caffeine contributes to our declining health. It gives us the same reactions that drinkers of regular coffee and black tea have experienced over the decades—reactions such as blood sugar imbalances, headaches, insomnia, anxiousness, mysterious sadness, depersonalization, chronic dehydration, kidney stones, weight gain years down the road, premature aging of the skin, adrenal fatigue, and even in some cases hair loss in women.

Paid-for studies will back the health benefits that are touted about high-quality chocolate and matcha tea, just as they have for black tea and coffee. These are guaranteed moneymakers for the industries because they're addictive. They're safe bets for investors. No one can easily quit their caffeine addiction. People are more likely to blame their health conditions on the one piece of fruit they ate in a week than they are on the chocolate or matcha tea they eat or drink every day. Keep this in mind if you're trying to recover from chronic illness. Don't let caffeine be the factor that holds you back.

Level 5

All Grains (except for millet and oats)

If you're asking yourself, "Why would I want to remove even gluten-free grains?" that's a very good question. It's not because it's a popular trend to remove grains from the diet. The misinformed concern is that they cause inflammation and are an unnecessary form of carbohydrate. Well, gluten-free grains do not feed pathogens, so we don't need to be concerned that millet, quinoa, brown rice, or oats would feed the common bacteria *Streptococcus* that everyone carries, unproductive bugs in the gut, or viruses such as EBV and herpes simplex—meaning that in truth, gluten-free grains do not cause inflammation.

No, there are other reasons to cut out all grains other than millet and oats when you're serious about healing. For one, grains can be too easy a food to rely on, taking up room on your plate and in your stomach that could be occupied by more nutrient-dense foods such as leafy greens and fruit. You're more likely to skip two or three healthy apples in the morning or a couple of bananas because you're eating a bowl of grains. While grains are nutritious, they don't offer the healing phytochemicals, antioxidants, and trace minerals of a pint of berries, a pair of apples, or a banana. Most importantly, grains don't offer antiviral, antibacterial compounds; these compounds found in fruits, herbs such as celery, leafy greens, vegetables, and sea vegetables are precious and help bring our lives back by reversing chronic illness. Grains are an easy filler for breakfast, lunch, or dinner, when other foods could be moving us forward faster with healing.

There's an even bigger reason to avoid grains: because of how they interact with fats. We don't tend to eat our grains without radical fat, or far removed in time from it. Think about it: oatmeal with peanut butter or almond butter, toast with avocado, granola with milk, protein bars, chicken sandwiches, pasta with oil. It's very rare to eat a grain dish as simple as, say, quinoa with steamed vegetables and no oil drizzled on top. Even when we do withhold fat from a snack or meal, it's usually not too long from when we ate a snack or meal that was rich in fat, so one fat-based food usually isn't out of the system by the time we're enjoying a grain-based food, even if they're hours apart. A breakfast of yogurt or eggs, for example, may still be digesting by the time we end up eating a lunch of quinoa salad. Why is this a problem? Insulin resistance. (By the way, quinoa is a healthy grain, although it is harder to digest than millet and oats. It's scratchy on the intestinal linings, which means it can bother people with intestinal tract disorders. For the purpose of keeping these cleanses as gentle and healing as possible for sensitive people, you will not see it recommended as a main staple in this book. I also want to recognize the debate about whether quinoa is a grain or a seed. We can call it either, because most grains are seeds, which is why you can sprout them.)

Throughout this book, you'll see me use the term *radical fat*. That's when the majority of a food's calories are derived from fat, whether healthy or unhealthy. (Ketogenic diets, for example, are based on radical fats.) Radical fats and grains both take a while to digest. Fats from chicken, avocado, bone broth, nuts and seeds, oils, butter, cream, milk, and more linger in the bloodstream as they go through their long absorption process, sometimes taking a full day to disperse, if not more. That translates to fats floating around in the bloodstream for hours. The complex carbohydrates of whole grains take less time to break down—they're usually gone within four to six hours, although that's still a long time—due to their density and the quantity you may have eaten. That's usually viewed as a positive, as they're considered slow-burning fuel.

Here's the issue: complex carbohydrates break down into sugars, and if there are fats in the bloodstream at the same time, well, then we've got fat plus sugar: the true cause of insulin resistance. Sugars attach themselves to insulin in order to enter cells so we can have energy, survive, and thrive. Fat interferes with this process. High blood fat prevents sugars from entering cells with ease because it absorbs some of the insulin and also gets in the way of the sugars binding to the insulin before that insulin weakens and dissipates. That causes more insulin to be produced, weakening the pancreas at the same time the fat in the blood clogs up the liver. Blood sugar instability can result. For example, your A1C could elevate, or you could get diagnosed with prediabetes or eventually diabetes. So if you're looking for that next level of healing, it's important that grains aren't present in your diet if radical fats are.

If you take away the radical fats, then the gluten-free grains work only in your favor. No insulin resistance can happen, although then we're back to the initial drawback of grains: the lower level of nutrition they offer compared to fruits, herbs, leafy greens, vegetables, and sea vegetables as well as grains' nonexistent level of antivirals and antibacterials. Fruit, by the way, is not a complex carbohydrate (unless it's a starch such as winter squash). Fruit's valuable sugar enters your bloodstream and organs quickly; many fruits are absorbed, assimilated, and used within one hour. If you're eating larger amounts of fruit—for example, if you eat one bunch of bananas in a sitting—that absorption could take two or three hours. Either way, fruit causes the least amount of resistance when it comes to sugar entering cells for fuel. If you have a lot of fat in your bloodstream, you may still have a little bit of insulin resistance with fruit, although not much, because insulin will attach to fruit sugar and bypass a lot of fat in the bloodstream to enter cells.

With grains, the absorption process is much more difficult if we're still eating radical fats. Trendy, high-fat diets of today such as ketogenic or paleo (whether plant based or animal protein based) lack understanding of this. They simply believe that grains cause symptoms, period. Creators of these diets don't realize that people's slightly swollen, lightheaded, foggy, and tired symptoms aren't a result of gluten-free grains causing inflammation; these symptoms come from digestive problems, liver issues, or low-grade viral and bacterial infections of bugs such as strep and Epstein-Barr virus. The combination of fats plus complex carbohydrates can contribute to all of this.

People often experience digestive issues from combining radical fats with complex carbs such as grains, and yet they rarely eat grains without fats. Think cheesy pasta, mac and cheese, pizza (that's a wheat crust plus cheese and oil), rice with butter, toast and avocado, oatmeal and peanut butter, or pork and rice. Fats and starches combined in the digestive tract put stress on the liver and pancreas, making it difficult for hydrochloric acid to do its job of breaking down grains in the stomach. That's because fats interfere with hydrochloric acid strength, and the liver has to produce more bile to break down fats while complex carbohydrates are in the way of the bile's job of dispersing fats. Other symptoms that can occur as a result are bloating, nausea, constipation, cramping, gastritis, and intestinal inflammation, all of them mistakenly blamed on grains and not on the fats consumed with them. So are the insulin resistance symptoms of sweating, hot flashes, mild dizziness, inconsistent energy, nagging hunger, swelling from slight water retention, and mild, intermittent tremors and shakes. If someone were consuming gluten-free grains with no radical fats in their diet whatsoever, it would be a whole different story.

Many people get along with fats and grains together just fine, most commonly if they're younger, because their system is strong and they don't have a lot of compromises. Their liver hasn't been too weakened over time yet by pathogens, high-fat or high-protein diets, toxic heavy metals, or a heavy toxic load, so the hydrochloric acid in their stomach is still partially strong, and their pancreas is still adequately strong too. Just because someone isn't exhibiting symptoms now doesn't mean weakness isn't building behind the scenes that could develop into a chronic issue because of the diet they're eating that's trending. Feeling fine in the moment isn't reassurance that everything is fine. For people looking to head off problems or people already experiencing chronic issues that they'd like to heal, removing all grains besides millet and oats from the diet is one way to further recover and strengthen. Another is removing or reducing radical fats at the same time.

(Do look for oats marked "gluten-free." Even though oats themselves are naturally gluten-free, growing and processing can sometimes contaminate them, so it's best to look for oats that were grown and processed with special care.)

Yet another step is to remove all grains from your diet while you're trying to move forward from a symptom or condition. This will give your digestive system a break and maximize the healing foods you have room for in every meal. You'll notice that millet and oats are okay in Days 1 through 3 of the Original 3:6:9 Cleanse and Days 1 through 8 of the Simplified 3:6:9 Cleanse. That's to give people who are new to removing foods from their diet some comfort foods. If you're really struggling with a condition and you're still very attached to grains, I would prefer you use millet. For even more healing, I'd prefer you remove grains altogether and try the Advanced 3:6:9 Cleanse.

All Oils
(including healthier oils such as olive oil, walnut oil, sunflower oil, coconut oil, sesame oil, avocado oil, grapeseed oil, almond oil, macadamia oil, peanut oil, and flaxseed oil)

It's not that some oils can't be healthy or hold benefits such as omega-3s and other nutrients. It's that oil, any oil, prevents full cleansing of the body. Oils have a hyper blood fat reception. That is, the blood fills up quickly with oil, much more quickly than if you were eating the whole food from which it came. Eating an avocado or a walnut, for example, is far different from consuming avocado oil or walnut oil. When you're eating an avocado or a nut on its own, your body processes it entirely differently.

Avocado, when we eat it in its whole form, lingers at the bottom of the stomach leading into the duodenum, taking its time to get broken down and dispersed by bile as it enters the small intestinal tract. The avocado's fat then gets absorbed into blood vessels in the intestinal lining that carry it up the hepatic portal highway into the liver, so it can get processed even more. The liver will store some of that fat so it's not all projected back up into the bloodstream on its way to the heart so quickly. Your liver will release the fat at a safe rate for your heart and brain.

On the other hand, when we consume oil that's been extracted from foods such as avocado, it's not a whole food anymore. Oil's hyper blood fat reception allows it to bypass the safety mechanisms built into our organs. As the oil enters our stomach, it drops quickly into the duodenum and small intestinal tract, faster than it would if it were a whole nut, seed, or avocado. In this process, oil bypasses the liver's responsibility altogether. Instead of the oil traveling up the hepatic portal highway into the liver, where it can be time-released to the rest of the body, because of its hyper blood fat reception rate, oil is forced to enter into blood vessels in the intestinal tract that fats from whole foods wouldn't normally enter. This raises the blood fat level more quickly and more aggressively. Oil instantly stops the body from cleansing because it lowers your oxygen, thickens the blood, traps toxins, and slows down the organs' ability to release poisons and toxins. The oil enters the bloodstream rapidly, causing spurts of excessive high blood fat that are highly unpredictable. Too much fat too quickly burdens the heart, so the adrenals are highly sensitized, ready to fire adrenaline as a blood thinner to protect the heart from being bombarded by fat that has released itself into the bloodstream too early—because as oil, fat doesn't get detained long enough through processing. All of this holds back the body's cleansing processes, which ultimately holds back healing. That's why, when you want to give yourself the best chance of moving forward from health challenges, you want to leave out oil.

Bonus

There is a "Bonus" level when it comes to protecting your health. For even better, faster results when healing, you can go beyond removing the main troublemaker foods from your diet. You can:

- **Cut out salt (and seasonings) entirely**

   Don't worry that leaving out even sea salt and Himalayan rock salt will somehow deprive you of nutrients. When you're eating a diet rich in fruits, vegetables, leafy greens, sea vegetables, and herbs, you get plenty of sodium naturally, along with minerals. And as you saw under "Excessive Salt," there are many good reasons to stay away from salt (and the seasonings that contain it) when you're trying to improve your health. Spices are fine as long as they're pure and free from salt and flavorings.

- **Avoid radical fats entirely**

   Cutting out radical fats is similar to cutting out salt in that you don't need to worry that you're missing out on nutrition. Again, fruits, vegetables, leafy greens, sea vegetables, and herbs provide all the beneficial omegas we need, at the perfect levels for our bodies to process when we're cleansing and healing. Read much more in "The Truth about Fat and Healing" in a few pages.

- **Limit or altogether avoid alcohol, natural and artificial flavors, nutritional yeast, citric acid, aspartame and other artificial sweeteners, monosodium glutamate (MSG), formaldehyde, and preservatives**

   Many people are sensitive to these ingredients, and while some of them can seem fun in the moment, their effects on our physical and emotional well-being aren't so enjoyable. Nutritional yeast, for example, is an MSG-contaminated ingredient—there's a reason why it's so addictive, with people pouring it on to flavor countless foods. It also has the potential to be an irritant to the digestive system and feed bugs such as unproductive bacteria.

THE TRUTH ABOUT FOOD COMBINING

If you've followed the food combining theories that are trending out there, please know that when you consume a radical fat and a sugar together, you're already in the process of causing health issues. Avoiding fat plus sugar should be your food combining focus. You saw prime examples of the trouble with fat plus sugar under "Eggs," "Pork Products," and "All Grains" in the previous pages. Insulin resistance is a primary concern with this combination.

Fat plus sugar: this is the true food combination to be wary of, and this is where food combining theorists are lost and unaware. Fat plus sugar also means fat plus starch and fat plus grain. It also translates to protein plus sugar, protein plus starch, and protein plus grain; that's because inside protein is fat. A doughnut—that's fat plus sugar. So is a cookie. And on the healthier side, oatmeal and peanut butter or coconut yogurt with fruit, maple syrup, and nuts and seeds: these are fat plus sugar. The real problem in the fat-plus-sugar equation is the radical fat, as we explored in the "All Grains" section.

If you're into plant proteins, there's a chance you may not break this true food combining rule. For example, you could eat rice and beans and leave off the butter, cheese, avocado, or oil. Spinach is a powerful protein that's not a radical fat, so spinach plus gluten-free grains makes a good combination too, unless you add oil, avocado, or an animal protein because that adds fat. It's these additions of fat to the starches (which our bodies break down into sugar) where it all goes wrong. The starches aren't the problem. The radical fats are.

If you're into animal proteins, then animal proteins plus leafy greens go well together. Grains plus animal proteins don't. It's the fat inside the animal proteins plus the sugar that the grains become in our body that causes the issue. Chicken plus rice doesn't work, for example, because of the fat inside the chicken combined with the starch of the rice—that's a food combining nightmare. Even experts on food combining theories are unaware that radical fats are the real food combining problem.

THE TRUTH ABOUT FAT AND HEALING

When anyone states that lowering fat in the diet isn't beneficial, it's pure speculation. Barely anyone today eats a diet low in fat. Even among health enthusiasts, whether plant based or not, it's very rare that someone leaves fat out of their diet or has eaten low-fat for long enough. There's no validity to the assertion that a no-fat or low-fat diet makes anyone susceptible to aneurysm, stroke, or other brain conditions—it's an empty assumption in line with the high-fat trend, not a conclusion drawn from human study. It's a wild dream someone influenced by popular opinion cooked up. There's nothing behind it.

The world is on a high-fat diet, and strokes, aneurysms, and embolisms abound. We're all still sick in this world. Millions of people worldwide from generations through the decades have demonstrated that eating high levels of dietary fat doesn't serve our health. A diet high in healthier fats is at least better than the standard. Nuts, seeds, olives, and avocados will lower some risks if they're in place of red meat, chicken, grease, oil, and lard. Brain conditions of any kind, including strokes, aneurysms, Alzheimer's, dementia, and Parkinson's, can improve when we rid our diets of processed foods, fast foods, and junk foods, which are high in problematic fats.

Someone who's eating certain fish along with olives, avocados, nuts, and seeds while keeping out fast foods and processed foods may say to themselves, "Whoa, I've found the Holy Grail," because they're feeling a difference from going off troublesome fats. What they don't understand is that you can go even further in reducing fats and as a result, lower your likelihood of these brain conditions and other diseases. High fat, even if it's good fat, can weaken and burn out your liver over time. This can, in turn, set you up for illnesses and diseases. Any form of fat thickens the blood. While fats from unhealthy, processed, fast foods cause thicker blood, healthy fats still thicken the blood. Either way, thick blood results in less oxygen being delivered to cells in the brain—because high blood fat suffocates oxygen out of the bloodstream—and that lack of oxygen to the brain ages the brain faster. The world is filled with aneurysms and strokes, and nearly everyone has been on high-fat diets, even healthy high-fat diets, long term. So you can't point to the handful of people who have been on fat-free diets long term and say that's where the problem is.

When we say "fat-free," we don't even mean devoid of all fats. No one's diet is ever entirely fat-free; it's impossible to be truly fat-free. Bananas have fat in them. Sweet potatoes have fat in them. Potatoes have fat in them. Mangoes have fat. So does butter leaf lettuce. All fruits, vegetables, leafy greens, sea vegetables, and herbs have beneficial omegas. Some plant foods such as figs, bananas, or butter leaf lettuce have a touch more natural fat occurring; some such as celery have barely a trace. Even when they're in trace amounts (sometimes especially when they're in trace amounts) our body can use these beneficial fats—and they're at low enough levels that they combine perfectly with the natural sugars in these foods. So when we remove radical fats from our diets—and again, by "radical fats," I mean foods where the main calorie source is fat—we're not depriving ourselves. When you're "fat-free"—that is, not eating radical fats—you're still getting the vital fats you need. When you eat some steamed potatoes (without butter, oil, or sour cream), for example, with lettuce of any kind, you're still going to get a small percentage

of fat in your diet, plenty to support your health. You don't have to go and eat a handful of mixed nuts to get healthy fats. You're already getting what you need.

No one's stopping their aneurysms by adding fat to their coffee. There's no study to prove it, and yet people have become convinced it will save them. And while hacking your coffee sounds like a great idea, the truth is that if you fill up your bloodstream with fat, you're going to cause more problems for your brain. Fats can be healthy and good for you—fats such as walnuts, sesame seeds, hemp seeds, and avocado, for example. I'm not arguing that these don't have benefits. You still don't want to overdo it. You want to keep your use of radical fats sparing, and you want to spread out those small amounts in any given week. Ideally, you're not eating radical fats every day.

The 3:6:9 Cleanse will help you get your head around how to do this, putting you in a rhythm of filling yourself with healing meals that are free from radical fats—and feeling what a difference that makes in your physical symptoms and even mood. Page through the recipes in Chapter 23 to see how fortifying food can be even without radical fats. If your condition is really difficult, you may want to be entirely free from radical fats for a while after the cleanse too, and wait until later to bring them back. (For more on this, see "Fat-Free beyond the Cleanse" in Chapter 19, "Critical Cleanse Dos and Don'ts.") The fat that's in fruits, vegetables, leafy greens, sea vegetables, and herbs takes the form of natural omegas at gentle enough levels that they won't overburden your liver, digestive system, and immune system. It's the perfect amount for your body to process when it's healing.

CHAPTER 8

Your Guide to Choosing a Cleanse

How do you choose among the cleanses in this book? The Original versus the Simplified versus the Advanced 3:6:9 Cleanse, for example—how do you know which to follow? Is it okay to jump right into one? Should you start by removing troublemaker foods with the Anti-Bug Cleanse first?

And how do you choose between a cleanse from this book and another cleanse in the Medical Medium series? If you're familiar with my work, you know that I offer at least one cleanse option in almost every book. Should you start with the 28-Day Healing Cleanse from *Medical Medium*? The 90-Day Thyroid Rehab from *Thyroid Healing*? Or the 3:6:9 Cleanse I first introduced in *Liver Rescue*?

As freeing as options are, I know that an abundance of them can also feel immobilizing. This book alone offers five basic choices—the Anti-Bug Cleanse, the Morning Cleanse, the Heavy Metal Detox Cleanse, the Mono Eating Cleanse, and the 3:6:9 Cleanse—with multiple paths you can follow within almost all of them. It also covers options for intermittent fasting, water fasting, and juice fasting for those who are enthusiasts of these practices. Where do you start? This chapter is here to help you figure that out for yourself.

Here are the main topics we'll explore:

- Overview of Cleanse Options
- The "Why" of Cleansing
- Choosing a Cleanse: Where to Begin in the Medical Medium Cleanse World
- The 3:6:9 Cleanse: Original versus Simplified versus Advanced
- Food Intolerances
- Pregnancy and Breastfeeding
- Children
- Liver Testing
- Heavy Metal Detox Testing
- Celery Juice: Powerful Medicine
- Counting Macros: The New Counting Calories
- Bulking and Cutting

A GUIDING QUESTION

As we consider which cleanse to select, we need to remember that throughout our lifetime, our body is going to change. When we first come to cleansing, we might have been dealing with a chronic illness that we've had for a long time, one that created a host of deficiencies along the way. And each year, we're exposed to different troublemakers. Sometimes our liver is toxic and sluggish and needs great care—it needs to be our focus and priority because its stagnancy has made our body so toxic. Sometimes we go through emotional exposures we didn't expect, and we find ourselves eating poorly and using a tremendous amount of adrenaline to get through hard times. Sometimes we're going along through life and we get exposed to a new pathogen that can weaken our once-strong immune system. We're ever changing, and life is not easy. One cleanse could be perfect for the moment we're living in now, while six months in the future, another will be the best option. That could keep shifting or repeating as the years go by.

Use this guiding question when choosing a cleanse option: What feels manageable for you right now? The cleanse you're actually going to do is the cleanse that's going to be most beneficial.

What may feel most doable in the moment is trying some time off from a few foods that are problematic for your health. If that's the case, turn to Chapter 15, "Anti-Bug Cleanse," and read about how taking a break from certain foods can give you relief. Trying out that cleanse, in which you select the level that feels right for you, may help you work up to the 3:6:9 Cleanse someday.

Or maybe you're traveling, and as much as you'd like to try the 3:6:9 Cleanse, it's simply not workable with your schedule. If that's the case, maybe the Morning Cleanse in Chapter 16 feels feasible enough to get you through until you have an open, stable stretch of nine days to really go for it with the 3:6:9.

Perhaps you're trying to help a family member with anxiety, depression, attention-deficit/hyperactivity disorder (ADHD), or Alzheimer's disease, and they're not enthusiastic about following guidelines at every meal. That's a time to rely on Chapter 17 for the Heavy Metal Detox Cleanse.

You may be in a very sensitive place digestion-wise. Before you can even think about juggling the different foods in the 3:6:9 Cleanse, you need to be able to process what you eat without pain or irritation. That's an excellent time to start with Chapter 18, "Mono Eating Cleanse," to give your body a gentle detox and help you heal your intestinal linings enough to one day branch out into the more vigorous 3:6:9 Cleanse.

Or maybe you're completely fed up with other chronic illness symptoms, your gut is functioning well enough, and you're ready for a change. You want to start moving the needle now. That's an ideal time to bring in the 3:6:9 Cleanse, whether Original, Simplified, or Advanced, for an overhaul.

And then, once you've completed the 3:6:9 Cleanse—as many rounds of it as you'd like—you may feel primed to take on the 28-Day Cleanse or the 90-Day Thyroid Rehab from my other books someday. If you're coming to this book having already completed one or more of the Medical Medium cleanses, congratulations! I mean that in all seriousness. Those cleanses have gotten you to a place where the 3:6:9 Cleanse can provide deeper healing.

Giving our bodies and minds what they need to heal is profound. Wherever you start, you will be changed by your experience. Then, when you come back to that guiding question of "What feels manageable right now?" your response might have changed.

THE SHORT ANSWERS

One answer is that you can't go wrong. Any Medical Medium cleanse prepares you for any other Medical Medium cleanse.

Another answer is that any version of the 3:6:9 Cleanse is nearly always an excellent place to begin. The 3:6:9 Cleanse is the most efficient cleanse and also the shortest, which makes it very doable. The 3:6:9 Cleanse goes directly to the heart of your health—which is actually your liver—and taps into its undiscovered rhythms in order to give your body a jump-start. By guiding your liver to release the deep-seated poisons and pathogens that have been hindering it, you open a gateway to healing for your whole self.

By the way, if you're wondering how the 3:6:9 Cleanse in this book is different from the Liver Rescue 3:6:9 in my book *Liver Rescue*, the answer is that the Original 3:6:9 Cleanse is the same as the Liver Rescue 3:6:9, with some upgrades. This book also offers the Simplified and Advanced 3:6:9 Cleanses, which are entirely new options.

It's your choice whether to go with the Original, Simplified, or Advanced—we'll get to that in a few pages. And you can take either the Original or Simplified 3:6:9 Cleanse to the next level, if you'd like, by integrating a heavy metal detox modification. You'll find information about that in Chapter 21, "Cleanse Adaptations and Substitutions." (The Advanced 3:6:9 Cleanse already incorporates heavy metal detox.)

Once you've completed your 3:6:9 Cleanse, you can repeat its nine-day cycle as many times as you'd like, choose one of the other cleanses for long-term healing or maintenance, or go back to your normal life. Any Medical Medium cleanse that you choose after the 3:6:9 Cleanse will be that much more effective because of the deep liver and organ work that the 3:6:9 structure accomplished. It sets you up to get even greater benefits from your healing practices afterward.

— OVERVIEW OF CLEANSE OPTIONS —

	PURPOSE	ESPECIALLY USEFUL FOR	LENGTH OF CLEANSE	WHERE TO FIND IT
ORIGINAL 3:6:9 CLEANSE — The upgraded Liver Rescue 3:6:9.	Uproot deep-seated toxins and pathogens so chronic symptoms and illnesses can finally heal.	Cleansing the liver and other organs of a lifetime of the troublemakers (poisons, toxins, and the viruses and bacteria that feed on them) responsible for creating chronic illnesses and symptoms such as heart palpitations, hot flashes, tingles and numbness, aches and pains, vertigo, dizziness, brain fog, migraines, anxiety, depression, bloating, fatigue, reproductive conditions, thyroid conditions, lupus, Lyme disease, RA, psoriatic arthritis, eczema, psoriasis, acne, UTIs, and so much more.	9 days (or repeated 9-day cycles)	Chapter 10
SIMPLIFIED 3:6:9 CLEANSE — Easier to accomplish, this option works at 70 percent of the strength and power of the Original.	Start healing by uprooting toxins and pathogens at a less intense level that's more manageable for a busy schedule.	High cholesterol, high blood pressure, fatty liver, arterial plaque, lymphedema, arthritis, insomnia, varicose veins, dark under-eye circles, acid reflux, constipation, IBS, dry skin, type 2 diabetes, headaches, migraines, and so much more. Because of its reduced strength, consider repeating more often than the Original to get the results you want.	9 days (or repeated 9-day cycles)	Chapter 11
ADVANCED 3:6:9 CLEANSE — An all-raw, fat-free option especially suited to those who have tried the Original 3:6:9 Cleanse or the 28-Day Cleanse and want to go further.	Reach a deeper cleanse state to take your healing to the next level when dealing with critical health conditions.	Health circumstances that you feel are impeding your well-being on a critical level.	9 days (or repeated 9-day cycles)	Chapter 12

OVERVIEW OF CLEANSE OPTIONS

	PURPOSE	ESPECIALLY USEFUL FOR	LENGTH OF CLEANSE	WHERE TO FIND IT
ANTI-BUG CLEANSE A top choice for maintaining progress after the 3:6:9 Cleanse or working your way up to it.	Give your body a break from taxing foods (you choose at what level) and make more room for healing foods so your system can repair itself.	Keeping a handle on pathogen-caused conditions such as autoimmune disease and all its symptoms. By removing foods that feed disease-causing viruses and bacteria from the diet, you'll prevent them from prospering and help interrupt the cycle of chronic health issues.	2 to 4 weeks or more (or adopt for life)	Chapter 15
MORNING CLEANSE Another top choice for maintaining progress after the 3:6:9 Cleanse or working your way up to it. Can be combined with Anti-Bug Cleanse.	Allow your liver and the rest of your body to continue their natural state of detox in the morning.	Strengthening hydrochloric acid, which improves digestion, and reducing fat levels in the bloodstream, which allows for higher oxygen content and deeper hydration.	2 weeks or more (or adopt for life)	Chapter 16
INTERMITTENT FASTING OPTION An option for those with an interest in intermittent fasting.	For intermittent fasting enthusiasts who want to improve their game and add celery juice into their lives.	Strengthening digestion, giving you more clarity, and potentially controlling weight gain—when applied correctly.	Intermittently as desired	Chapter 16
HEAVY METAL DETOX CLEANSE Can be combined with the Anti-Bug Cleanse or the Morning Cleanse, or integrated into the 3:6:9 Cleanse.	Responsibly free your brain and body from toxic heavy metals that threaten your ability to achieve optimal health.	Getting to the root of neurological issues such as ADHD, autism, anxiety, depression, Alzheimer's, dementia, memory loss, brain fog, focus and concentration issues, tremors, Parkinson's, tics, spasms, insomnia, sleep issues, fatigue, MS, lupus, autoimmune disease, and Lyme disease; plus skin conditions such as eczema, psoriasis, scleroderma, vitiligo, and rosacea.	3 to 6 months or more	Chapter 17 (see Chapter 21 for how to work heavy metal detox into the 3:6:9 Cleanse)

OVERVIEW OF CLEANSE OPTIONS

	PURPOSE	ESPECIALLY USEFUL FOR	LENGTH OF CLEANSE	WHERE TO FIND IT
MONO EATING CLEANSE An eating option that couldn't be simpler, for those times when your system needs calming.	Soothe a digestive tract that's irritated and inflamed and starve the pathogens causing it in order to heal the gut, allowing for better processing of food and assimilation of nutrients. At the same time, rule out foods that are harsh on the nervous system.	Recovery from food poisoning, digestive conditions, or periods of not being able to eat due to eating disorders, gastrointestinal disorders, or medical testing interference. Recovery from chronic, long-term food allergies and sensitivities. Mono Eating delivers ample amounts of glucose to the brain and other parts of the nervous system, allowing for repair of nerves throughout the body that viral neurotoxins* have clung on to and made hypersensitized and inflamed. This glucose delivery translates to relief from MS, fibromyalgia, ME/CFS, anxiety, and many other conditions for which viral neurotoxins are responsible. *Neurotoxins are byproduct that viruses such as EBV excrete when feeding on toxic heavy metals and other troublemakers in the body.	1 week or more at a time (can be used long term as needed)	Chapter 18
WATER FASTING For relief when your digestive system is critically overtaxed.	Navigate severe digestive issues in the short term.	Acute health conditions such as stomach flu, food poisoning, nausea, abdominal pain, gallbladder attacks, and appendicitis. Not recommended for neurological conditions and symptoms.	1 to 3 days	Chapter 19
JUICE FASTING An option for those with an interest in juice cleanses.	Short-term detox that protects the adrenals and liver in the process.	Quickly detoxifying the lymphatic system and alleviating stress on the pancreas, gallbladder, and liver. Quickly restoring hydration while taking away troublemaker foods that feed pathogens that create symptoms and conditions.	1 to 2 days	Chapter 19

THE "WHY" OF CLEANSING

Now for a more in-depth look at choosing a cleanse. When we're trying to cleanse the body, we need to think about what we're actually trying to remove. What do the words *detox* and *cleanse* mean? What are we trying to get out of our bodies? The cleanses out there in the world are very broad in how they talk about poisons and toxins, and how they talk about them coming out of your body. The word *detox* is thrown around so vaguely and generally that no one really knows what is exiting the system, if anything.

In the future, that word is going to be frowned upon. *Detoxification*: it draws attention to the toxins inside us. It makes you realize that toxification had to happen first, and then you start wondering about the origins of that toxicity. The last thing industries want is for us to be aware of their poisons and what they do to us and the need to cleanse them. If we stay unaware of the industrial poisons that contribute to keeping us sick, this eventually forces us to spend money to deal with the sickness, and that keeps the money machine going.

Chapter 3, "A Wake-Up Call to What's Inside Us," went into detail on what we should be trying to get out of our bodies—and what we should try to limit our exposure to in the first place. Here's a brief recap of what we have inside of us: for one, traces of industrialized chemicals that have saturated all of our organs. A wide variety of these chemicals were actually manufactured long before our time, passed down from generations before us via sperm and egg and then in utero. We have so many different types of these chemicals within us from industrial years past and present—we're quite the toxic society today.

So when we think about cleansing, we need to get granular. We need to think about extracting the toxic heavy metals, insecticides and other pesticides, fungicides, exhaust residue, household cleaners, air fresheners, scented candles, hairsprays, perfumes, colognes, and other chemicals from daily living that our tissue is riddled with. We need to think about all our organs, most critically our liver and our brain.

We also need to think about pathogens. One of the key reasons why we want to get these industrialized toxins out is so they don't feed pathogens inside us and create disease. That's the biggest problem: the more toxic, industrial chemicals and agents and poisons we have inside of us, the more food there is for the myriad viruses and unproductive bacteria that are the disease producers and creators. Different diseases are different combinations of pathogens plus toxins; when pathogens and toxins come into contact with each other inside our bodies, we're destined for some variety of symptom or condition.

What a gift we give our bodies when we send these specific troublemakers away. You'll notice that in the 3:6:9 Cleanse, and in any cleanse in this book, dietary fats are kept low. The idea is to thin out the blood. As you read in the first chapter, diets today—whether trendy eating plans or standard eating—nearly always include too much fat for the body to accomplish its daily detox measures. When you thin out the blood, poisons readily surface in tissue and enter the bloodstream freely. When you go a step beyond thinning the blood and add in foods with supportive nutrients and healing phytochemicals—and that's what any Medical Medium cleanse does—you give your cells the ability to carry toxins all the way out of the body and to start repairing the damage that pathogens and poisons left behind.

CHOOSING A CLEANSE: WHERE TO BEGIN IN THE MEDICAL MEDIUM CLEANSE WORLD

When someone is dealing with multiple chronic illnesses, it can be puzzling to decide where to begin with all of the Medical Medium information. As I mentioned, a useful place to start is the 3:6:9 Cleanse. With its efficient structure, the 3:6:9 can get someone stronger faster so that down the road, when applying another cleanse such as the 90-Day Thyroid Rehab from *Thyroid Healing*, that person will find it easier and more beneficial.

We need to keep in mind that we all have different combinations and varieties of pathogens, toxic heavy metals, and other troublemakers; emotional challenges, losses, and stressors; as well as different support systems and resources. Some of us haven't had a challenge yet or haven't faced a difficult struggle emotionally or even financially. So all of our differences play a role in how we feel and how our body works when looking for answers to heal. Blindly saying, "My body doesn't like that food," or, "That way of doing things isn't right for me but may be right for you," or, "That food doesn't work for me because my body's different, but you can do that food," doesn't take into account a key understanding: that our bodies function very much the same here on Planet Earth. The reason it may not seem that way is because of the different combinations of physical and emotional challenges we each face that challenge our health in different ways. We all stand to benefit from Medical Medium information.

I want to reiterate that you can't go wrong choosing a cleanse from the Medical Medium book series. You can't make a mistake. They are all good, and they can all help reverse disease.

Any Medical Medium cleanse prepares you for any other Medical Medium cleanse. And no matter what Medical Medium cleanse you choose, it will not be wasted time or energy for your healing process. Quite the contrary: it will get you moving forward.

Each cleanse is powerful for its own reasons, and each cleanse heals many aspects of the body—by trying the 90-Day Thyroid Rehab, for example, you're not neglecting your liver or brain. Look at the overview chart again, look through these pages, and see what makes the most sense for you at this moment in time. If the 28-Day Cleanse from *Medical Medium* speaks to you and you're comfortable with it, embark on it. And if the 3:6:9 Cleanse speaks to you—and it probably does, if you picked up this book—go ahead and embark on it. If you're looking for a longer-term cleanse, then do consecutive rounds of the 3:6:9 Cleanse, even choosing the Advanced if that feels right for your situation.

The 3:6:9 Cleanse effectively sets the stage for any other Medical Medium cleanse, so if you're open to where to begin, start with the 3:6:9. It's an ideal first cleanse to prepare you for the other cleanses, and it's also the most foundational cleanse. By that I mean that once you've experienced it, the 3:6:9 will always be there for you as a touchstone, a familiar landmark that's superiorly grounded.

By no means do you have to start with the 3:6:9 Cleanse, though. The other Medical Medium cleanses are grounded too. The reason I offer so many options is that choices matter with cleanses. Some of these cleanses are longer, some are shorter, some are flexible on time frame, some have a certain rhythm, and some have a special twist. Some focus on specific healing foods and some have wider parameters. Some give you suggestions to fit into your normal routine and some give you guidelines about what to eat all day. This is one time in life where your free will is not stifled, held back, or locked down.

You also have the freedom to change. We are constantly growing and evolving physically, emotionally, and spiritually, so we should be allowed to evolve in what variety of cleanse we want to try too. You may find that one cleanse speaks to you now, and months or a year down the road, another one you never expected ends up being your favorite. Some years we may travel more than others, some years we may spend more time at home, and some years we may spend more time at work, and that plays a role in our food prep options. Exploring the different cleanses is a spiritual experience. While the other Medical Medium cleanses are healing and life-changing in their own right, the 3:6:9

Cleanse is a home you can return to again and again when you come down off that mountain and need a place that sustains you. It's the cleanse of familiarity, the cleanse your heart and soul can root themselves to—because everyone needs that sense of being rooted at some point in their lives.

If you find yourself in a head cramp—*Should I do the cleanse from one chapter or another?*—release the blockage. Whichever cleanse you choose from this book or this book series is going to be the right one for you. Your angels know that your body needs to heal. The universe knows your body wants to heal. God knows your body is ready to heal. You will be guided right about where to begin, and in the future, whether that's a month from now or several months, you are free to choose another. The results you find with your healing process will help light the way.

——— **ORIGINAL CLEANSE UPGRADES** ———

If you're coming to this book from *Liver Rescue*,
you'll recognize the Original 3:6:9 Cleanse in Chapter 10
as the Liver Rescue 3:6:9 cleanse from that book.
You'll also notice that here, the cleanse features some upgrades,
so make sure to read that chapter, "Original 3:6:9 Cleanse,"
thoroughly. Also be sure to check out Part IV, especially Chapter 19,
"Critical Cleanse Dos and Don'ts," and Chapter 21,
"Cleanse Adaptations and Substitutions," for new insights.

THE 3:6:9 CLEANSE: ORIGINAL VERSUS SIMPLIFIED VERSUS ADVANCED

Say you decide that it's time to try the 3:6:9 Cleanse. How do you know whether the Original, Simplified, or Advanced is right for you? This brings us back to that guiding question: What feels manageable for you right now?

Does the idea of very specific guidelines appeal to you? Do you want to see faster results? Then you may like the straightforward nature of the Original 3:6:9 Cleanse.

What if you want a little more flexibility? Maybe you have a lot of responsibilities and want the option to eat a little more cooked food and slow down any possible healing reactions. That's a good time to opt for the Simplified 3:6:9 Cleanse.

Do you feel that you're in a critical place with your health? Have you already been eating pure for some time, or do you prefer an all-raw diet and want to take it to the next level? The Advanced 3:6:9 Cleanse is there to support you.

The Original 3:6:9 Cleanse actually starts out with a little more leeway during the first three days to help you ease into meal-by-meal eating plans, whereas the Simplified 3:6:9 gets right down to business by cutting out radical fats while providing more adaptability in the long run. That may be a factor in your decision, one way or another.

If you start the Original 3:6:9 and feel that it's too difficult to keep up with or you feel discomfort, it's perfectly okay to switch over to the Simplified 3:6:9 midway through. Someday, maybe you'll have a window to give the Original 3:6:9 another try. That's the beauty of the guiding question: "right now" is always going to change, so you never know where you'll be in the future.

Similarly, if you begin the Advanced 3:6:9 Cleanse and decide partway that the Original or Simplified would be more manageable this time around, that's fine. On the other hand, your motivation for staying on the Advanced 3:6:9 will probably be high, because this is the one you choose when you want deeper healing from more complicated health conditions. The seeker who is looking to move forward from months or years of pronounced chronic illness will usually find that the relief they experience with the Advanced keeps them eager to complete the full cleanse, if not several repetitions in a row.

FOOD INTOLERANCES

If you have food intolerances, you may worry about whether certain cleanses will work for you.

The first answer is that Medical Medium cleanses steer away from troublemaker foods. Depending on which cleanse you try, you'll either be limiting or removing the foods that are most disruptive to health—a break that will allow you to experience freedom from many food intolerances. On top of which, cleansing helps unload your liver of the burdens that cause many food sensitivities, which ultimately means more relief.

The second answer is that for the 3:6:9 Cleanse, which is the cleanse that calls for the most specific foods, there's an entire chapter on adaptations and substitutions so you can work around any sensitivities—that's Chapter 21.

The third answer is that if you're still concerned, that probably indicates you're nervous about eating fruit. When someone says they have a fruit intolerance, it probably means they have other food intolerances too. Fruit is the food that takes the hit because it's frequently under siege by professionals around the world for containing fruit sugar—a mistaken fear.

Food intolerances have to do with a sick liver. And if you never address that liver and work to heal or cleanse or rejuvenate it, how are you ever going to get ahead of your food intolerances, including what you may think of as a fruit intolerance? Discomfort with fruit is usually a warning sign that something else is really a problem. Fruit is so cleansing that it tends to get poisons and toxins moving and to push putrefied fat and protein out of the body, which can in turn result in healing reactions of bloating or rashing as your system sends them on their way. It's not that the 3:6:9 Cleanse or any other Medical Medium cleanse would be *causing* these problems. They're simply reactions to fruit's cleansing nature, and they would have been occurring before the cleanse anyway, whenever that person ate a piece of fruit.

The problems are already there and have been for longer than you've realized. The same is true when symptoms of illness surface outside of a cleanse: the underlying condition was developing long, long before it made itself known—it started at minimum months and usually years before symptoms appeared. Symptoms are signs of illness that showcase themselves long after a hidden imbalance has begun.

When fruit pushes the cleansing process along, poisons and toxins leave the liver and body, and it's possible to experience symptoms. You would likely have experienced these symptoms anyway, down the road, without fruit: as organs holding these poisons and toxins reached capacity and overflowed, for example, or if you exercised a little more vigorously than usual, dislodging "storage bins" of poisons and toxins that created symptoms three days later. Fruit has the power to move this all along more quickly, without our overdoing it with exercise or waiting for a toxin load to overflow. Fruit's cleansing nature forces whatever storage bins are filled with toxins to unload, helping send them out of the body to ease our suffering.

The symptoms we think of as fruit intolerance are not fruit's fault. When someone experiences these issues, they're going to keep getting that bloating or rashing no matter what their diet is, unless they stop and take care of their liver. Sometimes it can be inconsistent, at different times, with different foods—because again, with many food intolerances, it's not about the food; it's about the liver. If the reactions go away when someone eats a diet that keeps to little or no fruit, that doesn't mean the problem is completely gone and 100 percent fixed. It only hides the underlying problem: a sluggish, sick liver overburdened with the troublemakers we encounter in our everyday world. It's only getting worse behind the scenes, and keeping fruit out keeps away the messenger.

The way to heal the situation is to heal the liver, and that means cleansing. Exactly how to proceed with the 3:6:9 Cleanse depends on what your issues are. In Chapter 21, "Cleanse Adaptations and Substitutions," you'll find a modification that allows you to ease into the cleanse if your hesitance around fruit means you don't feel ready to try the full course. And if you're not ready to go near fruit yet, you still have an avenue: Chapter 18, "Mono Eating Cleanse," which includes non-fruit options. Or perhaps you feel ready to try the 3:6:9 Cleanse as it is, now that your mind is set at ease about fruit. If you experience some bloating or rashing on the 3:6:9 Cleanse, at least you're addressing the deep inner problem so that someday, you can be bloating and rash free.

When you have a thorn in your foot, while it may not be painless to pull it out—at least you've pulled it out. The same applies here. If you have a sick liver causing discomfort with fruit, you're better off addressing it to let the wounds finally heal.

PREGNANCY AND BREASTFEEDING

When you are breastfeeding, it's okay to go on the Original, Simplified, or Advanced 3:6:9 Cleanse, or any other cleanse in this book. They all help make breast milk cleaner by pulling impurities out of breast tissue.

If you are pregnant, know that both the Original and Simplified 3:6:9 Cleanses are extremely nutrient-dense. They are not only healing for your body; they are supportive and healing for a developing baby. While pregnant, you'll be more satiated if you modify the cleanse by repeating the Day 8 food plan for the ninth day, in place of the Day 9 protocol.

As far as the Advanced 3:6:9 Cleanse, if you want to try it while pregnant, bring it to the attention of your doctor(s). The likely reason you're interested in this variation is because of a symptom or condition you're facing during pregnancy, which means you're

already in contact with one or more physicians about that health struggle. Take these doctors' advice about whether the Advanced 3:6:9 is in line with what they recommend.

If you're dealing with symptoms or conditions that make you want to explore another cleanse in this book while pregnant, talk to the doctor(s) you're seeing about those health issues.

CHILDREN

It's okay for children to do either the Original, Simplified, or Advanced 3:6:9 Cleanse, with one key change: Adjust amounts according to what the child's mom or other primary caregiver knows about what the child is used to eating. That means reducing portions to what works for your kid's appetite. To help you determine the right serving sizes of celery juice, see the table on page 480. If Mom or another primary caregiver feels that Day 9 of the 3:6:9 Cleanse will be a challenge for their kid because it focuses on liquids, it's fine to repeat Day 8 instead.

The other cleanses in this book are perfectly fine for children too. All Medical Medium cleanses are kid-safe.

LIVER TESTING

Sometimes people wonder whether they need to cleanse in the first place, and they want a test that will indicate the answer. You don't want to wait for a test to tell you that you have liver issues before you decide to take care of your liver. Tests do not exist yet to detect liver issues early enough, at the precondition stage, when fatty liver is still the undiscovered *sluggish liver* or when a viral situation is starting to take hold in the liver.

Are there *any* indications when someone is in these early, undetectable stages of liver distress? Yes: symptoms. Specifically, many of the symptoms we brush off as normal parts of life are actually indicators of beginning liver trouble. That includes chronic constipation, bloating, dark under-eye circles, brain fog, flagging energy, unexplained weight gain, varicose veins, inflammation, insomnia, skin problems, food sensitivities, early aging, hot flashes, gallstones, heart palpitations, mood struggles, seasonal affective disorder (SAD), nagging hunger, reproductive issues (including PCOS, fibroids, and endometriosis), migraines, eczema, acne, vertigo, tingles, numbness, and many more that I covered in *Liver Rescue*. You could visit the doctor while experiencing any of these and hear that your liver is in perfectly good health, because medical communities don't yet have the training to interpret the symptoms of a liver that's starting to become overloaded, nor do they have the tools to diagnose liver problems that early.

Again, this is why it's not worth waiting to hear you have a liver issue before you think about unburdening your liver with a cleanse. We walk around with sick livers that have the potential to influence nearly any aspect of our health—with no one realizing it. Even someone who looks fit could have the unknown precondition *pre-fatty liver* that's causing unseen complications in the body. The beginning, undetectable stages of liver distress are ideal times to take action with a cleanse such as the 3:6:9.

If you are at a more pronounced stage of liver trouble, to the point where a blood test, imaging, or biopsy indicates a situation such as fatty liver, that doesn't mean it's too late to cleanse—not remotely. It only means you may have a longer road ahead of you. Even so, the relief you feel and results you see on the 3:6:9 Cleanse have the potential to be so rapid that they will give you a powerful sense of momentum to carry you along through healing.

HEAVY METAL DETOX TESTING

What about testing for toxic heavy metals? If you're trying to figure out whether heavy metal detox should be a concern for you, heavy metal testing is an option. Keep in mind, though, that this will only detect toxic heavy metals in the bloodstream that test makers know to look for at levels high enough to find. Even if your test results come back clean, you could still have toxic heavy metals in your system—plenty of them. Heavy metals don't always reside in the bloodstream. They're often hidden in organs such as the brain and liver, and testing fails to find them, even though the toxic heavy metal particles are inside us, however nanoscopic, creating trouble by making crevices in tissue, interrupting nerve signals, and taking that all further by reacting and oxidizing, sending corrosive runoff over critical organ tissue.

As with liver distress, we can more reliably figure out if we're dealing with toxic heavy metals through our symptoms. Examples include anxiety, depression, bipolar disorder, confusion, tics, spasms, brain fog, ADHD, Alzheimer's, Parkinson's, autism, eczema, psoriasis, rosacea, vitiligo, and Crohn's. Not that you want to wait for these either to tell you that it may be a good idea to try Chapter 17's Heavy Metal Detox Cleanse or to incorporate the heavy metal detox modification into your 3:6:9 Cleanse. Any time is a good time to be aware that the air we breathe, the water we drink, the prepared food we eat, the cosmetics we apply, the gas we put in our car, and the rain that soaks into our skin can bring us into contact with toxic heavy metals, and that it's worth pulling them out if we want to spare ourselves and our loved ones the tumult and heartbreak of toxic heavy metals' long-term effect on our health.

People sometimes worry about the side effects of heavy metal detoxing, and that's an important concern—when you're trying any other technique out there that claims to help you remove toxic heavy metals. As well-meaning as other methods are, they run the risk of dropping the metals they may pick up along the way in your system, and that's what causes reactions and side effects. In particular, chlorella and chelation formulas that contain chlorella can't be trusted to hold on to metals. In contrast, the heavy metal detox technique that you'll find in these pages is angelically put together to remove metals properly, with backup measures in place to keep a firm grip on the toxic heavy metals that are extracted throughout their entire path out of your body.

CELERY JUICE: POWERFUL MEDICINE

Fresh celery juice is a part of every cleanse in this book. It's a part of every herb and supplement list in Chapter 29, "The True Cause of Your Symptoms and Conditions with Dosages to Heal." It's in every book that I write. I even devoted a whole book to this medicinal tonic, because celery juice is that powerful.

With so many directions to go in the health world and so many approaches that sound convincing, it's easy to be thwarted from even giving celery juice a go. That's true for any Medical Medium information. There are people out there who say they've tried it, and discourage others from trying it, when the truth is that they only dabbled in it, and not for long enough to give it an honest try. It's like if you came to a bridge and someone standing there told you, "I've already crossed that. There's nothing on the other side." If you believed them, you'd never know that just a little bit farther on the other side of that bridge was a Garden of Eden. The person who warned you off never went far enough to discover it.

Try not to cheat yourself out of this amazing opportunity to heal because someone told you not to cross the bridge. Maybe that person wasn't sick enough to take the guidelines seriously, or maybe they were distracted by other approaches. Whatever their missteps might have been, it's easy to get discouraged before you even start, and for that to throw you off your healing trail.

As we'll explore in Chapter 24, "Living Words for Underdogs and a Note for Critics," there are the sick and there are the not-so-sick. The symptoms someone is dealing with do matter in how seriously they take healing protocols. For one person, it could be difficult to get out of bed each day, painful just to take a shower. Another person may complain about how hard they have it with their health, and yet they're able to travel and take a hiking vacation. These are different degrees of symptoms. It's entirely true that no matter how mild they are, symptoms do hold us back. A little eczema, some anxiety—these are frustrating. At the same time, someone in that situation is still able to live their life, and it's probably a pretty good one. That means they may not pay the same careful attention to following guidance correctly. They may be quick to cast away a powerful protocol when they lose interest. They may not be as motivated or committed as the person for whom survival is a moment-by-moment struggle. As an observer, it's very easy to get confused here. It's easy to assume that the person who says celery juice didn't work for them was in the same boat as the person who says it saved their life—it's easy to assume that they applied the guidelines properly and gave it more than a few days to start its work in the brain and body, when they really didn't.

Why is celery juice a part of every cleanse? Not because it's a cute little perk. It's there because it makes everything else work better. Celery juice enhances any Medical Medium cleanse and all that you're doing while you're on it. It helps you maximize the Heavy Metal Detox Smoothie benefits. It helps you maximize what you get out of any other cleanse recipe. That's the power and the difference of celery juice.

Whatever you're doing that's in service of your well-being, whether you're on a cleanse or not, celery juice taps into it and makes it more potent so that you can receive its full benefits. Celery juice will enhance any tools you're using that are providing benefits even at small levels. It enhances anything truly good and healthy in your diet.

Now, if you're eating foods or taking products that aren't beneficial, celery juice won't magically make them good for you. It *will* help work against those problematic items that feed viruses and unproductive bacteria and contribute to chronic illness—even the ones we wouldn't divulge to other people because it's human nature to share what we're proud of eating and hide what we know doesn't serve us. While it can't make junk food into health food, celery juice will at least help manage the effects of the foods you're not quite ready to give up yet. Celery juice is on your side.

SAVE YOURSELF FROM MISINFORMATION

As knowledgeable as health professionals are about other aspects of health, they lack the knowledge about what causes chronic illness in the first place. We need to recognize this to make progress.

On top of which, we can get distracted by the health enthusiasts out there who are fantastic at quickly spreading noise, articles, misinformation, and confusion on social media merely because it seems exciting. Health hobbyists are just starting to experience smaller symptoms and are at the beginning of their pathway to knowledge, driven at this stage by clicks and engagement while, unknowingly or knowingly, taking advantage of the rise of so many lost and confused chronic illness sufferers.

Keep all this in mind when a trend or theory out in the world makes you question the cleansing knowledge in this book. In earlier chapters of Part I, you found in-depth looks at three trends that get in the way of proper cleansing and healing; we deconstructed why the microbiome is not the answer to everything, why intermittent fasting is not the long-term solution for cleansing success, and why it's okay (and even vital) to toss the fiber when making fresh juice. To further illuminate how a popular practice can lead you away from the healing information you need, let's take a quick look here at the trends of bulking, cutting, and counting macros.

Counting Macros: The New Counting Calories

Counting calories has fallen out of favor as it becomes clear that it can lead to disordered thinking about food. In its place, counting "macros" (or macronutrients) is becoming popular. Now, young people (and older) are tracking how many grams of fat, carbohydrates, and protein are in everything they eat, and they're working to control their intake, meanwhile not acknowledging the most critical health-related parts of the food we eat: the phytochemical compounds, antioxidants, antivirals, antibacterials, trace minerals, and mineral salts. Because counting macros is more complex and customizable than counting calories, we're not supposed to think that it can get just as disordered. It's yet one more trend that's on track to mislead those who struggle with chronic illness. Among those in the fitness world and those outside it, many believe that it's more of a long-term solution. For your own protection and that of

your family, you need to know that it's not a long-term solution. It's got holes everywhere.

Bulking and Cutting

People often find themselves having trouble building muscle while keeping their bodies lean on a high-protein diet. This can be confusing, since so much messaging out there says that focusing on protein and eliminating or minimizing carbs is a secret to building muscle and getting fit. Somewhere along the way, the fitness community realized—though they won't admit it—that protein alone wasn't enough to build and sustain the lean muscle most desired. As a result, it's become a trend to engage in "bulking and cutting." That is, going through cycles of bringing excess calories (more than they burn or utilize) *with* a blend of protein, carbs, and fat (emphasis on protein) to gain body mass from their workouts and then, once they've gained what seems to be more muscle—yet in many cases is just a layer of swelling and toxic fat in and around the muscle—cutting back on calories with the goal of keeping the muscle and losing the fat they gained because they fear "fattening up." This keeps people in a vicious cycle. It's a big mistake in health right now. The goal should be the opposite: to not constantly have to minimize and maximize your calories to increase muscle mass. The gaining and losing weight strategy puts tremendous stress upon the body, especially the liver, and a weakened, stagnant, sluggish liver loses its ability to convert and store nutrients, which leads to nutrient deficiencies and accelerated aging later in life. This additional stress on the body can eventually show itself as cardiovascular issues, cholesterol imbalances, prediabetes, type

2 diabetes, unwanted weight gain, muscle tears, cartilage and joint wear and tear, kidney weakness, a weakened immune system, and more. If you end up with a whole different health issue down the line that's diagnosed as autoimmune, it can take a greater toll on your body because of the previous years of bulking and cutting.

The bulking theory is about increasing calories daily to create an abundance of fuel so someone can easily build larger amounts of muscle in a shorter period of time—all the while believing that the extra protein they're eating is building their muscles and that some of the carbs they're eating are getting stored as fat. Here's what's really happening: the extra carbs they're eating are what's actually building more muscle as they train hard. Meanwhile, the extra fat they're adding to what they don't realize is their already high-fat diet (they likely think it's only high in protein) creates an overload on the liver and causes the increased fat storage on the body.

There are normally two camps subscribing to the bulking theory. One camp purposely bulks up on unhealthy calories—for example, doughnuts, cakes, cookies, muffins, danishes, croissants, mac and cheese, pizza, ice cream, burgers, and oily fries—and they are unaware that it's not the carbs in these foods causing the increased fat buildup on the body; it's the radical fats within these unhealthier options. The other camp bulks up on what they believe are healthier options such as avocado toast, gluten-free pasta with oil-based sauces, nuts, seeds, nut butters, eggs, chicken, salmon, beans, rice with oil, hummus with tahini, oatmeal with peanut butter, and protein shakes made with almond butter, almond milk, oat milk, and a little bit of fruit. This camp believes that it's the beans, fruit, rice, and pasta causing the extra fat storage on the body, when what's really happening, once again, are the radical fats such as tahini, avocado, oils, and fat inside the eggs causing a person's body fat to increase. There's also a third camp that mixes and combines the foods that the other two camps eat.

The way to safely and more efficiently build muscle is to provide the proper levels of glucose to muscle cells along with ample trace mineral salts to help insulin attach itself easily to the glucose and drive it into muscle tissue for muscles to sustain themselves without atrophy when you're not working out and to grow when you can exercise. Lean muscle growth without fat gain cancels out the need to cut calories and engage in the cutting part of the bulking theory. Lowering fat is a critical part of building lean muscle.

As you know well if you follow my work, a high-protein diet (which translates to a high-fat diet) is hard on the body. At least it usually keeps people off processed foods, though, and encourages them to bring vegetables and leafy greens into their lives. When someone is eating both high-protein and high-carb, they tend to get more lenient with food, more likely to bring in those processed food items that aren't helping anybody.

What those who advocate bulking and cutting don't realize is that if they instead kept protein and fats low in the diet while bringing in carbs, they could build straight muscle without putting fat on the body that they then have to work to lose.

That's why you'll find that none of the cleanses in this book focus on protein and fat. Instead, they focus on the true sources of health and strength: fresh celery juice, leafy greens, vegetables, and what I call *critical clean carbohydrates* (CCC), those carbs such as fruit, squash, sweet potatoes, and potatoes that our bodies need to thrive. Are we really okay to cut back protein and fat? Yes—*more* than okay, even though conditioning to make us think otherwise is strong. You'll find further reassurance throughout this book, particularly in Chapter 19, "Critical Cleanse Dos and Don'ts."

People sometimes fear they'll lose muscle on a cleanse. Flipping through these cleanses and seeing that they don't include bulking, cutting, or counting macros may reinforce this fear. Worried they won't come out of a Medical Medium cleanse looking the way they want, they may think, *He doesn't know what he's talking about.* That's the old protein monster brainwashing darkness that came out of the 1930s, and it's going to trip people up from getting the help they need from this book—if they go into it uninformed. Don't let that be you. Don't write off the cleanses in this book because they don't incorporate bulking, cutting, or counting macros. You're in on the truth now: that precisely because they avoid the theories of bulking, cutting, and counting macros, these cleanses are the answer to building up your strength and vitality, at the same time they bring you back to health.

"You're about to engage with the profound nature
of cleaning and rejuvenating cells throughout the body
so you can have every opportunity
to recover and heal."

— Anthony William, Medical Medium

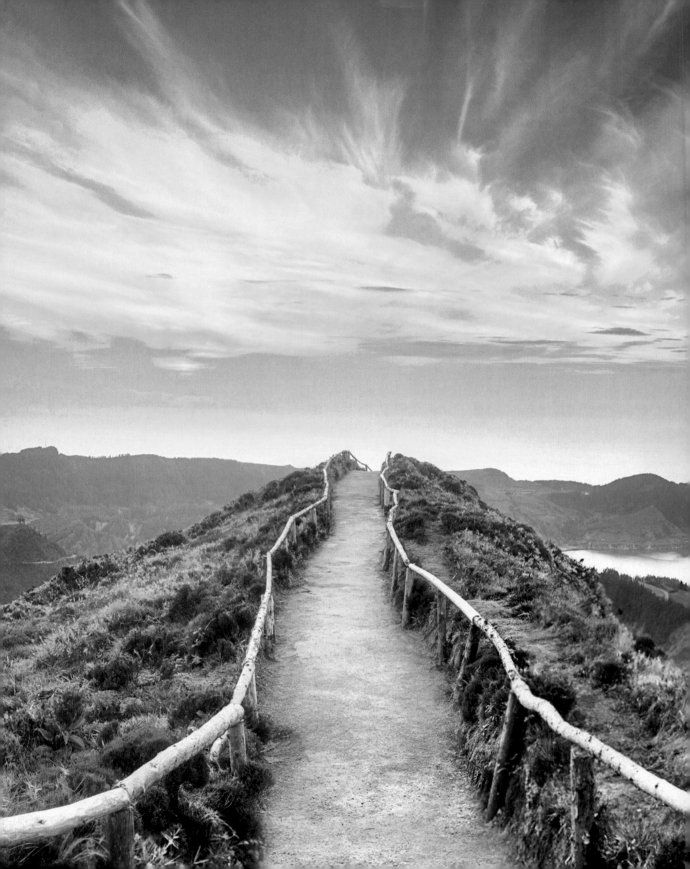

PART II

3:6:9 CLEANSE: LIFE PROTECTOR

CHAPTER 9

How the 3:6:9 Cleanse Works

You're about to engage with the profound nature of cleaning and rejuvenating cells throughout the body so you can have every opportunity to recover and heal.

THE 3:6:9 STRUCTURE

Whether you opt for the Original, Simplified, or Advanced 3:6:9 Cleanse, you'll begin with a three-day preparation phase, which I call *The 3*, and this is integral. You won't serve yourself by skipping ahead to the later days, because your body needs this gear-up time to benefit from everything that's to follow.

During the next three days, when you're in *The 6*, the internal cleansing begins. This is when your liver and other organs get to unpack some of their old "storage bins" of toxins (such as old pharmaceuticals, petrochemicals, plastics, and toxic heavy metals) as well as fats and viral waste matter they've been holding for months or years, getting to reach more deeply than they have throughout your whole life.

And during the final three days, when you're in *The 9*, your liver gets to let go, sending multitudes of troublemakers into your bloodstream for delivery out of your body to get you closer to your healing goals than ever before. It's the stage that completes the 3:6:9 Cleanse and the stage that helps you finally move the needle on your health.

If you're looking for a longer cleanse, it's more than okay to go back to the beginning and start again after you've completed one nine-day cycle of the Original, Simplified, or Advanced 3:6:9 Cleanse—you can keep repeating the nine days for as long as you'd like. For more guidance on this, see Chapter 13, "Repeating the 3:6:9 Cleanse," and Chapter 19, "Critical Cleanse Dos and Don'ts." Those chapters will also clear up questions about how to handle it if you need to stop the cleanse partway through for any reason.

The structure of this cleanse is not arbitrary. Aligning yourself with these three-day liver-care increments that add up to nine puts your body into a deep cleanse state. If you want to know more about the meaning behind the numbers, you'll find insights into their physiological significance in my book *Liver Rescue*. You'll also find a way to further tap into the numbers in "The Birthday Cleansing Secret" on page 217 of this book.

TIMING THE CLEANSE

The 3:6:9 Cleanse is designed to support you from Day 1, no matter where you are in life. If you're used to eating a pretty standard diet, don't worry that you need to work your way up to trying the cleanse—you don't need to spend a month removing troublemaker foods on the Anti-Bug Cleanse first or doing the Morning Cleanse or the Heavy Metal Detox Cleanse, although you're welcome to do so. Whatever you're used to eating on a daily basis, feel free to go straight into any version of the 3:6:9 Cleanse from there.

The exception is if you are extremely sensitive. If you are dealing with digestive difficulties that make it tough to process a variety of foods, then consider starting with the Mono Eating Cleanse instead. Refer back to Chapter 18 for a full explanation of how that works.

If you work Monday through Friday, a landmark way to approach this cleanse is to begin on a Saturday and end the next Sunday. That way you'll have the first weekend to ease into the eating plan as well as shop for ingredients and prepare food for the week ahead. Then you'll have the time and space of the second weekend to attend to the most potent days of the cleanse.

As the poisons and toxins are released, you may get waves of feeling a little tired or even emotional. The cleanse is not only physical; it can be a spiritual moment. When you're releasing poisons and toxins, you're releasing an older part of yourself. You're releasing the past. While those waves could happen at any time on the cleanse, prepare yourself especially for them to happen during the last three days. Before you even begin the cleanse, map it out. Choose a start date that will mean the

last three days arrive at a time when you can afford to be a bit more tired or emotional—that's one reason why I recommend ending the cleanse on a weekend. If your week is structured differently, or if your preference is to begin on another day for any other reason, then go ahead and start your 3:6:9 Cleanse whenever you'd like. It's about fitting it into *your* life and supporting *you*.

If you're coming directly from a standard diet—meaning you're used to various processed and fried foods or a fair amount of gluten, dairy products, and animal protein—and you feel inclined to launch directly into the Advanced 3:6:9 Cleanse, do be aware that it's going to be a much more radical change than starting with the Original or Simplified 3:6:9 Cleanse or another cleanse in this book first. That's not to make you fearful, only to prepare you for the fact that you'll be releasing a lot more poisons and toxins into the bloodstream than someone who was eating a purer diet before starting the Advanced. Your bloodstream will fill up rapidly with surface toxins from organs as well as from cells and tissue all throughout the body, while someone coming from a pure way of eating will be getting to mostly deeper toxins. That high volume of release will mean that you may want to build a little more downtime for yourself into all nine days of the Advanced 3:6:9 Cleanse.

ADRENAL PROTECTION

One of the beauties of the 3:6:9 Cleanse is that it protects your adrenal glands. Unlike so many cleanses that make you go hungry, forcing your adrenals to squeeze out excess adrenaline and putting your liver through even more strain in the process of mopping it up, the 3:6:9 Cleanse doesn't wreck these precious glands because it doesn't starve you.

If you remove food improperly—if you do a cleanse where food is removed without thought, consideration, or understanding of how your adrenal glands truly work—then your adrenal glands may react because they received no warning that food removal was going to happen. That reaction will come in the form of a continual release of adrenaline for the body to use as a replacement for blood sugar. This way, your organs remain stable and endure the unexpected lack of glucose from the new diet you're trying. The adrenals pay the price, though. Older keto and other high-fat/high-protein diets are an example of this; the removal of all carbohydrates always weakened and injured the adrenal glands, leaving a person with fatigue and low energy for months afterward.

If you're worried about hunger pangs on this plan, you can release your fear. The 3:6:9 Cleanse protects you and protects your adrenal glands. You don't need to limit yourself to tiny portions, and snack options are built into each version.

Even though the Original 3:6:9 Cleanse does lower dietary fat to take some burden off your liver and pancreas, it does so gradually, and to balance that, you get to fill yourself up with other delicious flavors. And even though the Simplified and Advanced 3:6:9 Cleanses do call for you to refrain from radical fats the entire time, you get to fill up to keep yourself grounded and satisfied. Plus the nutrient density of all three of these 3:6:9 food plans satiates on a deep cell level.

LIFELONG TOOLS: ORIGINAL, SIMPLIFIED, AND ADVANCED

As we explored in Chapter 8, "Your Guide to Choosing a Cleanse," the decision about whether to opt for the Original, Simplified, or Advanced 3:6:9 Cleanse comes down to a few factors, including how new you are to cleansing and where you are with your health. If you're dealing with only a couple of symptoms that aren't interfering with your everyday life, you may choose to go one direction. If you're facing multiple symptoms and conditions that are making your life difficult and you're in great need of cleansing, healing, and recovery, you may choose to go another. Your schedule is also likely to play a role. You're the expert on what your goals are and what feels doable right now. And remember, it's not all or nothing. No matter which cleanse version you choose now, the others will always be there for you to try another time. They're all lifelong tools available to you.

CHAPTER 10

Original 3:6:9 Cleanse

The purpose of the Original 3:6:9 Cleanse is to uproot deep-seated toxins and pathogens, opening the door to a future where it's possible to live free from your chronic symptoms.

When we're sick and struggling with prolonged symptoms, we tend to lose sight of what it was like to feel good. As the months and even years go by, we lose touch with what it was like to have more energy and less intrusive symptoms, or even not to have any symptoms at all. Some people have never known what it was to feel good, because they've been suffering since they were young. When symptoms rule our day, we can feel that good health is out of our control. The Original 3:6:9 Cleanse is a powerful way to put control back in your hands so you can finally move forward.

By cleansing the liver and other organs of the toxic troublemakers responsible for chronic health issues, the Original 3:6:9 Cleanse helps you begin to alleviate and even rid yourself of symptoms and conditions such as heart palpitations, hot flashes, tingles and numbness, aches and pains, vertigo, dizziness, brain fog, migraines, anxiety, depression, bloating, fatigue, reproductive conditions, thyroid conditions, lupus, Lyme disease, rheumatoid arthritis, psoriatic arthritis, eczema, psoriasis, acne, UTIs, and so many more. Without poisons and toxins and the viruses and bacteria that feed on them holding you back, life holds renewed possibility.

You have the right to heal. You deserve to feel strong and productive and to experience your body as a precious vehicle that can carry you through life with ease.

KEY CLEANSE NOTES

Keep these important notes in mind as you dig into this chapter:

Upgrades

As mentioned in Chapter 8, "Your Guide to Choosing a Cleanse," the Original 3:6:9 Cleanse is an upgraded version of the Liver Rescue 3:6:9 cleanse from my book *Liver Rescue*. Be sure to read the coming pages thoroughly so you can benefit from the updates—for example, so that you include celery juice on all nine days of the cleanse for an extra boost and add steamed zucchini or summer squash to your lunch on the first three days. Also check out Chapter 19, "Critical Cleanse Dos and Don'ts," where you'll find answers to common cleanse questions.

Recipes and Sample Menus

You'll find any recipes referenced here in Chapter 23. You'll also find sample menus outlining recipe options for every meal in Chapter 22.

Adaptations and Substitutions

If for any reason you can't eat or access any of the foods called for in the pages to come, or if solid foods are a problem for you, turn to Chapter 21 for a whole chapter's worth of modifications. There, you'll also find an option to incorporate the Heavy Metal Detox into this cleanse if you'd like.

——— THE 3: ORIGINAL ———

	DAY 1	DAY 2	DAY 3
UPON WAKING	16 ounces lemon or lime water	16 ounces lemon or lime water	16 ounces lemon or lime water
MORNING	Wait 15 to 30 minutes, then: 16 ounces celery juice Wait another 15 to 30 minutes, then: Breakfast and mid-morning snack of your choice (within guidelines)	Wait 15 to 30 minutes, then: 16 ounces celery juice Wait another 15 to 30 minutes, then: Breakfast and mid-morning snack of your choice (within guidelines), including: One to two apples (or applesauce)	Wait 15 to 30 minutes, then: 16 ounces celery juice Wait another 15 to 30 minutes, then: Breakfast and mid-morning snack of your choice (within guidelines), including: One to two apples (or applesauce)
LUNCHTIME	Meal of your choice (within guidelines), incorporating steamed zucchini or summer squash	Meal of your choice (within guidelines), incorporating steamed zucchini or summer squash	Meal of your choice (within guidelines), incorporating steamed zucchini or summer squash
MID-AFTERNOON	One to two apples (or applesauce) with one to two dates	One to two apples (or applesauce) with one to two dates	One to two apples (or applesauce) with one to two dates

	DAY 1	DAY 2	DAY 3
DINNERTIME	Meal of your choice (within guidelines)	Meal of your choice (within guidelines)	Meal of your choice (within guidelines)
EVENING	Apple (or applesauce) (if desired) 16 ounces lemon or lime water Hibiscus, lemon balm, or chaga tea	Apple (or applesauce) (if desired) 16 ounces lemon or lime water Hibiscus, lemon balm, or chaga tea	Apple (or applesauce) (if desired) 16 ounces lemon or lime water Hibiscus, lemon balm, or chaga tea
GUIDELINES	• Reduce your normal consumption of radical fats (nuts, seeds, oils, olives, coconut, avocado, animal proteins, etc.) by 50 percent, and wait to eat radical fats altogether (if desired at all) until dinnertime. While they are not a radical fat, skip beans entirely. • Avoid these foods: eggs, dairy, gluten, soft drinks, salt and seasonings, pork, corn, oils (including both industrial and healthier oils), soy, lamb, tuna and other fish and seafood (salmon, trout, and sardines are okay at dinner on Days 1 to 3), vinegar (including ACV), caffeine (including coffee, matcha, cacao, and chocolate), grains (millet and oats are okay on Days 1 to 3), alcohol, natural/artificial flavors, fermented foods (including kombucha, sauerkraut, and coconut aminos), nutritional yeast, citric acid, monosodium glutamate (MSG), aspartame, other artificial sweeteners, formaldehyde, and preservatives. • If you enjoy animal products, stick to one serving per day of lean, organic, free-range, or wild meat, fowl, or fish (salmon, trout, or sardines), eaten only at dinner for these first three days. • Focus on bringing in more fruits, vegetables, and leafy greens every day. Cook vegetables only by steaming or adding them to the soups and stews in the cleanse recipes in Chapter 23. Avoid baked and roasted foods for all nine days. • See the text to follow and Chapter 21 for substitutions and adaptations if any of the foods in the chart don't work for you. You'll find, for example, substitutions for dates and apples. • Eat the portions that are right for you. Scale back if you're overly full. • Stay hydrated by drinking about 1 liter (roughly 32 ounces, or 4 cups) of water during the day, in between your morning and evening lemon or lime water.		

THE 3: ORIGINAL

Understanding the "why" of all this is vital. To begin with, it's important to see the first three days of this cleanse like the countdown to taking the training wheels off a bike. It's not meant to be a drastic push—that wouldn't benefit you. Rather, it's the beginning of a cycle. Without this adjustment period, the full cycle of the cleanse can't be as effective or successful.

Bypassing The 3 is like showing up for a driver's test without being taught to start the ignition. It's a mistake that many of the man-made trial-and-error cleanses out there make, putting our organs in the hot seat and forcing them to perform under pressure with no preparation phase. Our organs can't operate with confidence in a situation like that. When it comes time to get going, it will be with hesitance, knowing that as sternly as the examiner instructs, "Begin"—as much as we may try to get our body to push the gas pedal and start cleansing—this whole enterprise isn't going anywhere because we didn't hand our body the keys.

In order to get past checking the mirrors and put ourselves onto the road of healing, the beginning of a cleanse especially needs to be kind to the body so it can usher out poisons and pathogens later on in the cleanse. We can't give our liver too much to handle right away or put it in a position where it's forced to give our brain and heart too much to handle. We need to offer it proper time and guidance, and that's the purpose of these first three days.

Upon Waking

- You'll start each of the three days simply: with **16 ounces of your choice of lemon or lime water.** (See Chapter 23 for the recipe with the proper ratio of lemon or lime to water. This isn't about squeezing 10 lemons into a glass of water.) If you prefer, go up to 32 ounces of lemon or lime water.

Tip

- If you'd like, you can add an optional teaspoon of raw honey to your lemon or lime water.

Morning

- Once you've finished your lemon or lime water, *wait at least 15 to 20 minutes, and ideally 30 minutes,* and then enjoy at least **16 ounces of celery juice** (recipe on page 276, or get it fresh from your local juice bar).

- After you finish your celery juice, *wait another 15 to 30 minutes,* and then enjoy the **breakfast of your choice,** within the guidelines in the table above and explained in more detail later in this chapter. Celery juice is a medicinal, not a caloric, drink, so do make sure to eat breakfast. That breakfast could be a fruit smoothie or some oatmeal. Find more inspiration in the recipes in Chapter 23 and the Original sample menus in Chapter 22.

- If you get hungry later on, go ahead and have a **mid-morning snack of your choice** that's free from radical fats and doesn't include any of the troublemaker foods listed in this chapter. Again, the recipes section will offer ideas. An apple is the easiest option.

- On **Day 2** and **Day 3,** make sure you snack on **one to two apples** at some point in the morning. You can eat the apples whole, cut them into slices, chop them up with other fruit, blend them into a smoothie, or even enjoy them as applesauce (raw or cooked). If apples don't work for you at all, have ripe pears. As a last resort, it's okay to drink freshly juiced apple juice instead. Apples can vary greatly in size, so you make the call about what amount feels right for you.

Tip

- An additional option is to enjoy the Heavy Metal Detox Smoothie as your breakfast in the morning—as long as you're not having the Heavy Metal Detox Smoothie to *replace* the morning apple(s) on Day 2 and Day 3. For more on incorporating heavy metal detox into your 3:6:9 Cleanse, see Chapter 21, "Cleanse Adaptations and Substitutions."

Lunchtime

- When you're ready for lunch, enjoy **the meal of your choice**, as long as it's free from radical fats and doesn't include any of the troublemaker foods listed in this chapter. Look to the recipes in Chapter 23 and Original 3:6:9 Cleanse Sample Menus in Chapter 22 if you need inspiration.

- Either as a side dish to your meal or incorporated into it, make sure you also eat at least **1 cup of steamed zucchini or summer squash** as part of your lunch.

Mid-Afternoon

- When you get hungry about one to two hours after lunch, snack on **one to two apples** (or equivalent servings of applesauce or ripe pears) with **one to two dates**.

Tips

- In Chapter 23, you'll find fun recipes for apples and dates.

- If the outlined snacks leave you hungry, snack on more apples.

- If you opt for store-bought applesauce, make sure it's free from additives.

- If you don't like dates or don't have access to them, good substitutes are a handful of mulberries (dried or fresh), raisins, grapes, or figs (dried or fresh), in that order. It's okay to chop or blend them up with the apples.

Dinnertime

- When you're ready to eat dinner, enjoy the **meal of your choice**, as long as it doesn't include the troublemaker foods from this chapter.

Tip

- This meal is your opportunity to eat an *optional* serving of lean animal protein (as long as it's not in the "avoid" foods list) or another form of radical fat such avocado, nuts, or seeds. You're not at all required to do so. If you want to take the cleanse to the next level, instead skip these dinnertime radical fats during The 3 to make it a fat-free cleanse.

Evening

- If you're hungry after dinner, turn to an **optional apple** (or applesauce or pear).

- An hour before you go to bed, get in another **16 ounces of lemon or lime water.**

- Also enjoy a pre-bedtime mug of **hibiscus, lemon balm, or chaga tea.**

Select one rather than blending them. It's okay to drink your tea at the same time as the lemon or lime water.

Tip

- It's also okay to add a teaspoon of raw honey to your nighttime lemon or lime water or tea.

THE 6: ORIGINAL

	DAY 4	DAY 5	DAY 6
UPON WAKING	16 ounces lemon or lime water	16 ounces lemon or lime water	16 ounces lemon or lime water
MORNING	Wait 15 to 30 minutes, then: 16 ounces celery juice Wait another 15 to 30 minutes, then: Liver Rescue Smoothie	Wait 15 to 30 minutes, then: 16 ounces celery juice Wait another 15 to 30 minutes, then: Liver Rescue Smoothie	Wait 15 to 30 minutes, then: 16 ounces celery juice Wait another 15 to 30 minutes, then: Liver Rescue Smoothie
LUNCHTIME	Steamed asparagus with Liver Rescue Salad	Steamed asparagus with Liver Rescue Salad	Steamed asparagus and brussels sprouts with Liver Rescue Salad
MID-AFTERNOON	At least one to two apples (or applesauce) with one to three dates (or substitutions) plus celery sticks	At least one to two apples (or applesauce) with one to three dates (or substitutions) plus celery sticks	At least one to two apples (or applesauce) with one to three dates (or substitutions) plus celery sticks
DINNERTIME	Steamed asparagus with Liver Rescue Salad	Steamed brussels sprouts with Liver Rescue Salad	Steamed asparagus and brussels sprouts with Liver Rescue Salad

	DAY 4	DAY 5	DAY 6
EVENING	Apple (or applesauce) (if desired) 16 ounces lemon or lime water Hibiscus, lemon balm, or chaga tea	Apple (or applesauce) (if desired) 16 ounces lemon or lime water Hibiscus, lemon balm, or chaga tea	Apple (or applesauce) (if desired) 16 ounces lemon or lime water Hibiscus, lemon balm, or chaga tea
GUIDELINES	<ul><li>Avoid radical fats (nuts, seeds, oils, olives, coconut, avocado, cacao, bone broth, animal proteins, etc.) entirely. Skip beans too.</li><li>Avoid these foods: eggs, dairy, gluten, soft drinks, salt and seasonings, pork, corn, oils (including both industrial and healthier oils), soy, lamb, tuna and all other fish and seafood, vinegar (including ACV), caffeine (including coffee, matcha, and chocolate), grains (including millet and oats now), alcohol, natural/artificial flavors, fermented foods (including kombucha, sauerkraut, and coconut aminos), nutritional yeast, citric acid, monosodium glutamate (MSG), aspartame, other artificial sweeteners, formaldehyde, and preservatives.</li><li>Instead, stick to the foods outlined in this chapter and the chart above. Cook vegetables only by steaming them. Avoid baked and roasted foods for all nine days.</li><li>See the text to follow and Chapter 21 for substitutions and adaptations if any of the foods in the chart don't work for you. You'll find, for example, substitutions for salads, asparagus, brussels sprouts, and smoothie ingredients.</li><li>Eat the portions that are right for you. Scale back if you're overly full.</li><li>Stay hydrated by drinking about 1 liter (roughly 32 ounces, or 4 cups) of water during the day, in between your morning and evening lemon or lime water.</li></ul>		

THE 6: ORIGINAL

During the middle three days of the cleanse, your liver gets a long-awaited breather from the need to produce large quantities of bile. Constant bile production mode is the state most everyone lives in due to diets high in fat—and the body's need to break down that fat. This normal rate of bile production tires out the liver, making it less likely to perform its daily cleansing duties. When the liver finally gets a break from producing volumes of bile, it can work on dislodging toxins that it's stored away in deep pockets over your lifetime. A liver that's capable of detoxifying poisons and restoring itself benefits your health on all levels; it becomes a backbone for recovering from chronic illness and other symptoms that won't go away—symptoms that could eventually develop into chronic illnesses if we don't care for our bodies with steps such as the 3:6:9 Cleanse.

Upon Waking

- Again, you'll start each of the three days with 16 ounces of your choice of lemon or lime water. If you prefer, go up to 32 ounces.

Tip

- If you'd like, you can add an optional teaspoon of raw honey to your lemon or lime water.

Morning

- Once you've finished your lemon or lime water, wait at least 15 to 20 minutes, and ideally 30 minutes, and then enjoy at least 16 ounces of celery juice.

- After you finish your celery juice, *wait another 15 to 30 minutes*, and then enjoy the **Liver Rescue Smoothie** (recipe on page 298). Make one serving or more, depending on how hungry you are, and have it whenever you'd like throughout the rest of the morning. Alternatively, enjoy the fruits from the smoothie recipe cut up together in a fruit bowl.

Tip

- An additional option is to enjoy the Heavy Metal Detox Smoothie later in the morning if you wish to follow the modification from Chapter 21—as long as you're not having the Heavy Metal Detox Smoothie to *replace* that first Liver Rescue Smoothie of the day.

If you'd like, make smaller servings of each so you have room for both.

Lunchtime

- On **Day 4** and **Day 5**, enjoy **steamed asparagus** with a **Liver Rescue Salad** for lunch.

- On **Day 6**, opt for **steamed asparagus** *and* **brussels sprouts** with a **Liver Rescue Salad** for lunch.

Tips

- You're welcome to eat the asparagus and/or brussels sprouts raw if you prefer—as in, for example, the Shaved Brussels Sprout, Asparagus, Radish, and Apple Salad or the Brussel Sprout Slaw recipes.

- Eat the vegetables either raw or steamed. Make sure that you don't roast them or prepare them with oil, cream, butter, vinegar, or salt during the Original Cleanse.

- If fresh asparagus and/or brussels sprouts aren't available, buy them frozen. If neither fresh nor frozen asparagus and/or brussels sprouts are available, substitute zucchini or summer squash.

- Either steam the vegetables just before your meal or prepare them ahead of time and enjoy them cold on top of your salad. You can also mash or blend the vegetables. See "Asparagus and Brussels Sprouts" on page 255 for more options.

- If raw salad doesn't work for you, whether because of the time it takes to eat or because of chewing or digestion difficulties, substitute the Liver Rescue Soup recipe for the Liver Rescue Salad. If even the soup feels like too much, substitute the Liver Rescue Juice recipe. Find further guidance under "Salads" in Chapter 21, "Cleanse Adaptations and Substitutions."

Mid-Afternoon

- When you get hungry after lunch, snack on at least one to two apples (or equivalent servings of applesauce or ripe pears) with one to three dates (or substitutions), this time adding celery sticks to go with them.

Tips

- Give yourself a hand by setting aside the afternoon celery sticks when you're prepping celery juice in the morning.
- If chewing celery is difficult for you, chop it up finely in the food processor or blend it with the apples.
- If that's not enough to fill you up and keep you going, you can eat additional apples during the afternoon.

Dinnertime

- For dinner on **Day 4**, enjoy **steamed asparagus** with a **Liver Rescue Salad** again.

- Dinner on **Day 5** is **steamed brussels sprouts** with a **Liver Rescue Salad**.
- And on **Day 6**, enjoy *both* **steamed asparagus** *and* **steamed brussels sprouts** with a **Liver Rescue Salad**.

Tip

- The same options apply as listed in the bullet points under "Lunchtime"—for example, it's okay to blend or mash your asparagus and/or brussels sprouts, eat them raw, substitute with zucchini or summer squash, or replace the Liver Rescue Salad with Liver Rescue Soup or Liver Rescue Juice from the recipes chapter. Read more in Chapter 21, "Cleanse Adaptations and Substitutions."

Evening

- If you're hungry after dinner, turn to an **optional apple** (or applesauce or pear).
- An hour before you go to bed, get in another **16 ounces of lemon or lime water**.
- Also enjoy a pre-bedtime mug of **hibiscus, lemon balm, or chaga tea**. Select one rather than blending them. It's okay to drink your tea at the same time as the lemon or lime water.

Tip

- It's also okay to add a teaspoon of raw honey to your nighttime lemon or lime water or tea.

THE 9: ORIGINAL

	DAY 7	DAY 8	DAY 9
UPON WAKING	16 ounces lemon or lime water	16 ounces lemon or lime water	16 ounces lemon or lime water
MORNING	Wait 15 to 30 minutes, then: 16 ounces celery juice Wait another 15 to 30 minutes, then: Liver Rescue Smoothie	Wait 15 to 30 minutes, then: 16 ounces celery juice Wait another 15 to 30 minutes, then: Liver Rescue Smoothie	Over the course of the day, consume: Two 16- to 20-ounce celery juices (one morning, one early evening; enjoy them 15 to 30 minutes apart from these other drinks) Two 16- to 20-ounce cucumber-apple juices (anytime) Blended melon, fresh watermelon juice, blended papaya, blended ripe pear, or fresh-squeezed orange juice (as many servings and as often as desired, as long as you consume them separately from each other) Water (as desired)
LUNCHTIME	Spinach Soup over cucumber noodles	Spinach Soup over cucumber noodles	
MID-AFTERNOON	Wait at least 60 minutes, then: 16 ounces celery juice Wait at least 15 to 30 minutes, then: One to two apples (or applesauce) plus cucumber slices and celery sticks	Wait at least 60 minutes, then: 16 ounces celery juice Wait at least 15 to 30 minutes, then: One to two apples (or applesauce) plus cucumber slices and celery sticks	
DINNERTIME	Steamed squash, sweet potatoes, yams, or potatoes with steamed asparagus and/or brussels sprouts plus optional Liver Rescue Salad	Steamed asparagus and/or brussels sprouts plus optional Liver Rescue Salad	
EVENING	Apple (or applesauce) (if desired) 16 ounces lemon or lime water Hibiscus, lemon balm, or chaga tea	Apple (or applesauce) (if desired) 16 ounces lemon or lime water Hibiscus, lemon balm, or chaga tea	16 ounces lemon or lime water Hibiscus, lemon balm, or chaga tea

	DAY 7	DAY 8	DAY 9
GUIDELINES	<ul><li>Continue to avoid radical fats (nuts, seeds, oils, olives, coconut, avocado, cacao, bone broth, animal proteins, etc.) entirely. Skip beans too.</li><li>Continue to avoid these foods: eggs, dairy, gluten, soft drinks, salt and seasonings, pork, corn, oils (including both industrial and healthier oils), soy, lamb, tuna and all other fish and seafood, vinegar (including ACV), caffeine (including coffee, matcha, and chocolate), grains (including millet and oats now), alcohol, natural/artificial flavors, fermented foods (including kombucha, sauerkraut, and coconut aminos), nutritional yeast, citric acid, monosodium glutamate (MSG), aspartame, other artificial sweeteners, formaldehyde, and preservatives.</li><li>Instead, stick to the foods outlined in this chapter and the chart above. Cook vegetables only by steaming them. Avoid baked and roasted foods for all nine days.</li><li>See the text to follow and Chapter 21 for substitutions and adaptations if any of the foods in the chart don't work for you.</li><li>Eat the portions that are right for you. Scale back if you're overly full.</li><li>Stay hydrated by drinking about 1 liter (roughly 32 ounces, or 4 cups) of water during the day, in between your morning and evening lemon or lime water. If the extra celery juice in the afternoon means you'd like to scale back on water a bit, that's fine.</li></ul>		

THE 9: ORIGINAL

Here we are: the moment your liver has been waiting for basically its whole life. That means it's the moment you've been waiting for too, because what makes your liver happy makes you happy. When your liver and other organs unburden themselves at this stage, you'll be amazed at the positive influence it can have on both your body and your mood. The ripple effect from here on out—the people who see the change in you, the further changes you're inspired to make in your life—will be profound and far reaching. Who knows whose lives you're going to touch with your improved health? Who knows what you'll get to do now?

Over the past six days, you've been warming up your liver's engine and building your body's reserves, getting them ready so that here in The 9, they'll have the power to drive out junk, garbage, and poison that your organs have been holding on to for years. This goes far beyond the Morning Cleanse's ability to process out daily waste. These liquid-heavy three days are completely new territory.

DAYS 7 AND 8

Upon Waking

- As usual, you'll start each day with **16 ounces of your choice of lemon or lime water.** If you prefer, go up to 32 ounces.

Tip

- If you'd like, you can add an optional teaspoon of raw honey to your lemon or lime water.

Morning

- Once you've finished your lemon or lime water, *wait at least 15 to 20 minutes, and ideally 30 minutes,* and then enjoy at least **16 ounces of celery juice.**

- After you finish your celery juice, *wait another 15 to 30 minutes,* and then enjoy the **Liver Rescue Smoothie.** Make one serving or more, depending on how hungry you are, and have it whenever you'd like throughout the rest of the morning. Alternatively, enjoy the fruits from the smoothie recipe cut up together in a fruit bowl.

Tip

- As before, another option is to enjoy the Heavy Metal Detox Smoothie later in the morning if you wish to follow the modification from Chapter 21—as long as you're not having the Heavy Metal Detox Smoothie

to replace that first Liver Rescue Smoothie of the day. Make smaller servings of each if you'd like.

Lunchtime

- Enjoy **Spinach Soup over cucumber noodles** for lunch (recipe on page 344). It's okay to blend the cucumber into the soup if you prefer.

Tips

- Make sure to enjoy the Spinach Soup raw rather than warming it up.

- It's okay to substitute mango or banana for the tomato in the Spinach Soup (just as long as you're not blending banana *with* tomato). You can also substitute butter leaf lettuce for the spinach. See more in Chapter 21, "Cleanse Adaptations and Substitutions."

Mid-Afternoon

- Enjoy another **16 ounces of celery juice** between lunch and dinner. Make sure to *wait at least 60 minutes after lunch* to drink it. After finishing your celery juice, *wait at least 15 to 30 minutes* to eat or drink anything else.

- Once you've had your celery juice and completed the short waiting period, snack on **one to two apples** or equivalent servings of applesauce (or pears) with **cucumber slices** and **celery sticks.**

Tip

- Feel free to make all your celery juice at once in the morning, setting aside this second serving in the fridge, if you don't have the time or inclination to fire up the juicer twice in one day. You can also get your celery juice fresh from a juice bar, ordering both servings at once and saving the second one for later.

Dinnertime

- For dinner on **Day 7**, enjoy **steamed winter squash, sweet potatoes (Japanese sweet potatoes are okay), yams, or potatoes** accompanied by **steamed asparagus and/or brussels sprouts** and an *optional* Liver Rescue Salad.

- For dinner on **Day 8**, enjoy your choice of **steamed asparagus and/ or brussels sprouts**, preferably both, with an *optional* Liver Rescue Salad.

Tip

- The same options apply as listed for lunch and dinner in The 6—for example, it's okay to blend or mash your asparagus and/or brussels sprouts, eat them raw, substitute with zucchini or summer squash, or replace the Liver Rescue Salad with Liver Rescue Soup or Liver Rescue Juice. It's also okay to blend or mash your steamed squash, sweet potatoes, yams, or potatoes; you can even blend them up with your asparagus, brussels

sprouts, and greens from your salad. Read more in Chapter 21, "Cleanse Adaptations and Substitutions."

Evening

- If you're hungry after dinner, turn to an **optional apple** (or applesauce or pear).

- An hour before you go to bed, get in another **16 ounces of lemon or lime water.**

- Also enjoy a pre-bedtime mug of **hibiscus, lemon balm, or chaga tea.** Again, select one rather than blending them, and feel free to drink your tea at the same time as the lemon or lime water.

Tip

- It's also okay to add a teaspoon of raw honey to your nighttime lemon or lime water or tea.

DAY 9

Upon Waking

- Start your day with 16 ounces of your choice of lemon or lime water. If you prefer, go up to 32 ounces.

Tips

- If you'd like, you can add an optional teaspoon of raw honey to your lemon or lime water.

Morning and Afternoon

- Once you've finished your lemon or lime water, *wait at least 15 to 20 minutes, and ideally 30 minutes*, and then enjoy at least **16 to 20 ounces of celery juice**.

- After you finish your celery juice, *wait another 15 to 30 minutes*, and then, over the course of the day, nourish yourself with **two 16- to 20-ounce cucumber-apple juices** at any time (aim for a 50-50 blend of cucumber and apple) and as much **blended melon, fresh watermelon juice, blended papaya, blended ripe pear,** or **fresh-squeezed orange juice** as you'd like whenever you get hungry (as long as you enjoy them separately from each other).

- Drink **water** throughout the day as desired. Ideally, add a squeeze of lemon or lime to your drinking water throughout the day. If plain water is all you can handle, that's fine. For more on water during the cleanse, see the general Original Cleanse guidelines following this section.

Tips

- If you've been following the Heavy Metal Detox modification, don't worry about the fact that you'll be skipping the Heavy Metal Detox Smoothie today. Day 9 is better focused on general flushing of toxins, plus you'll have enough remnants of spirulina, cilantro, barley grass juice powder, dulse, and wild blueberries left in your system to help remove any heavy metals that have been dislodged. Read more under "Heavy Metal Detox Modification" in Chapter 21, "Cleanse Adaptations and Substitutions."

- For more on cucumber-apple juice ratios and alternatives, see Chapter 21, "Cleanse Adaptations and Substitutions."

- When it comes to the blended melon, fresh watermelon juice, blended papaya, blended ripe pear, and fresh-squeezed orange juice, it's okay to change it up throughout the day—for example, you could drink blended melon in the morning, fresh-squeezed orange juice at midday, and blended papaya in the afternoon and at dinnertime. Or pick one and make that your staple throughout the day. It's your choice, as long as you don't blend them together or drink them together—for example, don't drink a melon-pear blend or drink blended papaya immediately followed by orange juice. Enjoy each separately and on its own.

- Melon digests best without other food in the stomach, so consider drinking any blended melon earlier in the day than blended papaya or blended pear. Try to avoid blended melon if you've already had blended papaya or blended pear during the day.

- Feel more than free to make or purchase all the fresh juice at a juice bar in the morning and save your later servings in the fridge.

- If you're very petite and can't get this much liquid in you, you can lower the serving sizes of the juices, as long as you don't underdo it. You want to make sure you get enough of those precious nutrients to support your body as it does its hard work of elimination.

Early Evening

- Drink at least **16 ounces of celery juice** in the early evening. Enjoy it *at least 30 minutes after* any blended fruit drinks and *at least 15 to 30 minutes* after any fresh juices or water.

- After finishing your celery juice, *wait at least another 15 to 30 minutes*. Following that waiting period, you're welcome to keep sipping your cucumber-apple juice, blended melon, fresh watermelon juice, blended papaya, blended ripe pear, fresh orange juice, or water as desired.

Evening

- An hour before bed, get in another **16 ounces of lemon or lime water.**

- Also enjoy a pre-bedtime mug of **hibiscus, lemon balm, or chaga tea** as usual. Again, select one rather than blending them, and feel free to drink your tea with your lemon or lime water.

Tip

- It's okay to add a teaspoon of raw honey to your nighttime lemon or lime water or tea.

ORIGINAL 3:6:9 CLEANSE GUIDELINES

General Guidelines

Follow these guidelines on all nine days of the cleanse.

Avoid Troublemaker Foods

Cut out the troublemaker foods from Chapter 7, "Troublemaker Foods." These are foods you'll want to leave out altogether for the entire nine days, unless noted otherwise:

- Eggs
- Dairy
- Gluten
- Soft drinks
- Salt and seasonings (pure spices are okay)
- Pork
- Corn
- Oils (including both industrial and healthier oils)
- Soy
- Lamb
- Tuna and other fish and seafood (salmon, trout, and sardines are okay for dinner on Days 1 through 3)
- Vinegar (including ACV)
- Caffeine (including coffee, matcha, and chocolate)

- Grains (millet and oats are okay Days 1 through 3)

- Alcohol

- Natural and artificial flavors

- Fermented foods (including kombucha, sauerkraut, and coconut aminos)

- Nutritional yeast

- Citric acid

- Monosodium glutamate (MSG)

- Aspartame and other artificial sweeteners

- Formaldehyde

- Preservatives

If you skipped Chapter 7, go back and check it out to understand the "why" behind avoiding these ingredients while you're on the cleanse. Keep that guide nearby for strength in the face of temptation. As delicious as it may be to sneak a slice of pepperoni pizza, that chapter will offer reassurance that you're doing the right thing by taking a break from certain foods while on the 3:6:9.

None of the troublemaker foods are on this list because it's trendy to take them out of the diet. Gluten, for example, isn't avoided because of today's conventional wisdom that gluten causes inflammation. It's for a much more specific reason that's important to understand. Even if you have already read that chapter, you may want to go back and give yourself a refresher while you're going through the cleanse. For further cravings support, turn to Chapter 25, "The Emotional Side of Cleansing."

Cutting out these foods is easier than it may sound—because you'll be so focused on fruits, vegetables, and leafy greens each day. Filling up on these nutrient-rich foods won't leave room for other tempting foods, and that will help curb cravings.

Steam (Don't Roast) Your Vegetables

Avoid baked and roasted foods for all nine days. While on the Original 3:6:9 Cleanse, cook vegetables only by steaming or adding them to soups and stews such as the recipes in Chapter 23. Baking and roasting tend to evaporate more of a food's water content, and while on the Original, it's important that foods retain a certain level of moisture, as it helps with the cleansing process. Baking and roasting are not bad by any means. Skipping them here simply improves the body's internal hydration mechanisms and ability to cleanse more toxins even faster.

Eat the Quantities That Are Right for You

Everyone is different, with unique calorie needs and appetite levels. Eat the portions that are right for you. Scale back if you're overly full. At the same time, the instinct on a cleanse is often to hold back on food. Don't let yourself get ravenous. Starving yourself will only work against the healing this cleanse is trying to accomplish.

In The 3, you increase your glucose intake in order to perk up your liver's and brain's functioning. In The 6, your organs need the foods from the chart and outline as diggers and cleaners so they can be ready for their time to shine: The 9. Stock up so you have an abundance of fresh, healing foods at your fingertips.

If the volume of food included in this cleanse feels like too much—for example, if two apples at a time feels uncomfortable—don't stuff yourself. At no point in this cleanse should you force food down the hatch if you're already full. For more on how to know how much to eat of what, see "Hunger and Portions" in Chapter 19, "Critical Cleanse Dos and Don'ts."

Stay Hydrated

Remember to keep yourself hydrated. **Each day, drink about 1 liter of water during the day in between your morning and evening lemon or lime water.** That's roughly equivalent to 32 ounces, or 4 cups. You're welcome to do more. If you feel you require more fluids at any point throughout the cleanse, don't hold back; allow yourself to improve your water levels.

Do avoid water with a pH above 8.0. This includes if you use an alkalized water machine—keep it set at a pH of 8.0 or below. Ideally, set it at 7.7; that's the best pH for drinking water. Water content with higher pH levels sits in the stomach until the digestive system can lower it to 7.7 to be released throughout the body. The same goes for water with a pH below 7.7—your body has to put energy into raising its pH. Drinking water at the ideal pH level prevents your digestive system from weakening.

On Days 1 through 8, you're welcome to sip Hot Spiced Apple Juice at any temperature (recipe on page 290) or coconut water (as long as it isn't pink or red and doesn't list "natural flavors" in the ingredients) throughout the day. That would be *in addition* to the liter of water.

With all of these beverages, do be mindful to space them out at least 15 to 30 minutes from your celery juice. If it's a day where you're drinking extra celery juice (for example, Day 7 or 8) and you'd like to scale back a bit on water, that's fine.

Additional Guidelines for Days 1, 2, and 3

As you go through Days 1 through 3, here are a couple more basic guidelines to follow:

Reduce Dietary Fat

Lower your dietary fat by at least half, and avoid radical fats altogether until dinnertime. Radical fats include nuts, seeds, avocados, oil, olives, coconut, bone broth, and all animal proteins. (Dairy products such as yogurt, milk, cream, butter, cheese, kefir, and whey protein are also radical fats. You're already cutting these out, because you're steering clear of all dairy during this cleanse.) Whatever amount of radical fat you eat on a typical day, cut it back by at least 50 percent.

By waiting until dinner to eat radical fats, you may be taking care of this already. Skipping your usual morning radical fats such as yogurt, nutty granola, avocado toast, buttered toast, bagels with cream cheese, smoothie with coconut milk or whey protein powder, bone broth, bacon, eggs, sausage, pancakes, waffles, chocolate, cacao nibs, or creamy coffee drinks already reduces your fat intake by a lot. Then you take it a step further by holding off on radical fats through lunchtime and midafternoon. That means you're avoiding foods that fall into both the healthier category and the less-healthy category, whether oil-based or creamy salad dressings; smoothies with nut butters; guacamole; hummus made with tahini or oil; vegetarian meat replacements such as hot dogs, sausages, and burgers; baked potatoes with avocado, oil, butter, sour cream, or cheese; BLTs; cheeseburgers; hamburgers; oil-based French fries; hard-boiled or other forms of eggs; salads with chicken, fish, or steak;

tuna fish sandwiches; crab cakes; peanut butter crackers; handfuls of nuts; or so many other common lunches or snacks that incorporate radical fats. This in turn means you're giving your body a break from all the work it takes to process the radical fats they contain.

If cutting out radical fats in the morning and afternoon alone doesn't bring your fats down by 50 percent for the day, then think about halving some of your normal dinnertime portions of radical fats and increasing your helpings of vegetables and leafy greens to compensate. If you're used to adding olives to dinnertime salads, for example, throw in half as many and add some chopped tomatoes and cucumbers instead. If you enjoy grilled salmon for dinner, serve yourself less than usual and heap your plate with leafy greens or steamed asparagus. Also be mindful of dressings, sauces, and dips, as they are often much higher in fat than we realize and often contain oil and other ingredients that you're avoiding on this cleanse. For satisfying dishes and snacks that aren't high in dietary fat, turn to Chapter 23, "Cleanse Recipes."

If you enjoy animal products, stick to one serving, eaten only at dinner. Make sure it's a serving of lean, organic, free-range, or wild meat, fowl, or fish (salmon, trout, or sardines) so that it has the best chance of supporting your health during these transition days.

One major reason to cut down on fats during The 3 is to give your liver a breather from relentless bile production so it can restore bile reserves. Freed up from processing so many fats, it can put its energy into getting you ready to detox.

Another reason is so you can get the glucose you need. Eating less fat allows your liver to absorb glucose better, and building up your glucose and glycogen reserves is vital for the liver's hard work to come of propelling poisons out of itself during The 9. As in the Morning Cleanse, potatoes, sweet potatoes (including Japanese sweet potatoes), yams, and winter squash are great, glucose-rich foods to eat during The 3 to build up fuel in your liver.

Eat More Fruits, Vegetables, and Leafy Greens

Focus on bringing in more fruits, vegetables, and leafy greens every day. By incorporating more of these healing foods into your snacks and meals in The 3, you're less apt to stay in old patterns and grab your normal, go-to items from the troublemaker foods list. The minerals, vitamins, and trace mineral salts in leafy greens and vegetables working together with the antioxidants and glucose in fruit are critical for stabilizing organs and replenishing cells. Another important aspect here is that fruits, vegetables, and leafy greens are foods that don't feed pathogens—and everyone is dealing with pathogens inside their bodies creating their symptoms.

Skip beans entirely during the 3:6:9 Cleanse. Beans are not a powerful cleansing food. While they are not a radical fat or a troublemaker food, their fat content is on the higher side compared to fruits, vegetables, and leafy greens. Staying off them will also ensure that the cleanse is as easy as possible on your digestive tract. It takes a stronger hydrochloric acid level to break down the proteins in beans, and most people are living with lower levels of hydrochloric acid, making beans harder to digest. Their stomach glands are tired, heavily worn, and in need of repair—repair that the celery juice in these cleanses helps to offer.

Additional Guidelines for Days 4, 5, 6, 7, and 8

As you go through the middle of the cleanse, here's what to remember on top of the general guidelines:

Avoid All Radical Fats

To support your healing, cut out radical fats entirely starting on Day 4. This means you're avoiding nuts, seeds, nut butters (such as peanut butter), nut milk, oil, olives, coconut, cacao, avocado, and animal products (including bone broth and dairy) entirely. At this point, if you consumed those fats, it would break the cleanse. It would be as if you were scrubbing dishes and someone dumped grease into your sink—requiring you to start over in order to truly get the plates clean.

For your liver to navigate The 6 (and The 9) successfully, it needs to be free from the interruption of being forced to backtrack and process radical fats. Your liver will still produce bile to keep your body functioning during this time; it just won't need to produce the same strength of bile for dissolving radical fats. By avoiding them, you allow your liver to use its energy to cleanse on a level it can't otherwise. Remember: it's very difficult for the liver to cleanse on a deep level while on a diet that's high in fat. This break from fats, combined with the bioavailable nutrient density of the foods you *are* eating, gives your body a profound opportunity to devote its energy to healing.

Reducing fats is also about the viscosity of your blood. If you have too much fat free-floating in your bloodstream, you slow down your body's ability to flush poisons and toxins—because the fat absorbs and holds on to toxins there, leading to pockets of toxic fat inside and around your body's organs. The goal during cleansing is to disperse deposits of fat (what people call fat cells)—to open them up so they can release the poisons, toxins, and old, stored adrenaline they contain to be sent out of your body. Continuing to eat radical fats during this period, which translates to having a high blood fat ratio inside your bloodstream, defeats the purpose of dispersing existing pockets of toxic fat.

By the way, if avocado is one of your favorites, enjoy it with dinner on the first three days of the cleanse. From Day 4 onward, you'll want to avoid it—because although avocado is indeed a fruit and is easier to digest than other radical fats, when you're cleansing the liver, even good, healthy, unique fats get in the way. You'll want to put avocado aside for now to keep from overburdening your liver and causing it to struggle when it's trying to cleanse.

And again, you'll continue to skip beans for all nine days of the cleanse. While beans are not a radical fat, their fat content is on the higher side compared to the cleanse foods, and they do give the digestive system extra work.

Devote Yourself to Fruits and Vegetables

Stick to fruits, vegetables, leafy greens, and herbs—specifically, the foods mentioned in this chapter and in the modifications and recipes it references. Also continue to avoid the troublemaker foods on pages 123 to 124—several of which are radical fats, so you'd be avoiding them anyway.

What does it mean to stick to the foods outlined for each meal? It means don't try to outsmart the cleanse. The specific foods are there for a reason: to help you heal. Trying to add other types of fruits to the smoothie, replace a salad with a smoothie or a smoothie with a salad, skip salad altogether, steam other veggies with the asparagus or brussels sprouts, snack on bananas in the evening, or sneak nutritional yeast or coconut aminos into your meal will too often mean that you miss out on what you really need for the cleanse to operate the way it should. If the steamed vegetable meals don't excite you, the sample menus in Chapter 22 will show you how to add some interest to your cleanse. Or if you have a specific problem with one of the cleanse foods, turn to Chapter 21, "Cleanse Adaptations and Substitutions." For example, if you have trouble eating salad, go ahead and blend it up into the Liver Rescue Soup, or make Liver Rescue Juice.

It may sound daunting to eat only fruits and vegetables. That's because we're used to such small servings of them. If one Liver Rescue Smoothie in the morning isn't enough, make another—or make a Heavy Metal Detox Smoothie. (See Chapter 21 for more on this modification.)

If salad doesn't seem like enough to satisfy you, that's probably because you're used to eating little side salads with limp greens and pale tomatoes. During the cleanse, make your salads robust by adding ample orange segments, ripe tomatoes, cucumbers, fresh greens, and other ingredients from the recipe on page 342. And remember to leave room,

because you're eating your Liver Rescue Salad along with steamed brussels sprouts and asparagus, which can be more filling than you'd expect.

If two apples don't satisfy you in the afternoon, eat another apple. If that's not enough, eat yet another apple. You don't need to worry about eating too many apples—unless your body tells you you're full. When that's the case, respect its limits.

Nourish your body with the specific foods (or their substitutes) that the cleanse mentions, and it will have untold benefits. Avoiding foods that take a little more work to digest is well worth the effort it takes to pass on them during this part of the cleanse. The nutrient density of the healing fuel you'll be eating instead is exactly what your body needs at this point.

Additional Guidelines for Day 9

Day 9: a day of liquids to send on their way any remaining poisons that the liver unearthed during The 6.

One important distinction that makes this day of fluids different from juice fasts or cleanses you might have tried before is that the blend of the celery, cucumber, and apple that you're getting throughout Day 9 has the right balance of mineral salts, potassium, and natural sugar to stabilize your glucose levels as your body cleanses itself of toxins. On this final day, when your body's working so hard to make you better, it's as important as ever to safeguard your adrenals—and that's just what Day 9's special tonics do.

Stick with Liquid and Blended

Devote yourself to the Day 9 cleanse beverages as outlined. At this stage of the cleanse, when your body is releasing larger amounts of poisons, viral and bacterial waste, and other troublemakers, it needs lower quantities of food and higher quantities of liquid-based healing solutions. These specific options provide critical balance as you flush out toxins.

By sticking to these cleanse beverages, you're aligning two critical pieces of the healing puzzle: (1) you're keeping the day fat-free and (2) you're removing a large percentage of digestive load. Even healthy, whole foods require some level of digestion, especially bulkier and cooked foods. With these particular light, raw, liquid and blended options, you give your body a rest from the normal digestive process it endures. In turn, this allows your body to use its reserves to flush and cleanse harmful toxins and poisons from your organs into your bloodstream and out of your kidneys and bowels.

Some special circumstances mentioned in this book call for repeating Day 8 rather than following the Day 9 plan. Or other life circumstances, such as unexpected travel that means you have less control over your food than you'd like, may lead you to stop the cleanse before reaching Day 9. In either case—whether you end the cleanse by repeating Day 8, or you have to stop the cleanse before you've finished a full nine-day cycle—don't worry about missing the Day 9 protocol. Every day of the 3:6:9 Cleanse that you complete takes you to that next level—however much you've completed, you've done an incredible amount of cleansing and you've only received gains.

Give Yourself a Rest

If you can, take it easy today. Think about saving certain commitments for another time. Maybe you can schedule Day 9 as a sacred rest day, or a day with at least some rest in it. If possible, set aside some down time, maybe even time for a nap. At minimum, be mindful of all your body's doing for you during this period. Take a moment to pause and think about your liver and other organs. This is the end of your liver's great big plunge into the depths of purification, and it's doing beautifully. You're succeeding in the healing process: rejuvenating yourself emotionally, physically, and spiritually by removing toxins and poisons and reducing pathogens and their waste. When you start freeing yourself of the burdens of symptoms and conditions, you head to a place of living your true potential as a healthy self and being.

REPEATING THE CLEANSE AND TRANSITIONING OUT

When you're ready to transition out of the 3:6:9 Cleanse, turn to Chapter 14 for special steps to make the adjustment easiest on your body.

As we'll cover in Chapter 13, "Repeating the 3:6:9 Cleanse," you may not be ready to transition out after only one cycle of the cleanse. If you're dealing with serious symptoms or illness, for example, or if you have a lot of weight to lose, you can take the cleanse longer term. You'll find detailed guidance on repeating the cleanse in that chapter. Whenever you decide to wrap up the cleanse, turn to Chapter 14 to help ease the transition.

CHAPTER 11

Simplified 3:6:9 Cleanse

The Simplified 3:6:9 Cleanse is helpful and powerful for both the beginner who's new to cleansing and the seasoned cleanser who wants a way to heal from chronic symptoms while balancing a demanding schedule.

Most people fall into patterns of reaching for the familiar and eating what has always offered comfort or convenience. Offering more flexibility and options than the Original, the Simplified reduces the emotional shock of changing course in order to heal from high cholesterol, high blood pressure, fatty liver, arterial plaque, lymphedema, arthritis, insomnia, varicose veins, dark under-eye circles, acid reflux, constipation, IBS, dry skin, type 2 diabetes, headaches, migraines, and so many other chronic health issues.

With fewer meal-to-meal changes and specifics, the Simplified is great to offer a family member or other dear one in your life who doesn't have the time or energy to focus on the details of the Original 3:6:9 Cleanse—that is, someone who prefers a more straightforward and at the same time versatile set of options. While the Simplified 3:6:9 Cleanse works at 70 percent of the Original, do not consider this the 3:6:9 for amateurs—far from it. This version still takes dedication and is extremely cleansing for anyone who wants to uproot toxins and pathogens. Not to mention that if you're more likely to start and stick with this than the Original, that's 70 percent more healing than you would have done. That could mean everything for your health and well-being.

KEY CLEANSE NOTES

Keep these important notes in mind as you dig into this chapter:

Recipes and Sample Menus

You'll find any recipes referenced here in Chapter 23. You'll also find sample menus outlining recipe options for every meal in Chapter 22.

Adaptations and Substitutions

If for any reason you can't eat or access any of the foods called for in the pages to come, or if solid foods are a problem for you, turn to Chapter 21 for a whole chapter's worth of modifications. There, you'll also find an option to incorporate the Heavy Metal Detox into this cleanse if you'd like.

——— THE 3: SIMPLIFIED ———

	DAY 1	DAY 2	DAY 3
UPON WAKING	16 ounces lemon or lime water		
MORNING	Wait 15 to 30 minutes, then: 16 ounces celery juice Wait another 15 to 30 minutes, then: Breakfast of your choice (within guidelines) and later, if desired: Apple (or applesauce)		
LUNCHTIME	Meal of your choice (within guidelines)		
MID-AFTERNOON	Optional: Apple (or applesauce) with one to four dates plus cucumber slices and celery sticks		
DINNERTIME	Meal of your choice (within guidelines)		
EVENING	Apple (or applesauce) (if desired) 16 ounces lemon or lime water Hibiscus, lemon balm, or chaga tea		

	DAY 1	DAY 2	DAY 3
GUIDELINES	• Avoid radical fats (nuts, seeds, oils, olives, coconut, avocado, cacao, bone broth, animal proteins, etc.) entirely. Skip beans too. • Avoid these foods: eggs, dairy, gluten, soft drinks, salt and seasonings, pork, corn, oils (including both industrial and healthier oils), soy, lamb, tuna and all other fish and seafood, vinegar (including ACV), caffeine (including coffee, matcha, and chocolate), grains (millet and oats are okay), alcohol, natural/artificial flavors, fermented foods (including kombucha, sauerkraut, and coconut aminos), nutritional yeast, citric acid, monosodium glutamate (MSG), aspartame, other artificial sweeteners, formaldehyde, and preservatives. • Instead, stick to fruits, vegetables, leafy greens, and (if desired) millet and oats. • For meal inspiration, check out the Simplified sample menus in Chapter 22. • See the text to follow and Chapter 21 for substitutions and adaptations if any of the foods in the chart don't work for you. You'll find, for example, substitutions for dates and apples. • For alternate amounts of celery juice if you're sensitive, see page 145. • Keep in mind that baking or roasting foods will slow down the detox. If you prefer lighter fare, steam your vegetables instead or cook them in the soup and stew recipes in Chapter 23. • Eat the portions that are right for you. Scale back if you're overly full. • Stay hydrated by drinking about 1 liter (roughly 32 ounces, or 4 cups) of water during the day, in between your morning and evening lemon or lime water.		

THE 3: SIMPLIFIED

As with the Original, understanding the "why" of all this is vital. To begin with, it's important to see the first three days of this cleanse like the countdown to taking the training wheels off a bike. It's not meant to be a drastic push—that wouldn't benefit you. Rather, it's the beginning of a cycle. Without this adjustment period, the full cycle of the cleanse can't be as effective or successful.

Bypassing The 3 is like showing up for a driver's test without being taught to start the ignition. It's a mistake that many of the man-made trial-and-error cleanses out there make, putting our organs in the hot seat and forcing them to perform under pressure with no preparation phase. Our organs can't operate with confidence in a situation like that. When it comes time to get going, it will be with hesitance, knowing that as sternly as the examiner instructs, "Begin"—as much as we may try to get our body to push the gas pedal and start cleansing—this whole enterprise isn't going anywhere because we didn't hand our body the keys.

In order to get past checking the mirrors and put ourselves onto the road of healing, the beginning of a cleanse especially needs to be kind to the body so it can usher out poisons and pathogens later on in the cleanse. We can't give our liver too much to handle right away or put it in a position where it's forced to give our brain and heart too much to handle. We need to offer it proper time and guidance, and that's the purpose of these first three days.

Upon Waking

- You'll start each of the three days simply: with **16 ounces of your choice of lemon or lime water.** (See Chapter 23 for the recipe with the proper ratio of lemon or lime to water. This isn't about squeezing 10 lemons into a glass of water.) If you prefer, go up to 32 ounces of lemon or lime water.

Tip

- If you'd like, you can add an optional teaspoon of raw honey to your lemon or lime water.

Morning

- Once you've finished your lemon or lime water, *wait at least 15 to 20 minutes, and ideally 30 minutes*, and then enjoy **16 ounces of celery juice** (recipe on page 276, or get it fresh from your local juice bar).

- After you finish your celery juice, *wait another 15 to 30 minutes*, and then enjoy the **breakfast of your choice**, within the guidelines in the table above and explained in more detail later in this chapter. Celery juice is a medicinal, not a caloric, drink, so do make sure to eat breakfast. Find more inspiration in Chapters 22 and 23,

where you'll find sample menus and various breakfast recipes.

- If you get hungry later in the morning, snack on **optional apples** (or applesauce or ripe pears).

Tips

- If you're sensitive, drink 8 ounces of celery juice in the morning instead of 16 ounces. For further information on celery juice amounts in the Simplified 3:6:9 Cleanse, see the guidelines later in this chapter.

- An additional breakfast option is to enjoy the Heavy Metal Detox Smoothie in the morning. For more on incorporating heavy metal detox into your 3:6:9 Cleanse, see Chapter 21, "Cleanse Adaptations and Substitutions."

Lunchtime

- When you're ready for lunch, enjoy **the meal of your choice**, within the guidelines in this chapter.

Tip

- Look to the sample menus and recipes in Chapters 22 and 23 for inspiration about what to eat at every meal.

Mid-Afternoon

- If you get hungry in the afternoon, snack on **optional apples** (or applesauce or pears), **one to** four dates, celery sticks, and cucumber slices.

Tips

- If you opt for store-bought applesauce, make sure it's free from additives.

- If you don't like dates or don't have access to them, good substitutes are a handful of mulberries (dried or fresh), raisins, grapes, or figs (dried or fresh), in that order. It's okay to chop or blend them up with the apples.

- Give yourself a hand by setting aside the celery sticks when you're prepping celery for juice in the morning.

- If chewing celery is difficult for you, chop it up finely in the food processor or blend it with the apples.

Dinnertime

- When you're ready to eat dinner, enjoy the **meal of your choice**, within the guidelines in this chapter.

Evening

- If you're hungry after dinner, turn to an **optional apple** (or applesauce or pear).

- An hour before you go to bed, get in another **16 ounces of lemon or lime water**.

- Also enjoy a pre-bedtime mug of **hibiscus, lemon balm, or chaga tea**. Select one rather than blending them. It's okay to drink your tea at the same time as the lemon or lime water.

Tip

- It's also okay to add a teaspoon of raw honey to your nighttime lemon or lime water or tea.

——— THE 6: SIMPLIFIED ———

	DAY 4	DAY 5	DAY 6
UPON WAKING	16 ounces lemon or lime water		
MORNING	Wait 15 to 30 minutes, then: 24 ounces celery juice Wait another 15 to 30 minutes, then: Fruit-based breakfast of your choice (within guidelines) and later, if desired: Apple (or applesauce)		

	DAY 4	DAY 5	DAY 6
LUNCHTIME	Meal of your choice (within guidelines)		
MID-AFTERNOON	Optional: Apple (or applesauce) plus cucumber slices and celery sticks		
DINNERTIME	Meal of your choice (within guidelines)		
EVENING	Apple (or applesauce) (if desired) 16 ounces lemon or lime water Hibiscus, lemon balm, or chaga tea		
GUIDELINES	• Breakfast: At this point, stick to fruit all morning, with optional leafy greens, celery, and cucumber to accompany it. Dried mango, dried figs, and dates are okay. • Continue to avoid radical fats (nuts, seeds, oils, olives, coconut, avocado, cacao, bone broth, animal proteins, etc.) entirely. Skip beans too. • Continue to avoid these foods: eggs, dairy, gluten, soft drinks, salt and seasonings, pork, corn, oils (including both industrial and healthier oils), soy, lamb, tuna and all other fish and seafood, vinegar (including ACV), caffeine (including coffee, matcha, and chocolate), grains (millet and oats are okay), alcohol, natural/artificial flavors, fermented foods (including kombucha, sauerkraut, and coconut aminos), nutritional yeast, citric acid, monosodium glutamate (MSG), aspartame, other artificial sweeteners, formaldehyde, and preservatives. • Instead, stick to fruits, vegetables, leafy greens, and (if desired) millet and oats. • For meal inspiration, check out the Simplified sample menus in Chapter 22. • See the text to follow and Chapter 21 for substitutions and adaptations if any of the foods in the chart don't work for you. • For alternate amounts of celery juice if you're sensitive, see page 145. • Keep in mind that baking or roasting foods will slow down the detox. If you prefer lighter fare, steam your vegetables instead or add them to the soup and stew recipes in Chapter 23. • Eat the portions that are right for you. Scale back if you're overly full. • Stay hydrated by drinking about 1 liter (roughly 32 ounces, or 4 cups) of water during the day, in between your morning and evening lemon or lime water.		

THE 6: SIMPLIFIED

During the middle three days of the cleanse, your liver settles into its long-awaited breather from the need to produce large quantities of bile. Constant bile production mode is the state most everyone lives in due to diets high in fat—and the body's need to break down that fat. This normal rate of bile production tires out the liver, making it less likely to perform its daily cleansing duties. When the liver finally gets a break from producing volumes of bile, it can work on dislodging toxins that it's stored away in deep pockets over your lifetime. A liver that's capable of detoxifying poisons and restoring itself benefits your health on all levels; it becomes a backbone for recovering from chronic illness and other symptoms that won't go away—symptoms that could eventually develop into chronic illnesses if we don't care for our bodies with steps such as the 3:6:9 Cleanse.

Upon Waking

- Again, you'll start each of the three days with **16 ounces of your choice of lemon or lime water**. If you prefer, go up to 32 ounces.

Tip

- If you'd like, you can add an optional teaspoon of raw honey to your lemon or lime water.

Morning

- Once you've finished your lemon or lime water, *wait at least 15 to 20 minutes, and ideally 30 minutes*, and then enjoy **24 ounces of celery juice**.

- After you finish your celery juice, *wait another 15 to 30 minutes*, and then enjoy the **fruit-based breakfast of your choice**, within the guidelines in this chapter. During The 6, breakfast should consist of fresh fruit, with optional leafy greens, celery, and cucumber to accompany it. Frozen fruit, dried mango, dried figs, and dates are also okay.

- If you get hungry later in the morning, snack on **optional apples** (or applesauce or ripe pears).

Tips

- If you're sensitive, opt for 16 ounces of celery juice instead of 24 ounces.

- As in The 3, one breakfast option is to drink the Heavy Metal Detox Smoothie.

Lunchtime

- When you're ready for lunch, enjoy **the meal of your choice**, within the guidelines in this chapter.

Mid-Afternoon

- If you get hungry in the afternoon, snack on **optional apples** (or applesauce or pears), **celery sticks**, and **cucumber slices**. (No dates this time.)

Dinnertime

- When you're ready to eat dinner, enjoy the **meal of your choice**, within the guidelines in this chapter.

Evening

- If you're hungry after dinner, turn to an **optional apple** (or applesauce or pear).

- An hour before you go to bed, get in another **16 ounces of lemon or lime water.**

- Also enjoy a pre-bedtime mug of **hibiscus, lemon balm, or chaga tea.** Select one rather than blending them.

It's okay to drink your tea at the same time as the lemon or lime water.

Tip

- It's also okay to add a teaspoon of raw honey to your nighttime lemon or lime water or tea.

THE 9: SIMPLIFIED

	DAY 7	DAY 8	DAY 9
UPON WAKING	16 ounces lemon or lime water		16 ounces lemon or lime water
MORNING	Wait 15 to 30 minutes, then: 32 ounces celery juice Wait another 15 to 30 minutes, then: Fruit-based breakfast of your choice (within guidelines) and later, if desired: Apple (or applesauce)		Wait 15 to 30 minutes, then: 16 ounces celery juice Wait another 15 to 30 minutes, then: Blended melon, fresh watermelon juice, blended papaya, blended ripe pear, or fresh-squeezed orange juice as desired, consumed separately from each other
LUNCHTIME	Meal of your choice (within guidelines)		Spinach Soup

	DAY 7	DAY 8	DAY 9
MID-AFTERNOON	Optional: Apple (or applesauce) plus cucumber slices and celery sticks		Wait at least 60 minutes, then: 16 ounces celery juice Wait at least 15 to 30 minutes, then: Fresh watermelon juice, blended papaya, blended ripe pear, or fresh-squeezed orange juice as desired, consumed separately from each other
DINNERTIME	Meal of your choice (within guidelines) that incorporates steamed asparagus and/or brussels sprouts		Asparagus Soup or Zucchini Basil Soup
EVENING	Apple (or applesauce) (if desired) 16 ounces lemon or lime water Hibiscus, lemon balm, or chaga tea		16 ounces lemon or lime water Hibiscus, lemon balm, or chaga tea
GUIDELINES	• Breakfast: On Day 7 and Day 8, you'll stick to fresh fruit all morning (frozen fruit is okay), with optional leafy greens, celery, and cucumber okay. On Day 9, follow this chart—you'll be consuming specific liquid and blended items all day. • Continue to avoid radical fats (nuts, seeds, oils, olives, coconut, avocado, cacao, bone broth, animal proteins, etc.) entirely. Skip beans too. • Continue to avoid these foods: eggs, dairy, gluten, soft drinks, salt and seasonings, pork, corn, oils (including both industrial and healthier oils), soy, lamb, tuna and all other fish and seafood, vinegar (including ACV), caffeine (including coffee, matcha, and chocolate), grains (millet and oats are okay), alcohol, natural/artificial flavors, fermented foods (including kombucha, sauerkraut, and coconut aminos), nutritional yeast, citric acid, monosodium glutamate (MSG), aspartame, other artificial sweeteners, formaldehyde, and preservatives. • Instead, stick to fruits, vegetables, leafy greens, and (if desired) millet and oats on Days 7 and 8. On Day 9, stick to the outlined items. • For meal inspiration, check out the Simplified sample menus in Chapter 22. • See the text to follow and Chapter 21 for substitutions and adaptations if any of the foods in the chart don't work for you. • For alternate amounts of celery juice if you're sensitive, see page 145. • Keep in mind that baking or roasting foods will slow down the detox. If you prefer lighter fare, steam your vegetables instead or add them to the soup and stew recipes in Chapter 23. • Eat the portions that are right for you. Scale back if you're overly full. • Stay hydrated by drinking about 1 liter (roughly 32 ounces, or 4 cups) of water during the day, in between your morning and evening lemon or lime water. If the extra celery juice means you'd like to scale back on water a bit, that's fine.		

THE 9: SIMPLIFIED

Here we are: the moment your liver has been waiting for basically its whole life. That means it's the moment you've been waiting for too, because what makes your liver happy makes you happy. When your liver and other organs unburden themselves at this stage, you'll be amazed at the positive influence it can have on both your body and your mood. The ripple effect from here on out—the people who see the change in you, the further changes you're inspired to make in your life—will be profound and far reaching. Who knows whose lives you're going to touch with your improved health? Who knows what you'll get to do now?

Over the past six days, you've been warming up your liver's engine and building your body's reserves, getting them ready so that here in The 9, they'll have the power to drive out junk, garbage, and poison that your organs have been holding on to for years. This goes far beyond the Morning Cleanse's ability to process out daily waste. These liquid-heavy three days are completely new territory.

DAYS 7 AND 8

Upon Waking

- As usual, you'll start each day with **16 ounces of your choice of lemon or lime water**. If you prefer, go up to 32 ounces.

Tip

- If you'd like, you can add an optional teaspoon of raw honey to your lemon or lime water.

Morning

- Once you've finished your lemon or lime water, *wait at least 15 to 20 minutes, and ideally 30 minutes*, and then enjoy **32 ounces of celery juice**.

- After you finish your celery juice, *wait another 15 to 30 minutes*, and then enjoy the **breakfast of your choice**, within the guidelines in this chapter. This time, breakfast should consist of fresh fruit *only*, with optional leafy greens, celery, and cucumber to accompany it. (Frozen fruit is fine. No dried fruit this time.)

- If you get hungry later in the morning, snack on **optional apples** (or applesauce or ripe pears).

Tips

- If you're sensitive, drink 16 ounces of celery juice in the morning and then drink your second 16 ounces of celery juice in the afternoon (spaced apart from other food and drink).

- As before, one option is to enjoy the Heavy Metal Detox Smoothie in the morning.

Lunchtime

- Enjoy **the meal of your choice**, within the guidelines in this chapter.

Mid-Afternoon

- If you get hungry in the afternoon, snack on **optional apples** (or applesauce or pears), **celery sticks**, and **cucumber slices**.

Tips

- If you're drinking a second serving of celery juice in the afternoon, make sure to *wait at least 60 minutes after lunch* to drink it. After finishing your celery juice, *wait at least 15 to 30 minutes* to eat or drink anything else.

- Feel free to make all your celery juice at once in the morning, setting aside this optional second serving in the fridge, if you don't have the time or inclination to fire up the juicer twice in one day. You can also get your celery juice fresh from a juice bar in the morning, ordering both servings at once and saving the second one for later.

Dinnertime

- Enjoy the **meal of your choice**, within the guidelines in this chapter, incorporating **steamed asparagus and/or brussels sprouts**, either as a side dish or as part of the main dish. See Chapter 22, "3:6:9 Cleanse Sample Menus," for meal ideas.

Tips

- If fresh asparagus and/or brussels sprouts aren't available, buy them frozen. If neither fresh nor frozen asparagus and/or brussels sprouts are available, substitute zucchini or summer squash.

- It's fine to chop up, mash, or blend the asparagus and/or brussels sprouts if you have trouble with solid foods.

- It's also fine to prepare the steamed vegetables ahead of time and eat them cold.

- If you prefer, the asparagus and/or brussels sprouts can be eaten raw instead of steamed.

Evening

- If you're hungry after dinner, turn to an **optional apple** (or applesauce or pear).

- An hour before you go to bed, get in another **16 ounces of lemon or lime water**.

- Also enjoy a pre-bedtime mug of **hibiscus, lemon balm, or chaga tea**. Again, select one rather than blending them, and feel free to drink your tea at the same time as the lemon or lime water.

Tip

- It's also okay to add a teaspoon of raw honey to your nighttime lemon or lime water or tea.

DAY 9

Upon Waking

- Start your day with **16 ounces of your choice of lemon or lime water**.

Tip

- If you'd like, you can add an optional teaspoon of raw honey to your lemon or lime water.

Morning

- Once you've finished your lemon or lime water, *wait at least 15 to 20 minutes, and ideally 30 minutes*, and then enjoy **16 ounces of celery juice**.

- After you finish your celery juice, *wait another 15 to 30 minutes*, and then enjoy the beverage of your choice from this list: **blended melon, fresh watermelon juice, blended papaya, blended ripe pear, or fresh-squeezed orange juice**. Sip as desired (as long as you enjoy them separately from each other).

Tip

- It's okay to change it up throughout the morning—for example, you could drink watermelon juice first and fresh-squeezed orange juice mid-morning. Or pick one and make that your staple. It's your choice, as long as you don't blend them together or drink them together—for example, don't drink a papaya-orange blend or drink watermelon juice immediately followed by blended pear. Enjoy each separately and on its own.

Lunchtime

- For your lunch, enjoy the **Spinach Soup** recipe on page 344. Since this is a day of all liquid and blended foods, skip the cucumber noodles or blend the cucumber into your soup.

Mid-Afternoon

- Enjoy another **16 ounces of celery juice** between lunch and dinner. Make sure to *wait at least 60 minutes after lunch* to drink it. After finishing your celery juice, *wait at least 15 to 30 minutes* to consume anything else.

- Once you've had your celery juice and completed the short waiting period, continue to sip **fresh watermelon juice, blended papaya, blended ripe pear, or fresh-squeezed orange juice** as desired, consumed separately from each other.

Tip

- Melon digests best without other food in the stomach, so you'll notice that blended melon doesn't show up in the afternoon list of beverages. If you want blended melon on Day 9, drink it earlier in the day, before any blended papaya, blended pear, or Spinach Soup.

Dinnertime

- Enjoy your choice of **Asparagus Soup** (recipe on page 392) or **Zucchini Basil Soup** (recipe on page 382). Skip any garnish.

Evening

- Get in another **16 ounces of lemon or lime water**.

- Also enjoy a pre-bedtime mug of **hibiscus, lemon balm, or chaga tea** as usual. Again, select one rather than blending them, and feel free to drink your tea with your lemon or lime water.

Tips

- It's also okay to add a teaspoon of raw honey to your nighttime lemon or lime water or tea.

SIMPLIFIED 3:6:9 CLEANSE GUIDELINES

General Guidelines

Devote Yourself to Fruits, Vegetables, and Leafy Greens

You'll rely on fruits, vegetables, and leafy greens to get you through all nine days of the Simplified 3:6:9 Cleanse. That means you're focusing on smoothies, fruit, salads, healing soups, and comfort foods such as sweet potatoes (including Japanese sweet potatoes), yams, regular potatoes, winter squash, and steamed broccoli, cauliflower, and asparagus.

Millet and oats are the exception—it's okay to include them in many of your meals. (Millet is the first choice. If you opt for oats, look for gluten-free oats.) Starting on Day 4, wait to have any millet, oats, or cooked vegetables until lunchtime or after. As you'll read about in a moment, you want to make your mornings fruit-focused by the time you reach The 6.

The recipes chapter at the end of Part IV will give you plenty of ideas about how to make this all work for you. It's worth it! By filling your snacks and meals with fruits, vegetables, and leafy greens, you're less apt to stay in old patterns and grab your normal, go-to items from the troublemaker foods list. The minerals, vitamins, and trace mineral salts in leafy greens and vegetables working together with the antioxidants and

glucose in fruit are critical for stabilizing organs and replenishing cells. Another important aspect here is that fruits, vegetables, and leafy greens are foods that don't feed pathogens—and everyone is dealing with pathogens inside their bodies creating their symptoms.

Skip beans entirely during the 3:6:9 Cleanse. Beans are not a powerful cleansing food. While they are not a radical fat or a troublemaker food, their fat content is on the higher side compared to fruits, vegetables, and leafy greens. Staying off them will also ensure that the cleanse is as easy as possible on your digestive tract. It takes a stronger hydrochloric acid level to break down the proteins in beans, and most people are living with lower levels of hydrochloric acid, making beans harder to digest. Their stomach glands are tired, heavily worn, and in need of repair—repair that the celery juice in these cleanses helps to offer.

It may sound daunting to eat only fruits and vegetables. That's because we're used to such small servings of them. Here, they're the main event. If salad doesn't seem like enough to satisfy you, that's probably because you're used to eating little side salads with limp greens and pale tomatoes. During the cleanse, make your salads robust by adding ample orange segments, ripe tomatoes, cucumbers, fresh greens, and other ingredients from the recipes such as the Liver Rescue Salad on page 342. And remember to leave room, because there are other great meal ideas in addition to salads, plus there are always opportunities for snacks between meals.

If an apple or two don't satisfy you for a snack, eat another apple. If that's not enough, eat yet another apple. You don't need to worry about eating too many apples—unless your body tells you you're full. When that's the case, respect its limits.

Nourish your body with the specific foods (or their substitutes) that the cleanse mentions, and it will have untold benefits. Avoiding foods that take a little more work to digest is well worth the effort it takes to pass on them during this part of the cleanse. The nutrient density of the healing fuel you'll be eating instead is exactly what your body needs at this point.

Avoid Radical Fats Entirely

To support your healing, cut out radical fats for all nine days. This means no nuts, seeds, nut butter (such as peanut butter), nut milk, oil, olives, coconut, avocado, chocolate, cacao nibs, dairy (including butter, cheese, milk, yogurt, kefir, and whey protein powder), bone broth, or other animal products. If you consumed those fats, it would break the cleanse. It would be as if you were scrubbing dishes and someone dumped grease into your sink—requiring you to start over in order to truly get the plates clean.

For your liver to navigate the Simplified 3:6:9 Cleanse successfully, it needs to be free from the interruption of being forced to backtrack and process radical fats. Your liver will still produce bile to keep your body functioning during this time; it just won't need to produce the same strength of bile for dissolving radical fats. By avoiding them, you allow your liver to use its energy to cleanse on a level it can't otherwise. Remember: it's very difficult for the liver to cleanse on a deep level while on a diet that's high in fat. The surprising bonus is that with radical fats out of your diet, you'll likely find food more satisfying than ever.

This break from fats, combined with the bioavailable nutrient density of the foods you *are* eating, gives your body a profound opportunity to devote its energy to healing. Without fat in your bloodstream blocking the absorption of glucose, your liver can build up the glucose and glycogen reserves that are vital for the hard work of propelling out poisons during The 9.

Reducing fats is also about the viscosity of your blood. If you have too much fat free-floating in your bloodstream, you slow down your body's ability to flush poisons and toxins—because the fat absorbs and holds on to toxins there, leading to pockets of toxic fat inside and around your body's organs. The goal during cleansing is to disperse deposits of fat (what people call fat cells)—to open them up so they can release the poisons, toxins, and old, stored adrenaline they contain to be sent out of your body. Continuing to eat radical fats during this period, which translates to having a high blood fat ratio inside your bloodstream, defeats the purpose of dispersing existing pockets of toxic fat.

By the way, even if avocado is one of your favorites, enjoy it *after* the Simplified 3:6:9 Cleanse. Although avocado is indeed a fruit and is easier to digest than other radical fats, when you're cleansing the liver, even good, healthy, unique fats get in the way. You'll want to put avocado aside for now to keep from overburdening your liver and causing it to struggle when it's trying to cleanse.

And again, you'll continue to skip beans for all nine days of the cleanse. While beans are not a radical fat, their fat content is on the higher side compared to the cleanse foods, and they do give the digestive system extra work.

Avoid Troublemaker Foods

Cut out the troublemaker foods from Chapter 7, "Troublemaker Foods." These are foods you'll want to leave out altogether for the entire nine days:

- Eggs
- Dairy

- Gluten
- Soft drinks
- Salt and seasonings (pure spices are okay)
- Pork
- Corn
- Oils (including both industrial and healthier oils)
- Soy
- Lamb
- Tuna and all other fish and seafood
- Vinegar (including ACV)
- Caffeine (including coffee, matcha, and chocolate)
- Grains (millet and oats are okay Days 1 through 8)
- Alcohol
- Natural and artificial flavors
- Fermented foods (including kombucha, sauerkraut, and coconut aminos)
- Nutritional yeast
- Citric acid
- Monosodium glutamate (MSG)
- Aspartame and other artificial sweeteners
- Formaldehyde
- Preservatives

If you skipped Chapter 7, go back and check it out to understand the "why" behind avoiding these ingredients while you're on the cleanse. Keep that guide nearby for strength in the face of temptation. As delicious as it may be to sneak a slice of pepperoni pizza, that chapter will offer reassurance that you're doing the right thing by taking a break from certain foods while on the 3:6:9.

None of the troublemaker foods are on this list because it's trendy to take them out of the diet. Gluten, for example, isn't avoided because of today's conventional wisdom that gluten causes inflammation. It's for a much more specific reason that's important to understand. Even if you have already read that chapter, you may want to go back and give yourself a refresher while you're going through the cleanse. For further cravings support, turn to Chapter 25, "The Emotional Side of Cleansing."

Cutting out these foods is easier than it may sound—because you'll be so focused on fruits, vegetables, and leafy greens each day. Filling up on these nutrient-rich foods won't leave room for other tempting foods, and that will help curb cravings. Plus, as you just read, the Simplified 3:6:9 Cleanse calls for avoiding radical fats altogether for all nine days. That automatically rules out dairy, eggs, lamb, pork, seafood, and oil from the list above, which means you would be skipping them anyway. That simplifies remembering what else to avoid.

Celery Juice

In the Simplified 3:6:9 Cleanse, you'll increase the amount of celery juice you consume every three days. This is a protective measure that works with the cleanse's 3:6:9 structure to encourage your liver and other organs to let go. The celery juice helps gather up the increased amounts of toxins your organs are releasing, bind onto them, and escort them out of your body.

The amounts are laid out in the cleanse charts and description you've already read. Here's another table to help you see what those increases look like:

	REGULAR	SENSITIVE
THE 3	16 ounces	8 ounces
THE 6	24 ounces	16 ounces
THE 9	32 ounces	32 ounces*

*As the cleanse description states, on Days 7 and 8, if you can't get the 32 ounces in you all at once, you can drink 16 ounces of celery juice in the morning and the other 16 ounces in the afternoon, spaced apart from other food and drink. Day 9 already divides the 32 ounces between morning and afternoon.

Breakfast

You'll also make some gradual changes with breakfast every three days in the Simplified 3:6:9 Cleanse:

	BREAKFAST	OKAY TO INCLUDE	WHAT TO EXCLUDE
THE 3	Breakfast of your choice	Fresh fruit Frozen fruit Dried mango, dried figs, dates, raisins Celery, cucumber, leafy greens Potatoes, sweet potatoes, yams, winter squash Millet or oats	Troublemaker foods Radical fats
THE 6	Fruit-based breakfast of your choice	Fresh fruit Frozen fruit Dried mango, dried figs, dates Celery, cucumber, leafy greens	Troublemaker foods Radical fats Cooked foods
THE 9	Fresh fruit breakfast of your choice	Fresh fruit Frozen fruit Celery, cucumber, leafy greens	Troublemaker foods Radical fats Cooked foods Dried fruit

When we're thinking about what to eat for breakfast, especially during a cleanse, hydration is key. In the morning, we're flooded with poisons and toxins that our liver and other organs have released overnight, so we want our initial meals of the day to have high water content to help flush them all out. On top of which, the cleansing process can be slightly dehydrating. Living foods—raw fruits, vegetables, herbs, and leafy greens and their juices—are the perfect solution; they have the water content we need. By working up to a breakfast of all fresh fruit (frozen fruit counts) over the course of the Simplified 3:6:9 Cleanse, we boost our bloodstream with fluids to help bind onto and remove toxins while flushing them out through our kidneys and intestinal tract. And because we're avoiding radical fats at the same time, we allow our body's natural cleansing to happen.

Here's another vital reason for a cleanse breakfast to focus on living foods: when our cells release poisons and toxins, it creates space within them for nutrients. Mineral salts, electrolytes, glucose, antivirals, antibacterials, antioxidants, healing phytochemical compounds, minerals, vitamins—these are healing nutrients for which our cells have been starving for many years. They're the very nutrients that fresh, water-rich fruits, vegetables, herbs, leafy greens, and their juices contain—and can drive into our cells now that space is available.

Stay Hydrated

Remember to keep yourself hydrated. Each day, drink about 1 liter of water during the day in between your morning and evening lemon or lime water. That's roughly equivalent to 32 ounces, or 4 cups. You're welcome to do more. If you feel you require more fluids at any point throughout the cleanse, don't hold back; allow yourself to improve your water levels.

Do avoid water with a pH above 8.0. This includes if you use an alkalized water machine—keep it set at a pH of 8.0 or below. Ideally, set it at 7.7; that's the best pH for drinking water. Water content with higher pH levels sits in the stomach until the digestive system can lower it to 7.7 to be released throughout the body. The same goes for water with a pH below 7.7—your body has to put energy into raising its pH. Drinking water at the ideal pH level prevents your digestive system from weakening.

On Days 1 through 8, you're welcome to sip Hot Spiced Apple Juice at any temperature (recipe on page 290) or coconut water (as long as it isn't pink or red and doesn't list "natural flavors" in the ingredients) throughout the day. That would be *in addition* to the liter of water.

With all of these beverages, do be mindful to space them out at least 15 to 30 minutes from your celery juice. If it's a day when you're drinking extra celery juice and you'd like to scale back a bit on water, that's fine.

A Note on Cooking Techniques

If you already eat a pure diet, then during the Simplified 3:6:9 Cleanse, you may wish to choose lighter recipes from Chapter 23 that include a lot of raw fruits, leafy greens, and vegetables, along with recipes for steamed vegetables, soups, or stews. Steaming or cooking in soups and stews preserves more water content. Baking and roasting food, while not bad by any means, does slow down detox because of the moisture that food loses while cooking with these techniques. The baked recipes in Chapter 23 still offer a fantastic and delicious choice for someone who is new to cleansing.

Guidelines for Day 9

Stick with Liquid and Blended

Devote yourself to the Day 9 cleanse items as outlined. At this stage of the cleanse, when your body is releasing larger amounts of poisons, viral and bacterial waste, and other troublemakers, it needs lower quantities of food and higher quantities of liquid-based healing solutions. These specific options provide critical balance as you flush out toxins.

By sticking to these cleanse liquids and blended items, you're aligning two critical pieces of the healing puzzle: (1) you're keeping the day fat-free and (2) you're removing a large percentage of digestive load. Even healthy, whole foods require some level of digestion, especially bulkier foods. With these particular light, liquid and blended options, you give your body a rest from the normal digestive process it endures. In turn, this allows your body to use its reserves to flush and cleanse harmful toxins and poisons from your organs into your bloodstream and out of your kidneys and bowels.

Some special circumstances mentioned in this book call for repeating Day 8 rather than following the Day 9 plan. Or other life circumstances, such as unexpected travel that means you have less control over your food than you'd like, may lead you to stop the cleanse before reaching Day 9. In either case—whether you end the cleanse by repeating Day 8, or you have to stop the cleanse before you've finished a full nine-day cycle—don't worry about missing the Day 9 protocol. Every day of the 3:6:9 Cleanse that you complete takes you to that next level—however much you've completed, you've done an incredible amount of cleansing and you've only received gains.

Give Yourself a Rest

If you can, take it easy today. Think about saving certain commitments for another time. Maybe you can schedule Day 9 as a sacred rest day, or a day with at least some rest in it. If possible, set aside some down time, maybe even time for a nap. At minimum, be mindful of all your body's doing for you during this period. Take a moment to pause and think about your liver and other organs. This is the end of your liver's great big plunge into the depths of purification, and it's doing beautifully. You're succeeding in the healing process: rejuvenating yourself emotionally, physically, and spiritually by removing toxins and poisons and reducing pathogens and their waste. When you start freeing yourself of the burdens of symptoms and conditions, you head to a place of living your true potential as a healthy self and being.

REPEATING THE CLEANSE AND TRANSITIONING OUT

When you're ready to transition out of the 3:6:9 Cleanse, turn to Chapter 14 for special steps to make the adjustment easiest on your body.

As we'll cover in Chapter 13, "Repeating the 3:6:9 Cleanse," you may not be ready to transition out after only one cycle of the cleanse. Because the Simplified 3:6:9 Cleanse works at 70 percent of the strength and power of the Original, consider repeating it more often to get the results you want. If you're dealing with serious symptoms or illness, for example, or if you have a lot of weight to lose, you can take the cleanse longer term. You'll find detailed guidance on repeating the cleanse in that chapter. Whenever you decide to wrap up the cleanse, turn to Chapter 14 to help ease the transition.

CHAPTER 12

Advanced
3:6:9 Cleanse

An all new version of the 3:6:9, the Advanced is for people who feel they are in critical health circumstances. You know best whether you fall into this category of a chronic issue impeding your health on a critical level, meaning that your symptoms interfere with your normal way of living and get in the way of experiencing life to its full capacity. The Advanced 3:6:9 Cleanse offers the opportunity to reach a deeper cleanse state for relief.

Still safe and gentle, the Advanced is more intense than the Original and Simplified in order to help you release larger quantities of toxins. People who are dealing with more critical issues are also dealing with more aggressive and antagonistic toxins built up in their systems, whether toxic heavy metals that have oxidized or neurotoxins and dermatoxins from viruses, and that's why they're so sick. The Advanced 3:6:9 Cleanse is here to sweep out the volumes of poison that are holding back that person who's hurting badly so it can quickly move them forward.

This cleanse is also for those who have tried the 28-Day Cleanse from *Medical Medium* and seen results from it, and want a version of the 3:6:9 that speaks to them. With special meals and a steady rhythm—it's the most straightforward of the 3:6:9 Cleanse versions—it allows those who resonate with eating all raw fruits and vegetables to tap into the 3:6:9 Cleanse like never before.

THE 3, THE 6, AND THE 9: ADVANCED

The meal options for the Advanced are the most streamlined of the 3:6:9. That's to help you find your flow as you navigate the cleanse meals and beverages while avoiding radical fats.

The main rhythm of this cleanse comes from the increases in celery juice, going from 24 ounces in the morning for the first three days to 32 ounces in the morning for the second three days to 32 ounces twice a day for the final three days. (And if you do the cleanse multiple times in a row, you up those initial 24 ounces to 32.) Leading your body through these gentle increases, combined with the specified nutrient-dense, easy-to-digest, fat-free, raw meals, gives your liver all the coaxing it needs to get ready for release on the signature Day 9.

In the Advanced 3:6:9 Cleanse, the body still moves through the shifts of The 3, The 6, and The 9 that you read about in the Original and Simplified, this time able to address the more potent toxins keeping somebody down. Those troublemakers could be neurotoxins and dermatoxins coming from viruses in the system, or they could be toxins that have built up in a person's body over months, years, or a lifetime.

As it moves through these stages, the Advanced equips us to release a greater load of toxins:

During The 3, the body adjusts to the cleanse, with our liver in particular getting a chance to gear up and trust that we're giving it an opportunity to help us heal. It's like warming up an engine.

During The 6, our body can move on to dislodging deep pockets of toxins that have been hindering our health and threatening our future.

And during The 9, our body can take the reserves it's been building since the beginning of the cleanse and put that power to work driving out junk, garbage, and poison that our organs have been holding on to for years.

If you've been struggling with your health long term and you've been losing hope that anything can help, know that the Advanced offers the chance for your body to start the process of repairing itself. Your body can heal. The Advanced 3:6:9 Cleanse will give it every opportunity to do so. Also consider looking at Part VI, "Knowing the Cause and the Protocol," to find out which supplementation can be applied to your condition after completing one or more rounds of the cleanse.

"The path of not knowing is not your path.
You don't have to be without the knowledge
of how to heal anymore."

— Anthony William, Medical Medium

	DAYS 1 TO 3	DAYS 4 TO 6	DAYS 7 TO 8	DAY 9
UPON WAKING	32 ounces lemon or lime water			
MORNING	Wait 15 to 30 minutes, then: 24 (or 32) ounces* celery juice Wait another 15 to 30 minutes, then: Heavy Metal Detox Smoothie and later, if hungry: Apple (or raw applesauce)	Wait 15 to 30 minutes, then: 32 ounces celery juice Wait another 15 to 30 minutes, then: Heavy Metal Detox Smoothie and later, if hungry: Apple (or raw applesauce)		Over the course of the day, consume: Two 32-ounce celery juices (one morning, one early evening; enjoy them 15 to 30 minutes apart from these other drinks) Two 16- to 20-ounce cucumber-apple juices (anytime) Blended melon, fresh watermelon juice, blended papaya, blended ripe pear, or fresh-squeezed orange juice (as many servings and as often as desired, as long as you consume them separately from each other) Water (as desired)
LUNCHTIME	Liver Rescue Smoothie or Spinach Soup (with optional cucumber noodles)			
MID-AFTERNOON	Optional, if hungry: Apple (or raw applesauce)		Wait at least 60 minutes, then: 32 ounces celery juice Wait at least 15 to 30 minutes, then: Apple (or raw applesauce) if hungry	
DINNERTIME	Kale Salad or Cauliflower and Greens Bowl or Tomato, Cucumber, and Herb Salad or Leafy Green Nori Rolls or Spinach Soup with optional cucumber noodles			

	DAYS 1 TO 3	DAYS 4 TO 6	DAYS 7 TO 8	DAY 9
EVENING	Apple (or raw applesauce) (if desired) 16 ounces lemon or lime water Hibiscus, lemon balm, or chaga tea			16 ounces lemon or lime water Hibiscus, lemon balm, or chaga tea
GUIDELINES	* If you are repeating the cleanse (starting over at Day 1 immediately after completing Day 9), increase your celery juice from 24 ounces to 32 ounces in the morning on the first three days. • Devote yourself exclusively to raw fruits, vegetables, and leafy greens—specifically, the ones outlined in the chart or recipes above. (Frozen fruit is okay.) • See the text to follow and Chapter 21 for substitutions and adaptations if any of the foods in the chart don't work for you. For example, you can substitute ripe pears for apples. • Find specific recipes in Chapter 23. When a smoothie or soup is listed, you can choose to eat the ingredients whole rather than blended if you prefer. Likewise, when a salad is listed, you can blend those ingredients if you wish. Apples or ripe pears can also be blended alone into pure, raw applesauce or pear sauce. • If you experience an intense cleansing effect from what seems to be the celery juice, reduce the amount by half and then work your way back up. • Avoid all radical fats (nuts, seeds, oils, olives, coconut, avocado, cacao, bone broth, animal proteins, etc.) entirely. Skip beans too. • Avoid these foods: eggs, dairy, gluten, soft drinks, salt and seasonings, pork, corn, oils (including both industrial and healthier oils), soy, lamb, tuna and all other fish and seafood, vinegar (including ACV), caffeine (including coffee, matcha, and chocolate), grains (including millet and oats), alcohol, natural/artificial flavors, fermented foods (including kombucha, sauerkraut, and coconut aminos), nutritional yeast, citric acid, monosodium glutamate (MSG), aspartame, other artificial sweeteners, formaldehyde, and preservatives. • Eat the portions that are right for you. Scale back if you're overly full. • Stay hydrated by drinking about 1 liter (roughly 32 ounces, or 4 cups) of water during the day, in between your morning and evening lemon or lime water. If the extra celery juice in the afternoon during The 9 means you'd like to scale back on water a bit, that's fine.			

DAYS 1 through 8

Upon Waking

- Start all nine days with **32 ounces of your choice of lemon or lime water.** (See Chapter 23 for the recipe with the proper ratio of lemon or lime to water. This isn't about squeezing 10 lemons into a glass of water.)

Tip

- If you'd like, you can add an optional teaspoon of raw honey to your lemon or lime water.

Morning

- On **Day 1 through Day 3**, once you've finished your lemon or lime water, *wait at least 15 to 20 minutes, and ideally 30 minutes*, and then enjoy **24 ounces of celery juice** if this is your first cycle of the cleanse. If you're doing multiple rounds of the cleanse in a row, then when you start over, increase your celery juice to 32 ounces in the morning on Days 1 through 3.

- On **Day 4 through Day 8**, once you've finished your lemon or lime water, *wait at least 15 to 20 minutes, and ideally 30 minutes*, and then enjoy **32 ounces of celery juice**.

- After you finish your celery juice each day, *wait another 15 to 30 minutes*, and then enjoy the **Heavy Metal Detox Smoothie** (recipe on page 300).

- If you get hungry later in the morning, snack on an **optional apple or ripe pear or two.** (It's fine to blend them into pure, raw applesauce or pear sauce. See recipes in Chapter 23.)

Tips

- For the Heavy Metal Detox Smoothie, you can choose to eat the ingredients whole rather than blending them. If so, mix the spirulina and barley grass juice powder into water and drink separately or mash them into banana.

- If you experience an intense cleansing effect (such as diarrhea) from what seems to be the celery juice, reduce the amount by half and then work your way back up.

Lunchtime

- Enjoy your choice of a **Liver Rescue Smoothie** (recipe on page 298) or **Spinach Soup with optional cucumber noodles** (recipe on page 344) for lunch.

Tip

- For either the smoothie or soup, you are welcome to eat the ingredients whole rather than blending.

Mid-Afternoon

- If you get hungry between lunch and dinner, snack on an **optional one to two apples** (or pure, raw applesauce, ripe pear, or pear sauce).

- On **Day 7 and Day 8**, enjoy another **32 ounces of celery juice** between lunch and dinner. Make sure to *wait at least 60 minutes after lunch* to drink it. After finishing your celery juice, *wait at least 15 to 30 minutes* to eat or drink anything else.

Tip

- Feel free to make all your celery juice at once in the morning, setting aside this second serving in the fridge, if you don't have the time or inclination to fire up the juicer twice in one day. You can also get your celery juice from a juice bar, ordering both servings at once and saving the second one for later.

Dinnertime

- For dinner, enjoy your choice of **Kale Salad** (recipe on page 356), **Cauliflower and Greens Bowl** (recipe on page 358), **Tomato, Cucumber, and Herb Salad** (recipe on page 360), or **Leafy Green Nori Rolls** (recipe on page 362).

- For any of these salads, you are welcome to blend the ingredients into a raw soup if you prefer. Alternatively, you can opt for **Spinach Soup with optional cucumber noodles.**

Tip

- If the dinner recipe you've chosen doesn't include raw asparagus, feel free to munch on a few pieces alongside your meal.

Evening

- If you're hungry after dinner, turn to an **optional apple** (or pure, raw applesauce, ripe pear, or pear sauce).

- An hour before you go to bed, get in another **16 ounces of lemon or lime water.**

- Also enjoy a pre-bedtime mug of **hibiscus, lemon balm, or chaga tea.** Select one rather than blending them. It's okay to drink your tea at the same time as the lemon or lime water.

Tip

- It's also okay to add a teaspoon of raw honey to your nighttime lemon or lime water or tea.

DAY 9

Upon Waking

- Start your day with **32 ounces of your choice of lemon or lime water.**

Tip

- If you'd like, you can add an optional teaspoon of raw honey to your lemon or lime water.

Morning and Afternoon

- Once you've finished your lemon or lime water, *wait at least 15 to 20 minutes, and ideally 30 minutes,* and then enjoy **32 ounces of celery juice.**

- After you finish your celery juice, *wait at least another 15 to 30 minutes,* and then, over the course of the day, nourish yourself with **two 16- to 20-ounce cucumber-apple juices** at any time (aim for a 50-50 blend of cucumber and apple) and as much **blended melon, fresh watermelon juice, blended papaya, blended ripe pear, or fresh-squeezed orange juice** as you'd like whenever you get hungry (as long as you enjoy them separately from each other).

- Drink **water** throughout the day as desired. Ideally, add a squeeze of lemon or lime to your drinking water throughout the day. If plain water is all you can handle, that's fine. For more on water during the cleanse, see the general Advanced Cleanse guidelines following this section.

Tips

- Don't worry about the fact that you'll be skipping the Heavy Metal Detox Smoothie today. Day 9 is better focused on general flushing of toxins, plus you'll have enough remnants of spirulina, cilantro, barley grass juice powder, dulse, and wild blueberries left in your system to help remove any heavy metals that have been dislodged. Read more under "Heavy Metal Detox Modification" in Chapter 21, "Cleanse Adaptations and Substitutions."

- For more on cucumber-apple juice, including ratios and alternatives, see Chapter 21, "Cleanse Adaptations and Substitutions."

- When it comes to the blended melon, fresh watermelon juice, blended papaya, blended ripe pear, and fresh-squeezed orange juice, it's okay to change it up throughout the day—for example, you could drink blended melon in the morning, fresh-squeezed orange juice at midday, and blended papaya in the afternoon and at dinnertime. Or pick one and make that your staple throughout the day. It's your choice, as long as you don't blend them together or drink them together—for example, don't drink a watermelon-papaya blend or drink orange juice immediately followed by blended pear. Enjoy each separately and on its own.

- Melon digests best without other food in the stomach, so consider drinking any blended melon earlier in the day than blended papaya or blended pear. Try to avoid blended melon if you've already had blended papaya or blended pear during the day.

- Feel more than free to make or purchase all the fresh juice at a juice bar in the morning and save your later servings in the fridge.

- If you're very petite and can't get this much liquid in you, you can lower the serving sizes of the juices, as long as you don't underdo it. You want to make sure you get enough of those precious nutrients to support your body as it does its hard work of elimination.

Early Evening

- Drink another **32 ounces of celery juice** in the early evening. Enjoy it *at least 30 minutes after* any blended fruit drinks and *at least 15 to 30 minutes after* any fresh juices or water.

- After finishing your celery juice, *wait at least another 15 to 30 minutes.* Following that waiting period, you're welcome to keep sipping your cucumber-apple juice, blended melon, fresh watermelon juice, blended papaya, blended ripe pear, fresh orange juice, or water as desired.

Evening

- An hour before bed, drink another **16 ounces of lemon or lime water.**

- Also enjoy a pre-bedtime mug of **hibiscus, lemon balm, or chaga tea** as usual. Again, select one rather than blending them, and feel free

to drink your tea with your lemon or lime water.

Tip

- It's okay to add a teaspoon of raw honey to your nighttime lemon or lime water or tea.

ADVANCED 3:6:9 CLEANSE GUIDELINES

General Guidelines

Follow these guidelines on all nine days of the cleanse.

Devote Yourself to Raw Fruits and Vegetables

Stick to fruits, vegetables, leafy greens, and herbs in their raw form—specifically, the foods mentioned in this chapter and in the modifications and recipes it references.

As always, the cleanse foods are here to help you heal. If you have a specific problem with one of the foods mentioned, turn to Chapter 21, "Cleanse Adaptations and Substitutions." For example, if you have trouble eating salad, go ahead and blend it up. Otherwise, stick to the recommendations in this chapter. You won't serve yourself by trying to outsmart the cleanse.

It may sound daunting to eat only fruits and vegetables. That's because we're used to such small servings of them. Here, they're the main event. If salad doesn't seem like enough to satisfy you, that's probably because you're used to eating little side salads with limp greens and pale tomatoes. The Advanced Cleanse recipes are robust, packed with flavor and nutrition to fill you up and ground you; at the same time, they digest easily so that your body can put as much energy as possible into healing.

Nourish your body with the specific foods (or their substitutes) that the cleanse mentions, and it will have untold benefits. Avoiding foods that take a little more work to digest is well worth the effort it takes to pass on them during this cleanse. The nutrient density of the healing fuel you'll be eating instead is exactly what your body needs at this point.

Avoid Radical Fats Entirely

To support your healing, cut out radical fats for all nine days. This means no nuts, seeds, nut butter (such as peanut butter), nut milk, oil, olives, coconut, avocado, cacao, bone broth, dairy (including butter, cheese, milk, yogurt, kefir, and whey protein powder), or other animal products. If you consumed those fats, it would break the cleanse. It would be as if you were scrubbing dishes and someone dumped grease into your sink—requiring you to start over in order to truly get the plates clean.

For your liver to navigate the Advanced 3:6:9 Cleanse successfully, it needs to be free from the interruption of being forced to backtrack and process radical fats. Your liver will still produce bile to keep your body functioning during this time; it just won't need to produce the same strength of bile for dissolving radical fats. By avoiding them, you allow your liver to use its energy to cleanse on a level it can't otherwise. Remember: it's very difficult for the liver to cleanse on a deep level while on a diet that's high in fat. The surprising bonus is that with radical fats out of your diet, you'll likely find food more satisfying than ever.

This break from fats, combined with the bioavailable nutrient density of the foods you

are eating, gives your body a profound opportunity to devote its energy to healing. Without fat in your bloodstream blocking the absorption of glucose, your liver can build up the glucose and glycogen reserves that are vital for the hard work of propelling out poisons during The 9.

Reducing fats is also about the viscosity of your blood. If you have too much fat free-floating in your bloodstream, you slow down your body's ability to flush poisons and toxins—because the fat absorbs and holds on to toxins there, leading to pockets of toxic fat inside and around your body's organs. The goal during cleansing is to disperse deposits of fat (what people call fat cells)—to open them up so they can release the poisons, toxins, and old, stored adrenaline they contain to be sent out of your body. Continuing to eat radical fats during this period, which translates to having a high blood fat ratio inside your bloodstream, defeats the purpose of dispersing existing pockets of toxic fat.

By the way, even if avocado is one of your favorites, enjoy it *after* the Advanced 3:6:9 Cleanse. Although avocado is indeed a fruit and is easier to digest than other radical fats, when you're cleansing the liver, even good, healthy, unique fats get in the way. You'll want to put avocado aside for now to keep from overburdening your liver and causing it to struggle when it's trying to cleanse.

And again, you'll continue to **skip beans entirely for all nine days of the cleanse.** Beans are not a powerful cleansing food. While they are not a radical fat or a troublemaker food, their fat content is on the higher side compared to fruits, vegetables, and leafy greens. Staying off them will also ensure that the cleanse is as easy as possible on your digestive tract. It takes a stronger hydrochloric acid level to break down the proteins in beans, and most people are living with lower levels of hydrochloric acid, making beans harder to digest. Their stomach glands are tired, heavily worn, and in need of repair—repair that the celery juice in these cleanses helps to offer.

Avoid Troublemaker Foods

Cut out the troublemaker foods from Chapter 7. These are foods you'll want to leave out altogether for the entire nine days:

- Eggs
- Dairy
- Gluten
- Soft drinks
- Salt and seasonings (pure spices are okay)
- Pork
- Corn
- Oils (including both industrial and healthier oils)
- Soy
- Lamb
- Tuna and all other fish and seafood
- Vinegar (including ACV)
- Caffeine (including coffee, matcha, and chocolate)
- Grains (including millet and oats in Advanced)
- Alcohol
- Natural and artificial flavors
- Fermented foods (including kombucha, sauerkraut, and coconut aminos)
- Nutritional yeast
- Citric acid
- Monosodium glutamate (MSG)
- Aspartame and other artificial sweeteners
- Formaldehyde
- Preservatives

If you skipped Chapter 7, go back and check it out to understand the "why" behind avoiding these ingredients while you're on the cleanse. Keep that guide nearby for strength in the face of temptation. As delicious as it may be to sneak a slice of pepperoni pizza, that chapter will offer reassurance that you're doing the right thing by taking a break from certain foods while on the 3:6:9.

None of the troublemaker foods are on this list because it's trendy to take them out of the diet. Gluten, for example, isn't avoided because of today's conventional wisdom that gluten causes inflammation. It's for a much more specific reason that's important to understand. Even if you have already read that chapter, you may want to go back and give yourself a refresher while you're going through the cleanse. For further cravings support, turn to Chapter 25, "The Emotional Side of Cleansing."

Cutting out these foods is easier than it may sound—because you'll be so focused on fruits, vegetables, and leafy greens each day. Filling up on these nutrient-rich foods won't leave room for other tempting foods, and that will help curb cravings.

Eat the Quantities That Are Right for You

Everyone is different, with unique calorie needs and appetite levels. Eat the portions that are right for you. You don't want to starve yourself, nor do you want to stuff yourself. You'll know what feels right quantity-wise. Stock up so you have an abundance of fresh, ripe, healing foods at your fingertips.

At no point in this cleanse should you force food down the hatch if you're already full. For more on how to know how much to eat of what, see "Hunger and Portions" in Chapter 19, "Critical Cleanse Dos and Don'ts."

Stay Hydrated

Remember to keep yourself hydrated. Each day, drink about 1 liter of water during the day in between your morning and evening lemon or lime water. That's roughly equivalent to 32 ounces, or 4 cups. You're welcome to do more. If you feel you require more fluids at any point throughout the cleanse, don't hold back; allow yourself to improve your water levels.

Do avoid water with a pH above 8.0. This includes if you use an alkalized water machine—keep it set at a pH of 8.0 or below. Ideally, set it at 7.7; that's the best pH for drinking water. Water content with higher pH levels sits in the stomach until the digestive system can lower it to 7.7 to be released throughout the body. The same goes for water with a pH below 7.7—your body has to put energy into raising its pH. Drinking water at the ideal pH level prevents your digestive system from weakening.

On Days 1 through 8, you're welcome to sip Hot Spiced Apple Juice at any temperature (recipe on page 290) or coconut water (as long as it isn't pink or red and doesn't list "natural flavors" in the ingredients) throughout the day.

Even if the Hot Spiced Apple Juice is warmed or the coconut water is pasteurized, it won't set back the healing and cleansing process of consuming raw foods. That's a personal choice. If you choose to reach for them, keep in mind that any you sip is *in addition* to the liter of water.

With all of these beverages, do be mindful to space them out at least 15 to 30 minutes from your celery juice. If it's a day where you're drinking extra celery juice (for example, Day 7 or 8) and you'd like to scale back a bit on water, that's fine.

Additional Guidelines for Day 9

Stick with Liquid and Blended

Devote yourself to the Day 9 cleanse beverages as outlined. At this stage of the cleanse, when your body is releasing larger amounts of poisons, viral and bacterial waste, and other troublemakers, it needs lower quantities of food and higher quantities of liquid-based healing solutions. These specific options provide critical balance as you flush out toxins.

By sticking to these cleanse beverages, you're aligning two critical pieces of the healing puzzle: (1) you're keeping the day fat-free and (2) you're removing a large percentage of digestive load. Even healthy, whole foods require some level of digestion, especially bulkier and cooked foods. With these particular light, raw, liquid and blended options, you give your body a rest from the normal digestive process it endures. In turn, this allows your body to use its reserves to flush and cleanse harmful toxins and poisons from your organs into your bloodstream and out of your kidneys and bowels.

Some special circumstances mentioned in this book call for repeating Day 8 rather than following the Day 9 plan. Or other life circumstances, such as unexpected travel that means you have less control over your food than you'd like, may lead you to stop the cleanse before reaching Day 9. In either case—whether you end the cleanse by repeating Day 8, or you have to stop the cleanse before you've finished a full nine-day cycle—don't worry about missing the Day 9 protocol. Every day of the 3:6:9 Cleanse that you complete takes you to that next level—however much you've completed, you've done an incredible amount of cleansing and you've only received gains.

Give Yourself a Rest

If you can, take it easy today. Think about saving certain commitments for another time. Maybe you can schedule Day 9 as a sacred rest day, or a day with at least some rest in it. If possible, set aside some down time, maybe even time for a nap. At minimum, be mindful of all your body's doing for you during this period. Take a moment to pause and think about your liver and other organs. This is the end of your liver's great big plunge into the depths of purification, and it's doing beautifully. You're

succeeding in the healing process: rejuvenating yourself emotionally, physically, and spiritually by removing toxins and poisons and reducing pathogens and their waste. When you start freeing yourself of the burdens of symptoms and conditions, you head to a place of living your true potential as a healthy self and being.

REPEATING THE CLEANSE AND TRANSITIONING OUT

When you're ready to transition out of the 3:6:9 Cleanse, turn to Chapter 14 for special steps to make the adjustment easiest on your body.

As we'll cover in Chapter 13, "Repeating the 3:6:9 Cleanse," you may not be ready to transition out after only one cycle of the cleanse. If you're dealing with serious symptoms or illness, for example, or if you have a lot of weight to lose, you can take the cleanse longer term. You'll find detailed guidance on repeating the cleanse in that chapter. Whenever you decide to wrap up the cleanse, turn to Chapter 14 to help ease the transition.

"Cleansing gives us back years of our life—
years we don't even know we've already lost and don't realize
we can gain back. This is your chance. Take it."

— Anthony William, Medical Medium

CHAPTER 13

Repeating the 3:6:9 Cleanse

Your liver knows what it's doing. On one cycle of the 3:6:9 Cleanse, it won't release a lifetime of toxins and accumulated fat—the strain on your system would be too great. Instead, your liver lets go of as much as it can safely and then keeps the rest until you can repeat the cycle. That's why it makes sense to do the 3:6:9 Cleanse more than once, whether consecutively or spaced out over days, weeks, or months: so you can continue to release what's holding you back in order to move forward.

FREQUENCY

After finishing one cycle of the 3:6:9 Cleanse, you may find you want to roll directly into another, starting over again at Day 1 and cycling through the nine days as many times as you'd like until your symptoms have moved on. If you're seeking more gradual changes in your health, you may find that you want to try the 3:6:9 Cleanse once a month instead, with some Morning Cleanses in between for maintenance. **It's ideal to try for at least one round of the 3:6:9 Cleanse every one to three months if you** **suspect you're dealing with a decent amount of troublemakers in your body.** Or you may find that one go-round gave you just what you were looking for at this time in your life. The choice is yours.

If you're symptom free and concerned with prevention, that's another instance where it's a good idea to try to get in a round of the 3:6:9 Cleanse every month, or at least every three months. This applies, for example, if you've seen family members develop illnesses and you're worried about the genetic cycle of what your parents and grandparents have been through catching up with you. Keep in mind that it's *not* our genes that make us sick—that's only what we're taught. The truth is that diseases in the family line come from toxins and pathogens passed down from generation to generation. We hold the power to stop that cycle by cleansing our inherited troublemakers and cleaning up our livers.

Life can pass by quickly, so have patience with yourself and do your best. If you find six months have passed and you meant to repeat the cleanse three months ago, don't spend time worrying or decide not to do the cleanse again because more time has passed than you intended. Go ahead and pick it back up, however long it's been.

BACK TO THE BEGINNING

Do start with Day 1 of the 3:6:9 Cleanse and follow it through to the end—unless life hands you unexpected interruptions; in that case, pick back up at Day 1 when you're ready rather than starting up again from the middle. And if you get through all nine days and decide to repeat the cleanse, in most cases, **go back to Day 1 and start over from the beginning.**

There are a few exceptions. In these specific circumstances, you wouldn't do the full nine days as they're laid out in the 3:6:9 Cleanse descriptions:

- Children trying the 3:6:9 Cleanse can repeat Day 8 rather than going on to the all-liquid-and-blended Day 9, if Mom or another primary caregiver feel that Day 9 will be a challenge.

- Repeating Day 8 in place of Day 9 is an option for someone who feels they are cleansing too fast.

- Repeating Day 8 in place of Day 9 is an option for someone who is pregnant. Consult with your doctor about what's best for you.

- For a special weight loss technique, complete one full round of the 3:6:9 Cleanse and then start over at Day 7. Keep repeating Days 7, 8, and 9 for any further rounds. Read more in Chapter 20, "Your Body's Healing Power."

- For those worried that the cleanse will bring on too-rapid weight loss for their circumstances, try Days 1 through 6 of the 3:6:9 Cleanse. If you'd like to do more than one round of the cleanse, keep repeating those first six days. That will help you heal to the point that you can reach a stronger, more stable physical place someday that has you more comfortable doing all nine days of the 3:6:9.

- For those who feel they have a food intolerance around fruit, try Days 1 through 3 of the Original or Simplified 3:6:9 Cleanse at least twice in a row. That will help prepare your body for the liver cleanse and put you on your way to experiencing lesser reactions.

DECIDING TO SKIP FATS

Here's another adjustment you can make: **you're welcome to eliminate radical fats altogether from the first three days of the Original 3:6:9 Cleanse.** By skipping the allowed dinnertime fats during The 3, you'll keep yourself in a heightened cleanse mode, and that's precisely what people are seeking when they ask to repeat the cleanse from midway through. (Note that the Simplified and Advanced 3:6:9 Cleanses keep radical fats out of all nine days anyway.)

It's fine to keep doing the Original 3:6:9 cleanse over and over like this, with no radical fats at all, if you're looking for that next level of healing. You're also welcome to skip the allowed fats during The 3 if you're coming to the cleanse fresh; it isn't an option just for those repeating the cleanse.

Or, if you're doing repeats, it's also fine to bring back the single serving of radical fat with dinner on those first three days whenever you start the cleanse over. It's up to you and how you're feeling.

HOW MANY ROUNDS?

There's no hard and fast rule for how many times to do the 3:6:9 Cleanse. It all depends on what state your health is in and how much healing you have to do. **Making the cleanse a regular part of your life, on whatever schedule works for you, is more important than focusing on how many rounds of the cleanse to do in total.** It's here for you as a lifelong tool.

Every time you do the 3:6:9 Cleanse, you're moving yourself forward. Every single time, you're accomplishing something great within your body. You may be someone with more toxins who's more viral, with more toxic heavy metals. While one round of the 3:6:9 Cleanse *will* offer healing and accomplish greatness within you, you may not experience those benefits quite yet. If that's the case, bring in the 3:6:9 Cleanse again. It's there for you to do repeatedly, as much as you need to, in order to get to that place of feeling better.

Many times, the 3:6:9 Cleanse will cleanse the underlying toxins and poisons that are making someone sick fairly rapidly, at the same time quickly killing some viruses and bacteria and slowly starving other pathogens of the toxic foods they like to eat. Even if the problem is fixed—meaning that the pathogen is killed off and the toxins are removed from your organs—you need more time to

heal because now it's time for the nerves, organs, tissue, and cells in the brain and body to recover, repair, and rejuvenate. Here, the proper supplementation can be very helpful. Turn to Chapter 29, "The True Cause of Your Symptoms and Conditions with Dosages to Heal," and find your issue in the list, and you'll see a brief explanation of what's behind it, along with which herbs and supplements can help your brain and body rebuild after you've extracted the troublemakers that were harming you and making you sick. (Also be sure to read Chapter 27, where you'll find critical guidance on supplementation.)

For example, if you were in severe body pain for years, with nerves that were seriously inflamed for a long time due to toxins and pathogens in the system, it could take months for the nerves to restore themselves, mend, and renew. That's not to say that your pain and suffering won't subside after the 3:6:9 Cleanse. Many people experience relief during or immediately after the cleanse. It's only to say that you shouldn't get discouraged if your tingles, numbness, neuropathy, aches and pains, vertigo, balance issues, dizziness, tics, spasms, burning skin, or other symptoms of inflamed nerves take time to calm down. After being chronically sick with them for years, you're an expert in the ups and downs of these symptoms. If you regularly apply the cleanses from this book, follow the individualized supplement recommendations from Part VI, and continue to keep the troublemaker foods from Chapter 7 out of your diet between cleanses, nerve damage can repair itself.

If you're someone who's been sick for a long time, repeating the cleanse is important because chronic illness is a sign that you have a lot of deep-seated toxins in the liver, whether pathogen-based, environmental, or toxic heavy metal–based. Repeating the 3:6:9 Cleanse is going to be extremely beneficial; with repetition, you should start to see results if you haven't seen them after doing it once.

CONSECUTIVE REPEATS OR BREAKS IN BETWEEN?

Whether you do multiple rounds of the 3:6:9 Cleanse in a row or you take breaks in between, repeating the cleanse is beneficial. Back-to-back repeats of the cleanse, or repeats of the cleanse with just a few days in between, are useful for deeper health conditions. These are people who need to cleanse a toxic, stagnant, sluggish liver overburdened with viruses, bacteria, toxic heavy metals, colognes, perfumes, hairsprays, plug-in air fresheners, scented candles, and so forth. Doing the 3:6:9 Cleanse over and over can be tremendously helpful in these cases.

On the other hand, you may be someone who's already got a pretty clean liver, who's not struggling with chronic symptoms or illness, in which case you may not feel a need to repeat it successively. Or you could be someone who does suffer chronically and is hypersensitive, who needs to take breaks in between repeats.

It's all about the individual—where you are with your health and how you feel. There is no "perfect." If you have the strength to do consecutive rounds, that's fine. If you're just as motivated to heal and yet need or want to take a week, a few weeks, or a month off between rounds, that's fine too. Gauge where you are and take it from there.

MORE TO KEEP IN MIND

If you're repeating the cleanse long term, **try not to get antsy and start straying from the cleanse guidelines.** Adding in different foods and drinks, even if they're healing options that you've read about in other Medical Medium books or other cleanses and health books outside of Medical Medium information, will distract from how this cleanse is meant to help you. For example, don't start swapping in cucumber juice for celery juice, unless you truly can't find or can't tolerate celery juice. Similarly, don't start distracting yourself with Liver Rescue Broth every day if you're on the Original or Advanced 3:6:9 Cleanse. With the exception of the specific adaptations and substitutions in the cleanse chapters and Chapter 21, stick with your chosen cleanse version as outlined, even long term.

One more exception is if you rely on ginger water or aloe water to address a physical need. It's okay to keep up with those during the 3:6:9 Cleanse, as long as you're spacing them out enough from the celery juice to give it time to work as it should.

Otherwise, get your variety from changing up your meals within the cleanse guidelines. Every version of the 3:6:9 Cleanse offers opportunities to customize meals to your taste, whether that's crafting different versions of the Liver Rescue Salad from the long list of ingredient options or choosing among the recipe options when a cleanse meal offers flexibility. You'll be thankful for the progress that comes from sticking to the guidelines.

CHAPTER 14

Transitioning out of the 3:6:9 Cleanse

Because every version of the 3:6:9 Cleanse protects your adrenals, you can get back to life afterward without feeling like all the energy's been squeezed out of you. In fact, you may be feeling so great that it will be easy to forget your body still likes TLC. If you're able, take a few extra steps to honor everything your organs have just done for you.

Whether you've done one cycle of the 3:6:9 Cleanse or many cycles in a row, these measures will help stabilize your system as it adjusts to coming out of the cleanse:

FIRST POST-CLEANSE DAY

- For your first post-cleanse day, **begin with the Morning Cleanse** from Chapter 16. You don't want to put your liver in shock by breaking your cleanse with bone broth, chocolate cake, pork, chicken, cheese, milk, or even yogurt or an egg white omelet;

liquids and high-quality glucose are more in line with what your liver needs at this point.

- In addition, see if you can **avoid radical fats** such as coconut, avocado, oil, olives, nuts, seeds, chocolate, cacao nibs, bone broth, dairy, and other animal products for the whole day.

- **Try not to use vinegar and salt.** If you really want them, use them sparingly.

- Instead, **focus on fruits, vegetables, and leafy greens** and recipes from Chapter 23 for your entire first day back. This is a great chance to use up any leftover potatoes, sweet potatoes, yams, winter squash, brussels sprouts, asparagus, and the like.

- If you can get **one celery juice** and **at least one apple** into your day, all the better.

SECOND DAY POST-CLEANSE

- On your second post-cleanse day, see if you can **try the Morning Cleanse again.**

- Continue to **use vinegar and salt** sparingly, if at all.

- Later in the day is a good time to reintroduce radical fats if you're missing them. **Stick to one serving of radical fats, either of animal protein–based or plant-based fats;** if you're a big fan of both, go with one little serving of each, and again, make it at the end of the day.

- **It's totally acceptable if you want to keep avoiding radical fats instead.** Staying off them for a longer period will continue some of the cleansing and allow you to keep getting positive results.

- Again, post-cleanse is still a great time to **turn to the recipes in Chapter 23 for meal and snack ideas** so you have healing options to support you as you continue on your path.

MORE TRANSITION OPTIONS

Incorporating the **Heavy Metal Detox Smoothie** into your transition from the cleanse is a great way to catch any leftover toxic heavy metals in your system. Whether or not you were incorporating the heavy metal detox modification from Chapter 21, "Cleanse Adaptations and Substitutions," into your Original or Simplified 3:6:9 Cleanse, bringing the smoothie into your post-cleanse life for a little while can be very beneficial. Ideally, drink the Heavy Metal Detox Smoothie in the morning for at least seven to fourteen days after the 3:6:9 Cleanse.

You're also welcome to use the cleanses from Part III, "Other Life-Saving Medical Medium Cleanses," as transition methods. For example, you could keep following the **Morning Cleanse** routine from Chapter 16 or **keep avoiding troublemaker foods** from Chapter 15, "Anti-Bug Cleanse," for as long as you'd like.

Keep in mind that some troublemaker foods feed the very bugs that make us sick. Pathogens such as EBV, shingles, HHV-6, HHV-7, herpes simplex 1 and 2, CMV, and other viruses, along with bacteria such as strep and *E. coli*, all prosper when we're eating foods these bugs like. When we keep those troublemaker foods out of our diet, the pathogens starve. As you'll see in more detail in Part VI, "Knowing the Cause and the Protocol," those viruses and bacteria are involved in the majority of chronic symptoms and conditions, so if you're dealing with a chronic health issue, the longer you keep out some or all of the troublemaker foods, the better.

That said, try not to become overwhelmed with this advice. These longer-term practices are only meant to empower you if you'd like to keep healing after the 3:6:9 Cleanse. The supplement lists in Part VI are also there to offer you individualized support.

No matter how you choose to proceed after completing the 3:6:9 Cleanse, know that you've succeeded already in so much cleansing and healing. You've moved yourself forward greatly.

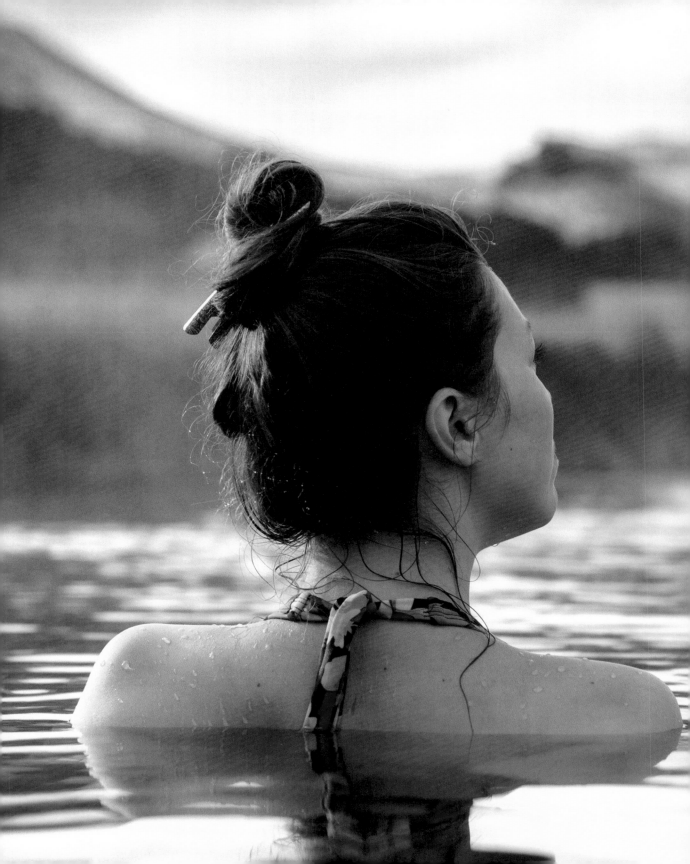

PART III

OTHER LIFE-SAVING MEDICAL MEDIUM CLEANSES

CHAPTER 15

Anti-Bug Cleanse

A very simple way to approach cleansing is to decide you're going to remove certain foods from your diet for a period of time in favor of more healing foods. That's because the goal of cleansing is to assist your body with flushing out toxins and starving bugs such as viruses and unproductive bacteria—and certain foods actively feed pathogens or make it difficult or almost impossible for certain varieties of toxins and poisons to exit your organs and bloodstream. It matters greatly which foods you remove. Awareness here is an important tool so you can succeed in your cleansing process. In Chapter 7, "Troublemaker Foods," you discovered what to avoid and why. This chapter will provide a structured plan for giving your body a break from those troublemaker foods.

THE ANTI-BUG CLEANSE

First, let's look at the basics of how the Anti-Bug Cleanse works.

What

- Drink at least 16 ounces of fresh celery juice on an empty stomach when you get up for the day. Wait 15 to 20 minutes, and ideally 30 minutes, after finishing your celery juice before eating or drinking anything else.

- Keep troublemaker foods out of your diet. In this chapter, you'll find a table of the troublemaker foods divided up into levels. You choose which level of foods to remove from your diet, depending on your state of health and how much progress you'd like to make. It's up to you whether that's Level 1, an intermediate level, or whether you feel ready to eliminate all the foods through Level 5. There are even bonus ingredients to watch out for if you're looking for the fastest, best results.

- Over the course of each day, drink at least 1 liter of water. That's roughly equivalent to 32 ounces of water, or 4 cups. Make sure to space it apart from the celery juice. Also, try not to drink your water at the same time that you're eating food. It's okay to sip coconut water, as long as it isn't pink or red and doesn't contain natural flavors, or the Hot Spiced Apple Juice recipe, at any temperature, from Chapter 23. Any coconut water or apple juice you sip would be *in addition* to your liter of water. (You're welcome to drink more than 1 liter of water. If you feel you require more fluids at any point throughout the cleanse, don't hold back; allow yourself to improve your water levels. Do avoid water with a pH above 8.0. To find out why, see Chapter 19, "Critical Cleanse Dos and Don'ts.")

How Long

- For the Anti-Bug Cleanse, remove the troublemaker foods from the level of your choice (and keep up with the celery juice) for **at least two weeks**.

- If you can, aim for one full month off the foods. You're also welcome to keep going past that for as long as you'd like.

Why

- Celery juice is a part of every day because it helps flush out old troublemaker foods from your system faster. It also assists with killing off bugs such as viruses and bacteria. (If you have no access to celery or can't tolerate it, turn to "Celery Juice" in Chapter 21, "Cleanse Adaptations and Substitutions.")

- These foods don't leave your system the moment you stop eating them. It takes some time for their byproducts to leave your system. Dairy, for example, floats around in your blood and lymph and clings to and accumulates along the walls of your small intestinal tract and colon. It takes 11 to 13 days for this dairy film to leave once you've eliminated the food from your diet. Gluten takes about 9 to 11 days to exit the blood, lymph, and gut. Eggs take about 7 to 9 days.

- That's not to mention the dairy, gluten, and egg particles in your liver. To get rid of those, it takes 90 days off dairy, gluten, and eggs. To varying degrees, most everybody's liver is stagnant and sluggish. Because this precious filter gets overburdened, overloaded, and congested, these particles need time to exit your liver.

- You may wonder why the 3:6:9 Cleanse is only nine days. That's because on the 3:6:9, you're doing so much else on top of removing troublemaker foods that you accelerate detoxification.

- By giving your body a chance to rid itself of troublemaker foods over 14 days (and ideally 28 days or more) on the Anti-Bug Cleanse, you give your blood, lymph, and intestinal tract a fresh start. This is extremely helpful for beginning to see improvements or maintaining progress in symptoms and overall health.

TROUBLEMAKER FOODS LIST

LEVEL 1	Eggs Dairy Gluten Soft drinks Be mindful of salt consumption
LEVEL 2	All of the above PLUS: Pork Tuna Corn
LEVEL 3	All of the above PLUS: Industrial food oils (vegetable oil, palm oil, canola oil, corn oil, safflower oil, soybean oil) Soy Lamb Fish and seafood (other than salmon, trout, and sardines)
LEVEL 4	All of the above PLUS: Vinegar (including apple cider vinegar) Fermented foods (including kombucha, sauerkraut, and coconut aminos) Caffeine (including coffee, matcha, and chocolate)
LEVEL 5	All of the above PLUS: Grains (millet and oats are okay) All oils (including healthier ones such as olive, walnut, sunflower, coconut, sesame, avocado, grapeseed, almond, macadamia, peanut, flaxseed)

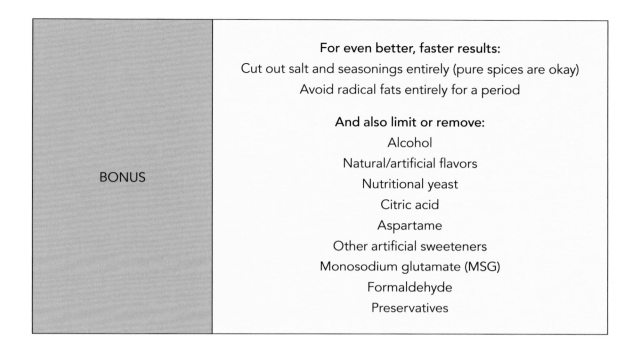

BONUS

For even better, faster results:
Cut out salt and seasonings entirely (pure spices are okay)
Avoid radical fats entirely for a period

And also limit or remove:
Alcohol
Natural/artificial flavors
Nutritional yeast
Citric acid
Aspartame
Other artificial sweeteners
Monosodium glutamate (MSG)
Formaldehyde
Preservatives

WHY TO REMOVE TROUBLEMAKER FOODS

For a refresher on the details of what makes these foods problematic for our health, page back to Chapter 7. Here, let's consider the foundations of why you'd want to give your body a break from the troublemaker foods:

Some foods are blood thickeners due to their fat content. They thicken the blood to such a degree that toxins stay suspended in the blood and never leave—until we cleanse. Our bloodstream is how toxins are eventually supposed to find their way to our kidneys and intestinal tract to be eliminated. When thick blood blocks that from happening, then in addition to staying suspended, some toxins go back into organs, fat cells, connective tissue, and even bones, which is unknown to medical research and science. "Storage bins" of fat in the body tend to hold on to highly toxic material such as old adrenaline, viral waste matter, and toxic heavy metals.

Some foods dehydrate your body, which also thickens the blood, contributing to dirty blood syndrome (read more about this condition in *Liver Rescue*). When you're chronically dehydrated on a deep level, it's almost impossible to achieve elimination of toxins from the organs, bloodstream, and body.

Some foods contribute new toxins to the body. You may be trying other beneficial measures such as celery juice or a cleanse in this book, and if you're keeping these foods in, you may find your progress stationary. Even as your other steps are trying to take toxins out, these foods are adding new toxins back into your system. It's like trying to bail out a boat that's taking on water.

Some foods feed bugs. Since viruses and unproductive bacteria are behind so many of the chronic symptoms and illnesses that hold people back in life, starving these pathogens is a priority if you want to safeguard your health.

By removing foods from each of those categories—blood thickeners, dehydrators, toxin contributors, and bug fuel—you gently allow your body to start to let go. And because certain toxins themselves feed viruses and bacteria, you're getting rid of yet another fuel source for those pathogens by cleansing toxins out. Removing both foods and toxins that feed pathogens is what makes this the Anti-Bug Cleanse. (Keep in mind that any other Medical Medium cleanse is antiviral and antibacterial too.)

Avoiding troublemaker foods doesn't guarantee you'll see an immediate shift in your health. For example, you could still be eating rich meals with high ratios of fats, or you may not be bringing in enough fruits, vegetables, and leafy greens to deliver healing nutrition to your body. If you're looking for more dramatic results, you can build on this chapter by incorporating the Morning Cleanse and Heavy Metal Detox Cleanse suggestions from the coming chapters at the same time. Or jump straight into the 3:6:9 Cleanse, which is designed to tap into your liver's natural cycles of cleansing for accelerated full-body benefits. Removing these troublemaker foods is a cornerstone of the 3:6:9 Cleanse.

If the Anti-Bug Cleanse is all you do for now, know that it's still an achievement. It's an amazing first step or ongoing life practice—you decide.

Informed Decisions

On the troublemaker foods list, you'll see that the foods are divided up by level, with Level 1 being the most important to remove if you want to make progress with your health. Which level you try is in your hands. You can always start with whichever feels comfortable now and work your way up to another later.

If you have a negative association with removing foods from your diet because of past diet protocols where food was eliminated—for example, for food allergy testing—please know that those were man-made programs. Their makers are unaware of what causes chronic illnesses such as autoimmune disease and how food plays a role. Those are guessing games that we don't play here. Only here will you find food empowerment and the ability to take control of your healing process using real knowledge. I recommend that you consider shifting your thinking from not being "allowed" to eat certain items to *choosing* not to for now. Because it truly is your choice. As I always say, I'm not the food police. This list is here so you can make informed decisions about what foods may prevent you from experiencing the health that you deserve.

Let's also be clear that none of the foods here are listed as problematic out of prejudice against a dietary belief system such as veganism, vegetarianism, plant-based eating, paleo philosophy, or the ketogenic theory. Nor is this cleanse about self-deprivation, starvation, or shame. The foods are listed solely because they pose the risk that you will not succeed with your cleansing and healing process.

An Opportunity to Heal

Leaving these foods out of your diet also creates an opportunity: to make your snacks and meals count for more. Instead of relying on foods that actively work against healing and detox, you'll now have room to bring in ingredients that work *with* your body. Feeling lost about what to eat? The recipes you'll find in Chapter 23 are full of ideas.

Cravings are natural. If you find yourself processing emotions, feeling left out in social situations, or missing favorite foods as you take a break from the items in the troublemaker foods list, turn to Chapter 25, "The Emotional Side of Cleansing." Also refer to Chapter 20, "Your Body's Healing Power." In both places, you'll find help with riding it all out so you can come out stronger on the other side.

A STEP FURTHER

If you want to take it a step further, you can expand your awareness beyond food. When you're putting so much care into what you do and don't put into your body, it makes sense to be mindful of pollutants that you may be breathing, bathing in, putting on your skin, or being exposed to in other ways.

You may want to revisit the guidance on this in Chapter 3, "A Wake-Up Call to What's Inside Us." While you can't control everything you're exposed to—you can't will a truck that's spewing heavy exhaust not to merge in front of you on the highway, for example, and you probably can't keep your neighbor from spraying pesticides on their lawn—you can make simple changes to limit or avoid many troublemakers. It's yet one more way to safeguard yourself when you're trying to cleanse.

"You just found something different. You found an escape hatch. And you found it for a reason."

— Anthony William, Medical Medium

CHAPTER 16

Morning Cleanse

No one likes to be rushed in the morning. What if you were prevented from following your morning routine? Is it important to you? What if you didn't have time to pick out an outfit, brush your teeth, take a shower, exercise, do your meditations, prayers, or affirmations, or whatever it takes to get you ready for the day? What if the moment you woke up, you were prevented from doing all of it because calls came through—important ones related to commitments, jobs, responsibilities, or friends or family members who needed your help or guidance in that very moment? You rely on your routine, a routine that starts your day on a good note.

What if you were interrupted every day of your life without fail? What if you never got your morning routine back and it never changed for the better? When we bombard our liver with the wrong food and liquid choices every morning, we unknowingly take away our liver's critical morning routine of ridding toxins. We compromise the very essence of our health and well-being. The consequences are far more serious than missing morning meditation or toothbrushing or exercise or phone time—or avoidance of your phone, if that's part of your routine. Our liver, other organs, lymphatic system, and bloodstream cannot cleanse or detox the troublemakers they're trying to discard when we don't let them.

Consuming radical fats such as bacon, eggs, milk, cheese, butter, yogurt, bone broth, avocado, chocolate, cacao nibs, nuts, nut milk, nut butters, and seeds in the morning—even mid-morning or late morning—thickens our blood just when our body is trying to complete its morning cleansing routine, and that means the blood becomes dirty with suspended toxins that can't leave the bloodstream. On top of which, we're often chronically dehydrated. When the liquids we consume are coffee, matcha tea, black tea, or energy drinks, that dehydrates us more, which further thickens the blood.

As a result of radical fats in our morning food and drinks, our liver overworks itself, creating an overload of bile to break down those fats. If we ate a dinner that was high in fat the night before, our liver was already struggling to process it while we were sleeping. That's on top of our liver working hard overnight to gather up and package poisons and toxins so they could be eliminated come morning. Every day that we bring fats into our morning with our early meals, we prevent our body from completing its natural detox routine.

On the other hand, every morning we work *with* our body by getting properly hydrated and keeping out radical fats, we guide ourselves toward healing. That's the purpose of the Morning Cleanse.

THE MORNING CLEANSE

This Morning Cleanse is an opportunity to allow your liver to perform its proper routine. If you're familiar with my book *Liver Rescue*, you'll notice that this cleanse aligns with the Liver Rescue Morning there, with an upgrade: it includes celery juice for even better results. Here are the Morning Cleanse guidelines:

What

- *Optional:* Drink 16 to 32 ounces of lemon or lime water upon waking. (See Chapter 23 for the recipe with the proper ratio of lemon or lime to water. This isn't about squeezing 10 lemons into a glass of water.) Wait 15 to 30 minutes, and then:

- **Drink 16 to 32 ounces of fresh celery juice on an empty stomach.** Wait 15 to 30 minutes before eating or drinking anything else.

- **Don't consume radical fats before lunchtime.** That means no nuts, seeds, peanut butter, any oils, coconut, avocado, cacao nibs, chocolate, ghee, milk, cream, yogurt, coconut yogurt, cheese, butter, kefir, bacon, eggs, bone broth, or any other animal proteins in the morning. They should all wait until lunch or after.

- **Keep out dried fruits and salt all morning** so you don't work against the cleanse.

- **Also stay hydrated, making sure that if possible, you choose juicy, water-rich fruits during the morning. Additionally, drink a minimum of 16 ounces of water or coconut water** (as long as it isn't pink or red and doesn't contain natural flavors) over the course of your morning, at some point after your lemon or lime water and celery juice.

- If you want to elevate the results you experience from the Morning Cleanse, also skip the troublemaker foods from Chapter 7 all morning—and ideally, all day.

How Long

- Follow the Morning Cleanse guidelines for at least **two weeks** at a time.

- Why not adopt the Morning Cleanse as a life habit, incorporating it into your daily routine alongside other practices like brushing your teeth?

Why

- As you read in Chapter 3, "A Wake-Up Call to What's Inside Us," we are walking around with many different toxins and pathogens inside our body, and we need to help them cleanse. The Morning Cleanse is a good way to be proactive and take preventative steps to help protect yourself from illness down the road.

- In addition to giving your liver a break, the absence of radical fats also helps you build up precious glucose reserves so that your muscles and nerves can receive the fuel they need to both strengthen muscles and restore nerve cells.

- As in the Anti-Bug Cleanse, you'll bring in celery juice every morning to provide sodium cluster salts to your cells and organs in order to help bind onto toxins, poisons, and pathogens and eliminate them out of the body. (If you have no access to celery or can't tolerate it, turn to "Celery Juice" in Chapter 21, "Cleanse Adaptations and Substitutions.")

Morning Cleanse Tips

- If you work a night shift, with your day starting in the afternoon or evening, then consider your "morning" the first

several hours after you've gotten up for your day.

- For this cleanse to give your body its needed break, the morning needs to be truly free from radical fats. That means no spoonful of peanut butter, no butter on your toast, no coconut oil or whey protein powder in your smoothie, no milk, no cheese, no coconut yogurt, no avocado toast, no cacao nibs or chocolate, and no almond butter or similar common morning foods.

- The ideal breakfast is a bowl of fresh fruit or a fruit smoothie—as long as that smoothie isn't blending in whey protein powder, peanut butter, almond butter, other nut butters, cacao powder or nibs, avocado, yogurt, dairy milk, nut milk, coconut milk, egg, or other sources of radical fat. See the smoothie recipes in Chapter 23. Keep your smoothie focused on fruit and, if you want them, leafy greens—just so long as the greens don't out-ratio the fruit. Without enough fruit in your smoothie, it won't keep you full enough, and you may find yourself tempted to reach for a handful of nuts or a protein bar to get you through your morning instead of honoring the guidelines of the Morning Cleanse.

- Steamed potatoes, sweet potatoes (including Japanese sweet potatoes), yams, winter squash, millet, or oatmeal are good options if you're looking for a cooked breakfast that will work within the Morning Cleanse guidelines—just as long as they aren't cooked in dairy milk, nut milk, or oil; served with cream, butter, or cheese; or topped with peanut or almond butter, seeds, nutty granola, cacao nibs, or other radical fats.

- It's fine and even good to snack throughout your morning, just so long as it's on fruit as your first choice or steamed potatoes, sweet potatoes (including Japanese sweet potatoes), yams, winter squash, millet, or oatmeal if you need a filling option in late morning.

- You'll find more breakfast ideas that support the Morning Cleanse in Chapter 23, "Cleanse Recipes."

INTERMITTENT FASTING OPTION

While I don't normally recommend intermittent fasting, this is an option for intermittent fasting enthusiasts. If you're going to try the technique, this is the proper way to do it. Please read more in Chapter 5, "Intermittent Fasting Revealed."

- Drink 24 to 32 ounces of lemon or lime water upon waking. (See Chapter 23 for the recipe with the proper ratio of lemon or lime to water.) Wait 15 to 60 minutes, and then:

- Throughout your morning, sip at least 32 ounces of celery juice. (You can work up to 64 ounces of celery juice if

you want more.) After you've finished your celery juice, wait at least 15 minutes, and then:

- Sip 16 to 32 ounces of lemon or lime water (with 1 teaspoon of raw honey added). You have the option of replacing up to 24 ounces of lemon or lime water with up to 24 ounces of coconut water. If so, find a coconut water that isn't pink or red and doesn't contain natural flavors.

That's it. Stick with lemon or lime water, followed by celery juice, followed by lemon or lime water (with raw honey) and/or coconut water. That means you're not reaching for coffee, matcha tea, energy drinks, or bone broth. I am not recommending that you run on caffeine and withhold food all day. It's best to eat within four to six hours of waking. This is a safer version of intermittent fasting. I would still prefer that you adopt the Morning Cleanse or one of the other cleanses in this book.

While my normal recommendation is not to treat celery juice as a meal replacement because it's not a calorie source (and therefore I usually say to follow it up with breakfast after 15 to 60 minutes), there are intermittent fasting enthusiasts out there who wonder how they can incorporate celery juice into their lives. This option is the answer.

This option fits within intermittent fasting because in the course of your morning, you're not adding any fat calories. When you intermittent fast, what you're really taking a break from are fats, and it's unknown that it's this break from fats that helps some people maintain or lose weight temporarily. (Again, refer to Chapter 5 for more on this.) And one of the real reasons that some people feel an improvement of energy and clarity when intermittent fasting is because energy that would normally go into digestive strength to break down fats in the morning is transferred to other body systems. There are more sustainable ways to lower the fats in your life for more lasting results, methods explored throughout this book.

The intermittent fasts that incorporate coffee with butter aren't giving your body true relief, because they're still bringing in fat, not to mention caffeine. Limiting your morning to lemon or lime water, a teaspoon of raw honey, celery juice, and optional coconut water limits calories and keeps out food, as intermittent fasters desire, while also doing what you really need to get results with your health: keeping fat out of your morning so your body can remain in its cleanse state from the night before. The option we've just reviewed gives you that respite from digesting fats. So does the Morning Cleanse and every other cleanse in this book.

"Spirit of Compassion has always said to me
throughout the years of helping so many people heal
that knowing the true cause of why you're sick is half the battle won.
Knowing what to do, what to take, and how to apply
those tools is the other half the battle won."

— Anthony William, Medical Medium

CHAPTER 17

Heavy Metal Detox Cleanse

Almost nobody believes they've been exposed to toxic heavy metals. If you're wondering if you have toxic heavy metals and where they could have come from, these suggestions may offer enlightenment:

Have you ever had a stick of gum that was wrapped in a foil wrapper? Have you ever used aluminum foil at a cookout, eaten from an aluminum takeout container, or used aluminum kitchen tools? Have you ever sipped seltzer, beer, or soft drinks from an aluminum can?

What about silver fillings? Many people have been exposed to mercury through metal amalgam dental fillings. Having them removed isn't as easy a fix as it sounds. The extraction process can re-expose someone to the mercury the fillings contain, because removal emits mercury vapor that can easily enter the bloodstream. That's why I recommend only having one silver filling removed per dentist's visit, and that's only if the silver filling is starting to fall apart or loosen or if there's a problem with the tooth.

Have you ever had a fluoride treatment? Even if not recently, have you had one at any point over the years, perhaps going back to childhood? The fluoride used for treatments is a byproduct of aluminum—a methyl-aluminum neurotoxin created

from manufacturing aluminum. Almost all of us have been exposed to it in one way or another, whether from fluoride treatments, toothpaste, or fluoridated tap water, and if we've had that exposure, it hasn't left our bodies unless we've taken the proper steps to remove it.

Speaking of tap water, town and city water supplies all have trace levels of toxic heavy metals such as lead, arsenic, copper, aluminum, and even mercury that are deemed safe enough for consumption without true knowledge of what happens when those trace metals accumulate in our system over time. Even if you use water filtration at home, you're exposed when eating out. Consider, for example, getting coffee at your favorite coffee shop. One cup of coffee made from the shop's tap water seems perfectly safe. So does one glass of tap water with tap water ice in a restaurant, or one cup of tea brewed with tap water, or one soda made from a soda fountain that's hooked up to an unfiltered water line. No one thinks about what happens after 10 years of stopping by for coffee every day, or drinking restaurant tap water several times a week—what that accumulation of lead, aluminum, mercury, arsenic, and copper can do inside your liver and brain. And what about the water you've used to bathe or brush your teeth? Have you ever used water that flowed through copper (or even lead) pipes that were leaching? You would be surprised how many houses and hotels have copper pipes with lead-based fittings.

Do you ever eat out, consuming food cooked with metal utensils scraping already scratched stainless steel pots and pans? Restaurants are one of the most common sources of toxic heavy metal exposure—not that it's the fault of the well-meaning people who run and work in restaurants.

People keep knives in their households for decades, continually sharpening them over time so that they get smaller and smaller. Did you ever wonder how your knives at home end up dull? The metal particles that made those once-sharp edges have found their way inside our food and inside our bodies. That's not to mention our worn silverware. Where do you think those metal particles went?

What about the tuna roll you've enjoyed from your favorite sushi bar or tuna melt from your local diner, or any other fish you've eaten? Or maybe you're eating grass-fed beef instead, so you think you're in the clear. Don't think beef is heavy metal–free. Toxic heavy metals fall from the sky every day and land on fields of grass on which cattle graze, and those toxic heavy metals end up in their meat. And never mind industrial-raised beef, which has more toxic heavy metals than grass-fed.

What about pharmaceuticals? All pharmaceuticals contain some variety of toxic heavy metal, whether aluminum, copper, or even platinum or mercury. From the simplest pharmaceutical to the most aggressive, there's always a toxic heavy metal about.

In the air we breathe, there are toxic heavy metals. They spew out of car exhaust in traffic, in the gasoline as it's burning. Toxic heavy metals fall out of the sky, from pesticides and herbicides in our local area and from DDT that drifts from continent to continent through the airstream. (DDT, other pesticides, and herbicides are major copper contributors.) Toxic heavy metals also drop down on us in the rain.

And you already read about even more toxic heavy metal exposures in Chapter 3, "A Wake-Up Call to What's Inside Us."

Truth is, many varieties of toxic heavy metals build up in us over time, and these are only some of the opportunities we have every day for collecting toxic heavy metals in our bodies. Toxic heavy metals are hidden and unseeable; it's impossible to witness that they reside within us. No technology has been created yet to truly determine the toxic heavy metals inside our organs. The need for such technology isn't even on research's and science's radar, so there's no intention to create this method of testing. Its development hasn't even been conceived of and isn't in the works. While direct exposure to a large amount of a metal such as lead can be detected in our bloodstream, that's an entirely different story from the toxic heavy metals that build up in our organs from year after year of exposure. Toxic heavy metals don't just float around in our bloodstream and leave. They sink deep into our tissue. This everyday type of toxic heavy metal accumulation is a great part of why our society is so sick today—and it should receive attention.

Instead, medical research and science tend to blame chronic illnesses on faulty bodies, genes, and the theory that the body can go haywire and attack itself. If science really looks into toxic heavy metals and brings the truth to light one day, it will mean a total revamp of our pharmaceutical system (because all drugs have toxic heavy metals in them) and an outcry of people who have been wronged by unnecessary exposure. You can imagine, then, that the reality of how often we encounter toxic heavy metals and what they do to us is going to remain hidden for the foreseeable future.

Rather than waiting for the world to catch up, it's in your hands to do something about toxic heavy metals now—by embarking on this detox to get them out of your system on a daily basis so you and your family can experience better health.

WHAT TOXIC HEAVY METALS DO TO US

Much as we may not want to believe it, we all have toxic heavy metals inside of our bodies. Mercury, aluminum, copper, lead, nickel, cadmium, barium, arsenic, and toxic calcium accumulate in different areas of different organs. The two most popular places that they gather are the brain and the liver.

Toxic heavy metals carry a disruptive charge that interferes with the electricity that travels through your brain. Neurotransmitter chemicals are meant to use the electrical neural highway there to carry information and life force to every cell in your brain. When toxic heavy metals such as mercury and aluminum are present, though, electrical impulses weaken as they hit these deposits. Electrical activity becomes diffused, and that leads to a host of symptoms and conditions that can develop over a lifetime. Brain fog, memory issues, confusion, anxiety, and depression are just a few. Toxic heavy metals in the brain can also lead to Alzheimer's disease, dementia, amyotrophic lateral sclerosis (ALS), Parkinson's disease, and even diagnoses such as bipolar disorder, mania, and schizophrenia.

It's not only the heavy metal deposits themselves that can be a problem. Toxic heavy metals also oxidize (picture rusting metal), releasing a discharge of heavy metal byproduct, which can travel to adjacent brain cells and affect more neurons, causing additional or worsened symptoms throughout the years. Heavy metals also interact with each other, becoming something more troublesome than what they already are when they stand alone. For example, when mercury and aluminum cross paths and touch each other, a highly toxic reaction occurs and they can both oxidize more rapidly. The result is a discharge causing neurological symptoms such as tremors, twitching, depression, anxiety, seizures, weak limbs, and memory loss.

At the same time, everyone has pathogens inside their bodies, ranging from many different strains and varieties of unproductive bacteria to many different strains and varieties of unproductive viruses. The Epstein-Barr virus, of which there are over 60 varieties, is a common one inside almost everyone. Here's why that's significant when it comes to the need to detox heavy metals: EBV has the ability to feed on toxic heavy metals in the body and then release a much more potent form of those metals as viral byproduct. Many toxic heavy metals sit inside the liver, which is also a popular place for viruses to reside. There, the heavy metals become an easy source of food for the viruses to continually feed on, and then release their poisons. These *neurotoxins* that viruses (such as EBV) expel after feeding on toxic heavy metals (such as mercury) create so many of the symptoms that sufferers of autoimmune disease experience. The neurological symptoms of fibromyalgia, MS, Lyme disease, RA, Hashimoto's, and ME/CFS, as well as stand-alone symptoms such as fatigue, aches, pains, tingles, numbness, vertigo, dizziness, tinnitus, eye floaters, nerve pain, neuropathy, heart palpitations, burning skin, and migraines—to name just a few—are a result of these neurotoxins.

By now you can see the value of getting toxic heavy metals out of your body. The Heavy Metal Detox Cleanse is critical for anyone struggling with the above symptoms and conditions and also critical for eczema, psoriasis, vitiligo, or any similar skin condition. Eczema and psoriasis are signs of someone dealing with an elevation of toxic copper inside the liver, where EBV is also present and feeding on the heavy metal, in this case creating an internal *dermatoxin* that medical research and science are unaware exists, let alone is involved in these conditions. The dermatoxin is pushed into the bloodstream, from which it surfaces to the derma and causes the patchy, scaly, itchy, rough, inflamed, or irritated skin that eczema, psoriasis, and dermatitis sufferers know too well. Vitiligo is an overload of aluminum in the liver, with a virus (usually HHV-6 and sometimes a variety of EBV) also present in the liver feeding on the toxic heavy metal and releasing a dermatoxin that destroys the pigment-forming cells in the skin.

Young children with levels of undetected mercury and aluminum inside the liver and brain often deal with attention-deficit/hyperactivity disorder (ADHD), difficulty regulating concentration and focus, learning differences, and behavioral issues. Obsessive-compulsive disorder, Tourette's syndrome, autism, and episodes of unwarranted anger and depersonalization are also a result of toxic heavy metals. Depression, anxiety, and insomnia are earlier-in-life signs of heavy metals too. If the toxic heavy metals in the brain that are causing any of these symptoms and conditions aren't removed and dealt with, toxic heavy metal accumulation and oxidation can lead to more serious issues: memory problems, dementia, Alzheimer's, or near-crippling OCD or schizophrenia.

So toxic heavy metals can create symptoms. Symptoms can, in part, shape who we are. They become a part of us as we have to live around them, act around them, work with or around them, and try to survive or thrive around them. Most people have toxic heavy metal symptoms that they have no idea are metal-related—it seems almost inconceivable. Once you work on removing heavy metals in yourself and your loved ones, though, and see what symptoms lift as a result, the changes you experience can reshape your life.

THE HEAVY METAL DETOX CLEANSE

Now let's look at the method for removing toxic heavy metals:

What

- Drink 16 to 32 ounces of lemon or lime water upon waking. (See Chapter 23 for the recipe with the proper ratio of lemon or lime to water.) Wait 15 to 30 minutes, and then:

- Drink 16 to 32 ounces of celery juice on an empty stomach. Wait at least 15 to 30 minutes, and then:

- Drink the Heavy Metal Detox Smoothie. You'll find the recipe on page 300. If you prefer, you can enjoy the smoothie ingredients separately instead of blending them—see "Smoothie Alternative" in a few pages.

- If you get hungry again before lunchtime, stick to snacking on apples (have more than one if you want). You're welcome to chop or blend your apples, create the raw Applesauce recipe in Chapter 23, go with cooked applesauce (as long as it doesn't contain additives), or opt for ripe pears if apples don't work for you.

- *Optional:* For even better results, take a look at the troublemaker foods list in Chapter 7 and start chipping away at it, seeing what foods there you'd like to avoid while you're on this cleanse. The fewer troublemaker foods in your diet, the more effective the Heavy Metal Detox Smoothie can be.

How Long

- Give this cleanse a **three-month** trial. Stick with the protocol every morning for 90 days to give it a real chance to make a difference in your life.

- If you can do it for six months or more, all the better, especially if you're dealing with disruptive symptoms and conditions.

- You can keep going past three to six months. If you're dealing with symptoms or an illness that metals could be contributing to, or if you're concerned about prevention, you have the option of doing the cleanse for a year or more to dig out deep-seated toxic heavy metals from the brain. It's also perfectly fine to adopt the practice of the Heavy Metal Detox Smoothie for life.

Why

- You'll start the day with lemon or lime water to prime the toxic heavy metals in your system to be more easily removed. It's imperative that you're hydrated enough that when the Heavy Metal Detox Smoothie starts uprooting metals and trying to remove them, you have adequate hydration to flush them out of your system. (If you're sensitive to lemons and limes, turn to Chapter 21, "Cleanse Adaptations and Substitutions," for guidance.)

- Celery juice comes next to loosen up metals, preparing them to be gathered up by the Heavy Metal Detox Smoothie. Celery juice also helps restore areas inside organs that have been damaged by toxic heavy metals, while the sodium cluster salts in celery juice help disarm the toxic charge of toxic heavy metals, making them less harmful. (If you have no access to celery juice or can't tolerate it, again, turn to Chapter 21.)

- The Heavy Metal Detox Smoothie is the main event here, the only heavy metal detox protocol available with the right combination of ingredients to extract deep-seated toxic heavy metals from your organs and round up free-floating metals and oxidative runoff that's also causing trouble, and carry it all safely out of your body. You'll find much more on how this works and why it's important in the pages that follow.

- If you're hungry later in the morning, apples are an excellent snack because they're a powerful medicinal cleansing food. The pectin in apples helps absorb bile coming from the liver into the intestinal tract—bile that may have traces of toxic heavy metals in it due to the Heavy Metal Detox Smoothie uprooting them from the liver.

- You're keeping your morning free from radical fats because you want to keep your blood from thickening so that the toxic heavy metals can detox more easily.

HOW THE HEAVY METAL DETOX WORKS

Removing toxic heavy metals from the body is kind of like playing the old medical children's game *Operation*. To be successful in *Operation*, you must grip a pair of tweezers and carefully remove tiny bones and organs from the cartoon body on the game board without hitting the sides of the cutouts—which sets off an alarm buzzer—or dropping the game pieces. It's all about having a steady hand. While extracting heavy metals is much more complex, the same idea of steadiness applies. For a heavy metal detox protocol to be effective, it's important that the tools and method you choose do not drop the toxic heavy metals along the way and cause disruption, which is the problem that other heavy metal "detox" protocols create. When you don't cleanse toxic heavy metals properly, you end up dropping the metals and losing the game.

Five Key Tools

There are suggestions out there in the alternative medicine world about toxic heavy metal chelation. Chlorella, for example, is often recommended to remove heavy metals from the body. Here's the truth: if this were *Operation*, chlorella would be setting off that alarm buzzer right and left. That's because chlorella does have the potential to dislodge some heavy metals—recklessly. When it does pick up toxic heavy metals, it drops them again soon and releases them into nearby tissue—which can guarantee old symptoms continuing, new symptoms beginning, or a combination of both.

Herbs such as garlic are sometimes recommended for removing toxic heavy metals. While at least garlic doesn't tend to drop metals along the way, that's mostly because it doesn't dislodge or remove toxic heavy metals too much in the first place. Its skill is in the intestinal tract. The sulfur compound in garlic creates an expectorant-like reaction, with mucus forming in a positive way around blood vessels inside the intestinal tract. This can, at best, sometimes loosen some toxic heavy metals there. Garlic is a standout in other ways. It's amazing for the immune system. It's simply not a specialty heavy metal detox tool.

Heavy metal detox is all about specialty tools—they're critical for doing it right. Without them, you're further away from removing these metals. The key ingredients of the Heavy Metal Detox Smoothie are:

- **Wild blueberries** (available frozen or as pure wild blueberry powder)
- **Spirulina** (find the correct kind in my supplement directory at www.medicalmedium.com)
- **Barley grass juice powder** (find the correct kind in my supplement directory)
- **Fresh cilantro**
- **Atlantic dulse**

The right bodily environment is also key for sending toxic heavy metals out of your organs, bloodstream, and eventually body.

Techniques you'll hear about elsewhere are too harsh and abrasive—and again, they drop metals along the way while still in the body. Some techniques can carry the heavy metals a little farther along in the body than others; nevertheless, they still let go too soon, allowing the metals to settle in the organs again. Being mindful of this means everything when we're trying to cleanse something that's been in our body since conception—and that's how it is with toxic heavy metals, because we first receive them passed down from the sperm and egg that created us, likely collected more in utero, and then continued to acquire them continually from early life through the present.

An Easter Egg Hunt

Not all toxic heavy metals in the body are difficult to reach. Some may be in the kidneys, so once they're dislodged from the kidneys' inside linings, they don't have far to travel to leave the body; we immediately urinate them out. It may take only one ingredient out of the five to completely dislodge these toxic heavy metals. Some toxic heavy metals are going to be in similarly easy-to-reach spots such as the small intestinal tract; it may only take two of the five ingredients to collect them and then carry them out safely all the way past the rectum through the elimination process. Some toxic heavy metals are in spots in the brain that are fairly accessible—you may only need three of the five ingredients to ensure that those metals are removed completely and travel the distance successfully. Then there are situations where toxic heavy metals have reached deeper tissue in areas of the brain and core of the liver and it's going to take four or all five ingredients to safely remove them from your body.

No matter what, you want to incorporate all five ingredients in your heavy metal detox whenever you can, because they're all there for each other as backup—and you don't know just how deeply toxic heavy metals and their debris might have settled themselves in your body. On top of which, you want the insurance policy of drinking celery juice to start your day, because its sodium cluster salts have the ability to loosen toxic heavy metals, preparing them for these five ingredients to lift them out.

This is all to say that there is no one hero of the Heavy Metal Detox Smoothie. Each ingredient has the potential to uproot heavy metals in the body, whether in easier-to-reach or unexpected places. It's like an Easter egg hunt, with each ingredient scouring your system on its own, like siblings let loose in the park for heavy metal "Easter eggs." The little sister is just as likely as the big brother to come back with a basket full of eggs, because it's all about where they happened to run. That is, if you think spirulina or cilantro is the real star of heavy metal detox, don't be surprised if as dulse happens to pass by, it sweeps up a critical deposit of toxic heavy metals that was causing a symptom that's been making life a struggle.

A Matching Game

As we covered at the beginning of this chapter, many different varieties of toxic heavy metals can take up residence in our bodies. That's another reason for the varied ingredients of the Heavy Metal Detox Smoothie—the ingredients have different degrees of carrying power for different toxic heavy metals. When you drink the smoothie, one ingredient will hold on to aluminum in your system more easily, whereas another will have more pickup power for copper or nickel, and another will do a better job with mercury. These are critical complexities that are not even considered by the makers of other toxic heavy metal removal modalities.

That's not to mention that we don't only walk around with stand-alone toxic heavy metals in our system. There are also alloys to consider—pockets of mercury and aluminum fused together, for example, or other metals that have found each other in our bodies and become one, as well as the corrosive, oxidative runoff that these metallic reactions create. Other heavy metal detox programs don't take this into account, because no one realizes this is what's happening in our bodies or that it's more difficult to dislodge and round up alloys (versus metals on their own) and alloys' debris.

Toxic heavy metal chelation processes can't just be thrown together. It takes a systematic structure to make sure that all the complexities of uprooting heavy metals are accounted for so that the toxic heavy metals actually leave the body. The true answer for tackling different toxic heavy metals in different combinations in different amounts in different areas of the body is here, in this Heavy Metal Detox Cleanse protocol. All five smoothie ingredients plus the insurance policy of celery juice's sodium cluster salts (and the bonus of drinking lemon or lime water first thing in the morning) are what will give you the results and peace of mind you deserve. (You can also make Heavy Metal Detox a part of the 3:6:9 Cleanse. See the end of this chapter for details.)

I'm really happy to see that the awareness I started sharing almost four decades ago about the toxic heavy metals we have within us and the need to detox them has kept growing. It's amazing to have gone from sharing at holistic dental conferences back then to where we are today. It's also important for you to know that this is the original source of the conversation around everyday toxic heavy metal detox, so you know that this is the original source of how to cleanse them properly.

HOW TO DEAL WITH MISSING INGREDIENTS

I know there will be days when the grocery stores in your area are out of cilantro, or when what they have in stock doesn't look fresh enough or you've run out of dulse or frozen wild blueberries. On those days, don't skip your Heavy Metal Detox Smoothie. Make it with whichever ingredients you do have. Make sure to incorporate spirulina, barley grass juice powder, and wild blueberry powder (keep this last one on hand for when you're out of frozen wild blueberries) to get yourself by until the other ingredients are available again.

If you have to miss a morning of the smoothie entirely, I understand. Try to consume the lemon or lime water, celery juice, apples, and other recipes from Chapter 23, "Cleanse Recipes," on any morning when you miss your Heavy Metal Detox Smoothie. Then add a day *with* the smoothie to the end of the cleanse to make up for any day you missed it in the middle. If, on the other hand, you eat a radical fat or troublemaker food, such as eggs, in the place of your missed Heavy Metal Detox Smoothie—or if you drink your Heavy Metal Detox Smoothie *and also* eat a radical fat or troublemaker food over the course of the morning—you'll need to add three extra days to the end of your cleanse.

SMOOTHIE ALTERNATIVE

You're not required to get the Heavy Metal Detox ingredients into yourself in smoothie form. While the Heavy Metal Detox Smoothie is the fastest, easiest way, it's not the only way. You also have the option of making sure you consume each of the five key foods over the course of 24 hours. For example, among your other snacks and meals for the day, you could decide to have 2 cups of wild blueberries with cut-up fruit in the morning, coconut water with a teaspoon each of spirulina and barley grass juice powder in the afternoon, and a salad that includes 1 cup of cilantro and 1 tablespoon of Atlantic dulse at dinner. (Another easy way to enjoy the spirulina and barley grass juice powder is to mash them into banana.)

If you opt for the Heavy Metal Detox Smoothie, your body has to do the least processing work, and toxic heavy metals will come out with less resistance. With this approach of separating and spacing out the Heavy Metal Detox ingredients, on the other hand, the body has to work a little harder to get heavy metals out. That's okay. If you don't like smoothies, don't have a blender, or for any other reason prefer this approach, it is still effective—and it's far superior to skipping the Heavy Metal Detox altogether. If you go this route of separating smoothie ingredients, still keep up with the lemon or lime water and celery juice first thing.

ADJUSTMENTS FOR CHILDREN

A child usually doesn't have the appetite for the full amount that the Heavy Metal Detox Smoothie recipe yields. To figure out the right portion for your child, think about when they're drinking a glass of apple juice—how much will they usually drink? Eight ounces? Ten or 12 ounces? Wherever you land, that's an appropriate amount of Heavy Metal Detox Smoothie to give your child. You can either reduce the recipe accordingly—for example, cutting it by half or two-thirds (making sure to keep the five key ingredients in there, in proportionate amounts)—or make the full recipe and drink the leftover that your child doesn't want. Or you can give them the ingredients separately within a 24-hour window, as in "Smoothie Alternative" above.

You can go ahead with the rest of the cleanse for your child too. It's fine to leave the lemon or lime water out for kids and also to reduce the amount of celery juice according to what feels right for your little one. See the table on page 480 for more guidance on celery juice amounts for children.

HEAVY METAL DETOX AND THE 3:6:9

It's possible to take your heavy metal detox to the next level by incorporating the Heavy Metal Detox Smoothie (or its separate ingredients) into the Original or Simplified 3:6:9 Cleanse. For guidance on what that looks like, read over the cleanse options in Chapters 10 or 11 and then turn to "Heavy Metal Detox Modification" at the beginning of Chapter 21, "Cleanse Adaptations and Substitutions."

And for the level beyond that, turn to Chapter 12, "Advanced 3:6:9 Cleanse." It already has heavy metal detox built into it, along with numerous other healing benefits.

CHAPTER 18

Mono Eating Cleanse

Mono eating can be an incredible technique for recovery from certain health issues. It has several applications, most notably for gut healing and food allergies. Mono eating saved my own life when I was a child suffering from food poisoning.

Figuring out what to eat when you're challenged with a digestive problem can feel impossible. So many people deal with celiac disease, colitis, Crohn's disease, irritable bowel syndrome (IBS), small intestinal bacterial overgrowth (SIBO), constipation, diarrhea, cramping, stomachaches, and bloating. They're at a loss about how to make food work for them as they flip-flop from trendy diet to trendy diet. This is understandable when you can't find answers about what's happening internally to cause your suffering in the first place. Diagnoses and labels of illnesses are not answers about their cause. So many people deal with undiagnosed stomach and intestinal issues too—a topic we'll cover later in this chapter. Diagnosed or undiagnosed, when no one can explain the discomfort occurring in the digestive tract, it makes many people fearful to even eat. For those who live day in and day out with gut trouble, whether it's given a name or not,

the idea of detoxing can feel out of reach. They need to know how to function and eat first.

An undiscovered aspect of many digestive issues is viral and bacterial activity. Both viruses and unproductive bacteria can embed themselves in the linings of the intestinal tract. There, these pathogens will feed on the troublemakers that pass by—pathogenic food ranging from eggs, dairy products, and gluten to toxic heavy metals. As bacteria thrive, they can irritate and inflame the linings, and as certain viruses thrive, they release neurotoxins that are highly allergenic to the intestinal nerve endings inside these linings. It's common for viruses and bacteria to live in the liver too; when viruses reside there, they often produce neurotoxins that can reach the digestive tract. Any of this can cause digestive discomfort, gastric spasms, intestinal spasms, excess gas, or even a case of ulcerative colitis. (Medical research and science are unaware that the shingles virus can cause a hemorrhaging of intestinal blood vessels.) In short, viral and bacterial activity can make the nerves attached to the intestinal walls extremely hypersensitive. This is what many are feeling as they eat and food travels through their digestive tract—they're feeling the food touch their intestinal walls and trigger off sensitive nerves that have become inflamed because of viral neurotoxins as well as bacterial activity.

Mono eating is all about addressing that dilemma. By "mono" we're not talking about mononucleosis, we're simply talking about "one." This way of eating is about eating very, very simply, sticking with only one or two (or sometimes three) specific foods in order to help your digestive tract recover. Among other benefits, the techniques that you'll find in this chapter are geared to bring life back to the stomach glands that produce gastric acid so your hydrochloric acid can restore itself in order to break down food. At the same time, these techniques improve your liver's condition. Most people's livers are stagnant and sluggish, filled with toxic troublemakers. Mono eating can cleanse the liver, restoring it so that its bile production can break down fats properly.

These plans are ideal for someone with a hypersensitive intestinal tract, because the food options are actually soothing as they move through the system. At the same time, these mono eating plans starve pathogens such as viruses and bacteria—which are so often behind gut disorders. Mono eating also offers your body a gentle detox, one that doesn't overwhelm your system.

For these reasons and more, mono eating can also be an invaluable technique for recovering from the flu, stomach bugs, food poisoning, food allergies or sensitivities, eating disorders, fasting, or ulcers, or when tremendous hardship or stress has put a strain on your digestion and made it difficult to process complicated meals. When you're going through any of these physical and emotional conditions, mono eating is here for you.

THE MONO EATING CLEANSE

Mono eating differs from the other cleanses in this book. While it does put your body into a gentle detox state and can act as a powerful mini cleanse when you want to give yourself a tune-up and heighten your senses, its main purpose is to help you get unstuck when you haven't been able to find a way forward with food. Getting yourself sorted with mono eating can allow you to try the other cleanses in this book later on, when your liver and digestive system have done some healing.

What

- *Optional:* Drink 16 to 32 ounces of lemon or lime water upon waking. (See Chapter 23 for the recipe with the proper ratio of lemon or lime to water.) Wait 15 to 30 minutes, and then:

- **Drink 16 ounces of fresh celery juice on an empty stomach in the morning. Ideally, work your way up to 24 and eventually 32 ounces of celery juice that you sip throughout the morning.** If you need to, you can split your celery juice into two servings, drinking 16 ounces in the morning and another 8 or 16 ounces later in the day. (And if you're really sensitive, you can start at 4 ounces of celery juice in the morning and then work your way up. If you really can't drink celery juice, you can start with pure cucumber juice at your desired amount.) The usual guideline applies: wait at least 15 to 30 minutes after finishing your celery juice before eating or drinking anything else.

- **Select one of the mono eating options on this page to eat in small meals throughout the day.** You can either have your first small meal in the morning or start eating around lunchtime, depending on your hunger level, how much celery juice you consumed, and what kind of fuel your mornings require. You'll stick with whichever food option you choose for the duration of your Mono Eating Cleanse, rather than selecting different options at different meals or on different days. For example, if you choose banana and lettuce, then stick to those all day long for every day you're doing the cleanse. That said, you're welcome to experiment a little with which option you like best before you settle into one.

- *Optional:* If you'd like another option in your day, you can drink pure cucumber juice in the afternoon. You don't have to, and this afternoon cucumber juice shouldn't replace your morning celery juice.

- **Keep out salt, seasonings, and spices.** For mono eating, simple is best. Also keep out the troublemaker foods from Chapter 7. That means you aren't adding items such as oil, butter, yogurt, tamari, or coconut aminos to your food. Stick to the specific food(s) of your chosen mono eating plan. Fresh lemon juice is fine for flavor.

- **Over the course of each day, drink about 1 liter of water** in addition to the optional lemon or lime water upon waking. That's roughly equivalent to 32 ounces of water, or 4 cups. Make sure to space it apart from the celery juice. Also, try not to drink your water at the same time that you're eating food. It's okay to sip coconut water during the Mono Eating Cleanse, as long as it isn't pink or red and doesn't contain natural flavors. Any coconut water you sip would be *in addition* to your liter of water. (You're welcome to drink more than 1 liter of water. If you feel you require more fluids at any point throughout the cleanse, don't hold back; allow yourself to improve your water levels. Do avoid water with a pH above 8.0. To find out why, see Chapter 19, "Critical Cleanse Dos and Don'ts.")

Mono Eating Options

Here are the possibilities when choosing a mono eating plan. Read more about each of these options later in this chapter. Also remember that whichever you choose, you'll start each day with celery juice as outlined above.

- **Banana** (with optional lettuce)

- **Papaya** (with optional lettuce)

- **Banana + papaya** (with optional lettuce)

- **Steamed potatoes** (with optional lettuce)

- **Steamed peas** (with optional lettuce)

- **Steamed winter squash + steamed green beans, brussels sprouts, or asparagus** (with optional lettuce)

How Long

- Try the Mono Eating Cleanse for **a minimum of one week** at a time.

- You can also use it long term as needed. For example, you may decide to continue the Mono Eating Cleanse for one to three months, six months, or even one to two years.

- Determining how long to mono eat is a different process for everyone. It depends largely on what condition you were in when you started and how much your body needed to heal. Keep in mind, for example, that if you have inflammation in your digestive tract, whether it's in the stomach, duodenum, small intestine, or colon—and remember, medical research and science and health professionals are unaware that this inflammation is caused by viruses, unproductive bacteria, and toxic heavy metals feeding them—it's going to take time to kill off the bacteria and viruses and restore your gut linings while improving your hydrochloric acid and strengthening your liver's bile production. While mono eating a choice such as bananas can get you to that place of getting better eventually, it's not likely to happen overnight if you have a more serious condition. On the other hand, many people with digestive problems do experience results overnight or at least within the first week. Hang in there with the mono eating, and don't get discouraged if you don't feel better

from the start. There's a lot of healing your body is doing behind the scenes, and the day is coming when you will start to see and feel the effects.

- Whenever you return to a more varied diet, **refer to the transition guidelines** at the end of the chapter.

Why

- **Celery juice is a vital part of the Mono Eating Cleanse** because it kills viruses and bacteria, which cause many digestive conditions, plus celery juice is critical for neurons and brain function. It also puts valuable, productive sodium into your bloodstream to keep you stable. It's important to drink enough celery juice on whichever plan you choose, starting at 4 ounces if needed and working up to 16 ounces and an ideal of 32 ounces per day, in order to help manage cravings. Celery juice's sodium cluster salts are what really help knock down cravings. Most cravings are for salt, and that's what can get us into trouble by prompting us to reach for foods that will hold us back. If you run out of celery one day or are still working your way up to the recommended amount, be prepared for the possibility of more cravings— you may need to accept that they're coming and ride them out. For more on what to do if you can't get or have celery, see Chapter 21, "Cleanse Adaptations and Substitutions."

- As you've already read, **mono eating is soothing to the digestive tract, starves the pathogens behind so many chronic conditions, and allows your body to enter a gentle detox state.** Its simplicity also allows your system to access nutrients like never before. Getting a break from trying to digest radical fats and complex meals gives your gut a reset that benefits your whole self.

- People don't know how truly food-sensitive they are. They're also unaware that they're consuming foods that feed the pathogens that cause their sensitivities to begin with, as we explored in Chapter 7, "Troublemaker Foods." Mono eating keeps out the foods that feed viral and bacterial problems, deplete hydrochloric acid, and weaken the liver—foods that people most of the time aren't aware are contributing to their discomfort—and that's part of how this technique offers relief. When you eventually go back to eating more foods, you'll be able to do so in a methodical way so that you can learn which foods are problematic for you and worth keeping out longer term.

- You'll read more about how each mono eating food option assists specific health situations later in this chapter.

WORRIED ABOUT DEFICIENCIES?

If you're concerned about deficiencies with mono eating, know that you *come into* the Mono Eating Cleanse with deficiencies. Everyone has deficiencies, whether they're living with digestive problems or chronic illness or even if they're walking around every day feeling fine, with few to no symptoms. So many people's digestive tract linings aren't functioning perfectly: inflamed, irritated, damaged linings from pathogens such as viruses and unproductive bacteria, along with other toxins (including toxic heavy metals) plus years of eating foods that are high in fat, not to mention processed foods, stand in the way of our full capacity for nutrient absorption. Everybody is walking around with deficiencies.

Mono eating properly is not going to create a deficiency. It will do the opposite. Not only will mono eating provide critically needed healing phytochemical compounds, antioxidants, trace minerals, mineral salts, antiviral compounds, and antibacterial compounds; the mono eating foods help restore damaged linings and starve viruses and unproductive bacteria that create damaged linings in the first place. At the same time, mono eating can help restore your hydrochloric acid, which will help you better break down proteins and other nutrients inside your food and kill off viruses and bacteria naturally, on your own. The Mono Eating Cleanse also helps restore your liver so that your bile reserves are strong and can once again properly break down fats. Also consider that the mono eating food options that you read about earlier are loaded with nutrients. These foods are more nutrient-dense and anti-pathogenic than any other foods you might have eaten in your life. By eating them individually in larger quantities, you're getting more nutrition than ever. All of these benefits combined reduce deficiencies. For more concerns, including concerns about protein and fat, see "Mono Eating Fear" near the end of this chapter.

Even if you go long term with the Mono Eating Cleanse, you will only improve deficiencies, not become more deficient. Eating the wrong way, with multiple wrong foods, while struggling with a digestive disorder that no one truly understands, will not repair deficiencies. Adding probiotics will not repair deficiencies. Talking about the microbiome will not repair deficiencies. Taking proper action toward healing the true causes of your injuries using foods that are highly nutritious is the way to protect yourself from becoming truly deficient so you can heal.

ALL ABOUT THE RIGHT FOODS

Mono eating is not about choosing any food out there to eat exclusively. It's about choosing one of the designated options listed in this chapter and using them correctly—options that are nourishing and soothing to the stomach and intestinal linings; not astringent, acidic, or irritating, or poky and jabby, the way nuts, seeds, and grains can be. If you were to pick a food to mono eat that wasn't in this chapter, you could upset your system more than if you weren't mono eating. Cranberries, blueberries, and grapes, for instance, are powerful medicinal foods. Yet if someone with weakened digestion and irritated digestive tract linings were to center their diet around them, they would probably experience discomfort, because these foods can be too tart and astringent. In the case of grapes and cranberries, the skins can be tough to process in quantity.

You'll sometimes hear health professionals out there recommend eating grapes and grapes alone. They don't realize that the astringency, acidity, and tartness of grapes can make someone with a digestive disorder even more uncomfortable. It's the wrong choice to mono eat. Mono eating grapes is an example of how someone took the mono eating food idea from Spirit of Compassion that I started delivering in lectures decades ago to both professionals and people trying to heal, and then turned around the concept and delivered it wrong on down the line. Here, you're reading about therapeutic mono eating for chronic illness from the original source, not someone who happened to like one or two foods and got into the habit of eating only that food for long periods of time.

So neither cranberries, nor blueberries, nor grapes are appropriate for mono eating, nor do they provide enough calories for long-term mono eating. Short term (meaning a day or two) with these medicinal fruits is okay, though not recommended for someone with chronic digestive discomfort or pain. These medicinal fruits all belong as snacks and ingredients in a more varied diet in order to access their healing benefits. The same goes for figs—an eating regimen should not be based on figs and figs alone. Their skins massage the intestinal tract, and as great as that is in moderation, it can become too aggressive if it's the only food you're eating. Raw cauliflower is also an amazing food to eat—healing and medicinal, it should be part of someone's diet if that diet incorporates a variety of foods. On the other hand, raw cauliflower and nothing else every single day is too fibrous for a very sensitive digestive tract. It's similar to how kale is incredible for the body and yet shouldn't be consumed in place of all other foods. Fibrous and stringy, kale is best eaten as one among many foods in your diet. The foods best for mono eating, while extremely healing and nutrient-rich, are gentler on a sensitive system.

We can't rely on what we've been *taught* about gentle foods to select what we mono eat. You don't want to mono eat eggs, for example—because as you've read, even though they don't seem irritating in the moment, they aggressively feed every pathogen in the body, both in the intestinal tract and in other organs and the bloodstream, making all of your digestive sensitivities worse and also, in the long run, worsening any other conditions with which you might have been diagnosed. Nearly everyone has pathogens inside their body waiting to feast on foods like eggs. These pathogens include strains and mutations of viruses of all kinds, such as EBV, HHV-6, CMV, herpes simplex 1 and 2, and shingles, as well as bacteria such as *Streptococcus*, *E. coli*, and *Staphylococcus*, plus every variety of unproductive fungus, yeast, and mold. Because eggs aren't fibrous, they may seem like a healthy choice to mono eat. In truth, they're quite the opposite.

(That said, if you happen to live somewhere on the planet where eggs are the only food available and you can't get a single potato or banana, or even peas, and you have no choice other than to mono eat eggs for a time, I completely understand. If a diet centered around eggs is your only chance at survival, then please embark on eating them. If you can, try to eat them with an herb or spice such as oregano, thyme, cinnamon, star anise, or cayenne pepper, which act as anti-pathogenics in the digestive tract to lessen the progression of anything that can occur from eggs feeding pathogens. Keep in mind that these spices can be harsh on someone with intestinal tract disorders and sensitivities.)

SUPPLEMENTS AND MEDICATIONS

For guidance on the use of supplements while on the Mono Eating Cleanse, turn to Chapter 27, "What You Need to Know about Supplements."

If you're on medication, please consult with your doctor about its use.

HOW TO CHOOSE A MONO EATING PLAN

Everyone is facing a different combination of varying pathogens, toxic heavy metals, and other toxins, so it may be difficult to figure out exactly which of these mono eating plans will work best for you. Don't get too hung up on the decision. All of them are helpful, and you're welcome to try any of them. The door is open for you to experiment until you find the one that you like the most. You may also find that as you read through the descriptions, one resonates more than the others as beneficial for your particular situation. Feel free to follow that instinct, so long as you keep to the guidelines of this chapter.

If you need time to adjust to the idea of mono eating for days, you can try one meal of it. For example, consider one dinner of plain steamed potatoes (with or without lettuce) or one breakfast of only bananas (with or without lettuce).

MORE ABOUT THE MONO EATING OPTIONS

Again, mono eating is not just about picking a food and eating only that for a while. There are specific healing options: banana, papaya, banana plus papaya, steamed potatoes, steamed peas, or steamed winter squash plus steamed green beans, brussels sprouts, or asparagus (all of them with the option to add lettuce).

In each case, you start the day with optional lemon or lime water and then fresh celery juice. A good way to structure the rest of your day is to enjoy your first serving of food mid-morning, if you're hungry. Somewhere in the afternoon, have another round of that same food. Then enjoy one last serving of that food for dinner—for a total of three "feedings" in the day. Alternatively, you have the option of four or five small "feedings" or meals in the day, or two small meals. As you'll read in more detail under "Serving Sizes," it's a good idea to experiment with smaller portions on the first day and work your way up after that if it feels like that amount of food didn't give you enough energy, or if you got too hungry. Not that you should under-eat on that first day. Basically, you don't want to sit down and eat five pounds of potatoes and then find yourself overstuffed. Also don't go too long without eating. Your blood sugar may drop and you may get shaky and moody or lose energy if you go too many hours without replenishing your glucose and mineral salts through one of these foods.

Now let's look at how these food options can help you:

Celery Juice

There's so much to say about the benefits of celery juice that I wrote a whole book about it called *Medical Medium Celery Juice: The Most Powerful Medicine of Our Time Healing Millions Worldwide*. You'll find answers to all your questions there.

Lettuce

It should go without saying that it's not advisable to mono eat lettuce as your only food in a day. Mono eating lettuce is not advisable because it doesn't have enough calories; lettuce on its own won't give you the fuel you need to get through the day. If you decide to include lettuce in your mono eating, you're opting for lettuce *in the same day as* your papaya, banana, potato, or steamed vegetables. You can eat it whole as a snack or side dish, use it as a salad base, wrap it around your food like a tortilla or taco shell, chop it up, or even blend it with your mono eating food choice.

Lettuce is self-limiting, so you can call the shots about amount. What I mean is, you could eat a handful of it periodically with your mono eating food, or you could eat a big bowl of lettuce if you desire. It's hard to overeat lettuce; you'll know when you're not in the mood to eat any more of it. If you're someone who's never in the mood to eat lettuce, then try washing some at the beginning of the day and keeping it easily accessible. With fresh lettuce ready and nearby, you may find yourself more likely to munch on some leaves of it.

If you can, look for butter leaf lettuce. It's the gentlest of all lettuces on the intestinal lining. Red leaf lettuce is another gentle option for the intestinal lining. They're both more soothing and easier to digest than anyone knows. If you're extra sensitive, stay away from mixed greens, unless that's all you can find. Many times, these mixes include pieces of kale, arugula, radicchio, and red cabbage that are good for us, though not as easy on someone who's sensitive and trying to mono eat. If you can only get mixed greens, try to pick out the pieces of lettuce or softer greens.

All lettuces are anti-pathogenic, meaning antiviral and antibacterial. Lettuces have chemical compounds that destroy and rid you of pathogens that are not supposed to be living inside your intestinal tract. (For more on how healing lettuce is for digestion, see "Salads" in Chapter 21, "Cleanse Adaptations and Substitutions.") Lettuces have traces of omega-3s, proteins that are extremely easy to assimilate and digest, and an abundance of trace minerals and mineral salts that are critical for building blood and supporting neurotransmitter function in the brain.

Banana

Bananas are useful for when you're on the go. They're easy to find and don't require any kitchen time, and for the most part, they're inexpensive. If you're concerned about bananas having too much sugar, fear not. The calories in a banana are not as high as you would think, and a banana is made up of more than just natural glucose. A banana also contains bioavailable protein, beneficial omegas, fiber, water, antioxidants, and healing phytochemicals such as potassium. High-potassium foods such as banana are extremely helpful for so many digestive system conditions; that potassium content is part of what makes banana mono eating so healing. Potassium helps regulate

heart function for cardiovascular health, feeds the central nervous system, and is helpful for nerve function in the digestive tract.

Bananas are also anti-pathogenic, and they're an incredible prebiotic as well—meaning, for one, that at the same time they help destroy and eliminate unproductive bacteria in the gut by binding onto it, they feed beneficial microorganisms there. When you're eating a food that doesn't feed pathogens (and none of the foods in this chapter do), you're already winning. Bananas' antiviral, antibacterial, antifungal properties are a bonus on top of that.

As you'll read about in a moment, this anti-pathogenic action is somewhat similar to potatoes. Bananas, though, have a different way of soothing the intestinal tract; they have a different effect on the digestive tract lining. Bananas have a "walk on water" quality that I call the *Jesus Effect*. This speaks to the way they move along the intestinal tract without touching the intestinal lining. The chemical compounds in banana become a film-like shield between the banana and the lining of the intestinal tract. While the nutrients in the banana (and other foods in the gut at the same time) can pass through the shield and absorb into your intestinal lining, as the banana breaks down, it doesn't rub on the intestinal lining. Its chemical compound coats and soothes the lining like a healing ointment.

It's up to you how you enjoy your bananas on this mono eating plan: whole, wrapped in lettuce leaves, blended in the food processor or blender, or mashed in a bowl with a fork. If you eat your bananas whole, make sure to chew them fairly well; don't just gobble them up and let them slide down. When you're dealing with digestive problems, it's good to start the breakdown process in your mouth by working the banana there before you send it down. If you go the blended route, don't add water—blend only the bananas. If you want some liquid, you're better off sipping water a little before or after eating your blended banana pudding. Try to avoid drinking it *with* the banana, though. When you have a compromised digestive system, you don't want to drink water at the same time you're eating food, or blend water into your food, unless you need to for some reason. Water dilutes the hydrochloric acid you need to process the food in that moment, so for maximum digestion, it's best on its own. Bananas are actually easier to digest than water, because bananas are more pH neutral and pH accurate for your stomach and intestinal tract. Most of the time, our water has a lower pH, making it a little harder to process than a banana. (Not that high-pH water is therefore beneficial. Refer to the note in Chapter 19, "Critical Cleanse Dos and Don'ts.") Coconut water is different (as long as it isn't pink or red and doesn't contain natural flavors), if you really need a little liquid with your food.

How Many Bananas?

Everyone has a different stomach and digestive system capacity, not to mention that bananas can grow in different sizes, so the number of bananas people consume on a banana Mono Eating Cleanse will vary. Some can only handle 6, 8, or 10 bananas in a day, whereas others could be eating more like 15-plus bananas a day. Men tend to be able to eat more bananas, and women, especially those who are petite or chronically ill, often can't get down as many. Some people have smaller stomachs, and some people's stomachs are a little more used to stretching and handling more food at once. It all varies, so the amount of banana

that it takes to get you through the day will be unique to you.

Don't be afraid of eating too many bananas because you're worried about too much sugar or too much potassium. You need ample amounts of glucose to function, keep muscles strong, replenish cells, and heal. Bananas are a perfect food when you're chronically ill to prevent muscle atrophy from not being capable of exercising to the degree that people normally can.

Banana Tips

Here are some more tips about banana mono eating:

Try not to consume bananas that are overripe, where the skin is completely brown. Also try not to consume bananas that are green or don't have any spots yet. You want bananas that have small brown dots on the skin yet are still mostly yellow and have some firmness to them.

Ripeness can be a little tough to discern sometimes, since there are different varieties of bananas that come from different farms in different places in the world. This can lead to some variability in ripeness indicators. For example, two bunches of bananas from different sources could have almost the same appearance and yet the fruit inside could be at different stages of ripeness. One indication that a banana is underripe is if you bite into it and get a fuzzy feeling on your tongue. Another is if you find the banana a little too hard or firm. Yet another sign it's not ripe yet is if the banana is hard to peel, with the skin kind of breaking as you try to remove it.

Successful banana mono eating means keeping on top of your banana supply so you always have bananas in the right stage of ripeness to support your healing. You may need to buy bananas a few times a week or consider asking your local grocer for a case of bananas so you have enough.

If you end up with too many ripe bananas to eat before they turn brown, it is okay to freeze them. I recommend that you do so by peeling your bananas and freezing the fruit in a reusable container. This is important, though: don't wait to freeze the bananas until they're *overripe*. That can be easy to do if you get a case of bananas and they all ripen at the same time and you suddenly realize a little too late that they're all over the hill. Still, freezing your bananas when the skins are completely covered in age spots or the fruit inside is mushy isn't helpful. They won't hold up well in the freezer, and when you thaw and blend them, the bananas will ripen even further—that's not great for you. Overripened bananas can be fermented. For a recap of why that's not ideal, refer to Level 4 in Chapter 7, "Troublemaker Foods."

If you freeze your bananas at peak, perfect ripeness, on the other hand, that's okay. Ideally, you're saving those frozen bananas to use once you've transitioned out of mono eating. Banana mono eating is best done with fresh bananas. That said, having a stock of frozen bananas can be a good anxiety reliever when you're mono eating bananas; knowing you have them there as backup is a great help when you're worried that you won't have enough ripe bananas on any given day. If you do need to pull out the frozen bananas as a last resort on your mono eating plan, thaw them before mashing or blending. Making banana "nice cream" (food processing frozen bananas until they're the consistency of soft-serve ice cream) is an okay one-off if you need some variety to keep yourself on track. Frozen banana is a little

harder to digest than thawed or fresh, though, and some people could experience digestive disruptions from it when they're sensitive, so you don't want to make it a whole day or consecutive days of frozen bananas. If you need to dip into your stock, mostly use them thawed.

People who say they get constipated from eating bananas are eating them underripe. The misguided belief that bananas are somehow better for you when they're green because the sugars haven't formed yet stems from a purposeful deception. There's a prejudiced belief system out there against fruit sugar, and even though some medical communities love this theory that fruit sugar is bad, it has no medical research or science to support it. It is merely a theory invented by misled professionals who fear fruit because they think all sugar is bad. The truth is that the less fruit you eat, the more you stay sick, because fruit helps us heal. Not that you should avoid the potato, pea, or steamed vegetable mono eating plans. They provide critical glucose as fruit does, and they'll help you heal to the point that you can start bringing fruit back into your life.

Even when not mono eating, it's not advisable to throw a green-skinned banana in a smoothie—because any food that isn't ripe is not very easy on the body systems. Anything unripe has a tannin that protects the fruit from insects and birds as it sits on the tree or shrub. As the fruit ripens, the tannin transforms into an antiviral, antibacterial compound to help us heal. This ripeness principle extends beyond fruit into the world of vegetables and herbs. With burdock root, you don't want to get it too early. With asparagus, if you let it go too tall, it will fern out. With dandelion greens, if you let them get too long, they're extremely bitter. Farmers who raise animals for consumption know best when their livestock are going to be agreeable to someone's palate too. The list goes on—there are best practices for harvesting and using every food, and when it comes to bananas, the best way to eat them will always be when they have yellow skins with small brown spots. (That is, as long as they're the textbook storebought variety of bananas. If you're lucky enough to get local varieties, their ripeness indicators can differ—it usually comes down to peel-ability.)

Papaya

If someone is having problems moving their bowels, then very helpful mono eating options are papaya, banana, or papaya plus banana. Papaya is useful for relieving constant, chronic, full-time constipation and is also good for someone who has lost their hydrochloric acid, with gastric strength virtually nonexistent. (That can look like extremely difficult digestion, with bloating, gastric pain, inflammation, cramps, spasms, acid reflux, hiatal hernia disruptions, or blockages from scar tissue or previous surgeries, or it may land you a diagnosis of an intestinal condition.) You can add in banana if your constipation is intermittent rather than continuous.

Whenever someone has gone through a period of not eating, whether from fasting, anorexia, or grave illness, blended papaya is like magic for the refeeding process because it offers ample calories, soothes nerves, is antiviral and antibacterial, contains trace minerals and beta-carotene, and digests so favorably. See the Papaya Pudding recipe on page 306. You're welcome to blend lettuce with the papaya.

It's important to use only papayas that aren't genetically modified. Look for Maradol papayas, a large variety that isn't GMO. Also make sure to eat only ripe papaya—you want the flesh to be spoonable. You can usually judge ripeness from the outside, when the skin gets some orange or yellow and yields like a ripe avocado under pressure from your thumb. As with bananas, think ahead so that you have a continual supply of ripening papayas. Many grocers that carry Maradol papayas will offer you the opportunity to purchase a case of them at discount so you can get the quantity you need to get through your days of mono eating.

Steamed Potato

Potato mono eating is ideal for someone who is dealing with loose bowels or bowel movements that are too frequent. Steamed potato on its own is also helpful for someone dealing with very low hydrochloric acid and low gastric acids. The potato is universally helpful—it's substantive enough to sustain someone who would normally rely on animal protein (such as eggs, chicken, fish, turkey, or beef) or plant protein (such as nuts, seeds, peanut butter, or tofu) as their calorie source and can't partake in those foods because of intestinal inflammation or other extreme sensitivities. Not only do potatoes have extremely easily assimilable protein; they're also rich in minerals such as potassium as well as the amino acid L-lysine to help reduce inflammation caused by pathogens. Potatoes are good for ulcers and burning stomach.

Sometimes people are told to be wary of potatoes because they're in the nightshade family. That word *nightshade* automatically triggers fear, so then people fear potatoes, worried that they have a sensitivity or allergy to them. Potatoes don't deserve this reputation, nor do they deserve to be in the fear zone because they're a source of carbohydrates. Theories such as nightshades causing problems were created by people guessing about what's wrong with other people when they have no idea what even causes chronic illness to begin with. Fears are created by guessing, and then once the rumor gets around, it becomes common "knowledge" that's completely misrepresented and wrong, and that misguides people. This also happens with sugar in fruit, lectins, oxalates, and many other food components that are shunned for no true scientific reason and that cause no harm. Nightshades fall into this category of a fear created by people in the industry who don't know what causes illness in the population. "Nightshade" and "carbohydrate" are very broad categories, and if we let ourselves be spooked by the terms, we'll deny ourselves the chance to heal. While yes, there are some wild herbal nightshade plants out there that are inedible, they are not the nightshade fruits and vegetables such as tomatoes, potatoes, eggplants, and peppers in our grocery stores. And while yes, there are some forms of carbohydrates such as processed wheat that aren't beneficial for your health, that doesn't make potatoes a problem. Potatoes can save people's lives. I've witnessed this over the decades.

It doesn't pay to avoid potatoes because they're a "white food" either. Do we consider an apple a white food, or a radish? Is a cherimoya a white food? When you crack into those, they're white inside, and yet we don't label them "white"; we know they're nutritious. The same goes for blueberries—a fruit named for its color—and when you look inside a cultivated blueberry, it's so white it's nearly clear. When you actually look at the potatoes at the store, you'll see piles of brown, yellow, purple, or red. Let that remind you that they don't belong in the "white food" category, a designation that should be reserved for refined foods such as white bread.

Do note that when we're talking about potato mono eating, we're only talking about plain and simple steamed potatoes. We're not talking about roasted potatoes or baked potatoes or boiled potatoes, as delicious as those can be at other times in your life, and certainly not fried potatoes, nor are we talking about steamed potatoes that include oil, butter, sour cream, or seasonings on top. While mono eating, it's okay to add some fresh lemon juice to your steamed potatoes for flavor. Keep spices away for mono eating. A really healing option for sensitive digestion is to eat your steamed potatoes wrapped in lettuce leaves or on a bed of lettuce. If you prefer not to eat the skins of potatoes because you think they're harder to digest, know that a steamed potato skin is actually easy to digest and packed with antiviral compounds and nutrients. If you're eating conventional potatoes, you can opt out of eating the skins if you desire. Don't eat a potato when its skin is green or it's growing sprouts.

Part of what has given potatoes their reputation is that they're almost always eaten with fats, in combinations that don't help us— whether fried in oil, whipped with butter and cream, or covered with bacon bits. Steamed potatoes with no added fats aren't even in our consciousness as an eating option, and yet it's the very option that can turn a life around. It's fine to eat your steamed potatoes warm or cold, whole or mashed or even pureed (as long as you're not mixing in dairy or other add-ins). If you do eat them whole, make sure to give them a good chew.

While sweet potatoes and yams are very healing, they aren't the best choice for mono eating. They have a lot of pulp in them that could feel very bulky. That often isn't the best for someone with digestive sensitivities. When it comes to mono eating, stick with regular potatoes.

Part of what makes steamed potatoes so healing is that they don't feed anything negative or toxic inside the body. They don't feed viruses, which are behind so much of the chronic illness in our world today (including intestinal illnesses), nor do potatoes feed unproductive bacteria, yeast, or mold. In truth, potatoes bind onto colonies of bacteria that are causing diverticulitis or prostatitis and carry them out past the colon; they can drive out strep, *E. coli*, staph, and unproductive funguses from the body. The chemical compounds in potatoes have a sticky, binding nature to them. It's not just the starch that causes this. As potato moves through the intestinal tract, pathogens cling and bind to the compounds and can't escape. Potatoes even help drive worms such as pinworms out of the rectum. For comparison, someone may not think they have an egg allergy, because we aren't taught to fear eggs, and meanwhile, the reality is that eggs feed every single bug we don't want in the intestinal tract and organs, serving as food for colonies of unproductive bacteria and multiple viruses. Potatoes feed no pathogens whatsoever. Instead, potatoes slow down pathogens and weaken them so that your immune system can get stronger and kill the pathogens more easily.

At the same time, potatoes are so easy on the digestive system, one of the most healing foods we have for the intestinal tract. So try not to be thwarted with the misinformation that potatoes are too high in sugar or carbohydrates, that they're going to feed *Candida* or anything else—that's not accurate. (Refer back to Chapter 4, "What about the Microbiome?" for more on *Candida*.) The potato mono eating plan is one that has revived people's digestive tracts and relieved symptoms from chronic diarrhea to bloating to gas to gastritis to constipation to acid reflux, and it has even alleviated symptoms of food poisoning and hiatal hernia. Soothing to the intestinal linings because they are gentle on the nerves inside the lining—they're non-abrasive—potatoes assimilate and digest easily, even with some of the worst digestive issues.

Steamed Peas

Steamed pea mono eating is excellent as a backup plan for someone who's not capable of finding or using banana, papaya, or potatoes. Gentle on the intestinal tract, though not as gentle as the other options, steamed peas do not feed pathogens. (None of the mono eating options do.) Peas contain easily assimilable healing phytochemical compounds and carbohydrates plus an abundance of chlorophyll that absorbs easily into the intestinal linings, where these components feed healthy cell growth and help restore mucus membranes when the intestinal tract linings have become scorched, scarred, injured, or damaged by excess adrenaline, toxic troublemakers, troublemaker foods, and pathogens.

Make sure you don't use pea protein powders. Always opt for fresh or frozen peas unless you're in a desperate situation and can only access canned peas. The best peas to use for mono eating are petite or baby peas (although, to be clear, we're not talking about baby food—just peas that are tender and small). Frozen peas will probably make your food prep easiest. If you have access to fresh, tender peas and you can shell enough to fill you up, that's certainly an option. Chances are, frozen peas will be most convenient. Do try to get organic peas if you have the option.

Steam the peas for as long as you'd like. If it feels best for your gut, you can steam them until they're very soft. If your digestive tract is less sensitive, you don't have to cook them too long if you don't want to. As with potatoes, you can steam all that you want for the day at once and set aside servings to eat cold, or reheat on the stove (without oil or butter), or you can steam them throughout the day as needed. If possible, please don't microwave your peas.

If you bring lettuce into your steamed pea mono eating, you could eat the peas on a bed of chopped lettuce as a salad or in lettuce "cups" like a taco, or you could eat the lettuce as a side dish to the peas. You could even puree your peas and lettuce together. Or you may not feel that lettuce is right for you at this time, in which case you can opt for celery juice in the morning and steamed peas on their own all day. Either way, remember that you're not topping those peas with butter, cream, any kind of oil, soy sauce, tamari, nutritional yeast, or even spices and so on. Fresh lemon juice is okay for flavor. The way to heal your gut is to eat simply.

Steamed Winter Squash + Steamed Green Beans, Brussels Sprouts, or Asparagus

This plan is for someone with a less sensitive intestinal tract who finds the concept of mono eating very challenging and needs a little more variety in their day to keep them interested. With the combination of winter squash plus steamed green beans, brussels sprouts, or asparagus (you'll select two of the three—more in a moment), you get a day packed with antioxidants, chlorophyll, sulfur-rich compounds, antiviral compounds, antibacterial compounds, beta-carotene, and vital glucose, all of which are great for restoring the liver and digestive tract while knocking down and even killing off pathogens. These foods help the liver produce bile and help restore nerves in the intestinal linings. They're gentle enough for mono eating, reliable, and easy to find.

Here's how it works with this option: after celery juice in the morning, you'll enjoy steamed winter squash up until dinnertime. That means some squash in mid-morning (if you're hungry), at lunchtime, and again in the afternoon. Whether you start in the morning or at lunchtime depends on your hunger level. As I mentioned at the beginning of this section, don't go too long without eating. Your mood and energy can drop if you go too many hours before your first meal of the day.

For dinner, select two of these three options on any given night: steamed green beans, steamed brussels sprouts, or steamed asparagus. That will give you that sense of choice and changing it up that you may like to prevent boredom with mono eating—although this is still serious mono-style eating and can really make a difference for almost any health condition.

Throughout the day, lettuces are also an option to accompany your steamed squash and vegetables.

A little more about that winter squash: butternut squash is the most common winter squash available, and that's one option. (Look for frozen butternut squash if cutting it up is too labor intensive.) Spaghetti squash, on the other hand, is generally not going to give you enough calories—you want a sweeter squash. Delicata, sweet dumpling, acorn, and kabocha squash (not to be confused with kombucha tea) are great options if you can get them. If you're sensitive, remove and discard the squash skins after cooking. If you have stronger digestion, you're welcome to eat the skins. Either way, steaming the squash is preferable to roasting or baking it. Remember to keep it free of butter, oil, and cream.

SERVING SIZES

The serving sizes you choose while mono eating depend on how much food you're used to eating normally. Are you accustomed to larger or smaller portions? That's going to influence what feels comfortable to eat when sticking with one or two foods at a time too.

For your first day of mono eating, it can be a good idea to experiment with smaller amounts of food. If you feel a drop in energy or you're distractingly hungry, then go ahead and eat a little more. This isn't about withholding food or undereating—not at all. Rather, the basic idea is that you don't want to jump straight into eating five pounds of peas or 20 bananas at once and overstuffing yourself. Because one of the main goals of mono eating is to help heal your digestive system, you don't want to tax your gut by overconsuming.

You're also not going to serve your healing process by starving yourself—which will only set you up to binge on a troublemaker food because you got so hungry.

Begin moderately and if you want, you have the option to increase as you go.

WHAT TO KNOW ABOUT MONO EATING

For the Gut

Even though mono eating is the most soothing technique available for the gut, people with sensitive intestinal tracts may still feel the food moving through and find themselves spooked, thinking that means they're not digesting it. If you experience some discomfort and you're following one of these plans to the letter, don't let yourself spiral with worry. When your intestinal walls and linings are inflamed, they can be hypersensitive as food brushes past. When those are gentle foods such as banana, papaya, lettuce, or steamed potatoes, peas, squash, green beans, brussels sprouts, or asparagus, they're not doing harm.

This may seem counterintuitive because maybe when you eat a piece of cheese or an egg, you don't feel any discomfort. That's deceiving. It's because cheese and eggs move through the body as soft goo, so they don't rub against hypersensitive nerves in that moment. They do feed the very bacteria, viruses, and even unproductive fungus that create inflammation in our intestinal tract, though, ultimately making that hypersensitivity worse. When you try to consume a healing food such as lettuce, you may feel a touch of discomfort as it touches those areas of intestinal lining inflammation and sends a signal through your nerve endings, and you may then decide to avoid lettuce because it feels like you're not digesting it (when indeed you are digesting the lettuce). You might decide to instead revert back to eating eggs and cheese (which contribute to your problem to begin with). It becomes a vicious cycle if you don't become aware of what's really happening and redirect by avoiding eggs and cheese and when you're ready, bringing lettuce into your life.

Gastroparesis

Gastroparesis is becoming more popular as a diagnosis, and yet what causes it remains mysterious to medical research and science. When someone is diagnosed with gastroparesis, it's extremely confusing, because it's all guessing. There's no true way to tell if there's paralysis in the stomach, duodenum, small intestinal tract, large intestinal tract, or rectum, unless someone sustained an actual physical injury or underwent a surgical procedure that injured nerve endings to a certain area of the digestive tract. In truth, many cases of gastroparesis are caused in the brain, with toxic heavy metals and pathogens causing brain inflammation that can minimize nerve strength in any areas of the digestive tract, resulting in a range of symptoms. Nerves around the intestinal linings can also become inflamed due to viruses such as EBV, shingles, and HHV-6 slowing down performance of the nerves' endings, in turn causing sluggish peristaltic action in the intestinal tract.

There are different levels of gastroparesis. If you're able to chew food and you're not bound to a feeding apparatus, mono eating can be extremely helpful for healing gastroparesis, allowing nerves to restore inside the digestive linings. The Mono Eating Cleanse also provides critically needed mineral salts and glucose to the brain so that neurons can strengthen and neurotransmitter activity can replenish, helping send signals to areas of the intestinal tract lining that are in critical need of peristaltic action. At the same time, these mono eating plans are antiviral, which means they can reduce low-grade viral infections that cause scar tissue and damage nerves inside the digestive linings and other areas of the digestive system. In essence, mono eating can retrain the digestive system, helping it align with the central nervous system and allowing someone to heal.

For Undiagnosed Gut Problems

As I mentioned earlier, issues with the digestive tract often go undiagnosed—circumstances where in truth, nerves in the stomach, duodenum, small intestine, and/or colon are hypersensitive due to pockets of inflammation caused by elevated bacterial or viral loads. This can bring tremendous discomfort, making it feel as if the digestive system can't process or assimilate food properly. Mono eating is an answer.

That's not even to mention the truth that the majority of people in the world live with a digestive problem that isn't visible: low hydrochloric acid. This means that they're not breaking down their proteins properly, so those proteins are rotting and putrefying inside the intestinal tract, creating a situation that eventually becomes bloating or distension in the upper and even lower GI. When food putrefies, it becomes food for unproductive bacteria. That can land someone a future SIBO or even Crohn's or colitis diagnosis.

Many people's stomachs are in terrible condition. Even if they don't realize it, someone's stomach lining could be in rough shape—covered with scar tissue, abraded, even bumpy. The stomach is an organ, and when it's been abused over a lifetime, it can weaken, both in its production of hydrochloric acid and in its flexibility. This can make it more vulnerable to pathogenic disturbances such as ulcers that are mostly created by bacteria.

Also, at the bottom of the stomach, on the way to the duodenum, a little pouch can form when rotting protein, fats, and other debris start to collect and weigh down this passageway. Doctors can't see that this happens, nor can they see how the stomach can start to deform as it stretches in one place and not the other because the connective tissue around the stomach has been saturated by toxins for so many years that it has started to stretch—and not uniformly. This can lead to hiatal hernia, stomach cramping, throat and esophageal spasms, acid reflux, and heartburn.

Mono eating takes someone off the train that's been leading them down this track and gives the stomach organ a chance to heal and rejuvenate. One day, the stomach can return to a point where it's strong enough and flexible enough, with its lining's damaged tissue mended enough, for it to function adequately.

For the Liver

When people struggle with digestive problems of any kind, whatever the symptoms may be, they all have one thing in common: a weakened liver that's not producing enough bile to break down fats properly. Filled up with toxins, poisons, and pathogens, that's a liver that has become stagnant or sluggish,

with a slower-moving blood supply, which is a problem for digestion because a weakened liver puts more stress on the digestive tract, including on the stomach glands that produce hydrochloric acid. All of these mono eating plans are liver-friendly, which then automatically helps the digestive tract and hydrochloric acid in the stomach.

For Food Allergies

The mono eating plans in this chapter are excellent for recalibrating and recovering from food sensitivities and allergies. In part, that's because limiting yourself to one of these plans keeps out troublemaker foods, which feed pathogens that cause the allergenic problem to begin with. With mono eating, your system gets a break from the toxic byproduct of pathogenic proliferation that results when troublemaker foods enter your system. In other words, viruses such as EBV love to feed on eggs, gluten, corn, milk, cheese, butter, all other dairy, and certain processed foods. And high-fat foods in general from both the plant and animal kingdom thicken the blood, which lowers oxygen in the bloodstream and weakens the liver, allowing viruses and unproductive bacteria to thrive. At the same time, those viruses are gobbling up the toxic heavy metals, pesticides, herbicides, and chemicals from conventional cleaning products, air fresheners, scented candles, colognes, perfumes, and more that we're exposed to on a daily basis. When viruses thrive like this, they excrete neurotoxins—neurotoxins that disrupt our system and can make us food-sensitive, even to foods that seem healthy. Bacteria such as strep proliferate in this environment too. By leaving out troublemaker foods, the Mono Eating Cleanse stops this cycle. The pathogens that cause food allergies and sensitivities begin to starve and die off, and that frees you up to start recovering.

DETOX EFFECT

At the same time that mono eating is a technique to get you through sensitivities, it is also a cleanse. While it won't clean out your liver to the degree that the 3:6:9 Cleanse will, the Mono Eating Cleanse can gently release mild levels of liver toxins while gently detoxing all other organs at the same time as the stomach, duodenum, small intestinal tract, large intestinal tract, and rectum. It provides a strong whole-body detox.

The mono eating options in this chapter are also, as we touched on before, anti-pathogenic: they're antiviral, antibacterial, antifungal, anti-yeast, and anti-mold. While you're mono eating any of these foods, pathogens will start to starve, and that has its own detox effect for the body. On top of offering physical benefits, this cleanse effect can also mean that mono eating has the potential to bring up cravings and emotional processing. To help yourself through it, check out Chapter 20, "Your Body's Healing Power," and Chapter 25, "The Emotional Side of Cleansing."

MONO EATING FEAR

When people learn about mono eating, sometimes they're afraid that it doesn't offer enough nutrients or variety. We can't go into mono eating with these fears—they stem from the misinformation that a meal that incorporates as many colors as possible is best for you. That fad doesn't take into account that

when someone is compromised, whether with an intestinal, liver, or pancreatic disorder; a chronic mystery digestive issue that doctors can't pinpoint and yet causes severe bloating, constipation, cramps, spasms, or burning pain; or even compromised with a blood sugar imbalance problem, mono eating can really move somebody forward. Moving forward is not about putting every single nutrient from every single food into your body—because when you're compromised, you can't process it all and put it all to use. Moving forward is about giving your body what it needs in this moment to tap into your natural ability to heal. You have the rest of your life to eat more foods. Right now, you're working on fixing what you're living with in the moment. Until you fix that, you won't be able to benefit from wide variety in what you eat.

The Food Rainbow

On the Mono Eating Cleanse, the larger amounts you're eating of a healing food such as papaya and the way your body benefits from that supersede the need for variety. If you're trying to get the entire rainbow on your plate, you're only getting tiny amounts of each food— one little piece of tomato in your salad, a couple of cucumber pieces, a few leaves of mixed greens. While it may give you the full spectrum, it's not like eating a whole bowl of heirloom tomatoes or a whole head of cauliflower in one sitting. Instead, you're spreading out your nutrients in little pieces of food. In some cases, that can work in the end. If your digestion isn't troubled, you may be able to go for it with a salad that's got that little piece of tomato, those couple bits of cucumber, a shred of grated carrot, two pieces of broccoli, a slice of red bell pepper, a sliver of avocado, and an orange slice (if you even allow yourself to eat fruit), with your slices of chicken breast on top. And then sometimes in our day-to-day lives, even when we're not mono eating, it's better to concentrate on the more powerful foods, and on having larger amounts of them. Snacking on 2 cups of wild blueberries, say, can be more useful than a tiny handful of wild blueberries among tiny handfuls of other foods, and that bowl of heirloom tomatoes can be more useful than half of a small tomato mixed up in your chopped salad that you didn't even finish at lunch.

If your digestion is poor, how much are you getting out of a diet that aims for the full spectrum? How many nutrients can your digestive system extract out of so many different little pieces when it's struggling to function at all? The truth is that when you're really compromised, larger servings of the specific, valuable healing foods offered in this chapter override the need for a little bit of this and a little bit of that. By focusing on meals of one or two (or three) of the healing foods in this chapter, you can really move forward.

Getting variety in your diet is not a race. It's not about getting everything possible in yourself within one day. Superfood powders with 50 ingredients are a prime example of how you lose out when you try to do that. When you scoop your tablespoon of powder blend, you're getting only a speck of each ingredient; that's virtually nothing. Variety should be a longer-term goal. You only have one stomach, and it can only hold so much food in a day. If you're aiming for a full-spectrum rainbow every 24 hours, you can actually get deficient, because weak digestion means you can only process some of those foods anyway. Plus troublemaker foods you're eating at the same

time could actually interfere with the absorption and assimilation of the valuable foods.

Even during months of mono eating one or two foods, you're getting more variety than you realize. On one visit to the grocery store, the bananas available may be from one farm. The next time you go, or when you visit a different grocery store, the bananas may be from a different farm, or from a different field at that same farm, and that translates to slightly different nutrient composition. The same goes for any of the other mono eating foods. One crop of Maradol papayas may be from one place, and the next time you buy a case of them, they may be from a different source. Even if you're exclusively mono eating potatoes and lettuce from the field next door to you, you'll get more than enough variety, because the soil composition changes over time.

When you mono eat, you get more nutrients than you may realize—more antioxidants, more trace minerals, more antivirals, more antibacterials, more healing phytochemical compounds, more vitamin C, more potassium, more mineral salts, more glucose—because you're eating incredibly nutritious foods in larger quantities than ever. Papaya is one of the most healing foods on the planet at this moment in time. Eating a good amount of it every day provides far more healing benefits than if you're so busy getting a rainbow of other foods in yourself every single day that you only eat one papaya every six months. And then after a few months of mono eating papaya and lettuce, you may feel that it's time to add in banana, or you may switch over to mono eating potatoes and lettuce for a period before you start reintroducing other foods. You'll get variety over time, and it will be variety that you can process, absorb, and assimilate and therefore benefit from on a profound level.

Celery juice is an important part of these mono eating plans too. It's an herbal medicine that's above a superfood, and making it part of your day while mono eating makes a world of difference. You could be someone who never drinks a glass of straight celery juice and yet eats a super diversified diet, and sickness can take over because the true underlying issue in the body that celery juice could have helped is never being addressed. If food variety is the key to health, why do so many people on what seem like healthy, varied ketogenic, paleo, or high-protein/high-fat vegetarian, vegan, intuitive eating, and plant-based diets still fall ill?

This is all to say that you can't walk into mono eating with the mind-set "I'm not going to get my nutrition." You'll deprive yourself of the possibility of healing. Instead, ask yourself how many people who eat a full spectrum of foods because they believe "everything in moderation" end up getting sick. The answer is a lot of people, including people who eat only unprocessed, whole foods. Those who bring in a variety of nuts, seeds, wild fish, organic fruits and vegetables, wild game, and grass-fed, unpasteurized animal proteins still fall prey to illnesses of all kinds, just like anyone else using any food belief system, because there's more to why we get sick than how much variety is in our diet or how balanced we think it is. We come into this world with different levels of pathogens and toxins that we've been exposed to already at conception, in the womb, and as newborn babies. On top of that, we collect more along the way from relationships and other avenues of easy exposure—and those poisons and pathogens are what cause our health problems throughout life. Addressing this truth is how we actually heal and protect ourselves.

We have to be careful that we don't harp on mono eating as being nutritionally deficient. One food can save someone's life when they're dealing with a mystery condition that doctors can't explain. When they're in the fetal position on the floor from gastric spasms that medical testing and various specialists haven't solved, or when they're dealing with mysterious vomiting, nausea, or gastritis that no gastroenterologist or other medical authority can illuminate, mono eating can turn their life around so that they can eat again without suffering, get the chance to heal, and move on with life.

What about Protein and Fat?

One question you have to be ready for when you're eating something like papaya for all your meals is "Where's your protein?" If you're someone who falls prey to the word *protein*—meaning that you give protein an elevated status and believe it's the answer in life—this most likely means you will be tempted to steer clear of mono eating and miss out on all its healing benefits. Or you can be ready for the question and know what to say back.

Remember these words: We live in a world that's eating an abundance of protein, and it's a very sick world. More and more people are eating more and more protein and only getting sicker. Does that make you think protein is the answer? Or do you think there could be another reason why people are getting sick?

When someone with chronic illness or symptoms of any kind goes to their health professional and the practitioner says, "Maybe you need more protein," does that make sense? It happens every day to millions of people. Shouldn't the practitioners say, "Let's take a look at other reasons you could be sick"? The truth is that everybody is dealing with pathogens, toxic heavy metals, other toxins, and deficiencies, and they're not being taught the correct foods to eat for healing. Protein isn't what's missing. The bioavailable amino acids, antioxidants, beta-carotene, glucose, mineral salts, antivirals, antibacterials, antifungals, trace minerals, and anti-aging phytochemical compounds in papaya, never mind celery juice or the other mono eating food options, are what offer true healing for conditions that make life unbearable—because they actually help stop the viruses and unproductive bacteria responsible for why so many people are sick. Protein doesn't do anything like that. Protein doesn't stop viruses or bacteria. Protein doesn't remove toxic heavy metals. Protein doesn't detox or cleanse the body. Protein doesn't nourish the central nervous system, neurotransmitters, or neurons. Protein doesn't recover or restore us after we've gone through hell with chronic illness.

Medical research and science don't actually have a grasp yet on any level of how much protein we need, what it actually does, or whether it's even beneficial. There's no technology that tracks protein as it enters the mouth, continues through the digestive system, and travels through the rest of the body—no technology to determine where it's going, what it's doing, or whether it's helping. The merit of protein developed as a theory and remains a theory, which means that when people talk about the best sources of protein, that's only theoretical, even though all the talk that you'll hear about protein can sound advanced. If medical research and science don't know what causes autoimmune and chronic illness, how would they know if protein is useful or not for

us, if it's what we need when we're chronically sick? They don't know what's wrong with us when we're sick, yet they're telling us we need protein when we're sick. The theory that protein is life's answer is, I'm sorry to say, nothing more than speculation and imagination. Even the most highly educated people don't have any idea what "protein" really means for our health—they haven't been given the tools to know—so don't let the topic intimidate you. In reality, you actually get enough protein while mono eating. These food options in this chapter provide your body with the most assimilable, bioavailable protein sources you need to keep you strong and vital.

People often worry about how much fat to eat too, especially as high-fat trends continue to gain attention. Well, we live in a world that's suffering while eating an abundance of fats. Does that make you think a high-fat diet is the answer either? It's not. The traces of beneficial fats that foods such as bananas, potatoes, papaya, and even lettuce contain are plenty to sustain your health, so you don't need to worry that any of these mono eating plans are problematic because they don't incorporate radical fats such as nuts, seeds, olives, or avocado. Any of these mono eating plans will give you the omegas you need. The truth is, it's an asset that mono eating is so low in fat—time off from radical fats helps balance out the large amounts of fat we've eaten at other times in life and gives the liver a rest from the immense burden of processing fat meal after meal after meal and in the process, burning out its bile reserves and weakening the pancreas. That rest for your liver (and pancreas) is a key part of healing with mono eating. (For more on fat, revisit Chapter 7, "Troublemaker Foods.")

Our Relationship with Food

Sometimes it's not protein or fat or variety of nutrients that people in your life worry about when you take up mono eating. Sometimes it's nervousness that you've become obsessed with food. If this kind of concern comes your way, comfort yourself with the knowledge that everyone is obsessed with food. Don't let anyone fool you into thinking they have it all together with eating and that food isn't the most important thing in their lives. Even if they say they don't think about food, that it's not their thing, that they simply eat when they feel like eating, see how they react if someone takes away the foods they like and replaces them with foods they don't like. It's all about food for everyone. No one's exempt from a fixation on food.

When someone who is struggling with a symptom or condition is using food to recover and heal, and they hear that they're obsessed with food, the person who calls them out is someone whose own symptoms and conditions aren't impeding their life yet. The doubter is obsessed with food themselves, only they're projecting their own fears about food onto the person who's actually talking about food and working with food every day to try to heal. No matter their background or what they eat or don't eat, food runs their life—again, everyone is obsessed with food. We have to be; it's the human condition to fixate on where the next meal is coming from. If we don't, if we actively avoid thinking about that next meal, we set ourselves up for unhealthy choices when we get too hungry, and that can lead to its own set of obsessive thoughts as we do a regretful postmortem on why we reached for that cookie or cupcake. We'll explore this all in more detail in Chapter 25, "The Emotional Side of Cleansing."

Is it possible to get so fixated on mono eating—because it was a lifeline when you were suffering—that fear stops you from bringing in other foods when it's time to move on? Sure. Just like it's possible to become fixated on cutting your grapefruit sections just so before putting sugar on top, or drinking coffee all day and then bingeing at night, or putting just the right amount of peanut butter on oatmeal, or dumping the crumbs from the cookie jar into a bowl to make sure they don't go to waste, or anything else to do with food. The key, as with any food fixation, is to bring awareness to it. Observe any hesitance in yourself to move on from mono eating, so you can see that fixation for what it is—a normal attachment to food that made you feel better.

What people who haven't tried mono eating don't realize is that if anything, the technique frees up your mental energy around food and can cut down on time in the kitchen. While you're on a mono eating plan, the puzzle of planning around endless ingredients and choices multiple times a day is replaced by radical simplicity. With that comes brain space you didn't even know you could have to focus on other areas of your life besides food. It's one of the secrets of mono eating—that it actually helps heal your relationship with food at the same time it helps heal your body.

Have freedom in knowing that you're not "other" for needing to devote mental resources to eating a certain way to heal yourself. As isolating as it can feel—because other people aren't always too vocal about their own food needs and hang-ups, even though believe me, they're there—you're not alone. Also have freedom in knowing that you aren't locked into mono eating forever. When your health improves, you'll start experimenting with adding in foods as you go along and leave mono eating behind. You'll find guidance on that transition process next.

TRANSITIONING FROM MONO EATING

You won't be mono eating for the rest of your life. Nor do you have to stop before you're ready—if you've been improving with the Mono Eating Cleanse, it makes sense that you may be afraid to change it up and risk losing ground.

Either way, the day will arrive when you're ready to go back to eating a more varied diet, whether you're eager or hesitant, whether that's after days or weeks or an extended period of months because you needed mono eating to address a more serious issue. There are considerations to make about when and how to navigate this transition. As much as you don't want to lock yourself into worrying that a mono eating plan is going to be for the rest of your life, believing you'll never be able to eat other foods, you also don't want to jump ship with abandon, reintroducing all sorts of new foods at once.

Maybe you're someone who wasn't experiencing any real symptoms and tried mono eating to improve your overall health and fine-tune your sense of taste so you could better appreciate different flavors. If that's you, start to diversify and bring in other foods at any time you'd like. Or maybe you're someone who was really suffering from a condition, and mono eating is how you found real healing. You're not trapped; you'll still be able to leave mono eating someday. Many times, you'll know yourself when the time is right.

The Right Time

When it is the right time, it's best not to go back to troublemaker foods. Instead, keep it simple and add one new (non-troublemaker) food you desire at a time. You can even decide to switch from one mono eating plan to another one long term, before you start introducing a big variety of foods. For example, if you've been on a potato and lettuce Mono Eating Cleanse for a long time and you're ready for a change and at the same time nervous about reintroducing too much, you can select another mono eating option from the beginning of this chapter instead.

How do you know you're ready to move on from mono eating? One way you can tell that your nerves are healing naturally is that you're gradually getting your life back. You're getting better than you were before. As you add in different foods, one at a time, you feel like your digestion is handling them well. You can see how far you've come from where you started.

Important Transition Guidelines

When you're ready to return to more foods, you don't want to dive into a steak dinner with fried onions and a buttered roll, with chocolate ice cream for dessert. You don't even want to dive into healthier radical fats right away. It's a good idea to take a little time to let your body adjust. That means:

- **Stay off radical fats for a little while.** As a reminder, radical fats include nuts, seeds, nut butters such as peanut butter, oil, coconut, avocado, cacao, chocolate, olives, bone broth, and other animal proteins. For how long depends on what condition you were in when you entered the Mono Eating Cleanse. Were you sick with a couple of mild symptoms, or were you in a really difficult situation? You can stay off radical fats for as long as you would like—don't have fear or panic that you're missing out on anything a radical fat offers. Try not to get confused or swayed by a well-meaning practitioner or article that states our brains need fats; that's based on propaganda and theories that have no scientific evidence behind them. Our brains are mostly made out of glycogen storage, and our brains run on glucose, which is a form of sugar. Without that sugar, our cells can't function; our central nervous system shuts down. So don't worry about rushing fats, and take your time with your healing process. The recipes in Chapter 23 will help you with meal and snack ideas. If you eventually want to reintroduce radical fats, avocado is the easiest on the digestive system. Start with a quarter of a ripe avocado, and eat it at the end of the day, along with a salad or steamed vegetables.

- **Also stay away from the full list of troublemaker foods** in Chapter 7. Especially if you were bad off before you started the Mono Eating Cleanse, stay off the troublemaker foods for good. Even if you weren't in a critical state before mono eating, try to keep them out of your diet.

You've Come So Far

Keep in mind that after the Mono Eating Cleanse, healthy fibrous foods (such as kale, red bell peppers, oranges, cauliflower, broccoli, and asparagus) or fat-based foods (such as salmon, nuts, seeds, nut butters, and gluten-free grains) that aren't on the troublemaker foods list may still cause some discomfort as you start to bring them back into your diet. Just because you're feeling discomfort doesn't mean these are bad foods. When people are healing, sometimes they don't realize how much they've improved. For example, they might have come to the Mono Eating Cleanse with extreme bloating, discomfort, lots of gas, and cramping. As they start to graduate out of mono eating, they may feel the new foods they introduce rub the linings of the digestive tract, or they may even feel very mild bloating. Even though the foods they're introducing aren't troublemaker foods, they may get spooked.

If this describes you, remind yourself how much better you are than before. You're more fine-tuned to your health than ever now, more aware of subtle sensitivities or subtle differences. The Mono Eating Cleanse gets you so comfortable with feeling better that when you make the transition, even though your digestion is far better than when you started—with stronger bile from your liver and hydrochloric acid from your stomach—you're more likely to feel your body's adjustments to different foods than ever before. Don't confuse that with how bad off you were prior to mono eating.

If you are worried about some subtle sensitivities even though you've come a long way, you can always go back to your comfort zone with the foods that felt good during mono eating. As much as you've improved, you may have leftover inflammation from leftover pathogens and toxins. It's normal to go back to mono eating for a bit as you start shifting your foods. Or you may want to experiment your own way with another mono eating food option from the beginning of the chapter as part of your transition. Or you may want to bring in multiple foods from this chapter and find a new comfort zone. Even if it isn't a straight path to return to a more varied diet, remember what a long way you've come with your healing process. You're in a much better place than you were before. You've brought yourself so far.

"Remember what a long way you've come with your healing process. You're in a much better place than you were before. You've brought yourself so far."

— Anthony William, Medical Medium

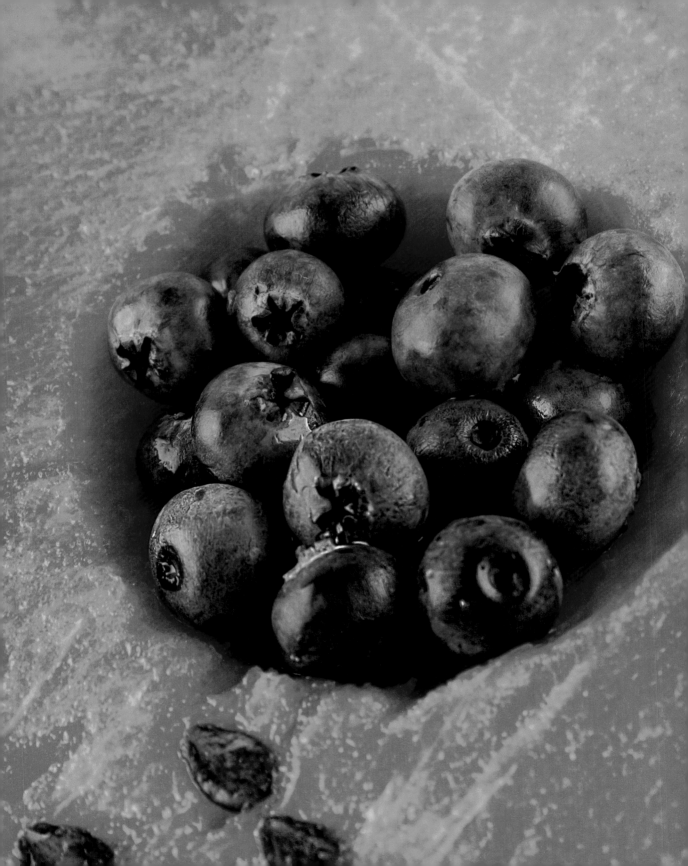

PART IV

THE INSIDER
CLEANSE GUIDE

CHAPTER 19

Critical Cleanse Dos and Don'ts

In this chapter, you will find powerful information about your cleansing process. Think of it as a care manual to help you become an expert on Medical Medium cleanses, with tips and answers to increase cleanse performance. It also goes beyond that. These are critical understandings and insights to make your cleanse a catalyst for change in your life.

Here's an overview of what's to come:

- This Is a Spiritual Cleanse

- When to Do the Cleanse

- The Birthday Cleansing Secret

- When to Eat on the Cleanse

- Cleanse Interruptions

- Water and Other Beverages

- Lemon Water

- Hunger and Portions

- Salt, Spices, Seasonings, Dulse, and Honey

- Supplements and Medications

- Children

- Pregnancy and Breastfeeding

- Gallbladder Issues

- Diabetes

- Organic versus Conventional

- Raw versus Cooked

- Fat-Free beyond the Cleanse

- Healing Reactions and Additional Detox Methods

- Water Fasting

- Juice Fasting and Juice Cleansing

THIS IS A SPIRITUAL CLEANSE

Any Medical Medium cleanse goes beyond the physical. The 3:6:9 Cleanse is a spiritual cleanse. So is every other cleanse in this book and this series. That's because they are not man-made. They come from above.

People often think, *Well, Medical Medium information got me to a point where I healed my symptoms. Now I need to go on my spiritual journey.* What they may not realize is that using the Medical Medium information to get better is the very genesis of their spiritual journey. As your body goes from twisted up, sick, and struggling to physically free, your soul is freed up too, and you're more easily able to continue your spiritual development. The same information that heals your body heals your soul.

I recommend that people look back a bit to see how far they've come, both physically and spiritually, after tapping into Medical Medium information. One of the greatest lessons in our spiritual development is to not take a miracle for granted. When you're struggling and suffering with symptoms and conditions, looking everywhere for answers and not getting them, and then those answers are given to you from above, you can't receive anything more spiritual than that. Just because there was a messenger involved does not mean these answers were man-made. And the answers here go so far beyond physical healing. Cleansing yourself of the true source of pain is the most spiritual healing there is. Healing your physical symptoms heals your soul.

We can't take the 3:6:9 Cleanse and the other cleanses in this book for granted, using them to heal our physical symptoms and then casting them aside so we can begin our spiritual journey in search of answers. We're already on our spiritual journey. Spiritual answers have already helped us cleanse; restored our confidence in our mental, emotional, and physical health; restored our soul; and allowed us to claim our free will to pursue whatever path we choose going forward. Always remember: Would we even be at this point of getting to move forward if it weren't for the spiritual development we'd already been through?

Keep in mind that any self-proclaimed expert who offers a course on the 3:6:9 Cleanse that incorporates health or cleansing content not sourced from Medical Medium information renders the cleanse null and void. The same is true if anybody tries to tie outside spiritual information to the cleanse—it will make it ineffective. These physical and spiritual cleanses rely on information that comes from the original source.

If you want to expand the spiritual nature of the 3:6:9 Cleanse or another cleanse in this book, apply the meditations from *Liver Rescue.* You'll also find support from the sunset meditation and other soul-healing techniques in *Medical Medium.*

WHEN TO DO THE CLEANSE

When it comes to choosing when to start the 3:6:9 Cleanse, the biggest deciding factor is what will work for you. Map out the nine days on your calendar and try to make sure that on that ninth day, you aren't going to be scheduled to the gills, since your body will be doing so much of its release work that day. And remember, it's best to plan for a couple of adjustment days once the cleanse is over to take a little time to reintroduce more food variety. In other words, you may not want to host a barbecue the day after you complete the cleanse.

THE BIRTHDAY CLEANSING SECRET

Now, there is a bigger picture, which has to do with your liver's cycle of renewal, a concept I introduced in *Liver Rescue.* Your liver renews itself on an ongoing, everyday basis. Just because your liver is generating new cells, though, doesn't mean they're clean cells. Polluted cells from the past contaminate new cells unless we're actively pulling out troublemakers such as viruses, viral byproduct and debris, toxic heavy metals, pesticides, air fresheners, scented candles, colognes, perfumes, and more.

If you don't remove the poisons from your system, there's always going to be a high level of contamination of new cells. Imagine, for example, that someone spilled cologne on a shirt you were wearing. Instead of washing the shirt, you hung it back in your closet. Now every fresh item of clothing that you put in your closet would get contaminated; it would pick up the scent and come out smelling like cologne. That's the same principle of how troublemakers can stick around in our livers for so long, getting passed along from contaminated cells to new ones. And it's the same principle of cleansing: to start fresh, you're going to want to give all the clothes in your closet a thorough wash—or to cleanse your cells of troublemakers—even if it takes a few rounds to get rid of the contamination.

In that spirit, any time is a good time to consider guiding your liver through the 3:6:9 Cleanse, because any time is a good time to put yourself on the path to a healthier liver, which is central to your well-being. Here's the bonus: every three years, we get a window when it's especially good to take care of our livers with the 3:6:9 Cleanse. Since birth, your liver has renewed itself in thirds every three years. Leading up to your third birthday, its routine cell renewal picked up speed for serious cell overhaul, regenerating a third of its working cells by about the time you turned three. Your liver renewed another third of its working cells leading up to your sixth birthday, and then it renewed the final third of its working cells leading up to your ninth birthday. As you were about to turn 12, it started all over again. This nine-year renewal cycle has continued and will continue for the rest of your life.

The key is to give your liver a chance to renew *clean, uncontaminated, healthy* cells. That starts with regular cleansing throughout the years, whether with the 3:6:9 Cleanse, Anti-Bug Cleanse, Heavy Metal Detox Cleanse, or any other Medical Medium cleanse. You can give yourself a special boost if, in the roughly three months leading up to a birthday that's a multiple of three, you're especially mindful to cleanse. (If you were born premature and underdeveloped, you have a few months to play with after your birthday.) If you're about to turn—just to name some random "three" birthdays—24, 39, 45, 51, 63, 78, 87, or 93, or if you're about to turn any other age that's a multiple of three, you're doing yourself a special service with the 3:6:9 Cleanse, with increased potential to feel a difference.

Are you seeing the spiritual nature of this too? When we're dealing with birthdays and numbers that cohesively work alongside our organs, it brings us into rhythm with the physical and spiritual clock of how we renew. This spiritual cleanse is not only about cleansing cells. It's about a spiritual algorithm and how numbers are involved with defining our human nature, how we were created, and how we can heal. That increases cleansing's power of spiritual development and rebirth.

The 3:6:9 Cleanse maximizes the mind-body connection, helping you bring together your mind, body consciousness, and physical body. It connects you to the very essence of what everybody who's seeking any kind of spiritual insight is seeking: it connects you to who we are.

For extra support when you're not cleansing over those few months before a "three" birthday, consider sipping more celery juice, eating a little less fat, avoiding the troublemaker foods from Chapter 7 when you can (especially the top-level foods), bringing in more fruit for antioxidants, antiviral and antibacterial compounds, trace minerals, and critically needed glucose; staying more hydrated; and bringing in the Morning Cleanse on a more regular basis.

WHEN TO EAT ON THE CLEANSE

When you're thinking about how to time your meals and snacks during these cleanses, the most important point to remember is to enjoy your celery juice on its own and give it time to do its work. In the morning, that means waiting 15 to 30 minutes after drinking lemon or lime water before starting your celery juice and then waiting at least another 15 to 30 minutes after finishing your celery juice before you start your breakfast. If you're someone who gets shaky without food first thing, or you feel you need some calories at that time of morning, be sure to add a little raw honey to the lemon or lime water that you drink upon waking.

When you're drinking a second serving of celery juice in the afternoon, wait at least 60 minutes after lunch to start sipping it, and then wait 15 to 30 minutes after finishing your celery juice before you dig into any snacks. I know it's not fun or easy to keep track of that timing guidance around celery juice. It *is* worth it—taking care with celery juice timing has a profound effect on its ability to help you.

As for when or how to space out your other food and drink during the day, there are no real rules. If you have preexisting digestive system sensitivities, then you have the freedom during this cleanse to keep going with the meal spacing that works for you. For example, if you always find it tough to get food in yourself first thing in the morning, you don't have to force a smoothie down right away; you can take some time letting your body adjust to the day before you reach for it. Alternatively, you could be someone who needs food early; in that case, get your lemon or lime water (with raw honey, if desired) and celery juice in yourself first thing (still remembering to space them out) so that you can get to breakfast as soon as possible. Whatever chronic digestive problem you're used to dealing with, whether a finicky, delicate, emotional digestive tract that feels like it doesn't want to cooperate, or constipation that you can alleviate by eating at certain times, work with how you're feeling in the moment. Adapt the personalized strategy that you've developed for daily survival so that you use it during the cleanse too, eating and drinking when it's comfortable for you.

If you're not someone who deals day in and day out with sensitive digestion, then after you've gotten through the specific lemon or lime water and celery juice guidelines first thing in the morning, you're also free to eat and drink when it's comfortable for you. There's no need to go to extreme lengths to space out every drink, snack, and meal because of a belief system you learned somewhere, nor is there any real benefit to an exacting approach. For example, if you find yourself eating dinner late at night because you were strictly spacing out meals all day, you won't do yourself any favors with the lost sleep that results. Ease up on yourself as you go about your day and pay attention to what meal timing works for you.

CLEANSE INTERRUPTIONS

If you need to stop the cleanse partway through, don't worry—nothing bad will happen. This is a cleanse that is liver-worthy and liver-friendly. It is built with automatic protections so that there are no negative ramifications for your body.

There are a lot of different cleanses out there in the health world and a lot of theories about how these cleanses could go wrong—theoretically—if you have to stop midway. There's a lot of folklore and fear in this area. Let's remember that those are man-made cleanses, with no accurate understanding of how to safely and properly cleanse the human body. The makers of man-made cleanses have no idea what causes chronic illness in the first place. Keep that in mind.

With the 3:6:9 Cleanse, whether Original, Simplified, or Advanced—and with the other cleanses in this book—you can put all that fear aside. These cleanses are made for the human body. They come from above, with answers about what causes chronic illness built into the cleanse information. They are here to work with your life, and sometimes life is unpredictable. If you start the cleanse and then circumstances prevent you from going more than three or four days this time, there's no harm done. Only positive healing can occur as a result of those three or four days—you advanced your liver and your body more than you would have if you hadn't tried to start. While of course the goal is to get

through all nine days of the 3:6:9 Cleanse, nothing negative can come of stopping.

As you read in Part II, the way the 3:6:9 Cleanse is structured, your liver doesn't really start flushing out the poisons until the last three days of the cleanse—and most of that flushing happens on the final day: Day 9. That means that if you stop the cleanse at Day 2, all you're doing is stopping your body from fortifying itself to let go. If you stop at Day 5, you're only stopping when your liver is starting to build up more strength and uproot poisons and toxins—and that's perfectly fine and healthy. Even if you stop at Day 8, when you've truly started to cleanse, that's fine. You can stop at any point, and the only effect is that you've gotten yourself further along in the healing process.

If you do find yourself in this position of needing to stop mid-cleanse, you don't need to take extra measures like drinking excessive amounts of water afterward. Instead, it's ideal if you can drink some lemon or lime water the next morning and then get through the Morning Cleanse protocol from Chapter 16—at least skipping fats until lunchtime—to help flush poisons. You don't need to do anything special beyond that. Unlike other cleanses out there, the 3:6:9 Cleanse is safe. So is any other Medical Medium cleanse. (For more on the backlash of the reckless cleanses out there, refer back to Chapter 1, "Cleanses from Above.")

When you're ready to try the 3:6:9 Cleanse again, don't pick up where you left off. You do need to go back to the beginning of the cleanse and start over at Day 1.

It's different if you're on the Anti-Bug Cleanse, Morning Cleanse, Heavy Metal Detox Cleanse, or Mono Eating Cleanse. On these, if you get interrupted for a day, you don't need to go back to Day 1. Rather, add three days to the end. For example, if you're doing the Heavy Metal Detox Cleanse for three months and on one morning in the middle, you eat oatmeal with peanut butter, a protein shake, an egg and cheese sandwich, or a bagel with cream cheese, add three days at the end so that it goes from 90 days to 93. If you're doing the Anti-Bug Cleanse for three weeks and you eat a troublemaker food in the middle, add three days so that what would have been 21 days becomes 24.

And remember this: getting through Day 1 alone of any cleanse is a major accomplishment. One day of being compassionate to your liver and working with its healing processes—and what that means for your brain and the rest of your body—means you're succeeding. Even one day of the Morning Cleanse is helpful and important. Don't let guilt cloud your mind. You will make other opportunities to try again, and the more you try, the more momentum and your healing process will carry you through. For now, you've done something really special for yourself.

WATER AND OTHER BEVERAGES

As I've mentioned before, if you already rely on aloe water or ginger water for physical relief, it's okay to keep doing them during the 3:6:9 Cleanse (or any other cleanse in this book), as long as you drink them spaced out enough from the celery juice (15 to 30 minutes apart) for celery juice to do its work. When a cleanse calls for lemon or lime water and you can't do lemons or limes, it's okay to do ginger water instead. Don't add aloe water or ginger water to the cleanse just because, though—you're doing enough with the other drinks and foods.

Cucumber juice should only be used as a replacement for celery juice in the 3:6:9 Cleanse,

not as an addition. Remember that as healing as cucumber juice is, it doesn't offer what celery juice does. While following any of these cleanses, try to focus on celery juice.

And as logical as it may sound to sip Liver Rescue Broth all day during the 3:6:9 Cleanse, save it for after (unless it's listed as an ingredient in one of the lunch or dinner recipes you're using from Chapter 23). Complicating the cleanse with any more options than what's already outlined runs the risk of distracting you from what you really need. It doesn't pay to try to outsmart the cleanse.

As far as water goes while cleansing, how much should you drink? Try to get in 1 liter of water (roughly equivalent to 32 ounces, or 4 cups) over the course of the day. That's not counting any morning lemon or lime water, evening lemon or lime water, or evening tea—this liter of water is in addition to those, something you drink between meals and snacks as you go about your day. Feel free to squeeze some lemon or lime into that drinking water. (More on lemon water in a moment.) As ever, be mindful not to drink the water too close to drinking the celery juice—make sure you space them at least 15 to 30 minutes apart.

If a liter of water feels like too much, even spread out every few hours, don't force it all down. On the other hand, if you're used to drinking more water and you still have enough appetite for the cleanse foods, it's okay to drink more than 1 liter during the day. The bottom line is that you don't want to get dehydrated on the cleanse and you also don't want to drink so much water that you eat less and get into trouble.

As we covered in "3:6:9 Cleanse," avoid water with a pH above 8.0. That's true whether you're cleansing or not, and it applies whether or not you use an alkalized water machine. The ideal pH for drinking water is 7.7. Water with higher or lower pH levels sits in the stomach until the digestive system can adjust the pH before releasing it throughout the body, and that takes precious energy that your body could devote to healing. Drinking water at the ideal pH level prevents your digestive system from weakening.

Lastly, while on the 3:6:9 Cleanse (or another cleanse in this book) it's fine to sip coconut water—as long as it doesn't contain natural flavors and isn't pink or red. Pink to red means it's old coconut water that has oxidized, although you wouldn't know because the coloring is marketed as a good thing. For any cleanse other than Mono Eating, it's also fine to sip Hot Spiced Apple Juice (at any temperature, made from the recipe in Chapter 23). Keep in mind that any coconut water or Hot Spiced Apple Juice would be *in addition* to the liter of water during the day, not in place of any of that water.

LEMON WATER

There's a misconception that lemons are bad for your teeth—that lemons' acidity can weaken your enamel or cause gum issues. This is a theory that has developed over recent years with no research, science, or studies to support it. Dentists' chairs globally are filled with people with dental issues, and these people aren't eating lemons all day long or drinking lemon water. Teeth and gum problems are the result of mineral deficiencies, trace mineral deficiencies, antioxidant deficiencies, and many other phytochemical compound deficiencies. We come into the world with deficiencies. Millions of children have tooth problems right from the start because they were born with trace mineral deficiencies, and these children have not been

drinking lemon water since birth. It has nothing to do with lemons or lemon water.

When you're in the dentist's chair getting root canals or cavities drilled and filled or teeth pulled, it's not because you've dedicated your life to eating, drinking, or juicing lemons in any way. It's those years of nutrient deficiencies leading to weakened enamel. It's putrefying proteins and rancid fats caked along the linings of your gut, shielding pathogens that are feeding on this hazardous material and outgassing ammonia, which rises up to your teeth. It's a stagnant, sluggish liver producing lower bile reserves, allowing fats to go rancid in the first place. It's weakened hydrochloric acid in your stomach from worn-out stomach glands, allowing proteins you're eating to rot. It's coffee drinks eroding teeth for years by making the enamel nutrient-deficient and wispy-thin, allowing bacteria to create cavities with ease. It's troublemaker food choices that feed pathogens that, again, produce ammonia, which seeps into teeth and can destroy them as the years go by. It's viruses such as herpes simplex, shingles, and EBV that inflame nerves in the jaw, gums, and teeth, causing them to ache, hurt, and feel sensitive, especially when a beverage you're drinking is hot or cold. No matter which of these factors is the true cause of your dental issue, it's easy (and mistaken) to blame the lemon water you've been drinking for the last day, week, or month. If you're coming to any of these cleanses with fear about lemon water or lemons, you've been misled. That misinformation saturates both alternative and conventional health outlets every day, and it cheats you out of true healing. Lemon (and lime) water cleanses, flushes, destroys, and kills unproductive bacteria, and this leads to a healthier oral environment.

Another reason that teeth can fall apart over time is previous fluoride treatments from years before, weakening the enamel of the teeth. Fluoride is an aluminum byproduct that does not help teeth; it hurts teeth. This speaks to a larger point: as problems develop with your teeth now, it's not necessarily from what you're doing in the moment. The tooth problems that the dentist is telling you about today started years and years ago.

Lemons aren't anyone's favorite food. They're one of the foods people consume the least of—and when someone does eat lemon, it may be in a lemon bar, lemon cake, or lemon tart. It's not the lemon in baked goods that gets our teeth in trouble. It's the milk, eggs, cream, butter, and gluten. If someone's chewing on a fake, synthetic lemon candy every day, or a fake, synthetic lemon gum, I'm sure that's not helpful for their teeth. That has nothing to do with squeezing a half or whole lemon into a large glass of water or squeezing a half a lemon onto your salad. Vinegar doesn't help people's teeth, yet that's a top contender for a food that's in most people's diets. Vinegar is an ingredient in so many recipes and on everyone's salads, and the truth is that it can hurt and hinder enamel. There are very few people who consume lemons on a daily basis. Very few people drink lemon water even on a monthly basis. And very few people even get a lemon in them once a year in some shape or form. So when it comes to lemons, I recommend that you persevere in spite of the misinformation. Let's not blame lemons as the reason that hundreds of millions of people are at dentists' offices getting their teeth worked on. That confusion will only rob you of a powerful tool to cleanse and heal. Move forward with your healing and override your fear of lemons.

HUNGER AND PORTIONS

If you're finding the 3:6:9 Cleanse to be too much food, it's okay to reduce some portions. With the Liver Rescue Salad, for example, you can cut the recipe in half, scaling back how many toppings you include and cutting the base from 8 cups of greens to 4 cups of greens. Otherwise, how much you scale back a given meal or snack really depends: What quantities are you used to eating?

Do be mindful when eating less than the recommended amount of food. Are you cutting back portions so much that you're going to be hungry later and feel the need to reach for something you shouldn't during the cleanse? Fruits, vegetables, and leafy greens are lighter and not as dense as many other foods due to their high water content, even when cooked, and high fiber content. They're somewhat airy, with almost an expansive quality to them. If we're used to eating a hard-boiled egg on a piece of toast in the morning or a piece of cheese, it can take some adjustment to get used to eating a little more food and what fullness feels like when we're focused on fruits, vegetables, and leafy greens.

Also know that when your body is detoxing poisons, your blood sugar can drop because your body uses glucose for strength so it can have the energy and reserves to release poisons. Sugar in your bloodstream doesn't stop your body from detoxing. This makes it that much more important that you consume enough during this cleanse. These cleanses are designed to protect your adrenals because without glucose in your bloodstream, your adrenals will release adrenaline to act as a glucose replacement to keep you functioning and not crashing—and you pay a price for that. If you veer from the recommendations, though—meaning you don't eat enough or don't eat often enough—you could start detoxing a little too quickly, causing your blood sugar to drop and your adrenals to suffer. All that will do is counteract the healing you're trying to accomplish with the cleanse. So remember: keep yourself nourished while cleansing! If someone feels sicker after trying another cleanse out there in the health world, one reason is that it weakened or even injured their adrenal glands. Meanwhile, they'll be told that they're feeling sicker because they detoxed. The truth is that the strain that cleanse can put on their adrenals could be so great that it has them suffering for months afterward.

If you're finding a Medical Medium cleanse to be too *little* food, it's okay to increase portions to whatever your liking is. One exception is that single serving of animal protein that's allowed during dinner on the first three days during the Original 3:6:9 Cleanse—continue to stick with only one serving of it on those days, and continue to limit any other radical fats to dinnertime too, with your overall fat consumption reduced by at least 50 percent.

To feel fuller, up the amounts of recommended fruits, vegetables, and leafy greens. Take apples for example. On the Original 3:6:9 Cleanse, if you're still hungry after, say, the afternoon snack of one to two apples, one to three dates, and celery sticks on Days 4 through 6, first ask yourself where the hunger is coming from. Is it an emotional hunger? Or is it because the day before, you missed some of the foods on the cleanse—had you gotten into a cleanse mind-set where you didn't eat enough? What about lunch? Did you eat a few pieces of lettuce with a handful of brussels sprouts, or did you make your salad with

nourishing toppings and eat it with enough brussels sprouts or asparagus to feel full? If you have been eating enough and your afternoon snack still leaves you hungry, that's okay. In that case, eat or blend up another apple or two with more celery if desired—you'll only get better more quickly. (Do limit yourself to the number of dates called for in each version of the 3:6:9 Cleanse—as beneficial as they are, you want to make sure you leave room for water-rich foods. With too many dates, you could fill up so much that you miss out on the other healing foods.)

That same thinking goes for the other meals and snacks on the cleanse. Take it bit by bit, asking yourself where your hunger is coming from, and if it feels like a need for more calories, increase how much you eat. An easy place to do this in the Original 3:6:9 Cleanse is with the smoothie in the morning. It's perfectly fine and good to make a whole extra Liver Rescue Smoothie to drink mid-morning or to make a supplemental Heavy Metal Detox Smoothie, as you'll read more about in Chapter 21, "Cleanse Adaptations and Substitutions."

Hunger is complex, and sometimes the desire to eat more isn't the body's cry for more calories. Sometimes hunger is a stress response or, as you can read about more in the chapter "Mystery Hunger" in *Liver Rescue*, a liver deficient in glucose. Ultimately, the 3:6:9 Cleanse will help you with both.

While you're on the cleanse, though, and your body is still healing, how do you know what "enough" is in general? Well, if you're someone who never feels quite satisfied no matter what you're consuming, keep that in mind here, so you don't overdo it—say, by eating so much asparagus or brussels sprouts that you know you'll be in discomfort later. Instead, start with a dish of asparagus or brussels sprouts, and see how you feel after eating them with your salad. If you need more after that first serving, add more—or else set aside any extra for a future meal. Hold on to your common sense and take a break when you're satisfied enough and know you've eaten a reasonable amount.

"Satisfaction" can feel different on this cleanse than it does in everyday life. If you're used to eating heavy foods, for example, or lots of grains or radical fats, it may be an adjustment to discover what it feels like to fill up on water-rich fruits and vegetables instead. Everyone's experience is different. For some people, it's the most full and satisfied they've ever been. For others, cravings are going to surface. (Read more about cravings in Chapter 25, "The Emotional Side of Cleansing.") Keep this in mind: While on this cleanse, your liver and body are being satisfied in ways they've never been. They're getting what they need in order to get toxins out and nutrients in. That's eventually going to translate to greater hunger satisfaction and maybe even a whole new relationship with food.

One more concept to keep in mind: If the reason you need more food is because you're very active, do be mindful to take it easy on at least the final day of the 3:6:9 Cleanse. On Day 9, your body is doing a lot of critical work, and staying on all liquids is what supports this work. To honor that, take a break from cardio or other intense exertion.

SALT, SPICES, SEASONINGS, DULSE, AND HONEY

During a Medical Medium cleanse, we need to be mindful about flavoring our food. Here are some guidelines:

Salt: On the 3:6:9 Cleanse and any other cleanse in this book, stay away from even the highest-quality salt. Feel free to squeeze lemon (or lime or orange) on anything and everything for the flavor and mineral salts that citrus contains.

Spices: Cinnamon, cayenne pepper, and similar pure spices are okay to add to your food during the 3:6:9 Cleanse, as long as they're not mixes that have salt or flavoring added. Black pepper is okay too, if you're used to it and like it, although some people find it an irritant. Skip spices during the Mono Eating Cleanse.

Seasonings: Stay away from other seasonings while cleansing. Too often, they have salt, nutritional yeast, flavors, or other hidden ingredients. Avoid soy sauce, tamari, nama shoyu, and coconut aminos too. Stick to pure spices.

Atlantic dulse: This salty Atlantic sea vegetable is also an excellent alternative to salting your food. It's okay to have up to one small, compact handful of Atlantic dulse per day on any 3:6:9 Cleanse version. Dulse is okay on any cleanse in this book other than the Mono Eating Cleanse.

Raw honey: On the 3:6:9 Cleanse, it's okay to have 1 teaspoon of raw honey in your morning lemon or lime water, 1 teaspoon in your nighttime tea or lemon or lime water, as well as the raw honey in any cleanse recipes. For all the other cleanses in this book, raw honey is okay too—up to 1 tablespoon per day.

SUPPLEMENTS AND MEDICATIONS

Here's the most important point about supplementation and cleansing: do not take non–Medical Medium recommended supplements. Popular supplements such as fish oil and collagen, for example, will interfere with your healing.

You'll find a wealth of information about helpful supplementation in Part VI, "Knowing the Cause and the Protocol." Whether to take these supplements or not during a cleanse is up to you—read more in Chapter 27, "What You Need to Know about Supplements." If you're staying on Medical Medium–recommended supplements on the 3:6:9 Cleanse, you'll most likely find it best not to take them on Day 9, when you'll be enjoying so many liquids.

With the other cleanses in this book, you can bring in supplements as you would in your everyday life, as long as they're the specific supplements listed in Chapter 29, "The True Cause of Your Symptoms and Conditions with Dosages to Heal." Find more detailed guidance on supplementation, whether you're cleansing or not, in Chapter 27 too.

If you're on medication, please consult with your doctor about its use.

CHILDREN

In Chapter 8, "Your Guide to Choosing a Cleanse," we covered that all Medical Medium cleanses, including all versions of the 3:6:9 Cleanse, are kid-safe. Mom or another primary caregiver should make the call about what portions are right for your child, reducing amounts to suit your child's appetite. You'll find a table with celery juice amounts for children on page 480.

On the 3:6:9 Cleanse, if Day 9's liquid-focused plan seems like it will be a challenge for your child, you can have them repeat Day 8 instead.

PREGNANCY AND BREASTFEEDING

Also mentioned in Chapter 8, "Your Guide to Choosing a Cleanse," the Original and Simplified 3:6:9 Cleanses are extremely nutrient-dense options when you're pregnant, supportive and healing both for your body and for a developing baby. You'll find both cleanse versions more satiating while pregnant if you repeat Day 8 in place of the Day 9 protocol.

If you want to try the Advanced 3:6:9 Cleanse while pregnant, that's probably an indication that you're dealing with a symptom or condition, which means you're already talking to your doctor about that health struggle. Ask for your doctor's advice about whether the Advanced 3:6:9 Cleanse is in line with what they recommend.

If a health struggle has you wanting to explore another cleanse in this book while pregnant, also ask your doctor(s) for their advice.

When you are breastfeeding, any version of the 3:6:9 Cleanse, and any other cleanse in this book, is okay. It will help pull impurities out of breast tissue, leading to cleaner breast milk.

GALLBLADDER ISSUES

Is it okay to do the 3:6:9 Cleanse, or any other cleanse in this book, if you no longer have a gallbladder? Yes. When someone has had their gallbladder removed, taking care of the liver should be top of mind, and nothing cares for the liver like the 3:6:9. A stagnant, sluggish, problematic, diseased liver that's lost its bile production is far more problematic than not having a gallbladder. The 3:6:9 Cleanse involves eating, and a cleanse that includes eating is always good for someone who doesn't have a gallbladder, because foods low in fat help dilute and sop up the continual flow of bile so that the bile doesn't become irritating to the gut linings. Most importantly, the 3:6:9 Cleanse dramatically lowers or eliminates radical fats (depending on which version you choose), and it's fats that call for the liver to produce an overabundance of bile; a constant diet of high fats constantly prompts the liver to churn out large amounts of bile, and that can be irritating to someone without a gallbladder. The less fat consumed in the diet, the more beneficial for, frankly, anyone—especially someone missing their gallbladder. With a break from radical fats, your liver can get healthy and strong, less stagnant and sluggish, because it gets a reprieve from constant bile production mode.

DIABETES

If you are an insulin-dependent diabetic and interested in the 3:6:9 Cleanse, talk to your doctor about how to make it work. The cleanses in this book are safe for diabetics; they're geared to help cleanse toxins out of the liver, which can improve someone's diabetic condition for the better. Everyone is different, though. Some people have more control over their diabetes and others have more difficult cases to manage. Consult your doctor about what will work with your individual protocol and medications. Also refer to Part VI,

"Knowing the Cause and the Protocol," for a list of supplements specifically for diabetes.

ORGANIC VERSUS CONVENTIONAL

While organic foods are preferable, it's completely understandable if you don't have the access or resources to get organic and you need to use conventional instead.

RAW VERSUS COOKED

If you're raw and plant based, you can continue to eat raw by selecting the Advanced 3:6:9 Cleanse. Keep in mind that any raw diet you already follow probably includes radical fats, dehydrated foods, salt, and other add-ins such as apple cider vinegar, so the Advanced 3:6:9 Cleanse is not the same as what you're already doing. Don't look down on the Advanced as easy or beneath you because you already eat raw. It's still very much a cleanse.

If, on the other hand, you avoid raw food because you associate it with digestive discomfort, so you're wary of raw cleanse dishes such as the Liver Rescue Salad and other cleanse salads, consider this:

(1) Discomfort that we associate with raw food often has to do with items that are tough to digest. Raw carrots, for example, are what we think of when we think of raw vegetables, and they aren't always the easiest to process. The same is true for raw zucchini. While zucchini noodles are quite popular and a great alternative to wheat on other days, raw zucchini can be a little tough on the stomach, and the farther along we are on a cleanse, the easier on the gut we want to go, so the body can put its energy into elimination. There are many more gentle options, such

as cucumber noodles and lettuce, and those are the foods the raw cleanse dishes in this book highlight.

(2) Sensitive nerve endings in the digestive tract are another reason people sometimes have reservations about raw food. As we will cover in Chapter 21, "Cleanse Adaptations and Substitutions," lettuce brushing against the linings of the colon is easy to mistake for trouble digesting it. In truth, that lettuce is helping heal those nerve endings in the long run, so it's on your side.

And if raw foods are an issue for you for any other reason, whether allergies or chewing, then as you'll see in Chapter 21, there are plenty of modification options for you.

FAT-FREE BEYOND THE CLEANSE

What if you feel so great taking a break from radical fats while on the 3:6:9 Cleanse that you want to avoid them for weeks, months, or even years? Is there a reason to go back to eating radical fats? These are great questions that come up often. Answer: it's absolutely fine to avoid radical fats in day-to-day life, and you aren't missing out nutritionally.

As you read in Chapter 7, "Troublemaker Foods," the reality is that there are naturally occurring fats in nearly every fruit, vegetable, leafy green, sea vegetable, and herb. In a small handful of dulse, there's a bit of fat. In butter leaf lettuce, in potato, in banana, in green beans, and on and on, you'll find traces of fat, all of it much better able to serve your health than when you consume radical fats in large portions. So you're not missing out. You can go "fat-free"—by which I mean

avoiding radical fats such as nuts, nut butters, seeds, oils, olives, coconut, avocado, and animal products—long term, for a lifetime if you want, and you won't be missing out on nutrients. Beneficial omegas are in countless foods, including berries, mangoes, lettuces, other leafy greens, and more.

There are only so many foods a person can eat. Is the person who eats nuts and seeds also regularly getting every fruit and vegetable for every possible nutrient? Not even that—is the person who eats nuts and seeds getting a complete variety of nuts and seeds, with chia seeds and flax seeds and hemp seeds and every other nut and seed under the sun laid out on their table, or is it always the same walnuts on their granola or peanut butter on their oatmeal? No one circulates through every food and gets everything.

Inundating ourselves with variety isn't the answer. You can get more nutrition from eating only a handful of different foods in a day versus eating the entire rainbow of foods in one day. There's only so much room in a day, an appetite, a schedule to get so many foods into ourselves. The person who doesn't eat radical fats has more room for more nutrient-dense foods—that is, fruits, vegetables, leafy greens, herbs, and sea vegetables—to fill their plates. These foods contain critically needed healing phytochemical compounds, antioxidants, antivirals, antibacterials, trace minerals, bioavailable protein, and mineral salts that don't come from radical fats. That usually means they're getting a wider array of nutrition over time than someone on fats.

What's concerning is the person who excludes fruit altogether. Think of these critical nutrients they're missing out on from foods such as watermelon, banana, wild blueberry, and papaya if they turn instead to chicken or a handful of walnuts. Think of all the beta-carotene and multitudes of other nutrients someone is getting, on the other hand, when they sit down for a meal of two or three mangoes and some leafy greens. That's powerful.

(Never be concerned, by the way, about getting too much beta-carotene from fruits such as mango and papaya. You can never get too much of it; beta-carotene is one of the most important aspects of skin health and anti-aging.)

HEALING REACTIONS AND ADDITIONAL DETOX METHODS

While cleansing, it's easy to get into a frame of mind where you want to heighten the cleanse effects as much as possible by trying other techniques at the same time. Infrared sauna, yoga, bodywork—should you turn to these during the 3:6:9 Cleanse? For reasons you'll read much more about in Chapter 20, "Your Body's Healing Power," you're best off keeping yourself focused on the cleanse. Your body is doing a lot on the 3:6:9, and giving it anything new to juggle isn't the ideal approach.

In that chapter, you'll also find support to guide you through any detox symptoms, which I call *healing reactions*, that may arise as you cleanse. Not everyone feels physical effects while cleansing. If you do, though, it's natural, and it helps to understand what's going on beneath the surface. Further, it's natural when changing up your food, even for one meal or one day, for emotions or cravings to surface. You'll find insights into how to navigate that side of cleansing in Chapter 25, "The

Emotional Side of Cleansing." And again, as this is a spiritual cleanse, you may want to bring in the meditations from *Liver Rescue*. They're incredible for emotional support.

WATER FASTING

Water fasting from one to three days is an option for acute health conditions—for example, for food poisoning, gallbladder attacks, or possible appendicitis. I don't recommend water fasting past three days; it takes a toll on the body, more so than water fasting professionals believe.

There's a good chance you're going into a water fasting program with a chronic health condition. If your health condition is neurological on any level, water fasting works against your condition instead of helping it. A neurological condition can range from chronic migraines to body pain to burning sensations on the skin to neuropathy to tingles and numbness, weak limbs, brain fog, anxiety, depression, twitches, tics and spasms, OCD, bipolar disorder, and so many more. I strongly advise against water fasting with an anxiety condition. Water fasting is also not good for people with posttraumatic stress symptoms (also known as PTSD) or any kind of emotional injury, because it can be a difficult emotional experience all on its own to stop eating. It's emotional enough for many people to stop foods that aren't good for us such as eggs, pizza, coffee drinks, matcha, and lots of chocolate, never mind to stop everything altogether. Water fasting can even trigger old emotional injuries into high gear, putting a person back in that mental space of when they experienced the injury.

When you do choose to water fast, there's always the question: Are you water fasting properly? Are you consuming enough water on your water fast? If you are, it has to be just water. And distilled water is not good for water fasting; it doesn't have enough minerals or trace minerals within it, so water fasting with distilled water can lead to a severe electrolyte crisis, especially for someone struggling with any kind of neurological condition. I'm not totally against water fasting. It is a useful tool at times. It's not a strong, foundational healing and cleansing tool to embark on long term to help you recover from symptoms and conditions and move forward. Breaking a water fast is when a lot of mistakes are made—which food they choose, how much they consume. Water fasting also has an addictive and obsessive quality to it, where once you've passed a certain number of days, you're almost afraid to start eating.

If you do choose to water fast, stick to a one- to three-day timeline. Drink a 16-ounce glass of water every hour, starting from when you wake up and continuing until you go to sleep. Make sure you're not driving. Make sure you're not running around doing errands. Make sure you are in a safe place, and if possible, you have a coach to communicate with via the phone or Internet. A 24-hour water fast is a good standard for when you have an acute condition that warrants it—if you're dealing with lots of nausea you've never had before or abdominal pain, or if you caught the stomach flu. If you're really committed to water fasting to give your digestive system a vacation, you can experiment and try it one day a month. Whenever you break a water fast, don't jump into normal eating right away. Break your water fast with the Morning Cleanse from Chapter 16.

JUICE FASTING AND JUICE CLEANSING

If you feel the need for a juice fast or juice cleanse, I recommend one to two days of celery-cucumber-apple juice. Start each day with 16 to 32 ounces of lemon or lime water, follow that up 15 to 30 minutes later with 32 ounces of celery juice, and after another 15 to 30 minutes, you can start sipping your celery-cucumber-apple juice. Make each juice 16 to 20 ounces, and drink one every two hours for the rest of the day. If you want, you can add a touch of ginger, spinach, or kale as you're juicing. Consume nothing in between each celery-cucumber-apple juice besides water, preferably a 16-ounce glass of water an hour after each juice. Keep life low-key during your juice fast—don't overextend yourself, and rest when needed. While one to two days of this juice fast can be very helpful, I still recommend doing the other cleanses in this book to really help heal, detox, and cleanse the organs in your body.

I don't recommend long-term juice fasts or juice cleanses. Long term, they don't cleanse the liver and detox the body properly, because they eventually start to place stress on your body systems. While the celery-cucumber-apple blend provides the perfect balance to stabilize your glucose levels short term, going past two days on the juice leads to a lack of glucose that starts weighing heavily on areas that really need it: your brain, your liver, and your heart. A long-term juice fast or juice cleanse also doesn't provide enough calories to sustain you and keeps your blood sugar too low, so your detoxing works against you as your adrenals start doing a lot more work to fill in for blood sugar. This constant pumping of adrenaline (also called epinephrine) can give you a false high. It's the reason people on extended juice cleanses can experience moments of high energy—that's the adrenal glands clicking in after two days to release adrenaline as a mechanism to protect you. You don't want to put your adrenals in this position; it backfires. As the excess adrenaline enters the brain, it starts to break down neurotransmitter chemicals, saturate neurons, and saturate the liver, and it is corrosive to the nervous system overall. By the time you're on the fifth, sixth, or seventh day of juice fasting, you're running on adrenaline. Is this better than running on coffee all day long and not eating? Yes, it's better. If you want to cleanse, though, and you want to cleanse properly, you don't want long-term juice fasting.

If you see this section of the book and say, "Ah, juice fasting! Just what I wanted to do," and then you go to the Internet to look up juice programs, know that you're not going to be embarking on something as helpful as you're told it is. If you've done a juice fast before and you've experienced benefits, I'm more than happy to hear that. Other issues can appear with your health down the road because of that long-term juice fast, though—weakened adrenals, for example, and a stagnant, sluggish liver because it had to soak up all that adrenaline during your juice fast. A juice fast or juice cleanse sometimes irresponsibly detoxes too many toxins, which don't leave your system and get reabsorbed back into your liver.

The maximum length for a juice fast or juice cleanse is three days. Past the three-day mark, you're venturing into glucose deficiencies, neurotransmitter and electrolyte imbalances, stress upon your liver, and weakening of your adrenals. Anywhere between one to three days can be helpful, as long as you follow the guidelines from the first paragraph of this section: lemon or lime water followed by celery juice followed by celery-cucumber-apple juice (and water) for the rest of the day.

"Empowerment is having answers.
It's knowing that your body is not attacking itself.
It's knowing that your genes or hormones are not responsible
for your sickness, that you are not a faulty person.
It's knowing that you're not a bad person either, and that
you didn't create your illness with your mind-set and emotions."

— Anthony William, Medical Medium

CHAPTER 20

Your Body's Healing Power

Even as a Medical Medium cleanse is offering relief in many ways—relief that we can either feel immediately or will experience down the road a little—life can still hand us its usual challenges. For example, maybe a relationship will expose us to a new bug, or we'll forget to wash our hands before eating and we'll find ourselves with the sniffles. Maybe we'll take an emotional hit from a conflict with someone close to us, and we'll find ourselves feeling down or even experiencing a physical symptom such as a stomachache. Maybe we'll be eating at a friend's house or restaurant as a last hurrah before a cleanse, and we'll pick up food poisoning that kicks in just as we start the cleanse. It can be easy to mistake these challenges for cleanse-caused problems.

In truth, these challenges are not the cleanse's fault. They're not our fault either. They're part of the reality that life isn't perfect. And that's fine! We can't control everything coming at us. While it is possible to experience mild healing reactions from the cleanses in this book—that is, physical and emotional signs of detox, which we'll get to in this chapter and Chapter 25, "The Emotional Side of Cleansing"—it's just as possible to run into normal hassles, annoyances, and obstacles. For people who are chronically ill, these tend to create more disruption. For example, going to the store and trying on clothing that was treated with fungicides, or buying new clothes and not washing them properly before wearing them, could make someone itchy and irritable if they're chemically sensitive. It would be easy to blame those symptoms on a Medical Medium cleanse, when they're entirely unrelated.

The same goes for heightened stress at work or in the home; financial issues; exposure to mold, pesticides, or herbicides; or similar situations that occur just before or during a cleanse. Everyone is sensitive to different stressors, some of which they may not even realize are triggers for physical or emotional trials. Try to maintain this awareness. Try not to blame your cleanse or lose faith in cleansing. If you do, you'll block yourself from accessing this profound path to healing.

WHAT TO EXPECT WHEN YOU'RE CLEANSING

Your cleanse experience will be unique to you. Each time you cleanse will also be unique. The cleanses in this book, and especially the different versions of the 3:6:9 Cleanse, were created to be there for all your differences—because in so many ways, we are not all the same. Emotionally, physically, and spiritually, your experience and how you're going to feel may not be like how someone else feels after completing such a powerful healing process. And your experience the first time you try the 3:6:9 Cleanse may not be the same as when you try it again, or again after that. Try to leave room for those different experiences from person to person and cleanse to cleanse.

More Detox Measures

If you're a fan of other detox measures or modalities, hold off during your cleanse. As beneficial as healing arts such as infrared sauna, yoga, chiropractic treatment, massage, and acupuncture can be, try not to introduce any of them during your cleanse if they're new to you—or if you're bringing them back after time away. If you're used to getting weekly massages or acupuncture or going to yoga at least once a week, it's okay to continue during the cleanse. What I don't want you to do is say, "Okay, I'm doing this 3:6:9 Cleanse. Let me jump into a sweat lodge"—or hit a sauna or jump into a hot spring or head to a retreat center or start a spinning class or take a yoga class for the first time—because chances are, you're going to tire yourself out and stress your body while you're doing the cleanse. Or, and this is just as important, I don't want you to say, "I'm

starting this 3:6:9 Cleanse. Why don't I *restart* the yoga practice I stopped months ago?"

I know it can be tempting to try to juggle some different healing practices when you start a cleanse. You've probably cleared a little space in your life and gotten yourself into that cleansing mind-set, so it makes sense to want to go into full-on self-care mode. The best self-care you can give yourself is to relax and focus on the 3:6:9 Cleanse.

One reason is that healing practitioners are likely to give you other recommendations while you're on the cleanse, such as suggesting certain foods or supplements, and that can throw you off course. Here you are on track with the 3:6:9 Cleanse, and you visit a new acupuncturist, for example, who says, "Why aren't you on fish oil?" If that leads you to start taking it halfway through the 3:6:9 Cleanse, you'll throw off the whole cleanse with the practitioner's well-meaning and misled advice.

Another important reason not to start introducing or restarting practices during the cleanse is that as you're processing out toxins and poisons, your body is trying to find balance. If you haven't done yoga in two years and you decide to do an hour of it, or if you haven't had a massage in a long time and you decide to get one while you're cleansing, you may throw off that equilibrium your body is trying to find. Say you strain a muscle while doing yoga for the first time in a long time—now your body has to dedicate part of its immune system's precious reserves to repairing and healing the injury so inflammation reduces, even if it's mild. Any modality, however beneficial, stands to tax your body's immune system as it adjusts, and that takes away from your body being able to do what it needs to do as it follows through on the cleanse to the letter.

Weight

Our weight isn't nearly as straightforward as we've been led to believe. If you have extra weight on your body and don't find it coming off as quickly as you'd like on the 3:6:9 Cleanse, that's not a sign that the cleanse isn't working for you. Know this: your body is using its energy reserves on other, more important aspects of your body that need to be healed, versus shedding a few pounds in the moment. The weight loss can come later. Organ repair and central nervous system repair start first. This doesn't mean your body hasn't started the weight loss process. In truth, as fat cells disperse, if they're toxic fat cells, then the body produces a little more water to hold on to the toxins being released so they can be safely cleansed out of your body.

Most people are filled with retained water and compacted stool. Basically, their colons are packed, even if they're on what they believe is a healthy, balanced keto, paleo, plant-based, vegetarian, or vegan diet. They've got 7 to 8 pounds of extra stool, sometimes even more—as much as 10 or 14 pounds if they've been on a standard, conventional diet; others have only 5 to 6 pounds of extra stool in them if they've been on a somewhat pure diet. Everyone's intestinal capacity is different too. Some small intestines are narrow and some colons are extra large, with pockets. Then there's swelling and fluid buildup (edema) from a lymphatic system overburdened by toxic waste. Some people are swollen with 5 to 10 pounds or even 20 or more of water weight, and water weight can look like fat.

The 3:6:9 Cleanse will have many people eating lighter than usual. Even though you should eat the quantities you need to feel full, the foods themselves are water-rich and packed with glucose, bioavailable protein, antivirals, antibacterials, trace omegas, trace minerals, antioxidants, and healing phytochemical compounds, and that's going to encourage your body to let go. Especially at the end of the 3:6:9 Cleanse, you'll be eating lighter, so when you go to the bathroom, you'll be releasing much of what's in the intestines as well as the fluid buildup. That's part of what results in weight loss.

If you're someone who's not really swollen with a lot of water retention or backed-up stool and you don't have a lot of fluid to lose, you may not see immediate weight loss, because first your body needs to get properly hydrated. That is, you could be someone who ate very small portions before starting the cleanse, maybe due to discomfort or emotional struggle, and who didn't drink fresh juices and smoothies or eat fresh, juicy fruits. Instead, maybe you were on caffeine to give yourself energy, sipping lots of coffee drinks, which left you chronically dehydrated because caffeine is a diuretic. When you go on a Medical Medium cleanse, then, because you're getting more fiber and pulp and you're getting hydrated for the first time, your weight loss may not show itself on the scale right away, even though you are losing fat cells.

Someone else could lose the weight quickly because they do have a lot of water retention and edema, plus they're coming into it with lots of impacted, backed-up stool. The timing is going to be different for everyone. Many times, I've seen people who were constipated rapidly drop 5 to 10 pounds or even 18 to 20 pounds when they switched over to the cleanse foods because they eliminated backed-up stool.

Here's how much the extra matter that accumulates in our gut factors into weight: Say the morning after skipping dinner, you wake up, go to the bathroom, eliminate your lunch and breakfast from the day before, and weigh yourself. The scale could show you're five to seven pounds lighter than the next day, when you weigh yourself in the morning after eating dinner the previous night. That's perfectly natural and healthy. It's because in the morning, your evening meal is still being processed in your gut.

Now say you eat dinner, maybe a big dinner, wake up the next day, and eliminate yesterday's breakfast and lunch. Then you go ahead and have your morning coffee, bagel, avocado toast, oatmeal, eggs, or smoothie; you follow it up with lunch; and then you visit the doctor's office around 1 or 2 P.M. If you're weighed there, you could be 7, 8, 9, or even 12 pounds heavier than the morning after you skipped dinner, because you're still carrying around three meals' worth of food plus liquids.

Again, this is perfectly normal—and it confuses a lot of people who weigh themselves at different times during different cleanses. It can even incite a kind of weighing frenzy if someone hears from the doctor, for example, that they're at one weight one day versus "Oh, you're eight pounds lighter," or six pounds lighter, or six pounds heavier another day, all of it varying because the readings are from different times of day after consuming different fluids and eating different types of meals that are at different stages of digestion. If you needed one more sign in life that it's not worth basing your self-worth on the number on the scale, this is it. There is no one number anyway; it's constantly changing, and so are you—and that's exactly as it should be.

By the way, those examples are all if someone is eliminating fully and regularly. When most people visit the bathroom, it's not yesterday's meals they're eliminating. They may still be processing food from two or three days ago without even realizing it—that's some of the extra stool I'm talking about that people carry around. The other extra stool that people carry is impacted on the sides of the intestinal walls. When you try one of the cleanses in this book, particularly the Original or Advanced 3:6:9 Cleanse, that impacted stool starts loosening up and moving through so it can finally exit your body and leave you lighter.

Worries about Weight Loss

What if you follow the cleanse to a T and you don't lose as much weight as you'd like, meaning that your body still has some healing to do? Or what if after the cleanse, you start gaining weight back—which can happen if you return to eating food that's not great for your body, as fluid and stool retention start back up again, with the potential to add another one, three, five, or more pounds on the scale?

The solution in both cases—whether you want to lose more weight or you want your weight loss to be more lasting—is to repeat the cleanse, the details of which we'll cover soon. This is important: don't try to outsmart any Medical Medium cleanse by deciding to starve yourself while you're on it. Starving yourself—holding off on meals because your mind-set is that you're on a cleanse and you want weight loss—will reduce your calories and maybe show a difference on the scale in the short term, yet it won't ultimately accomplish what you're trying to accomplish. Instead, it will put your body into adrenaline-production mode. That will both counteract what the cleanse is trying to do—a liver saturated in adrenaline is one of the factors that can contribute to weight gain in the first place—and set you up to make troublemaker food choices when the hunger catches up with you. On top of which, excess adrenaline scorches your neurotransmitters, which can trigger emotional hunger.

The Square One Rule

Another reason that it can take your body a bit of time to release excess weight is that your body has a pushed-too-far built-in protection mechanism. When your liver is stagnant and sluggish and filled up with toxins and pathogens, your body is constantly acclimating to and compensating for your individual toxin levels, constantly adjusting to try to keep your weight level. At a certain point, the liver becomes so saturated that your body can't keep its balance anymore, and workouts and standard diet changes aren't enough to keep the weight off. That's when you may try a more drastic diet or workout routine. Here's the drawback: when you're losing weight by manipulating your body systems, using adrenaline as the trigger and causing a crisis, that's a false result that's only temporary because it wasn't done in a healthy way. Everyone has their own unique trip switch when it comes to how far the body will let itself be pushed in these cases.

Here's what I mean: We can make a mistake one time—that is, we can try a technique that manipulates the body systems—and the body forgives us. Once we've realized the technique isn't sustainable and we've let it go, the body adjusts itself back to a new starting line, one that is not as helpful as where we were before we made the mistake. When we make a mistake two times—we try another adrenaline-heavy technique—the body forgives us again and goes back to yet another starting line, one that is less helpful than the previous. If we make a mistake three times, the body still forgives us and takes us back to a new starting point, this one not as helpful as any before. Most of the time, our body gives us these three allowances for making mistakes.

Sometimes, it only has two allowances or even one allowance to give. It all depends upon a person's toxic levels and pathogens, along with the condition of the liver and adrenal strength.

After the three (or two or one) allowances the body has to give, the pushed-too-far mechanism kicks in to protect you. It's a trip switch for your body to protect itself—because there is a cost to the mistakes we make as we try to lose weight or search for better health. In truth, we're constantly making mistakes. That's not our fault; it's because there are so many modalities, techniques, and belief systems out there that are all theories that are not good for us, and how are we supposed to know they're not serving us when we're told that they're sanctioned and sensible? The reality is that there isn't a single health professional who truly knows why people gain weight. It's only theories about macros, calories, metabolism, and how much you exercise, and when all else fails, they theorize that your genes must be the reason you have weight on you. Really, there is a cause, and there is a health issue behind a struggle with weight. When the blame is on the person, though, we will continually be lost. We will keep moving on to the next theory and the next theory, and this will cause more and more damage, more and more emotional and physical harm to the ones who are struggling with their weight. We *are* harmed by these theories, even though we have to go into denial that a technique or diet or modality harmed us in any way.

One common mistake is the weight loss advice to hit the gym for two hours a day, with no one realizing that doing so can burn out the adrenals, especially if someone's already living with adrenal fatigue. When you push the adrenal glands harder and harder, they can weaken, causing even more weight gain later on. People who go no-carb and eat nothing but protein and fat to try to lose weight rapidly don't realize how much harm this process does. While yes, they are removing processed foods, which can be helpful in the short term, there's always a price to be paid for a diet of high-fat/high-protein foods. No one is free from the trouble that cutting out carbs causes for the body—the glucose deprivation of the brain and organs, and the stress upon the liver and adrenals from the increase of fat in the diet.

As we test out these different misconceptions, our bodies forgive us and bring us back to square one, with damage done. Take note: "square one" could mean gaining back weight. That is, if you lost weight recklessly by cutting out carbs based on a guessing-game theory that wasn't created around what your body has to endure or why you'd even gained weight to begin with, then it may mean you put weight back on as your body tries to bring you back into balance. And remember, there's that three-allowance (or sometimes two- or one-allowance) limit. At a certain point, our body will hold its ground, and it may have some extra weight on it when it reaches this stage—the stage where the safety switch has been tripped and our body doesn't give in to the mistakes we make in our trial-and-error efforts to make ourselves healthier. Our body doesn't trust our decisions; it doesn't trust us anymore—which again, even if we haven't picked the best food choices and even if we overeat, isn't our fault.

Keep in mind that there always seem to be people who can get away with eating anything without gaining weight . . . until years later. What's happening in the moment when they seem to be untouchable is that toxins and pathogens haven't caused a stagnant, sluggish liver and other health conditions as early in life. Their high-fat diets haven't caught up with

them—yet. They're in the same boat, susceptible to the same chronic mistake factor that can be involved with our health-making attempts on so many levels. It's only that timing that hasn't brought them to the same place yet.

If you haven't made a lot of mistakes while seeking help and you have weight to lose, weight should come off while you're on the 3:6:9 Cleanse. If you *have* been led to make a lot of mistakes in trying out different theories, weight loss options, and diets that weren't beneficial, your body is likely to have lost trust and may hold its ground by keeping some weight on for a little while longer before it allows change to occur. In this situation, I recommend doing the Original or Advanced 3:6:9 Cleanse multiple times, and even multiple times in a row, where after completing all nine days, you go back to Day 1 and start over again. As you'll see in the next section, you could also consider starting over at Day 7 after your first round.

After you wrap up your repetitions of the 3:6:9 Cleanse, I also recommend a low-fat or preferably no-fat policy long term: for 90 days minimum. When I say "low-fat" or "no-fat," I'm referring to limiting or cutting out radical fats such as avocado, nuts, seeds, nut butters, cacao, chocolate, oils, chicken, beef, bone broth, and fish. As we've covered, you'll still get all the beneficial fats you need from foods such as fruits and vegetables, so you don't need to worry on the nutrition front. I also recommend saying no to the troublemaker foods from Chapter 7, as they are a sure way to gain weight.

I know that removing radical fats may sound like a radical approach. What it does is allow your body to trust you again. You could even decide to cut out radical fats for 90 days *before* your cycles of the 3:6:9 Cleanse *and* 90 days after. That's a way to really engage your body's trust.

Your body's trust may come quickly as your liver begins to rejuvenate, something radical fats do not let it do. After you start your second consecutive 3:6:9 Cleanse, you'll usually start to lose weight more rapidly. Or the trust may take a bit of time, and that's why it serves you to stay off radical fats long term. Trust depends on how much your body has been through, how many mistakes it's encountered that weren't liver-friendly or adrenal-friendly. It also hugely depends on how bogged down, burdened, toxic, and problematic your liver is. If your liver is filled with pathogens and toxins—and you may not realize it is—cleansing could take longer to alleviate your liver of toxin levels, because your body could be releasing those toxins more slowly to protect you. That means everything in the long run, so try to have patience. As you restore your body's trust in you, you'll find your trust in your body start to restore.

And as you think about weight loss, also consider that theories about what makes an "ideal body" are personal preferences based on what someone has been conditioned to think is acceptable or not, weight-wise. The world doesn't understand frame sizes in the context of water weight versus body fat. It's all guesswork out there. How can anyone know what's truly standard when no one knows what causes sickness or weight gain to begin with? What about when some women lose their period after they start eating really well? Is that bad or good? It's all guessing, and the guesses usually blame low body fat. What about when a women loses her period and has body fat? Standards are thrown around and created by nothing other than guesswork. As long as chronic illness remains a mystery, who knows what is really healthy or not and what the body needs? That's why the cleanses in this book come from above: to take the guessing games out of how to take care of yourself.

Repeating the 3:6:9 Cleanse for Weight Loss

If you feel your weight is not yet where you'd like it to be for your health, I recommend repeating the 3:6:9 Cleanse. The Original and Advanced 3:6:9 Cleanses are the most likely to give you results in this area. You have a few choices in how you do that:

- As soon as you finish Day 9 of one complete 3:6:9 Cleanse, you can start the cleanse over from Day 1, cycling through as many times as you'd like; or

- As a technique to really focus on reducing weight, as soon as you finish Day 9 of one complete 3:6:9 Cleanse, you can start over at Day 7 and keep repeating those last three days as much as you'd like; or

- You can go back to your normal life after one cycle of the 3:6:9 Cleanse and then fit a cycle of the cleanse into your life again the next month and the month after that and so on. In between your rounds of the 3:6:9 Cleanse, do the Morning Cleanse each day, stay off troublemaker foods entirely, and consider holding back radical fats periodically.

Whichever option you choose will allow you to keep getting healthier and healthier, rejuvenating your liver, detoxing poisons, restoring nerves, and helping every organ in your body heal. That's what sets you up to bring the edema down, release the impacted stool from your intestines, release and disperse unwanted fats and toxic lymph fluid, and lose more weight.

Worries about Rapid Weight Loss

Some people are in the opposite boat, concerned about losing too much weight. If that's you, we need to think about it from a few different angles. How much does your concern have to do with a number on a scale? How much does it have to do with how you look? How much does it have to do with how you feel? In some cases, a person who's been chronically ill is missing muscle from not being able to exercise, and that lack of muscle mass is what makes them appear thin. Rebuilding their health is what they need to work on first, and slowly. Once their symptoms (for example, fatigue or body pain) are improved, they can then start to use their muscles more and more each day, doing basic tasks and chores, and they can even get to a point of being able to exercise and build muscle again rather than trying to focus on eating a lot more food.

Sometimes it's the case, especially with men, that they don't realize they have a lot of swelling, with a layer of toxic fluid and a thin layer of fat over all their muscles. When the body starts healing, that swelling may start to dissipate quickly as the toxic fluid cleanses from the body. If you were used to being bigger, at a higher, more robust weight, this process can be confusing. The reality is that you had gotten comfortable with being toxic and swollen.

In some cases, a person is naturally petite and small-framed, used to getting told how thin they are when that's just how they're built. This can create insecurity around their weight. Some people have a history of disordered eating, so when they try to heal themselves by eating better and they end up losing some toxic water weight, compacted stool, or fat, alarm bells can ring for those who care about them, which can in turn trigger the people who are trying to heal. Some have suffered emotional harm from others' comments about their weight, whether because others thought they were carrying too much weight or not enough. This applies pressure and can also cause fear that they're making the wrong decisions in trying to heal.

With all of this, it can be very difficult to balance perception of weight and body size versus what's really going on with your body in the moment—it's hard to see when you're in it. This book is about getting rid of your symptoms, your sickness, your illness that you're struggling with. When you're healthier, you can build muscles faster and more easily. You can get your life back on track. You can get your confidence back. You can become more secure and at ease with your natural weight where it is.

How hungry are you? Are you withholding food, eating only one or two bananas and one or two potatoes a day, with various fruits and juices, and feeling hungry and losing weight? Are you never hungry, eating very little because of that, and dropping weight? People do get into situations like these, where they need to be careful to eat enough. They need to be continually mindful to remember to eat during the cleanse.

One important part of all this to remember is the backed-up stool that most everyone carries around in their guts. Particularly with the Original or Advanced 3:6:9 Cleanse, someone is apt to become 5 to 10 pounds lighter fairly rapidly over the course of the cleanse as they go to the bathroom and eliminate accumulated stool. In other words, don't panic if you see your weight go down markedly at first. Recall that scenario where you're getting weighed at the doctor's office midday—and showing up a few pounds heavier than at another time of day. Our weight fluctuates greatly based on how much food and liquid are inside us at a given moment, which is exactly as it should be. We need to remember this so that we don't get too obsessive over the number on the scale. The 3:6:9 Cleanse is balancing and will help you reach that place of healing where you can build the muscle you want to build.

If someone is underweight, then the way to handle the Original or Advanced 3:6:9 Cleanse is to cycle through the first and second three days of the cleanse—that is, to do Days 1 through 6 (The 3 and The 6)—and to save the final three days (The 9) for a time when they've recovered their health enough and feel confident enough to do all nine days. If you're trying this approach, you can cycle through Days 1 through 6 however many times you want, by which I mean once you've completed Day 6, you can go right back to Day 1.

You can also try Days 1 through 6 once, wait a couple of weeks, do Days 1 through 6 again, and keep up with that schedule until you eventually feel ready to do all nine days together.

There's no rush in getting to all nine days of the 3:6:9. With each repetition of those first six days of the cleanse, you will still be releasing toxins, starving pathogens, cleansing and healing your organs, and preparing your liver to get out even more poisons when the time is right. You will still be healing.

Bowel Movements

It is perfectly normal to experience increased bowel movements on the cleanses in this book. The 3:6:9 Cleanse especially provides more hydration and fiber than you likely get in day-to-day life, and the daily celery juice restores your hydrochloric acid and liver function while killing pathogens that are highly toxic, which can in turn improve your bowel movements. Plus the pitaya in the Liver Rescue Smoothie tends to move through your system quickly because it can have a mild laxative effect.

You won't experience constipation for the first time in your life on these cleanses. If you do experience constipation, it's an indication that you came to the cleanse with constipation, or that you've experienced it before. In that case, it's not unusual to experience constipation while on the cleanse, as your intestinal tract is still in the process of recalibrating and healing.

HEALING REACTIONS

When we're cleansing or detoxing the body, we have to remember the basic truth that we're dealing with poisons, different poisons that have accumulated in our systems in different quantities for everyone. Some varieties are more toxic than others. Some people have experienced more exposure in daily life: for example, spilling gasoline on their hands while mowing the lawn or pumping gas; or regularly breathing in harmful household cleaners, air fresheners, colognes, perfumes, or scented candles; or frequently coming into contact with pesticides, herbicides, fungicides, or even indoor insecticides in the home.

I can't tell you how many times I've heard the story of someone who saw a bug skittering across the kitchen counter and in response, grabbed a can of bug killer and sprayed the spider or ant right there on contact, on a food surface, while also inhaling it and getting the spray on their skin. We live in a world with constant exposures like this. These poisons build up in our bodies, and we walk around with more of them inside us than anyone realizes.

The same goes for pathogens. We all walk around with multiple viruses and bacteria that eventually feed on these toxins that build up in our bodies. This combination is what begins causing our first set of symptoms that we walk around with and that starts us off looking for answers.

So again, when we talk about getting better, we're talking about battling quite a lot. It can take our bodies time to let go of toxins and kill pathogens and repair the damage that's been done for years. How that process works and looks can be different for everyone. Sometimes letting go looks like immediate relief from your symptoms. Sometimes it takes a little more time, and we need to know that this is okay too.

Remember, before you decide that any discomfort you're feeling on the 3:6:9 Cleanse (or any other cleanse in this book) is the cleanse's fault, it's important to ask yourself a few questions: Is this part of a natural rhythm with a preexisting symptom? Did you experience a trigger that had nothing to do with the cleanse? Was anything in your life inconsistent? Did you catch the flu right before the cleanse and think the cleanse caused your symptoms? Did you experience an emotional blow or stressful event right before the cleanse? Were you exposed to air freshener, perfume, or cologne in a ride service car just as you were beginning the cleanse? Were the foods you were eating before the cleanse troublesome—were you pushing the envelope, and now it's catching up with you?

That last question is important: Did you party before you started the cleanse? Ninety percent of people who start any cleanse give themselves extra leeway beforehand, drinking and eating foods they know they won't be able to eat soon, foods they wouldn't even normally eat, as a last hurrah before buckling down. Whether premeditated or without thinking, people eat a few farewell meals and then hop into a cleanse and forget about it. When a symptom arises—which can even happen four or five days into it—they don't realize it's a direct result of their pre-cleanse party period, not a detox symptom. As you read in Chapter 7, "Troublemaker Foods," these party drinks and foods stick around in our bodies.

It's all too easy to blame anything that crops up during or after the cleanse on the cleanse itself—just as it's all too easy to blame any symptom on anything new in your life, rather than on the old problems that have been building and building out of sight. When someone gets their very first migraine, for example, whatever they did that day becomes etched in their mind as the cause. If they happened to try coconut for the first time in years and the migraine came on that day, the coconut will become the fall guy. Or maybe someone was about to get their very first migraine when they started the 3:6:9 Cleanse—it was coming anyway—and the cleanse is the easy target for blame. They don't realize that migraines are caused by a complex interaction of multiple issues that have been building in the body, and that really, their migraine came on because their liver had been becoming stagnant and sluggish, causing the body to become too toxic over time. As you'll read about soon, sometimes on a certain level—even subconsciously—you feel a symptom coming on and start the cleanse when you get that internal signal. The cleanse certainly wasn't the cause; it was your instinctive measure to give your body extra care to get through it. A Medical Medium cleanse is there to help you heal and bring you that much closer to getting any symptoms out of your life.

If all your ducks are in a row, none of the above explains your symptom, and you really feel that what you're experiencing is from the cleanse, then know that it's a healing reaction—a sign that the cleanse is digging out a lot of poisons and killing off pathogens. As the cleanse is cleaning out your liver and other organs, some toxins are touching on nerves and surfacing to the skin on their way out of your body. The symptoms this causes are generally mild, since any Medical Medium cleanse is designed to create a very controlled release. If you're filled with a lot of toxins, though, and your healing reaction reaches a point of too much discomfort, you can always stop the cleanse, take a break, and restart it another time. If it was the Original 3:6:9 Cleanse you tried, give the Simplified 3:6:9 Cleanse a try when you're ready and then come back to the Original 3:6:9 Cleanse later. If it was the Advanced 3:6:9 Cleanse you tried, then go back to the Original. Or you can always try the Mono Eating Cleanse.

Throughout this process, it helps to be able to interpret what your body is doing, and that's why this section on healing reactions is here for you. Besides interpretations of what common healing reactions mean, you'll also find explanations of when a particular experience is *not*

a healing reaction and instead a sign that your body still has some healing to do.

Flare-Ups and Emotional Episodes

While on the 3:6:9 Cleanse, if you experience a flare-up of any sort of symptom or condition that you're used to dealing with, first ask yourself how often your flare-ups occur at other times. Whether acne, eczema, fibromyalgia, tinnitus, aches and pains, fatigue, or any other issue, how frequently do you struggle with these bouts? Have you paid attention along the way, documenting when they arrive? Do they occur every 10 days, every two weeks, every month? If your eczema acts up during the 3:6:9 Cleanse, it could just be one of your natural cycles of flare-ups—and doing the cleanse diligently and often enough will ultimately help those cycles die down.

If you experience a symptom flare-up on or after the 3:6:9 Cleanse and it doesn't coincide with your normal flare-up timing, then we need to consider the next set of questions. Have you experienced any triggers lately? In the week before you started the cleanse, was anything emotional occurring in your life? Were you up against intense stress? Did you give yourself a pre-cleanse party period, and now it's catching up with you?

Say you've determined that this isn't one of your normal symptom flare-up cycles, and you can't think of any other possible trigger. Then yes, it does so happen that some people experience the symptoms of preexisting health problems as healing reactions while the cleanse addresses the underlying issues.

A skin condition such as eczema or psoriasis is a useful example here. With milder varieties, it's not common for a flare-up to occur in relation to the cleanse, because the 3:6:9 Cleanse eliminates toxins from the liver and body in such a controlled manner. If someone has dealt with a long-term severe struggle with eczema or psoriasis, on the other hand, and has perhaps taken medication to help them survive it, then they could experience a skin flare-up after the cleanse. That's because these pronounced skin conditions are a sign of an overload of toxins inside the liver, and when dermatoxins especially start flooding out, even in a measured way, sensitive skin can become irritated. When this happens, it's important to keep in mind that you're one step closer to getting to the finish line of eventually healing your eczema, psoriasis, or other skin condition, as so many have before by using Medical Medium information.

With flare-ups, we also need to consider the pathogenic side. When we're starving viruses of the foods they like to consume, they can become desperate. Previously, they were comfortable in our body, in an environment that was supportive of them. It's not our fault that pathogens were thriving; it's because we're taught to eat certain foods and at the same time not taught why we're sick or what causes the illnesses of our time. When someone doesn't have a certain pathogen and they're eating a standard, "normal" food, they feel like a normal person. When someone has a virus or bacteria and they're eating that same food, they can keep getting sicker and sicker because they're feeding that pathogen with that food, and they're completely unaware of what's happening. Instead, it's the confusion of "Well, that other person can eat that same food and not experience an effect. Why can't I?" That's if a person even realizes they're affected by a food. And if they do realize it, they may guess

it's an allergy or a sensitivity and blame their body rather than pointing to the food itself as a troublemaker. At any rate, pathogens become comfortable in an environment where they're fed, and when you take food away from the pathogens, there can be an uproar. Our medical system doesn't yet have these answers about food, so it isn't yet capable of delivering this critical information so we can protect ourselves.

It's not unlike disturbing a beehive. Viruses and unproductive bacteria that have colonized certain organs or other parts of our body are happy when they can grow and proliferate and live a life cycle. And when we change that environment by taking away their fuel, they become desperate. They go searching for food and even need to draw on the storage deposits of food they've rationed away inside their cells and our organs. When we starve a bacterium or virus—and that's what we do on the 3:6:9 Cleanse—it cannot live long. The pathogen's colonies often start to die off quickly, and as a result, we can temporarily develop a symptom we've experienced before from that same pathogen. When it's a toxic virus, one that's filled with a food source such as mercury, egg protein or hormone, or a toxic chemical it's found inside our liver, then when it's not being fed anymore and starts to die, it's going to release that poison. Some viruses even explode as they die off. And that poison release is what can instigate symptoms we experienced when the pathogen was alive and releasing those same poisons as neurotoxins.

So if you're someone who's susceptible to shingles pain, which comes from the neurotoxins created by the shingles virus family, and you go on the 3:6:9 Cleanse and start killing off shingles virus cells because you've taken their food sources away, that virus is going to start dying off and can release the same poison it did when it was thriving. As your body carries the viral poisons out, they can touch nerves or surface to the skin as shingles pustules, making it seem that the virus is active again when in truth it's a sign of die-off.

Another important point is that before the virus cells die off on the cleanse, they start scrambling and looking for fuel. To propel them on this search for food, they need to use up whatever energy source they have stored inside them, and that means they expel and release that poisonous energy source as they move along. It's like how, if you needed to get up off the couch and go running down the street, you'd start sweating and probably need to go to the bathroom before too long because the movement got everything moving inside of you too. When you starve a pathogen, it needs to get up off the "couch" where it's been happily chilling out in a comfortable environment, and it needs to go running down the "street"—basically, your bloodstream— looking for resources. On this race for survival, the virus is going to expend energy and excrete enormous amounts of poison. Even though it will eventually die off, the poison it expels on its search for food can mean that you experience a small flare-up. That flare-up can just translate to being more tired, with less energy and maybe a little swelling and a little more neurological pain.

That's if someone has been viral for quite a while and they've built up and stored a lot of viral toxins. Take note that not everybody experiences pathogenic die-off symptoms. Everybody has different varieties of bugs, and a lot of bugs are not so toxic. That is, you certainly don't need to go into the cleanse with

fear in your heart. You could easily be someone with milder varieties of bugs or toxins who doesn't feel the effects of them leaving the body. If, on the other hand, you happen to be someone who experiences the confusion of a mild flare-up during or after the cleanse, return to this section to reassure yourself that what your body is going through is normal— and that any temporary discomfort is a healing reaction, not a cause for worry.

If you experience your normal bouts of fatigue, brain fog, or other symptoms you've had before, or if your current symptoms continue during the cleanse, that doesn't mean you're not healthier after the cleanse or that you're not closer to getting rid of the symptoms altogether. Sometimes it takes more than one cycle of the 3:6:9 Cleanse to expel enough poisons, toxins, viruses, and unproductive bacteria so that you can eventually be symptom free.

Also keep in mind that if you're going through any sort of flare-up, even if you haven't experienced the symptoms in a long time, it means the underlying issue or illness that's causing the symptoms never disappeared altogether. Or it's possible that you've picked up a new bug along the way, and now you're experiencing new symptoms that are similar to what you've had before. Either way, the cleanse is necessary to work on getting to the root of that condition so that it doesn't turn into a deeper disease down the road. The cleanse is working to help you heal and rid pathogens. It can take some time to tame a virus so you can heal. When you're between cycles of the 3:6:9 Cleanse, there's supplementation to assist with so many different chronic symptoms, conditions, and illnesses. This extra measure is often needed to help you heal and repair, especially from a viral situation, which is why you'll find that Part VI, "Knowing the Cause and the Protocol," is entirely devoted to herb and supplement lists for health issues.

What about an emotional episode? Is that normal after the 3:6:9 Cleanse? It can be, for the same reasons that a flare-up can be. It's not normal to have an episode of anxiety, depression, or mania that's any worse than what you've experienced before, though, not unless you happened to experience emotional confrontation or challenge before, during, or after the cleanse, or unless you went through an unexpected loss or difficult emotional stress. Instead, episodes will be milder due to cleansing's improvement of poison, toxic heavy metal, and viral neurotoxin levels. For example, your episodes of anxiety could even be completely gone after the cleanse.

It's also not normal as a result of any Medical Medium cleanse to experience the onset of anything new. If during or after the 3:6:9 Cleanse or any other cleanse in this book, you do develop a symptom you've never had before, it was already on its way. It's common when you're dealing with chronic health issues for newer symptoms to pop up along the way. The cleanse didn't bring the symptom on or bring the symptom on sooner. It was a coincidence of timing or—here's a truly important point—on some level, you could have felt the symptom coming on, and that's what could have subconsciously prompted you to start the cleanse when you did, to give your body some extra care. You'll read more about this in the next section. You don't need to worry that the cleanse somehow caused your problem; what a Medical Medium cleanse does is protect you from future symptoms while supporting you through anything in the present.

Sniffles, Coughs, Sinus Infections, Migraines, Sties, UTIs, Sore Throat, Tongue Coating, and Fatigue

It may just so happen that you develop an acute symptom such as a sniffle, cough, sinus infection, migraine, sty, UTI, sore throat, tongue coating, or fatigue during or after the 3:6:9 Cleanse. This isn't because the cleanse caused the symptom or made you sick. Rather, what often happens is that someone has that intuitive, instinctive feeling that something is going wrong in the body, and they get the sense that it's a good time to try a cleanse. Maybe you read the 3:6:9 Cleanse section a month ago and then one day out of the blue, it occurs to you that you should begin. It may not be so out of the blue. Whether entirely subconsciously or on a slight physical level, in some way that feeling of coming down with something influenced you. It was going to come anyway, and an internal instinct kicked in to try to protect yourself with the cleanse, like feeling the need to prepare before a storm.

This intuition is one we've had inside us for thousands of years. It's the same instinct that would have kicked in to send you down to the riverbank to bathe the day that bad bacteria started festering on your body, even if you didn't know it. Bathing—cleansing ourselves on the outside—is an inherent urge we have when we feel we need extra help in some way. So is cleansing from the inside out.

In our modern world, the flu goes around 24/7 everywhere on the planet. So do other bugs we can pick up eating out at restaurants or using public restrooms or sharing utensils, plates, and cups. We're susceptible to picking up and passing on bacteria and even viruses in intimate relationships. And before we feel the onset of any of these bugs, before we show any symptoms, our body sends us messages. Usually, those messages make us drink a little more water or herbal tea—or start a cleanse.

This book could have been sitting on your shelf for months, and one day you pick it up and decide to try out the 3:6:9 Cleanse. If along the way, you start to come down with flu-like symptoms, a sinus infection, a migraine, or the like, know that it wasn't the cleanse that caused it. Rather, the cleanse is here to help you through it.

Chemical Sensitivities

If you're chemically sensitive, you're most likely already dealing with an abundance of toxins, plus viral toxins such as Epstein-Barr neurotoxins. I share in detail about chemical sensitivities in *Liver Rescue*, and in Part VI of this book, I offer a list of supplements to help with healing from them. Before you even start cleansing the poisons, you're already sensitive in so many ways. For example, if you brush your teeth with a toothpaste that has a little too much essential oil and you're chemically sensitive, you may experience irritated linings in the mouth. People with chemical sensitivities have a hard time dealing with both synthetic and even the most natural chemicals in many cases because the system is so overburdened— there's no room for any kind of additional exposure. Again, that's life before you've even started to cleanse.

Some people are more chemically sensitive than others, so how they experience cleansing will be different. And because of the unique variations of toxins that different people carry, how those toxins affect someone as they come

out of the liver and out of other cells in other organs will vary. For some, it may play a role in increasing a symptom temporarily. The 3:6:9 Cleanse is geared for the most sensitive people, though. No version of the cleanse is harsh, pushing all poisons out at once. Rather, it allows poisons to leave gradually—and to actually leave the body instead of getting reabsorbed and causing more trouble later.

Because the cleanse is so gentle, if you experience an upsurge of chemical sensitivity symptoms during it, there's a good chance that there's an outside cause that happened to coincide. What else were you doing in the days and hours leading up to the symptoms? Did you breathe in some diesel fumes when you walked past a truck in a parking lot? Did you try a new toothpaste? Did you go into a store that had scented candles or plug-in air fresheners or cologne or perfume in the air? Did a neighbor get a pesticide treatment around their house, condo, or apartment building when you had your windows open, and you unknowingly breathed in the chemicals? Did a delivery person whose arms were covered in cologne drop off a package at your home, causing your front entryway to reek of chemicals from the smell of the box? Did you get new clothes that have been treated with fungicides? Have you been driving a car that secretly harbors mold, taking more rides in it than usual? Did you try a new makeup or hair care product? Did you spend a few hours chatting with friends whose clothes smelled heavily of scented detergent or fabric softener—and your flare-up occurred the next day? There are endless factors like these that we need to consider before blaming the 3:6:9 Cleanse.

Is it possible for the 3:6:9 Cleanse to cause some sort of chemical sensitivity flare-up? Yes, a mild symptom could arise—and if so, it would be a detox symptom, a positive sign of healing and release. This is the gentlest cleanse there is for someone with chemical sensitivities because it takes such careful care of the liver. The 3:6:9 Cleanse and the other cleanses in this book help rid chemical sensitivities. If you don't feel ready to try the full nine days of the 3:6:9, you can always do a shortened version—see the "Back to the Beginning" section of Chapter 13, "Repeating the 3:6:9 Cleanse" for options. Or the Mono Eating Cleanse from Chapter 18 is an excellent option for you.

Edema, Water Retention, and Swelling

If you're already sensitive to swelling of any kind—such as lymphedema, in which lymphatic vessels fill and expand with fluid, creating distension, bloating, or swelling in various regions of the body, whether the ankles, calves, legs, hands, breasts, arms, face, or abdomen—then it's a sign of a liver that's highly toxic, inflamed, sluggish, and stagnant from various poisons it has collected in order to protect you. When someone is especially viral, they become more susceptible to swelling as well, often gaining weight, much of it water retention.

The liquid of lymphedema and water retention is not clear water. It's a pus-like, opaque fluid that has filled the lymphatic system and organs, and it's a direct result of pathogenic activity in the body. Many of the over 60 varieties of EBV, for example, produce a lot of viral byproduct. That triggers the body to produce fluid to trap the byproduct in order to protect that person from experiencing, for instance, more neurological or fibromyalgia symptoms. Even in certain more serious situations, that fluid is produced to try to save your life.

When this fluid was first produced it was clear, and once it trapped the toxins, that's when it changed its color. This fluid retention can be sporadic. It could be more pronounced at different times of the month or week. It could happen every two weeks or every day. It could be down in the morning, increasing all day long, and up at night, especially if someone is sensitive to gluten, eggs, dairy products, corn, or even too much salt.

All of this plays a role if someone is trying any of the Medical Medium cleanses such as the 3:6:9 Cleanse, or any other cleanse, for that matter. If someone already deals with edema, they may see their swelling come and go while on a cleanse. Sometimes, if the liver is very toxic, with a lot of viral byproduct built up, the body may produce more fluid to protect you as a safeguard while the cleanse sends poisons, toxins, and viral waste matter out of the liver and flushes them out of the body. For the person experiencing the resultant swelling, this can be confusing. It can seem as though the cleanse is not working or that you're moving backward. In truth, it's a healing reaction.

If you want to manage your water retention in between cycles of the Liver Rescue 3:6:9, then take yourself off all the troublemaker foods from Chapter 7 both before and after the 3:6:9. This will starve the pathogens and allow poisons and toxins to continue to leave the body with ease. Once you've been off the foods for long enough, you'll start to experience swelling less and less.

Bloating

Most often, the Medical Medium cleanses *alleviate* bloating. If you do experience any bloating while on one of these cleanses and never had bloating before, it can be an indication of unproductive bacteria in the gut dying off. It could also be the result of the cleanse purging the liver of toxins that then have a slight inflammatory effect on the intestinal tract on their way out. Once you've gotten through this healing stage, you're likely to start experiencing less bloating post-cleanse.

You may be someone who experienced bloating before your cleanse. In that case, it's going to take time to restore your hydrochloric acid, bring your bile reserves to a stronger capacity, and kill off the bacteria causing your bloating. Try to have patience with it and remember that you've started healing already.

Upset Stomach or Nausea

As with everything else on this list, an upset stomach or nausea while cleansing is not by default a result of the cleanse. In the 3:6:9 Cleanse, there's the flexibility in the foods to consider. That is, during the first three days of the Original 3:6:9 Cleanse and during almost all of the Simplified 3:6:9 Cleanse, you have license to choose some of your own foods. Did you try to push the boundaries and reach for a troublemaker food that could have disrupted your digestion?

Also important to consider is whether you happened to pick up a stomach bug before you started a Medical Medium cleanse, or if you've been eating out during the cleanse and could have picked up food poisoning that way—or if you ordered something out that seemed healthy and, unknown to you, had a troublemaker ingredient. We need to keep an eye on even prepared food from the natural foods store. These prepared foods often have MSG-based ingredients such as nutritional yeast, seasonings, and natural flavors. Also be mindful about canola oil

when eating out. Kitchens often use an oil blend that they label as only "olive oil."

When someone experiences nausea on the 3:6:9 Cleanse and it's not from the above, then it's someone who already deals with nausea periodically in life, which is often caused by viruses and toxic heavy metals inflaming the vagus nerve. The cleanse wouldn't cause nausea—not unless somebody is cranky and truly detests the food on the cleanse, which is unusual. Rather, someone with nausea on the cleanse is someone who's already sensitive. Perhaps they're triggered by food smells or by fragrances and cologne. That could continue on the cleanse, although it's not the cleanse's fault. In truth, the 3:6:9 Cleanse can help alleviate conditions such as nausea over time.

As far as upset stomachs go, if there's no chance you've picked up any sort of bug or pushed boundaries in the food department or had an emotional confrontation or emotional moment, then what you may be feeling are sensitive nerves in the digestive tract. When lettuces or other leafy greens and raw vegetables brush past these nerves in your gut while they are still healing, you may feel some discomfort. An important point to remember is that those foods are actually providing nutrients to help the nerves heal, and that gentle brushing is helping clean up the intestinal tract. You may still find it's too much bulk for you right now, in which case you can consider blending up your various meals, as the cleanse guidance outlined.

If you start the Original or Advanced 3:6:9 and experience discomfort—whether stomach upset or nausea, whether from a bug you picked up or any other reason—it's fine to switch over to the Simplified 3:6:9 partway through. You can also stop the cleanse altogether and try to address what's going on by using the Mono

Eating Cleanse. Once you're feeling better and feeling ready, you can give any version of the 3:6:9 Cleanse another try.

Abdominal Discomfort

While cleansing, people occasionally experience discomfort in the general area of the liver and worry about what this means. One possibility when this happens is that somebody has a sensitive region in their small intestinal tract or colon that happens to be close to the liver. It may be a "hotspot" they contend with throughout their days in normal life, and while they're cleansing, that ache, pain, or other symptom has come to awareness because they've started tuning in to their body more. The underlying reasons for these types of hotspots vary. They can happen because of bacteria such as *E. coli* or *Streptococcus* inflaming the colon. The small intestinal tract can also become inflamed from pathogens such as viruses and bacteria. And these bugs cause gas to be produced that moves around the intestinal tract, triggering sensitive hotspots by putting pressure in areas that are inflamed, which can cause intestinal spasms and cramping. Most everyone is dealing with gas production. Pathogens and their toxic byproduct can inflame nerves around the organs and intestinal tract too. Because these problems all take time to address and heal, someone could still be feeling discomfort from any of them while cleansing. Ultimately, the cleanses in this book are going to move you toward relief from these hotspots.

There are also reasons why someone may feel actual liver discomfort while cleansing. The 3:6:9 Cleanse wakes up the liver. Many people's livers are so stagnant and sluggish that they're practically asleep—they've had to shut

themselves down in order to stay alive. A liver that's filled with poisons, toxins, and fat deposits struggles too much otherwise, overusing energy and heating up. Blood doesn't move through it freely, clearly, and easily. Previous diets haven't fed it with what it needs to recharge, so the liver tries to preserve and sustain itself by going into what's basically sleep mode as it performs the critical functions that keep you alive and breathing in order to protect you. When you start the 3:6:9 Cleanse, it's like you're waking that sleeping giant. You're saying to your liver, "Hey, it's safe to cleanse now. I'm about to give you what you need to restore yourself so you can recharge." And as though it were a mighty old lion waking up from a nap in the middle of a hot day and doing a big stretch and yawn and shaking its body out a little, your liver comes to life. That purging liver starting to realize it's allowed to cleanse is a new sensation to many people. And when they first become aware of it, they could identify it as discomfort. An awakening liver also means that its cells start to regenerate and renew themselves, including the cells that create bile. That liver cell renewal alone can cause a gentle spasm. It's like an old engine rumbling and sputtering as it sparks back to life.

Hemorrhoids

As I mentioned in "Bowel Movements," when you change your diet by going on a very healthy cleanse, you may find yourself eliminating more often. If you're someone with preexisting hemorrhoids, going to the bathroom more than usual—and passing poisons and toxins that are barreling out of the liver and leaving through the urinary and intestinal tracts—can cause an already inflamed rectal area, where veins and mucus membranes are sensitive, to flare up.

Often people have a certain rhythm of going to the bathroom. If they only move their bowels once a day, hemorrhoids may be kept at bay. Suddenly, eating more fruits, vegetables, and leafy greens means more fiber and enzymes moving food along, expelling poisons from the liver, and sweeping it all out of the colon, and that can translate to bowel movements a couple of times a day or more. While that won't aggravate hemorrhoids for everyone, when it does, those inflammatory poisons and toxins that you're passing are the reason.

This is temporary, because you're getting rid of the very poisons that have been residing in you and causing flare-ups on and off, causing constipation over the years, and causing you to strain on the toilet and hemorrhoids to worsen. The 3:6:9 Cleanse can eventually move you to the point of not flaring up old hemorrhoidal tissue. Once the inflammatory poisons and toxins have passed from your liver and intestinal tract, hemorrhoids really can be a thing of the past—on top of which, you can find yourself going to the bathroom with ease and not running into constipation, and that alone can make enough of a difference to give you relief.

Dizziness

Some sensitive people may feel a bit of lightheadedness or mild dizziness on Day 9 of the 3:6:9 Cleanse. When that happens, it's usually because someone is not so used to eating lightly, and at the same time, they're detoxing and flushing poisons out of the body. Some people have a higher load of toxins to flush out. Some people have been chronically ill for a long time, with sensitive central nervous systems and high anxiety, and they're cleansing a lot of poisons such as viral neurotoxins, other viral byproduct, pathogens, toxins, and toxic heavy metals, which inflame the vagus and phrenic nerves and are mainly responsible for vertigo and dizziness.

This is why I recommend staying low-key and close to home on Day 9 of the 3:6:9 Cleanse. Plan ahead so that it's not a day when you have a bunch of errands or a full day of work on your plate. Most hypersensitive individuals tend to spend more time at home and gauge their calendars wisely anyway. They know how to make their schedules fit their needs, so protecting Day 9 as a chance for downtime while they're eating lighter should come as a natural choice.

Aches and Pains

Other than the possible viral or neurological flare-up symptoms we covered, it's not typical to develop aches and pains as a healing reaction on Medical Medium cleanses. It's important to remember that not everything you experience while on the cleanse is a result of the cleanse. An ache or a pain is likely to be preexisting—that is, you're likely to have experienced that ache or pain before. Keep in mind that it's even possible to be in the process of developing a viral infection from a bug you were exposed to months or even years ago, and that the viral infection is creating inflammation in the nerves that's causing aches and pains. It's ideal that you've started the Medical Medium cleanse, then, because it will help you address the underlying bug. Also remember that aches and pains can come up from normal, day-to-day causes such as lifting heavy grocery bags, heavy bags of garbage, or packages delivered to your home, or from adjusting a piece of furniture in your house or deciding to exercise for the first time in quite a while.

Headaches

If you're already prone to getting headaches and migraines, you could get one while cleansing if you experience any of your normal triggers. As with aches and pains, headaches will only occur on a Medical Medium cleanse if they're already a part of your life; a bad headache isn't a symptom of detox.

Dry Skin

Dry skin while detoxing—is this normal? For this answer, we need to break it all down a bit.

First, when the liver is stagnant and sluggish, filled with neurotoxins and other viral byproduct, dry skin can occur as a resulting symptom. Sometimes it just so happens to occur on a cleanse—and it was going to happen anyway because those viral toxins were poised to spill over and cause dry skin. (As toxins exit the liver, sometimes they don't all leave the bloodstream fast enough, and some of these toxins enter the derma and try to leave through the skin.) That is, there are individuals who were heading for dry skin without realizing it.

There are also individuals who start a cleanse just as they're beginning to experience dry skin in their life, or they've already been getting dry skin because their liver is filled with toxins. And keep in mind that chlorinated water, indoor heat, and weather conditions such as cold, heat, humidity, and dry air all play a role in increasing skin irritations that can result in dry skin. Starting a cleanse at the same time the weather changes and brings drier air could be that perfect storm that creates the symptom of dry skin that just so happens to coincide with when you start the cleanse. The cleanse will get

the blame—because again, we tend to blame our problems on anything new.

Sometimes it's not entirely a coincidence that dry skin occurs on the cleanse. While the cleanse isn't the *cause* of the dry skin, it has sped up the process of viral toxins surfacing through the skin, so the symptom occurs earlier than it would have otherwise. Because the toxins are surfacing as part of a detox process, this is ultimately serving you; the goal is that after you get through this, your skin will be more hydrated than it would have been if you hadn't tried the 3:6:9 Cleanse or another Medical Medium cleanse in this book.

On occasion, someone will go through the cleanse, lose a little weight, feel better in different ways, and move on—and then two or three months later, develop dry skin. Because the cleanse wasn't all that long ago, they may wonder if it was the cleanse that somehow brought it on. When this happens, the reality is that the dry skin was coming anyway, and the cleanse prevented it from being worse.

In cases of eczema, psoriasis, dermatitis, rosacea, vitiligo, and similar skin conditions, the cleanse is not causing them to worsen. These conditions mainly occur as the result of dermatoxins produced by a virus in the body that's feeding largely on toxic heavy metals. As we examined under "Flare-Ups and Emotional Episodes," the 3:6:9 Cleanse can flush out those dermatoxins from the liver, causing them to surface to the skin as someone goes through their healing process. This elimination brings someone closer to minimizing the symptoms of their skin condition, to healing, and to experiencing more hydrated skin, as you can see on all the healing stories on social media.

CHAPTER 21

Cleanse Adaptations and Substitutions

As you go through the 3:6:9 Cleanse, try to stick to the foods as outlined. That's especially important in the Original and Advanced 3:6:9 Cleanse, where foods are laid out meal by meal. Try to follow what the cleanse offers rather than switching it up because you decide to drink more juice than is recommended or to eat bananas after dinner or steamed veggies as a snack before bed.

All of that said, I don't want you to panic if there are any foods in the cleanse you can't access or enjoy. In cases where following the letter of the law doesn't work when it comes to each specified food, adaptations and substitutions are available to you, and we'll explore those later in this chapter.

There's also one way to augment the Original or Simplified 3:6:9 Cleanse if you're interested, and that's with the Heavy Metal Detox Modification. (No need to augment the Advanced 3:6:9 Cleanse, which already incorporates heavy metal detox.) Let's look at that modification first.

HEAVY METAL DETOX MODIFICATION

If you're concerned about cleansing toxic heavy metals specifically, first, know that as part of addressing a broad group of troublemakers, the 3:6:9 Cleanse will help you eliminate some heavy metals—and not just any cleanse would do that. Most importantly, any version of the 3:6:9 gets other poisons and toxins out of the liver so that you can more successfully detoxify toxic heavy metals afterward. Freed up from other troublemakers following the cleanse, your liver and other parts of your body will be able to deliver deeper pockets of metals for extraction—pockets that you couldn't have gotten to before. So one option is to complete the Original or Simplified 3:6:9 Cleanse as outlined and then turn to the Heavy Metal Detox Cleanse in Part III, knowing that it can be more effective than ever.

Another option is to choose the Advanced 3:6:9 Cleanse, which has heavy metal detox built into it.

And yet another option is the following modification that incorporates targeted heavy metal detox into the Original or Simplified 3:6:9 Cleanse.

How the Modification Works

In the morning, drink the Heavy Metal Detox Smoothie (recipe in Chapter 23). It's as easy as that. It's your choice whether to add the smoothie to Days 1 through 8 or to start it at The 6—that is, to drink it on Days 4 through 8. In either case, hold off on the Heavy Metal Detox Smoothie on Day 9 and stick to the protocols as outlined. (More in a moment.)

If you're on the Original 3:6:9, this doesn't mean you should drink the Heavy Metal Detox Smoothie *instead* of the Liver Rescue Smoothie. Rather, drink it *in addition* to the Liver Rescue Smoothie. A good option would be to have the Heavy Metal Detox Smoothie mid-morning, after you've had the Liver Rescue Smoothie. If you don't have room for full servings of both over the course of the morning, you could make each smoothie a little smaller than the recipe. You don't need to space out the smoothies from each other—it's okay to drink your Heavy Metal Detox Smoothie just after your Liver Rescue Smoothie if you'd like.

See Chapter 17, "Heavy Metal Detox Cleanse," for how to handle missing ingredients. There's also an option to eat the smoothie ingredients separately rather blending them, which that chapter explains.

How to Handle Day 9

Don't worry about the fact that you'll be skipping the Heavy Metal Detox Smoothie on Day 9 of the 3:6:9 Cleanse. On that day,

it's not about removing heavy metals specifically. It's about removing everything that's ready to leave the liver and other organs at this point. It's about pushing all these poisons, toxins, dissolved fats, and old storage pockets of adrenaline out of the liver's cells and the body's bloodstream and guiding them out of the kidneys and intestinal tract. This will naturally include toxic heavy metals that have been loosened in the cleansing process and that have already started to leave thanks to your Heavy Metal Detox Smoothies on other days. And *because* of those recent smoothies, you'll still have remnants of the five key ingredients of spirulina, cilantro, barley grass juice powder, Atlantic dulse, and wild blueberries in your system—enough remnants to remove any dislodged toxic heavy metals on Day 9. So remember, in order to cleanse your bloodstream as intended, hold off on the Heavy Metal Detox Smoothie on Day 9 and concentrate on the fluid-focused Day 9 protocol from whichever version of the 3:6:9 Cleanse you selected.

(The exception is if you're repeating Day 8 of the 3:6:9 for any of the reasons mentioned in Chapter 19, "Critical Cleanse Dos and Don'ts." In that case, it's fine to keep the Heavy Metal Detox Smoothie in your morning. It's specifically when you're following the Day 9 liquids that you'll want to skip the smoothie.)

FOOD AND RECIPE ADAPTATIONS AND SUBSTITUTIONS

It's not always possible to access the foods specified in the 3:6:9 Cleanse, or you may have a concern about chewing, digestion, or food sensitivity. Keep reading for guidance.

Fruit

Some people feel they have a food sensitivity around fruit. Keep reading for specific insights into apples that will help illuminate your more general hesitance around fruit. Also find specific smoothie ingredient substitutions under "Liver Rescue Smoothie" in a few pages.

If you're still hesitant, remember that in Chapter 13, "Repeating the 3:6:9 Cleanse," you found guidance on repeating Days 1 through 3 to help your body start healing enough that you can bring in more fruit again to benefit from its cleansing power. For much more on what's behind concern around fruit, see the chapters "Chemical and Food Sensitivities" in *Liver Rescue* and "Fruit Fear" in *Medical Medium*.

Apples

If you avoid apples for any reason, there are options for you. First, if it's because you have difficulty chewing apples—for example, due to trigeminal neuralgia, temporomandibular joint dysfunction (TMJ), or a dental situation—you're welcome to chop them up in a food processor or blend them into a raw applesauce. Or sometimes people have trouble with raw apples and find that cooked apples work fine. In that case, make yourself some simple cooked applesauce or buy some in a jar—just make sure that if it's store-bought, you select high-quality organic applesauce with no additives such as citric acid, added sugar, or natural flavors.

There are cases where someone feels they can't stand applesauce. They'd like to chew the apples and can't for physical reasons; they'd like to eat the apples blended and can't due to an emotional aversion. In that specific circumstance, you could do fresh apple juice as a replacement. Know this, though: this isn't like celery versus celery juice (where juicing celery unlocks all the benefits to make it work best). With apples, the pulp and the pectin are part of what make the fruit so healing. Plus, if you rely on juicing apples, you'll get hungry—you won't get the satiation effect that's important to keep you going on the cleanse. Say someone brings bagels into the office during your 3:6:9; you may end up eating a bagel because your empty stomach is telling you they're irresistible—and that will mean needing to start the cleanse over from Day 1. If you had eaten an entire apple, with all the pulp, pectin, and juice it contains, there's a good chance you would have snubbed the bagel. Substitute fresh apple juice for the apple snacks in the cleanse only as a last resort—if you can't tolerate whole apples, applesauce, or ripe pears (the last of which you'll read about in a moment).

In the 3:6:9 Cleanse, you're welcome to eat as many apples as you'd like. If two apples don't fill you up in the afternoon, eat three or even four. People sometimes wonder if they can overdo it—if there's a limit to how many apples they should eat. The answer is that the only way you can eat too many apples is if you're forcing them down, making yourself uncomfortable. Apples are self-limiting, meaning that they're hard to overeat. Even with the sweetest, juiciest varieties, you'll get a pretty clear signal from your body of "That's all the apple I can fit in right now." Let that be your guide.

Some apples are too tart to eat in quantity. For example, Pink Ladies sometimes get sour, dry, or hard. Similarly, Granny Smiths are usually not juicy or sweet enough for this cleanse—you'll get sick of them too quickly. Fujis, though, can be excellent, as can so many other types of apples out there, including varieties that may be specific to your region. Actively seek out different types of apples until you find at least one you really like. Head to the grocery store or farmers' market, look at the piles of colorful varieties available, pick some up and examine them, read the descriptions, and see what appeals to you. Try not to get pigeon-holed into eating one type of apple—try different apples. Find the most palatable apples you can—everyone has different tastes. Eating them should be enjoyable, not a chore.

If your favorite apple happens to be a red-skinned apple, you are in luck, because red-skinned varieties contain some of the most beneficial antioxidants and antiviral, antibacterial phytochemical compounds available from apples. Red-skinned apples also happen to be sweeter in most cases, so once again, you're in luck. The extra glucose in red apples can even be more helpful for your liver when it's depleted of its glucose reserves from years of a high-fat diet.

Keep in mind that sometimes, people fear apples because they were told they have an apple sensitivity, when the truth is that allergy testing is often not accurate. As a result of a fallible allergy test, a well-meaning practitioner will commonly give a patient a whole list of items they're allergic to, with apples on that list, when the reality is that the person has never reacted to apples in their life. If that sounds like you—that is, you've always felt fine eating apples, and you're only avoiding them because you've been told to—try not to deny yourself the healing opportunity that apples can offer.

If you do react to apples, period, then opt for ripe pears instead during the cleanse. This will take a little planning—you may have to shop a few days before you start The 3 so that you have soft enough pears by the time you need them, and then you may need to replenish your stock partway through the cleanse to make sure they're ripening on schedule. Ripe pears will offer easier digestion than unripe ones.

At the same time, know this: In truth, apple sensitivities trace back to someone biting into an apple covered with wax and pesticides that hadn't been washed off first. When that happens, the tongue will instantly pick up on the chemicals, and sensitive trigeminal and vagus nerves, which connect with the mouth, will trigger a reaction that may include itchiness, tingles, numbness, or a burning sensation. Chemically sensitive people who've experienced this often have to stay away from apples for a little while and then may find that if their nerves calm down after a few months, they can try an organic apple, peeled if needed, without having a reaction.

Asparagus and Brussels Sprouts

As you read in the Original 3:6:9 Cleanse chapter, you can substitute zucchini or summer squash for asparagus or brussels sprouts if needed.

Here are a few more notes on asparagus and brussels sprouts:

If you have difficulty chewing, try mashing, food processing, or blending your steamed or raw asparagus or brussels sprouts (or zucchini or summer squash). You can even blend them together with the Liver Rescue Soup ingredients (or simply the greens from the soup) and then sip the mixture.

Alternatively, you can boil your asparagus or brussels sprouts (or zucchini or summer squash) in some water or Liver Rescue Broth and then blend them together for a hot soup variation. That's a very basic option. If you'd like proper recipes, see Asparagus Soup or Brussels Sprout Vegetable Soup in Chapter 23.

If you're highly sensitive and don't feel you can handle any of the above alternatives, it's okay to juice your asparagus or brussels sprouts. In that case, follow the Liver Rescue Juice recipe.

Blended Melon, Fresh Watermelon Juice, Blended Papaya, Blended Ripe Pear, and Fresh-Squeezed Orange Juice

These foods are varied enough that you should be covered for your Day 9 blended options. It's up to you whether you want to pick one and sip on that all day, or if you want to try, say, blended melon in the morning and blended papaya later in the day. If you're going to mix it up, do be mindful not to blend them with each other (no orange juice–pear blends, for example). Enjoy each on its own.

If you want a little green with your fruit, you are welcome to blend these with barley grass juice powder or spirulina. Don't experiment with other powders, though. And in the case of papaya, while blending a few papaya seeds with the fruit can be beneficial at other times, hold off during the 3:6:9.

Dates

If you don't enjoy dates, you don't have access to any, or you want to mix up the routine, mulberries (dried or fresh), raisins, grapes, and figs (dried or fresh), in that order, can all stand in for dates as beneficial liver warmers. You can swap in a handful of whichever you choose to substitute for the dates. It's okay to

chop or blend them up with the apples you'll be snacking on at the same time.

Celery and Cucumber Snacks

For the celery stick snacks that go along with the apples on certain days, it's okay to substitute extra cucumber if you're low on celery. Likewise, you can use extra celery sticks in place of cucumber when needed. And remember, if chewing celery (or cucumber) is difficult for you, you're welcome to chop it finely in the food processor or blend it up with the apples.

Celery Juice

If you can't access celery to make celery juice and you can't get fresh, pure celery juice from your local juice bar, don't despair. Cucumber juice is the ideal substitute in this case. While it can't offer the specific healing benefits that celery juice does, it does have unique benefits such as hydration to support your health. Treat it the same way you would celery juice—make it pure (cucumber only) and drink it on an empty stomach, apart from other food and drink.

Ginger water, aloe water, and lemon or lime water are alternatives if you can get neither celery juice nor cucumber juice.

Cucumber-Apple Juice

As you read in Part II, "3:6:9 Cleanse," the rule of thumb with this Day 9 cucumber-apple juice that's called for in the Original and Simplified is to make it a 50-50 blend. If you prefer apple over cucumber or vice versa, it's okay to make it a 75-25 blend, favoring whichever of the two you like better. And if raw apple doesn't work for you, you can make it a cucumber-pear juice instead.

It's not the end of the world if you do straight cucumber juice. While it will be lacking in calories, you can get glucose and calories from the blended fruit that you're drinking the rest of Day 9.

And if for some reason you can't find cucumbers, look for fennel bulb as a replacement in your cucumber-apple juice.

Hibiscus, Lemon Balm, or Chaga Tea

If there is a specific reason why you can't do hibiscus, lemon balm, or chaga tea—for example, you are under a doctor's orders to avoid herbs or you feel physical discomfort when you drink them—it is okay to skip the evening tea during the cleanse.

If, on the other hand, you want to skip over the tea-drinking part of the cleanse only because you don't much like the flavor of hibiscus, lemon balm, or chaga or you're not in the mood, you should keep going with the tea. Find the one you think is most palatable and drink a mug of it before bed. (You can add a teaspoon of raw honey if desired.) You may find that after a day or so of adjustment, you start to enjoy it more than you expected.

Lemons and Limes

If you have any fear about lemons and acidity, go read "Lemon Water" in Chapter 19, "Critical Cleanse Dos and Don'ts." It will set your mind at ease about lemon or lime water, especially as it relates to dental health.

If for some reason lemons or limes don't work for you or you can't access them, you can

make ginger water instead in the morning and evening or opt for plain water.

If you'd like, you're welcome to add a teaspoon of raw honey to your morning lemon or lime water.

As an alternative to lemon or lime (or orange) juice on your Liver Rescue Salad, try adding chopped fruit from the toppings list in that recipe for flavor in place of dressing.

Salads

Sometimes people have difficulty chewing raw vegetables. In that case, you're welcome to pulse your salad in the food processor until it's finely chopped or blend the ingredients together to make blended salad. That's what the Liver Rescue Soup recipe is: an easy blended salad for anyone who needs it during the Original or Simplified 3:6:9 Cleanse (or in everyday life).

If you're on the Advanced 3:6:9 Cleanse, you're welcome to take the ingredients of the Kale Salad; Cauliflower and Greens Bowl; Tomato, Cucumber, and Herb Salad; or Leafy Green Nori Rolls and blend them into a raw soup as well, or you can select Spinach Soup as your meal.

Those are also helpful approaches for people who feel they have trouble digesting raw vegetables, or "roughage." If you're on the Original 3:6:9 Cleanse and really highly sensitive, you can even make the raw Liver Rescue Soup recipe instead of the Liver Rescue Salad, with the option of blending the steamed asparagus and/or brussels sprouts called for in your meal into the Liver Rescue Soup. And as a last resort on the Original 3:6:9 Cleanse, it's okay to juice the salad ingredients using the Liver Rescue Juice recipe and get the nutrients in yourself that way. When your digestion is that compromised, you may prefer to start with the Mono Eating Cleanse from Chapter 18.

Note that some slight discomfort when digesting raw vegetables isn't necessarily a sign that you need to avoid them. As I covered in the "Food Sensitivity Secrets" section of *Liver Rescue*, it's easy to have a fearful response when different foods rub the intestinal linings, touching sensitive nerves and causing discomfort. Someone may say, "I can't eat lettuce—I react—but eggs, cheese, or bread feel good." The irony is that lettuce actually helps massage intestinal linings, loosening debris and other pockets of waste matter so they can be eliminated, without providing viral fuel, while eggs, cheese, and gluten feed pathogens such as the Epstein-Barr virus, resulting in more neurotoxins and eventually creating more chemical and food sensitivities. Eggs, cheese, and bread feel good going down because they travel down the middle of the intestinal tract, turning into smooth, liquefied glue. Lettuce, on the other hand, starves EBV. Part of lettuce's magic lies in brushing the intestinal linings, yet with irritated nerve receptors there, it can easily feel like you're having a reaction to it. Ultimately, lettuce soothes nerves; the milky substance in its core has an overall tranquilizing, sedative effect.

Liver Rescue Smoothie

These substitutions and adaptations will specifically address the Liver Rescue Smoothie. For questions on the Heavy Metal Detox Smoothie, see Chapter 17, "Heavy Metal Detox Cleanse."

If you're not a fan of banana, you can substitute Maradol papaya or leave out an extra fruit altogether and simply blend pitaya with the other ingredient(s) in the smoothie option you choose.

If you have no access to pitaya or have a strong aversion to it, you can resort to wild blueberries in its place or, in a pinch, blackberries, regular cultivated blueberries, or frozen cherries. In order to get the healing benefits your liver needs, you want to make sure you get those anthocyanins into yourself one way or another.

If you're experiencing the mild laxative effect that pitaya can sometimes offer (which makes it an amazing food for constipation) and you're not in the mood for that laxative effect, cut down the portion of pitaya you use in the smoothie and increase the portion of banana or papaya.

If you prefer not to blend the fruits, it is okay instead to enjoy the fruits from the smoothie recipe cut up together in a fruit bowl.

If you usually like to add powders and supplements to your smoothies, it is okay to add the supplements you'll find in Part VI of this book, specifically barley grass juice powder and spirulina. Stick to the recommended supplements, though. Don't add protein powders (including whey protein powder), flax oil, collagen, coconut oil, moringa powder, nuts, seeds, nut butters, cacao nibs or powder, almond milk, coconut milk, hemp milk, oat milk, goat milk, yogurt, or any other common smoothie add-ins.

Although it may be tempting to start throwing additional fruits in your smoothie, it's best to stick with the recipes and these substitutions unless you have no other options. Keeping your smoothie simple will help the main ingredients deliver their potency in full.

Spinach Soup

The basic ingredients of the Spinach Soup recipe in Chapter 23 are spinach and tomatoes. If spinach doesn't work for you, it's okay to substitute butter leaf lettuce. If tomatoes don't work for you, there are a couple of options. First, you can use mango instead. If you're having trouble finding fresh, sweet mangoes, buy frozen mango chunks instead and thaw them. Alternatively, you can substitute bananas for tomatoes—as long as you're sure not to blend bananas *with* tomatoes, because those two foods don't digest well together.

On Day 9 of the Simplified 3:6:9 Cleanse, skip cucumber noodles when serving the Spinach Soup. Otherwise, the suggested way to serve Spinach Soup on other days is over cucumber noodles—that is, very thin slices of cucumber, made using a spiralizer or julienne peeler. That's to add some fun and crunch to the meal. (For a note on why I don't recommend zucchini noodles instead, see "Raw versus Cooked" in Chapter 19, "Critical Cleanse Dos and Don'ts.") Can you blend the cucumber into the soup instead of eating it as noodles? Absolutely.

Winter Squash, Sweet Potatoes (including Japanese Sweet Potatoes), Yams, and Potatoes

If for some reason none of these options work for you as Day 7 dinner on the Original 3:6:9 Cleanse, substitute with brussels sprouts that you steam until they are so soft that a fork goes right through them.

"You're still here.
And with the life ahead of you, you can choose
to be part of a powerful healing movement."

— Anthony William, Medical Medium

CHAPTER 22

3:6:9 Cleanse Sample Menus

"What person, health professional or otherwise,
has the right to claim that you're not on a balanced diet,
or to offer a balanced diet, when they're in the
dark along with the rest of medical research and science
as to why someone is sick and how they can recover?
It's merely a guessing game of removing processed foods
and bringing in vegetables, nuts, and seeds, and that's
not an answer. Before anyone can weigh in with authority
on a balanced diet, they need to understand chronic illness."

— Anthony William, Medical Medium

ORIGINAL: THE 3

	DAY 1	DAY 2	DAY 3
UPON WAKING	16 ounces Lemon or Lime Water	16 ounces Lemon or Lime Water	16 ounces Lemon or Lime Water
BEFORE BREAKFAST (at least 15 to 30 minutes later)	16 ounces Celery Juice	16 ounces Celery Juice	16 ounces Celery Juice
BREAKFAST (at least 15 to 30 minutes later)	Raw Apple Banana "Oatmeal"	Pitaya Smoothie Bowl	Fruit Cereal
MORNING SNACK	Optional, if hungry: Apple or Applesauce	One to two apples or Applesauce	One to two apples or Applesauce
LUNCH	Potato Salad + Steamed Zucchini or Summer Squash	Tomato, Cucumber, and Herb Salad + Steamed Zucchini or Summer Squash	Cauliflower Sushi + Steamed Zucchini or Summer Squash
AFTERNOON SNACK (one to two hours after lunchtime)	One to two apples or Applesauce with one to two dates	One to two apples or Applesauce with one to two dates	One to two apples or Applesauce with one to two dates
DINNER	Sweet Potato and Zucchini Stew + Leafy Green Salad	Curried Cauliflower and Peas	"Cheddar" Broccoli Soup + Leafy Green Salad
ONE HOUR BEFORE BED	Apple or Applesauce (if hungry) + 16 ounces Lemon or Lime Water + Hibiscus Tea	Apple or Applesauce (if hungry) + 16 ounces Lemon or Lime Water + Hibiscus Tea	Apple or Applesauce (if hungry) + 16 ounces Lemon or Lime Water + Hibiscus Tea

ORIGINAL: THE 6

	DAY 4	DAY 5	DAY 6
UPON WAKING	16 ounces Lemon or Lime Water	16 ounces Lemon or Lime Water	16 ounces Lemon or Lime Water
BEFORE BREAKFAST (at least 15 to 30 minutes later)	16 ounces Celery Juice	16 ounces Celery Juice	16 ounces Celery Juice
BREAKFAST (at least 15 to 30 minutes later)	Liver Rescue Smoothie	Liver Rescue Smoothie	Liver Rescue Smoothie
MORNING SNACK	Optional, if hungry: Liver Rescue Smoothie or Heavy Metal Detox Smoothie	Optional, if hungry: Liver Rescue Smoothie or Heavy Metal Detox Smoothie	Optional, if hungry: Liver Rescue Smoothie or Heavy Metal Detox Smoothie
LUNCH	Steamed Asparagus + Liver Rescue Salad	Steamed Asparagus + Liver Rescue Salad	Either Shaved Brussels Sprout, Asparagus, Radish, and Apple Salad or Steamed Asparagus + Steamed Brussels Sprouts + Liver Rescue Salad
AFTERNOON SNACK (one to two hours after lunchtime)	Raw Mini Apple Pie Tarts + Celery sticks	Apple Pie Filling + Celery sticks	Apple Cinnamon Stuffed Dates + Celery sticks
DINNER	Asparagus Soup + Liver Rescue Salad	Lemon Garlic Steamed Brussels Sprouts + Liver Rescue Salad	Steamed Brussels Sprouts and Asparagus in Maple Cayenne Sauce + Liver Rescue Salad
ONE HOUR BEFORE BED	Apple or Applesauce (if hungry) + 16 ounces Lemon or Lime Water + Chaga Tea	Apple or Applesauce (if hungry) + 16 ounces Lemon or Lime Water + Chaga Tea	Apple or Applesauce (if hungry) + 16 ounces Lemon or Lime Water + Chaga Tea

ORIGINAL: THE 9

	DAY 7	DAY 8	DAY 9
UPON WAKING	16 ounces Lemon or Lime Water	16 ounces Lemon or Lime Water	16 ounces Lemon or Lime Water
BEFORE BREAKFAST (at least 15 to 30 minutes later)	16 ounces Celery Juice	16 ounces Celery Juice	Over the course of the day: Two 16- to 20-ounce Celery Juices (one morning, one early evening) + Two 16- to 20-ounce Cucumber-Apple Juices (anytime) + As many servings and as often as desired: Melon Smoothie or Papaya Pudding or Pear Sauce or Watermelon Juice or Fresh-Squeezed Orange Juice + Water (as desired)
BREAKFAST (at least 15 to 30 minutes later)	Liver Rescue Smoothie	Liver Rescue Smoothie	
MORNING SNACK	Optional, if hungry: Liver Rescue Smoothie or Heavy Metal Detox Smoothie	Optional, if hungry: Liver Rescue Smoothie or Heavy Metal Detox Smoothie	
LUNCH	Spinach Soup with Cucumber Noodles	Spinach Soup with Cucumber Noodles	
AFTERNOON SNACK (one to two hours after lunchtime)	16 ounces Celery Juice + (at least 15 to 30 minutes later) Apples with cucumber and celery	16 ounces Celery Juice + (at least 15 to 30 minutes later) Apples with cucumber and celery	
DINNER	Butternut Squash Noodles + Liver Rescue Salad (if desired)	Steamed Asparagus + Steamed Brussels Sprouts + Liver Rescue Salad (if desired)	
ONE HOUR BEFORE BED	Apple or Applesauce (if hungry) + 16 ounces Lemon or Lime Water + Lemon Balm Tea	Apple or Applesauce (if hungry) + 16 ounces Lemon or Lime Water + Lemon Balm Tea	16 ounces Lemon or Lime Water + Lemon Balm Tea

Refer to Chapter 10, "Original 3:6:9 Cleanse,"
for the full description of this cleanse.

WHAT TO EAT AND DRINK

- Eat the portions that are right for you, remembering not to go ravenous. At no point should you be forcing food either.
- Stick to the foods as outlined in the recipes specified above and the cleanse guidance in Chapter 10.
- If you enjoy animal products, stick to one serving per day of lean, organic, free-range, or wild meat, fowl, or fish (salmon, trout, or sardines), eaten only at dinner for these first three days.
- Stay hydrated by drinking about 1 liter (roughly 32 ounces, or 4 cups) of water during the day, in between your morning and evening lemon or lime water. In addition, you're welcome to sip on Hot Spiced Apple Juice at any temperature (recipe on page 290) or coconut water (look for one without natural flavors).

WHAT NOT TO EAT AND DRINK

- For the first three days, limit radical fats (nuts, seeds, oil, olives, coconut, avocado, animal proteins, etc.)—if desired at all—to dinnertime, lowering your normal amount of fats by at least 50 percent. For the rest of the cleanse, avoid radical fats entirely. Skip beans for all nine days too.
- Avoid these foods entirely during the cleanse: eggs, dairy, gluten, soft drinks, salt and seasonings, pork, corn, oils (including both industrial and healthier oils), soy, lamb, tuna and all other fish and seafood (salmon, trout, and sardines are okay at dinner on Days 1 to 3), vinegar (including ACV), caffeine (including coffee, matcha, cacao, and chocolate), grains (millet and oats are okay on Days 1 to 3), alcohol, natural/artificial flavors, fermented foods (including kombucha, sauerkraut, and coconut aminos), nutritional yeast, citric acid, monosodium glutamate (MSG), aspartame, other artificial sweeteners, formaldehyde, and preservatives.

SUBSTITUTIONS AND MODIFICATIONS

- Follow the recipe instructions, making substitutions only as outlined in Chapter 21, "Cleanse Adaptations and Substitutions." If you prefer simpler snacks or meals, refer to Chapter 10, "Original 3:6:9 Cleanse," for general food guidance. For example, in place of a dish such as Steamed Brussels Sprouts and Asparagus in Maple Cayenne Sauce, you can enjoy simple steamed brussels sprouts and asparagus.
- If you can't access fresh or frozen asparagus or brussels sprouts, use steamed zucchini and/or summer squash in their place.
- Cook vegetables only by steaming or adding them to cleanse recipe soups and stews. Avoid baked and roasted foods for all nine days.
- If you don't have time to eat salads, you don't like them, you have difficulty chewing, or you have sensitive digestion, feel free to make the Liver Rescue Soup in place of the Liver Rescue Salad. If even that feels like too much, substitute the Liver Rescue Juice.
- If apples are a problem for you due to a sensitivity, enjoy ripe pears instead.
- Find further substitution guidance in the cleanse description in Chapter 10 and in Chapter 21, "Cleanse Adaptations and Substitutions."

——— SIMPLIFIED: THE 3 ———

	DAY 1	DAY 2	DAY 3
UPON WAKING	16 ounces Lemon or Lime Water	16 ounces Lemon or Lime Water	16 ounces Lemon or Lime Water
BEFORE BREAKFAST (at least 15 to 30 minutes later)	16 ounces Celery Juice	16 ounces Celery Juice	16 ounces Celery Juice
BREAKFAST (at least 15 to 30 minutes later)	Wild Blueberry Porridge	Spaghetti Squash Hash Browns	Banana Oat Cookies
MORNING SNACK	Optional, if hungry: Apple or Applesauce	Optional, if hungry: Apple or Applesauce	Optional, if hungry: Apple or Applesauce
LUNCH	Stuffed Butternut Squash	Sweet Potato Tots + Leafy Green Salad	Warm Spiced Roasted Vegetable Salad
AFTERNOON SNACK (one to two hours after lunchtime)	Optional, if hungry: Apple Cinnamon Stuffed Dates + Celery sticks and cucumber slices (if desired)	Optional, if hungry: Apple Pie Filling + Celery sticks and cucumber slices (if desired)	Optional, if hungry: Raw Mini Apple Pie Tarts + Celery sticks and cucumber slices (if desired)
DINNER	Mini Potato Cake Pizzas + Leafy Green Salad	Butternut Squash Falafels + Leafy Green Salad	Zucchini Lasagna + Leafy Green Salad
ONE HOUR BEFORE BED	Apple or Applesauce (if hungry) + 16 ounces Lemon or Lime Water + Hibiscus Tea	Apple or Applesauce (if hungry) + 16 ounces Lemon or Lime Water + Hibiscus Tea	Apple or Applesauce (if hungry) + 16 ounces Lemon or Lime Water + Hibiscus Tea

SIMPLIFIED: THE 6

	DAY 4	DAY 5	DAY 6
UPON WAKING	16 ounces Lemon or Lime Water	16 ounces Lemon or Lime Water	16 ounces Lemon or Lime Water
BEFORE BREAKFAST (at least 15 to 30 minutes later)	24 ounces Celery Juice	24 ounces Celery Juice	24 ounces Celery Juice
BREAKFAST (at least 15 to 30 minutes later)	Apple Cinnamon Smoothie	Mango Smoothie Berry Parfait	Liver Rescue Smoothie
MORNING SNACK	Optional, if hungry: Apple or Applesauce	Optional, if hungry: Apple or Applesauce	Optional, if hungry: Apple or Applesauce
LUNCH	Chunky Sweet Potato Fries with Spinach Pesto	Roasted Red Pepper and Tomato Soup + Liver Rescue Salad	Potato and Herb Stuffed Peppers
AFTERNOON SNACK (one to two hours after lunchtime)	Optional: Hot Spiced Apple Juice or Apple(s) with cucumber and celery	Optional: Hot Spiced Apple Juice or Apple(s) with cucumber and celery	Optional: Hot Spiced Apple Juice or Apple(s) with cucumber and celery
DINNER	Portobello Stew + Steamed Asparagus or Steamed Zucchini or Summer Squash	Carrot, Zucchini, and Potato Patties + Leafy Green Salad	Potato Pizza Boats + Leafy Green Salad
ONE HOUR BEFORE BED	Apple or Applesauce (if hungry) + 16 ounces Lemon or Lime Water + Chaga Tea	Apple or Applesauce (if hungry) + 16 ounces Lemon or Lime Water + Chaga Tea	Apple or Applesauce (if hungry) + 16 ounces Lemon or Lime Water + Chaga Tea

SIMPLIFIED: THE 9

	DAY 7	DAY 8	DAY 9
UPON WAKING	16 ounces Lemon or Lime Water	16 ounces Lemon or Lime Water	16 ounces Lemon or Lime Water
BEFORE BREAKFAST (at least 15 to 30 minutes later)	32 ounces Celery Juice	32 ounces Celery Juice	16 ounces Celery Juice
BREAKFAST (at least 15 to 30 minutes later)	Heavy Metal Detox Smoothie	Watermelon Fries	Melon Smoothie or Watermelon Juice or Fresh-Squeezed Orange Juice
MORNING SNACK	Optional, if hungry: Apple or Applesauce	Optional, if hungry: Apple or Applesauce	
LUNCH	Zucchini and Summer Squash Stir-Fry over Cauliflower Rice	Sweet Potato Noodles with Garlic, Red Pepper, and Asparagus + Leafy Green Salad	Spinach Soup
AFTERNOON SNACK (one to two hours after lunchtime)	Optional: Hot Spiced Apple Juice or Apple(s) with cucumber and celery	Optional: Hot Spiced Apple Juice or Apple(s) with cucumber and celery	16 ounces Celery Juice + (at least 15 to 30 minutes later) Papaya Pudding or Pear Sauce
DINNER	Brussels Sprout Vegetable Soup + Liver Rescue Salad	Lemon Asparagus with Roasted Tomato and Spinach Salad	Asparagus Soup or Zucchini Basil Soup
ONE HOUR BEFORE BED	Apple or Applesauce (if hungry) + 16 ounces Lemon or Lime Water + Lemon Balm Tea	Apple or Applesauce (if hungry) + 16 ounces Lemon or Lime Water + Lemon Balm Tea	16 ounces Lemon or Lime Water + Lemon Balm Tea

SIMPLIFIED 3:6:9 CLEANSE REMINDERS

Refer to Chapter 11, "Simplified 3:6:9 Cleanse,"
for the full description of this cleanse.

WHAT TO EAT AND DRINK

- Eat the portions that are right for you, remembering not to go ravenous. At no point should you be forcing food either.
- Stick to the foods as outlined in the recipes specified above and the cleanse guidance in Chapter 11.
- For breakfast, work your way up to a fruit-based breakfast by The 6 and fresh fruit breakfast (with frozen fruit okay) by The 9. See page 145 for further guidance.
- Note the celery juice increases every three days. For alternate amounts if you're sensitive, see the table in Chapter 11.
- Stay hydrated by drinking about 1 liter (roughly 32 ounces, or 4 cups) of water during the day, in between your morning and evening lemon or lime water. In addition, you're welcome to sip on Hot Spiced Apple Juice at any temperature (recipe on page 290) or coconut water (look for one without natural flavors).

WHAT NOT TO EAT AND DRINK

- Avoid radical fats (nuts, seeds, oil, olives, coconut, avocado, cacao, bone broth, animal proteins, etc.) entirely for all nine days. Skip beans for the entire cleanse too.
- Avoid these foods entirely during the cleanse: eggs, dairy, gluten, soft drinks, salt and seasonings, pork, corn, oils (including both industrial and healthier oils), soy, lamb, tuna and all other fish and seafood, vinegar (including ACV), caffeine (including coffee, matcha, and chocolate), grains (millet and oats are okay on Days 1 to 8), alcohol, natural/artificial flavors, fermented foods (including kombucha, sauerkraut, and coconut aminos), nutritional yeast, citric acid, monosodium glutamate (MSG), aspartame, other artificial sweeteners, formaldehyde, and preservatives.

SUBSTITUTIONS AND MODIFICATIONS

- Follow the recipe instructions, making substitutions only as outlined in Chapter 21, "Cleanse Adaptations and Substitutions." If you prefer simpler snacks or meals, refer to Chapter 11, "Simplified 3:6:9 Cleanse," for general food guidance.
- If you already eat what you feel is a clean diet, you may wish to choose recipes that include a lot of raw fruits, leafy greens, and vegetables; steamed vegetables; or the soup and stew recipes. While there are many baked recipes included in the Simplified sample menu plans to provide variety and inspiration, keep in mind that baked recipes will slow down the detox. They are still a fantastic and delicious choice for someone who is cleansing for the first time.
- If you don't have time to eat salads, you don't like them, you have difficulty chewing, or you have sensitive digestion, feel free to blend them.
- If apples are a problem for you due to a sensitivity, enjoy ripe pears instead.
- Find further substitution guidance in the cleanse description in Chapter 11 and in Chapter 21, "Cleanse Adaptations and Substitutions."

ADVANCED 3:6:9 CLEANSE SAMPLE MENUS

	THE 3	THE 6	THE 9	
	DAYS 1 TO 3	DAYS 4 TO 6	DAYS 7 TO 8	DAY 9
UPON WAKING	32 ounces Lemon or Lime Water	32 ounces Lemon or Lime Water	32 ounces Lemon or Lime Water	32 ounces Lemon or Lime Water
BEFORE BREAKFAST (at least 15 to 30 minutes later)	24 (or 32) ounces* Celery Juice	32 ounces Celery Juice	32 ounces Celery Juice	Over the course of the day: Two 32-ounce Celery Juices (one morning, one early evening) + Two 16- to 20-ounce Cucumber-Apple Juices (anytime) + As many servings and as often as desired: Melon Smoothie or Papaya Pudding or Pear Sauce or Watermelon Juice or Fresh-Squeezed Orange Juice + Water (as desired)
BREAKFAST (at least 15 to 30 minutes later)	Heavy Metal Detox Smoothie	Heavy Metal Detox Smoothie	Heavy Metal Detox Smoothie	
MORNING SNACK	Optional, if hungry: Apple or Applesauce	Optional, if hungry: Apple or Applesauce	Optional, if hungry: Apple or Applesauce	
LUNCH	Spinach Soup with or without Cucumber Noodles	Liver Rescue Smoothie	Spinach Soup with or without Cucumber Noodles	
AFTERNOON SNACK (one to two hours after lunchtime)	Optional, if hungry: Apple or Applesauce	Optional, if hungry: Apple or Applesauce	32 ounces Celery Juice + (at least 15 to 30 minutes later, only if hungry) Apples	
DINNER	Kale Salad or Cauliflower and Greens Bowl	Tomato, Cucumber, and Herb Salad	Leafy Green Nori Rolls or Spinach Soup	
ONE HOUR BEFORE BED	Apple or Applesauce (if hungry) + 16 ounces Lemon or Lime Water + Hibiscus Tea	Apple or Applesauce (if hungry) + 16 ounces Lemon or Lime Water + Chaga Tea	Apple or Applesauce (if hungry) + 16 ounces Lemon or Lime Water + Lemon Balm Tea	16 ounces Lemon or Lime Water + Lemon Balm Tea

Refer to Chapter 12, "Advanced 3:6:9 Cleanse," for the full description of this cleanse.

WHAT TO EAT AND DRINK

- Eat the portions that are right for you, remembering not to go ravenous. At no point should you be forcing food either.
- Stick to the foods as outlined in the recipes specified above and the cleanse guidance in Chapter 12. You'll be consuming exclusively raw fruits, vegetables, and leafy greens for all meals and snacks. (Frozen fruit is okay.)
- Stay hydrated by drinking about 1 liter (roughly 32 ounces, or 4 cups) of water during the day, in between your morning and evening lemon or lime water. In addition, you're welcome to sip on Hot Spiced Apple Juice (recipe on page 290) at any temperature or coconut water (look for one without natural flavors). If the extra celery juice in the afternoon starting on Day 7 means you'd like to scale back on water a bit, that's fine.

* See page 152 for details on morning celery juice amounts during The 3.

WHAT NOT TO EAT AND DRINK

- Avoid radical fats (nuts, seeds, oil, olives, coconut, avocado, cacao, bone broth, animal proteins, etc.) entirely for all nine days. Skip beans for the entire cleanse too.
- Avoid cooked foods for the whole cleanse.
- Avoid these foods entirely during the cleanse: eggs, dairy, gluten, soft drinks, salt and seasonings, pork, corn, oils (including both industrial and healthier oils), soy, lamb, tuna and all other fish and seafood, vinegar (including ACV), caffeine (including coffee, matcha, and chocolate), grains (including millet and oats), alcohol, natural/artificial flavors, fermented foods (including kombucha, sauerkraut, and coconut aminos), nutritional yeast, citric acid, monosodium glutamate (MSG), aspartame, other artificial sweeteners, formaldehyde, and preservatives.

SUBSTITUTIONS AND MODIFICATIONS

- Follow the recipe instructions, making substitutions only as outlined in Chapter 21, "Cleanse Adaptations and Substitutions."
- When a smoothie or soup is listed, you can choose to eat the ingredients whole rather than blended if you prefer. Likewise, when a salad is listed, you can blend those ingredients if you wish.
- If apples are a problem for you due to a sensitivity, enjoy ripe pears instead. Apples or ripe pears can also be blended alone into pure, raw applesauce or pear sauce.
- If you experience an intense cleansing effect from what seems to be the celery juice, reduce the amount by half and then work your way back up.
- Find further substitution guidance in the cleanse description in Chapter 12 and in Chapter 21, "Cleanse Adaptations and Substitutions."

CHAPTER 23

Cleanse Recipes

When preparing juices and other recipes with apples, cucumbers, and other fruits and vegetables that have edible skins, you can keep the skins on if a recipe does not specify and the items are organic, or you're welcome to peel them. If they're conventional, peel and discard the skins—or if you can't peel the conventional fruit or vegetable for any reason, wash it with vigor before using.

LEMON OR LIME WATER

Makes 1 serving

While it sounds simple, don't overlook lemon or lime water as a powerful part of your daily routine. This easy hydration source takes only a moment to prepare, is extremely beneficial for everyone, and brings your water to life!

½ **lemon or 2 limes, freshly cut**

16 ounces (2 cups) water

Squeeze the juice from the freshly cut lemon or limes into the water, straining seeds if necessary.

Wait at least 15 to 20 minutes and ideally 30 minutes after you finish drinking your lemon or lime water before you consume your celery juice or anything else.

TIPS

- If you prefer 32 ounces (4 cups) of lemon or lime water upon rising, that's a great way to give yourself extra hydration and cleansing support. Simply double the recipe and enjoy.

- In your daily life, it's best to drink at least two or more 16-ounce lemon or lime waters over the course of a day. A great routine is to drink one upon rising, another in the afternoon, and another one hour before bed.

- If you have any concerns about lemon water, turn to Chapter 19, "Critical Cleanse Dos and Don'ts," for reassurance about lemon water and dental health.

- Limes vary in size and juiciness. If your limes are dry, use two limes per 16 ounces of water, as the recipe calls for, to get enough juice. If your limes are big and juicy, you may only need half of a lime.

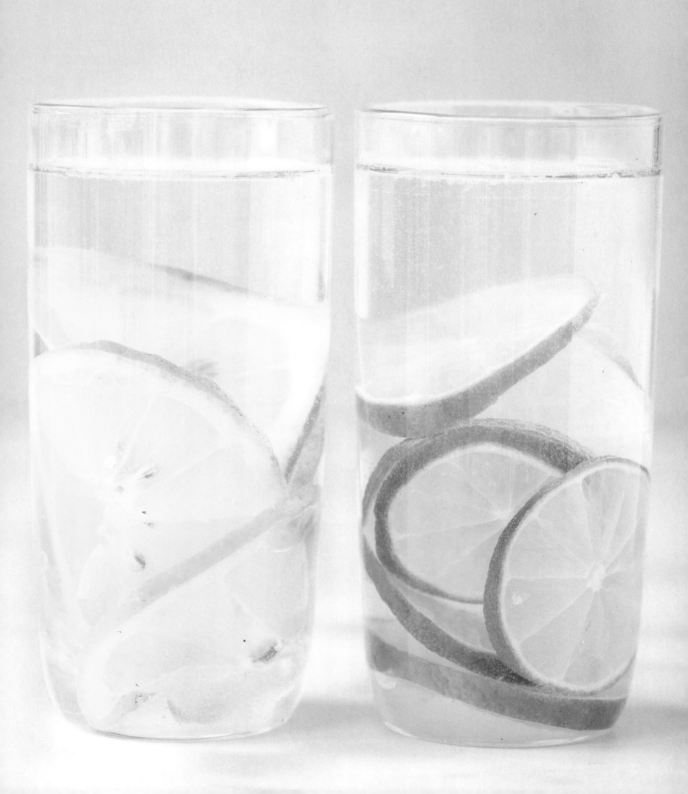

LEMON, GINGER, AND HONEY WATER

Makes 1 serving

This Lemon, Ginger, and Honey Water is refreshing and hydrating. It's the perfect drink to begin your day, enjoy as an afternoon pick-me-up, or sip over the course of the day. (If you're starting your day with it, try it 15 to 20 and ideally 30 minutes or more before or after your celery juice.) When you drink this healing tonic upon waking, it will help your liver flush out toxins it's collected for release throughout the night while giving your liver and body the critical hydration and glucose it needs to begin your day.

1 to 2 inches fresh ginger
2 cups water
½ lemon, juiced
1 teaspoon raw honey

Grate the ginger into 2 cups of water. Allow the water to steep for at least 15 minutes and ideally longer. You can even leave it steeping in the fridge overnight if you wish. When you're ready to drink it, strain the ginger out of the water, add the lemon juice and raw honey, and stir well.

TIPS

- As an alternative to grating the ginger, try chopping it into a few small pieces and squeezing them in a garlic press—it will act like a mini juicer. Be sure to take out the "pulp" from the press afterward, chop it finely, and add it to the water to steep. As instructed above, strain before drinking.

- It can be helpful to prepare a big batch of ginger water in advance to sip as desired. For best results, add the raw honey and lemon just prior to consuming.

- It's important to use raw honey for this recipe. You won't receive the same healing benefits from heated, processed honey.

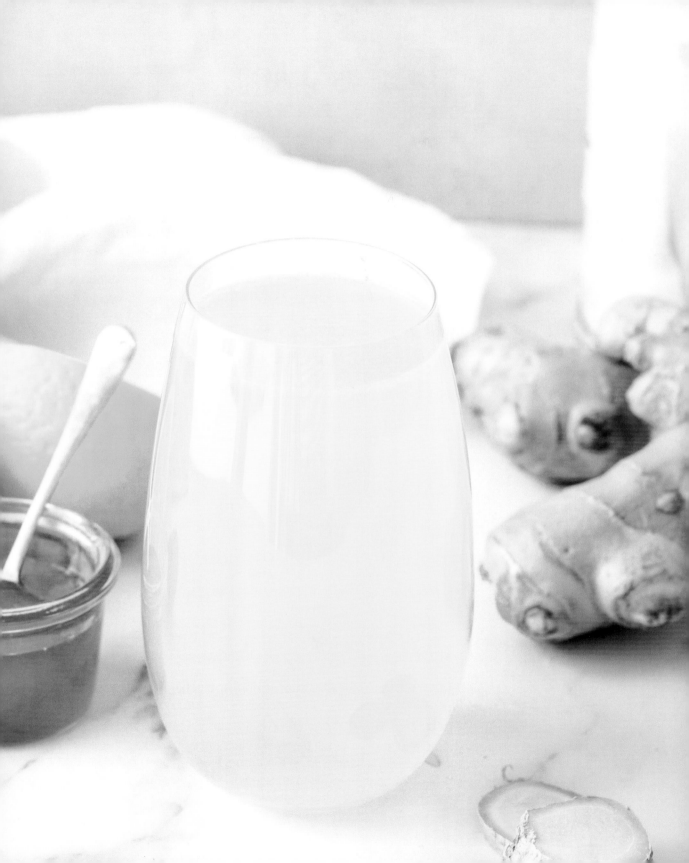

CELERY JUICE

Makes 1 serving

This simple herbal extraction has an incredible ability to create sweeping improvements for all kinds of health issues when consumed in the right way. That's why celery juice is an important component of the 3:6:9 Cleanse and every other cleanse in this book. It's an ideal way to start your day even when you're not on a cleanse.

1 bunch of celery

Trim about a quarter inch off the base of the celery bunch, if desired, to break apart the stalks.

Rinse the celery.

Run the celery through the juicer of your choice. Strain the juice if desired to remove any grit or stray pieces of pulp. Drink immediately, on an empty stomach, for best results. Wait at least 15 to 30 minutes before consuming anything else.

If you don't have a juicer, you can make celery juice in a blender. Here's how:

Trim about a quarter inch off the base of the celery bunch if desired to break apart the stalks. Rinse the celery. Place the celery on a clean cutting board and chop into roughly 1-inch pieces. Place the chopped celery in a high-speed blender and blend until smooth. (Don't add water.) Use your blender's tamping tool if needed. Strain the liquefied celery well; a nut milk bag is handy for this. Drink immediately, on an empty stomach, for best results. Wait at least 15 to 30 minutes before consuming anything else.

TIPS

- Steer clear of putting additional ingredients such as lemon, apple, ginger, or leafy greens in your celery juice. While these are wonderful foods, celery juice only offers its full benefits when consumed alone.

- If you're not going to be able to drink your full batch of celery juice right away, the best way to store it is in a glass jar, with a sealed lid, in the fridge. Freshly juiced celery retains its healing benefits for about 24 hours. It does lose potency by the hour, so drinking it more than 24 hours after it's made is not recommended.

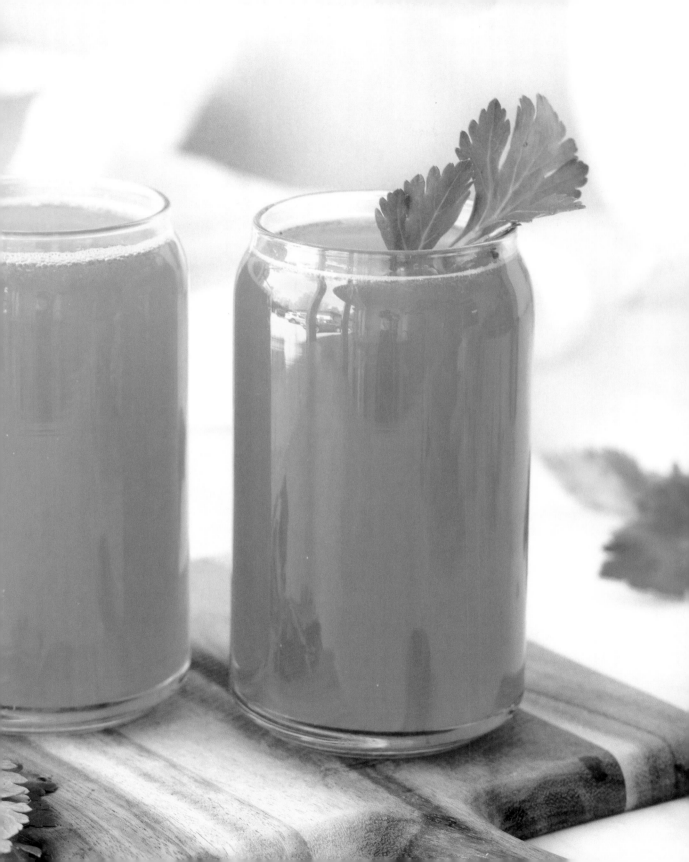

CUCUMBER JUICE

Fresh cucumber juice is an alternative rejuvenation tonic. Highly alkalizing and hydrating, cucumber juice has the ability to cleanse and detox the entire body. Its mildly sweet flavor makes it easy to drink.

2 large cucumbers

Rinse the cucumbers and run them through the juicer of your choice. Drink immediately, on an empty stomach, for best results.

If you don't have access to a juicer, here's how you can make it instead:

Rinse the cucumbers, chop them, and blend them in a high-speed blender until smooth. (Don't add water.) Strain the liquefied cucumber well; a nut milk bag is handy for this. Drink immediately, on an empty stomach, for best results.

TIPS

- Fresh cucumber juice is a good alternative to celery juice if you're not able to find celery or you really struggle with the flavor of celery juice. While cucumber juice is an incredible healing drink, it does not offer the same healing benefits as celery juice, though, so it's important to include celery juice daily as much as possible. For most people, the taste of celery juice becomes more enjoyable with consistent consumption.

- Steer clear of putting additional ingredients such as lemon, apple, ginger, or leafy greens in your cucumber juice. While these are wonderful foods, cucumber juice offers the most benefits when consumed alone.

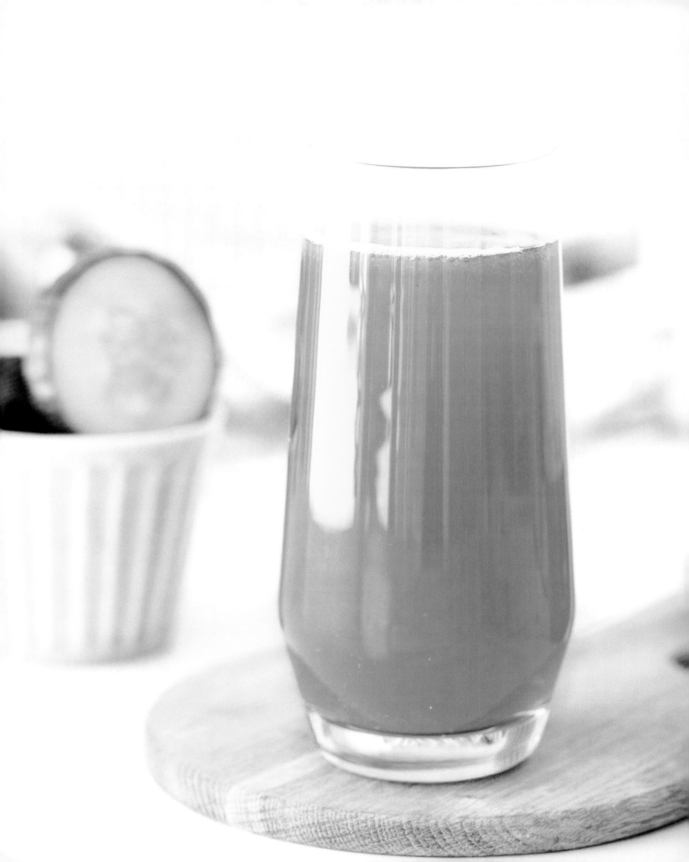

CUCUMBER-APPLE JUICE

Makes 1 serving

This delicious juice is so easy to drink that you might find yourself craving it regularly. The cucumber and apple work together to deeply hydrate and gently cleanse your body, making it a key part of Day 9 of the Original and Advanced 3:6:9 Cleanse.

1 large cucumber

3 apples

Run the ingredients through a juicer. Enjoy immediately for best results. Store any leftover juice in an airtight container in the fridge.

Alternatively, chop all of the ingredients and then blend them together in a high-speed blender (don't add water) until liquefied and then strain through a nut milk bag or cheesecloth.

TIPS

- The ideal ratio of cucumber to apple juice in this recipe is about 50:50, yielding about 16 ounces of juice. Feel free to adjust the amounts of cucumber or apple as needed based on their size.

- If you don't like cucumber as much, you can use more apple. If you don't like apple as much, you can use more cucumber.

- Red-skinned apples have the highest nutrient content, so try to use apples of any red-skinned variety when possible.

- If you need an alternative to apples, substitute pears.

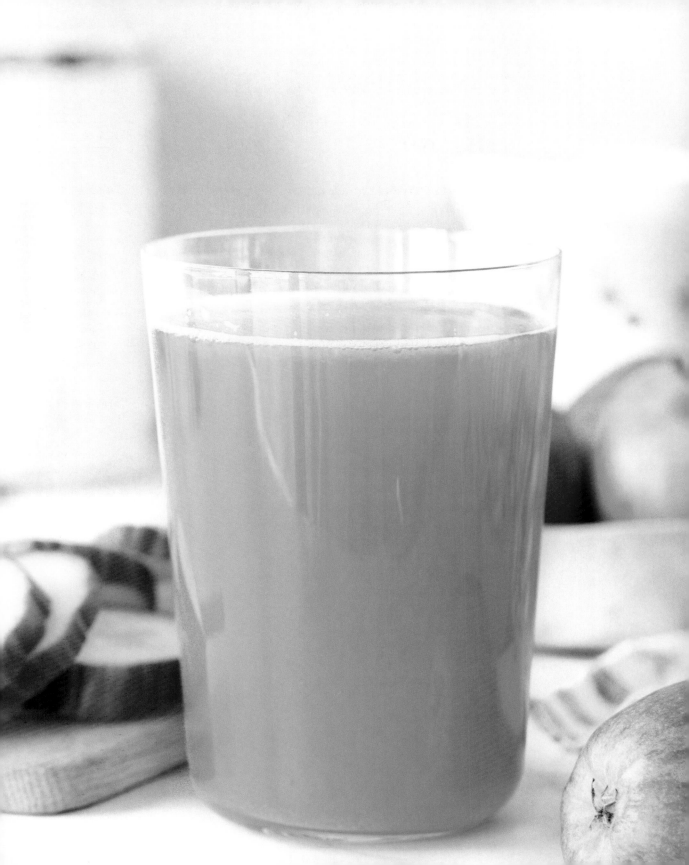

GREEN JUICE

The surprisingly pleasant and mellow flavor of this all-green juice makes it easy to drink, while its healing properties deeply nourish, balance, and energize you.

5 stalks celery
1 medium-sized cucumber
¼ cup parsley, tightly packed
1½ cups spinach, tightly packed, or 2 cups chopped romaine lettuce, tightly packed

Run all the ingredients through the juicer. Enjoy immediately for best results. Store any leftover juice in an airtight container in the fridge.

Alternatively, chop all of the ingredients and then blend them together in a high-speed blender until liquefied (don't add water) and then strain through a nut milk bag or cheesecloth.

TIPS

- Enjoy this recipe as it is, or feel free to add extra spinach or romaine.

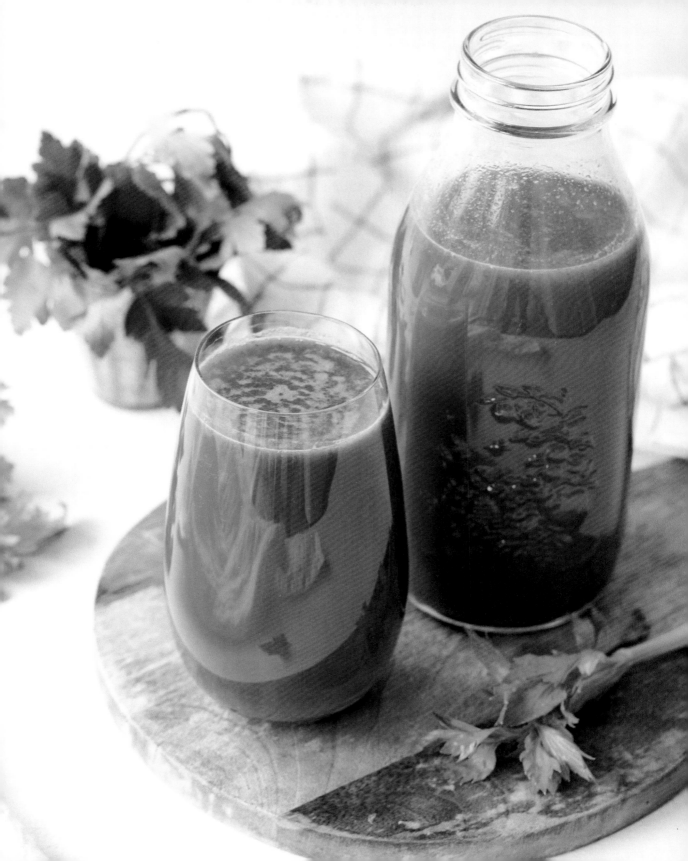

LIVER RESCUE JUICE

Makes 1 to 2 servings

Liver Rescue Juice is the perfect option for anyone with severe digestive issues who finds eating fibrous salads or soups uncomfortable or challenging. You can enjoy this refreshing juice instead of Liver Rescue Salad and Liver Rescue Soup during the 3:6:9 Cleanse as needed.

VERSION 1
With Asparagus

3 medium-sized red apples

1 cup fresh cilantro, loosely packed

2 cups spinach, tightly packed

1 pound asparagus, ends trimmed

1 cucumber

VERSION 2
With Brussels Sprouts

3 medium-sized red apples

1 cup fresh cilantro, loosely packed

2 cups spinach, tightly packed

2 pounds brussels sprouts, ends trimmed

1 cucumber

VERSION 3
With Asparagus and Brussels Sprouts

3 medium-sized red apples

1 cup fresh cilantro, loosely packed

2 cups spinach, tightly packed

1 pound brussels sprouts, ends trimmed

½ pound asparagus, ends trimmed

1 cucumber

Run the ingredients through a juicer. Enjoy immediately for best results. Store any leftover juice in an airtight container in the fridge.

Alternatively, chop all of the ingredients and then blend them together in a high-speed blender until liquefied (don't add water) and then strain through a nut milk bag or cheesecloth.

TIPS

- This is a great juice to make a part of your regular lifestyle, whether you are doing the 3:6:9 Cleanse or not. It makes for a wonderful second juice after your morning celery juice or a great pick-me-up in the afternoon.

- If you need an alternative to apples, substitute pears.

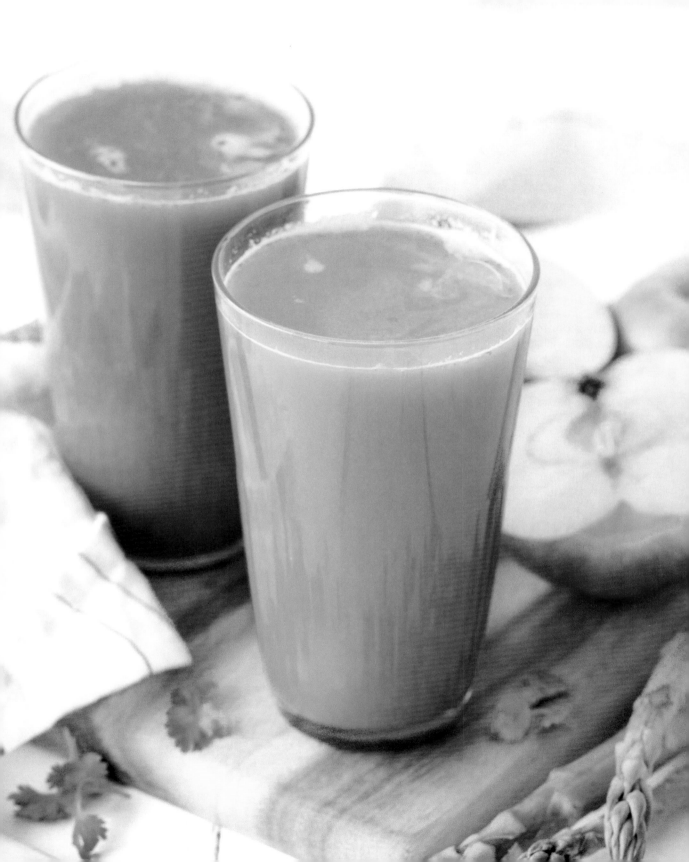

WATERMELON JUICE

Makes 1 to 2 servings

When it comes to sweet, refreshing juices, it doesn't get much better than fresh watermelon juice. Watermelon juice is deeply hydrating and cleansing, making it a perfect juice to enjoy in the morning, 15 to 20 and ideally 30 minutes or more after your celery juice. All melons are special, so you can also try juicing other melon varieties to find your favorite.

1 small watermelon (about 4 pounds), cubed (or substitute the same amount of any other melon)

Run the watermelon through a juicer. Pass through a fine-mesh sieve to remove any remaining pulp (if needed). Serve immediately.

Alternatively, blend the melon in a high-speed blender until liquefied and then strain through a nut milk bag or cheesecloth.

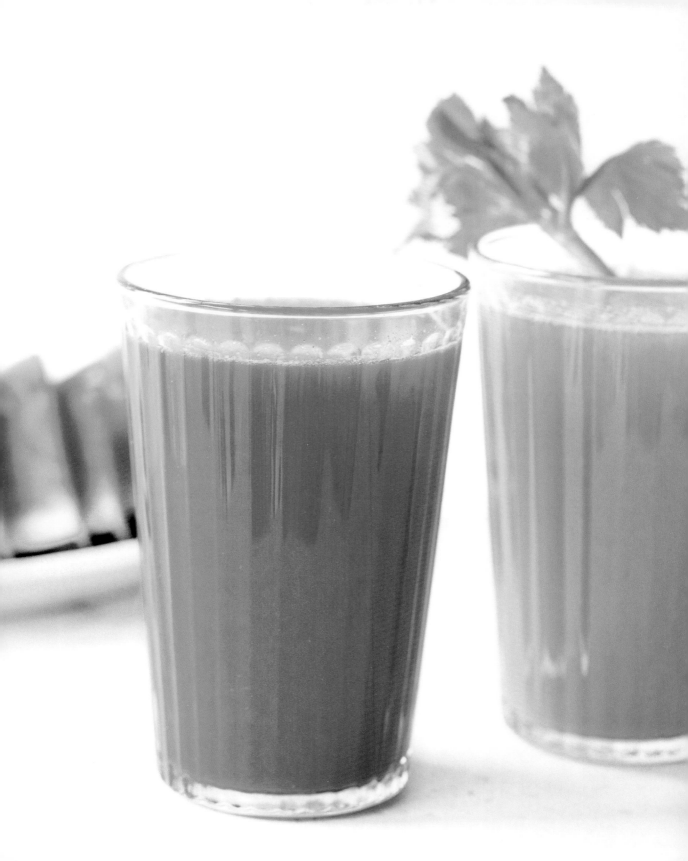

FRESH-SQUEEZED ORANGE JUICE

Makes 1 to 2 servings

When made fresh and consumed within 30 minutes, orange juice offers a vast array of antivirals, antibacterials, vitamins, minerals, antioxidants, and healing phytochemicals. Enjoy this healing juice to bring more sunshine into your day.

10 oranges

If you are using a hand-held citrus reamer, cut the oranges in half and twist the flesh of the oranges on the reamer to extract the juice and pulp.

If you are using an electric juicer, peel the oranges and pass them through the machine. Serve.

TIPS

- If the oranges are very firm, roll them on the countertop with your palm before cutting open or peeling. This helps break up the individual segments, releasing more juice.

- If you prefer pulp-free orange juice, use a strainer to remove the pulp before serving.

- If you can't drink your orange juice within 30 minutes, store it in a glass jar with an airtight lid in the fridge. It's best to consume the juice within a few hours and at most, within 24 hours.

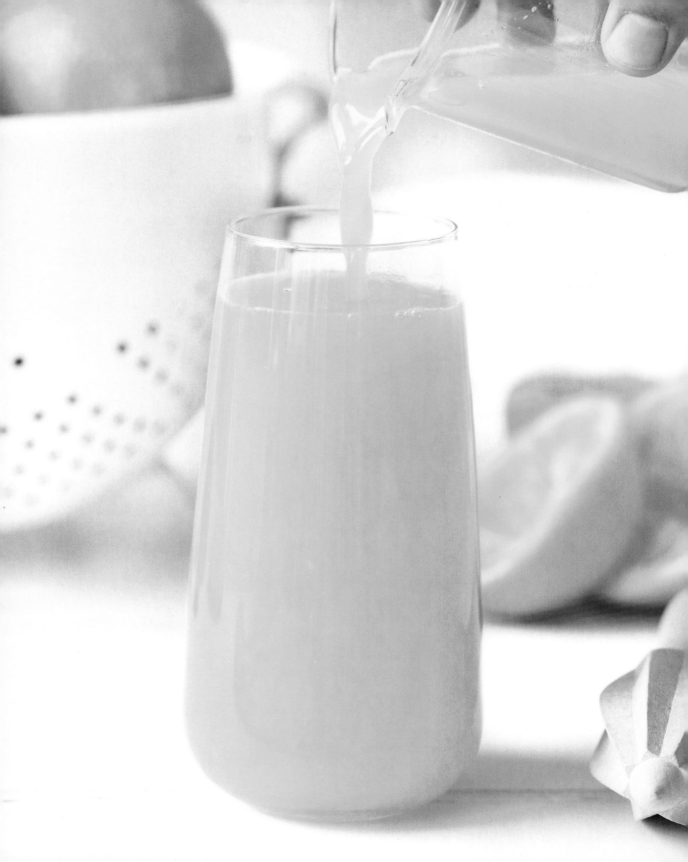

HOT SPICED APPLE JUICE

Makes 2 to 3 servings

For a big mug of pure comfort packed full of healing spices in a delicious base of apple juice, look no further than this delicious Hot Spiced Apple Juice. You may find this recipe quickly becomes a weekly staple. When it goes down warm or hot, this beverage is very soothing and relaxing for the liver. If you'd prefer to enjoy this as a cold drink, there's an option for that too!

10 apples, cored and chopped (yields 3 cups of juice)

¾ teaspoon ground cinnamon

½ teaspoon ground ginger or 1 teaspoon finely grated fresh ginger

Pinch of ground nutmeg (optional)

Pinch of ground cloves (optional)

½ teaspoon grated orange peel

Juice the apples using an electric juicer.

Add the cinnamon, ginger, nutmeg, cloves, and orange peel to the juice.

If you are serving the juice cold, let it infuse for at least 10 minutes. Strain through a fine-mesh sieve and serve.

If you are serving it hot, place the juice in a small saucepan and heat until simmering. Turn the heat off and infuse for 5 to 10 minutes. (If you can avoid heating it up in the microwave, that's ideal.) Strain through a fine-mesh sieve and serve.

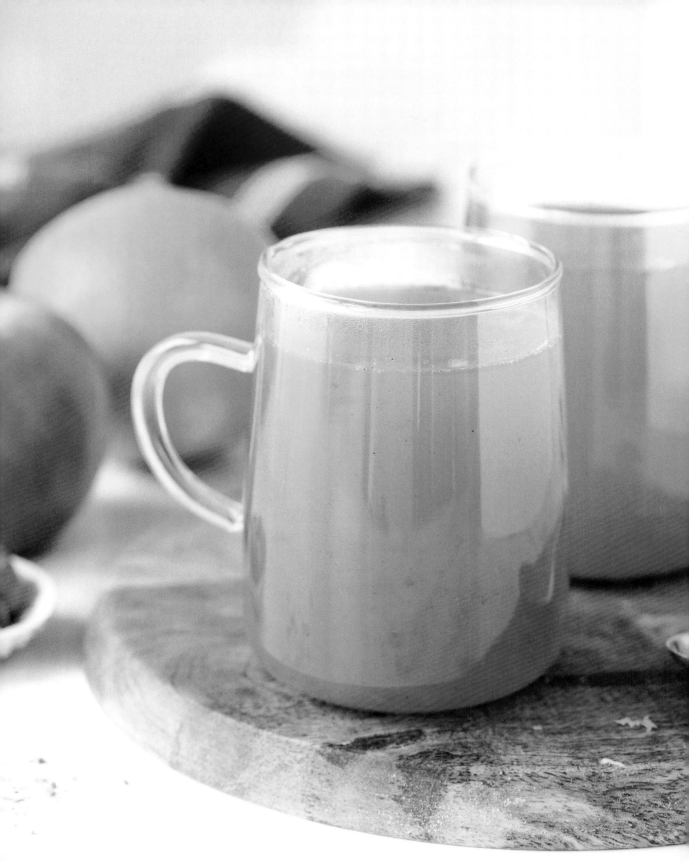

HIBISCUS TEA

Hibiscus tea is even more healing than it is beautiful and vibrant. The unique anthocyanin compound that gives hibiscus its red coloring helps rejuvenate the liver, making it a preferred choice for the 3:6:9 Cleanse.

1 tablespoon dried hibiscus or 2 hibiscus tea bags

1 cup water

1 teaspoon raw honey (optional)

Place the hibiscus in a mug or teapot. Add boiling water and steep for 10 to 15 minutes. Stir in raw honey (if using). Strain (if needed) and serve.

TIPS

- It's important to steep the tea for the full 10 to 15 minutes in order to receive enough of the healing benefits of the herb.

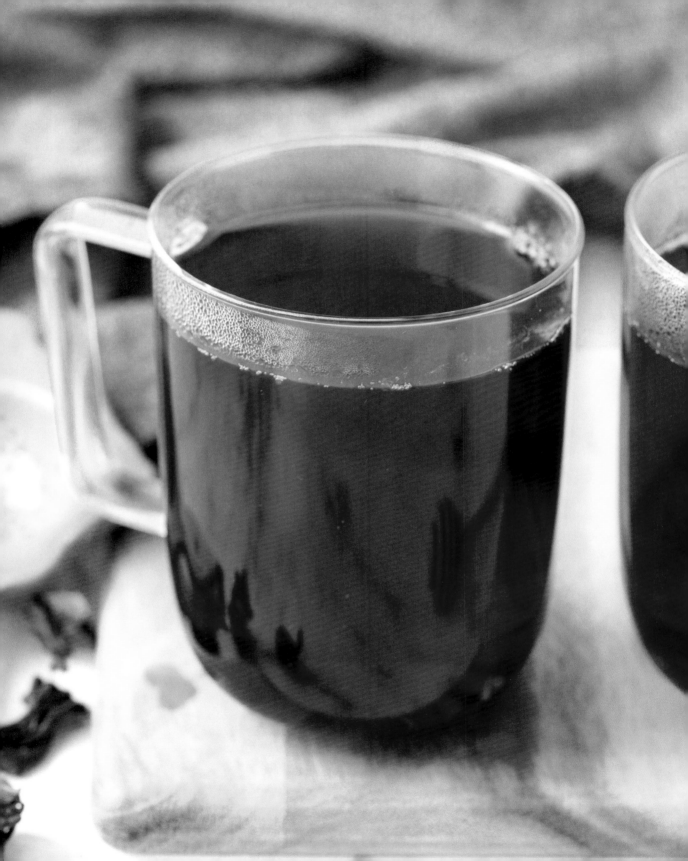

LEMON BALM TEA

Lemon balm tea is a favorite all-rounder for its healing properties and its taste. It makes a light, refreshing tea you can enjoy even more knowing that this special herb works to kill off viruses and other pathogens in your system. It also calms the nerves of the liver, leading the organ to become less spasmodic, agitated, and angry.

1 cup hot water

2 tablespoons fresh or 1 tablespoon dried lemon balm or 2 lemon balm tea bags

1 teaspoon raw honey (optional)

Place the lemon balm in a mug or teapot. Add boiling water and steep for 10 to 15 minutes. Stir in raw honey (if using). Strain (if needed) and serve.

TIPS

- It's important to steep the tea for the full 10 to 15 minutes in order to receive enough of the healing benefits of the herb.

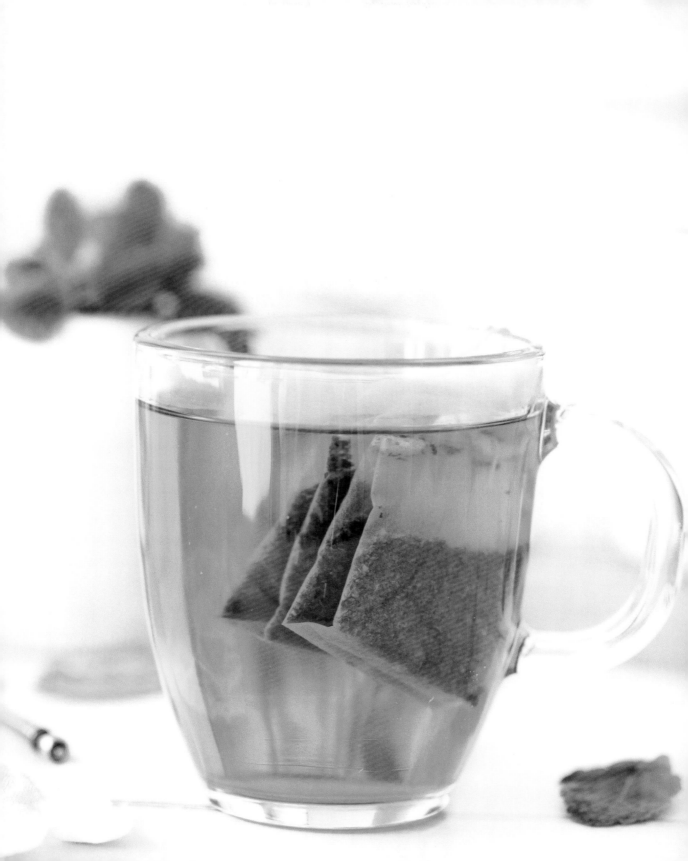

CHAGA TEA

This powerhouse healing mushroom makes a rich, earthy tea with a flavor that some feel is reminiscent of coffee. Adding raw honey will help drive the medicinal properties of the chaga deeper into hard-to-reach places, enhancing body system functions.

1 cup hot water

1 teaspoon chaga powder

1 teaspoon raw honey (optional)

Place the chaga powder in a mug. Add boiling water and stir well. Add raw honey (if using) and serve.

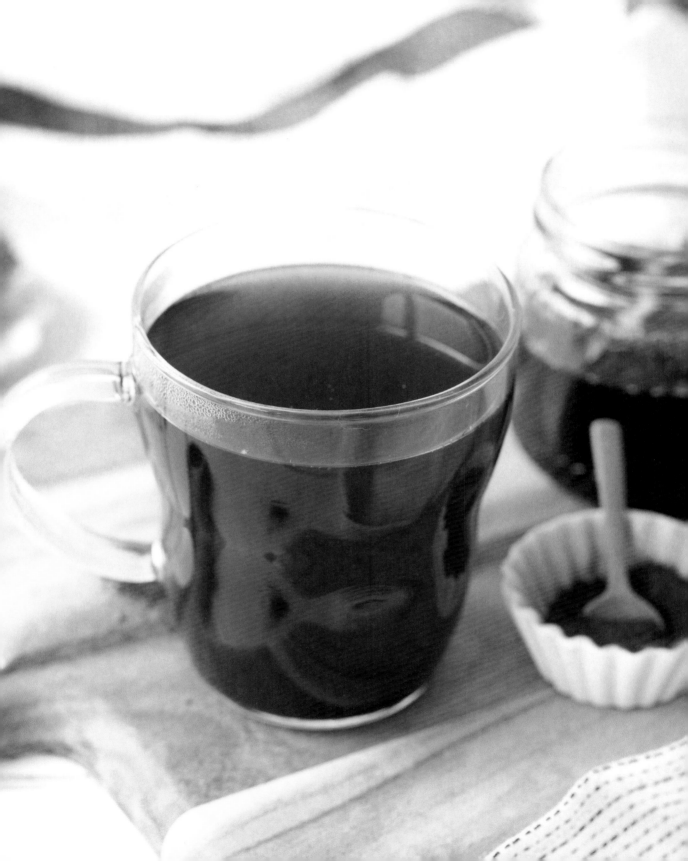

LIVER RESCUE SMOOTHIE

The first smoothie option below is a fast, simple, antioxidant-rich tonic to add to your life for deep liver healing. The second smoothie option is a light, cheery alternative that brings together greens and fruit. If you've never thought of adding sprouts to your smoothie before, now is a perfect time to try it out. They're powerful and mild, and they blend perfectly into this smooth, tropical treat.

OPTION A

2 bananas or ½ Maradol papaya, cubed

½ cup fresh, 1 packet frozen, or 2 tablespoons powdered red pitaya (dragon fruit)

2 cups fresh or frozen or 2 tablespoons powdered wild blueberries

½ cup water (optional)

OPTION B

1 banana or ¼ Maradol papaya, cubed

1 mango

½ cup fresh, 1 packet frozen, or 2 tablespoons powdered red pitaya (dragon fruit)

1 celery stalk

½ cup sprouts (any variety)

½ lime

½ cup water (optional)

Combine all ingredients in a blender. Blend until smooth. If desired, stream in up to ½ cup of water until desired consistency is reached.

TIPS

- If you'd like to include the Heavy Metal Detox Smoothie (see the next recipe) in the 3:6:9 Cleanse, you can drink a smaller serving of the Liver Rescue Smoothie and then later in the morning enjoy a smaller serving of the Heavy Metal Detox Smoothie too.

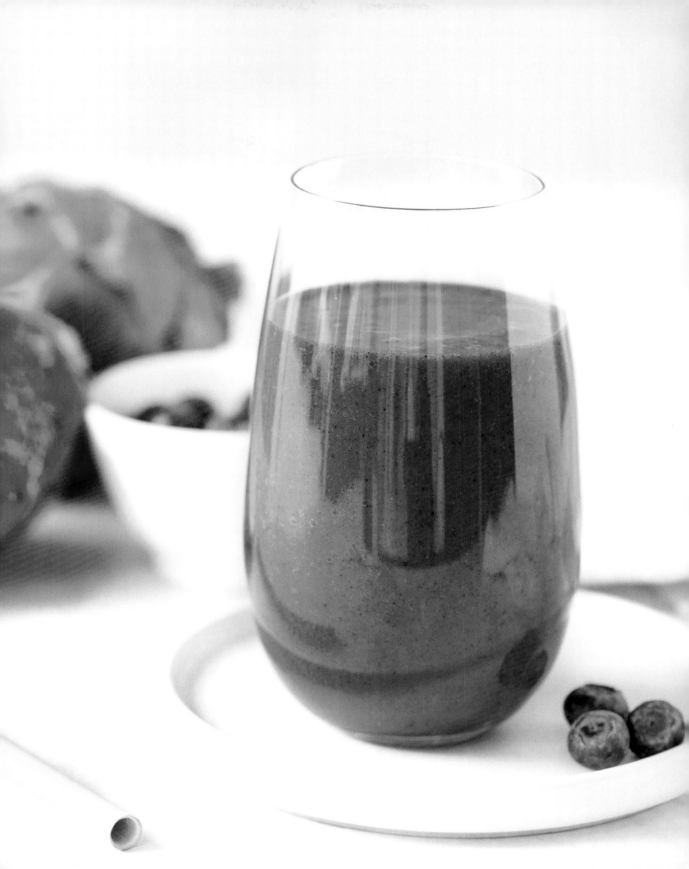

HEAVY METAL DETOX SMOOTHIE

Makes 1 serving

This smoothie is a perfect and powerful combination of the five key ingredients for safely detoxifying toxic heavy metals from your brain and body. It's an honorable, life-giving blessing to help reverse so many symptoms.

2 bananas

2 cups frozen or fresh wild blueberries or 2 tablespoons powdered wild blueberries

1 cup fresh cilantro

1 teaspoon barley grass juice powder

1 teaspoon spirulina

1 tablespoon Atlantic dulse

1 orange

½ to 1 cup water (optional)

Combine the bananas, wild blueberries, cilantro, barley grass juice powder, spirulina, and Atlantic dulse with the juice of one orange in a high-speed blender and blend until smooth. Add up to 1 cup of water if a thinner consistency is desired. Serve and enjoy!

TIPS

- If the barley grass juice powder and spirulina make the taste too strong for you, start with a small amount of each and work your way up.

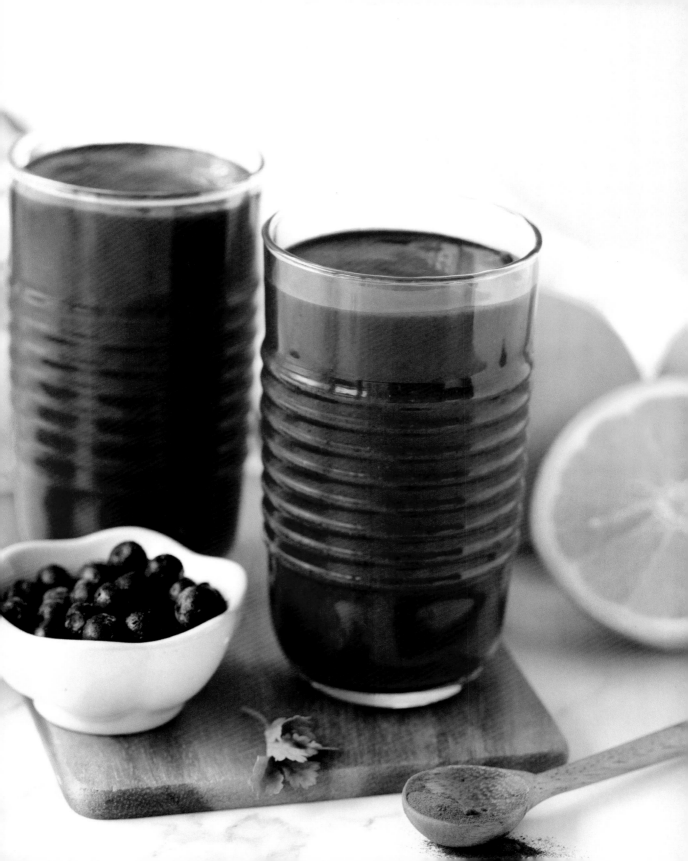

MELON SMOOTHIE

Makes 1 serving

This recipe is simplicity at its best! Choose any variety of melon and blend it alone into a delicious, sweet nectar that couldn't be easier to digest. No matter which melon variety you pick, it will offer your body incredible healing benefits.

3 to 4 cups cubed melon, such as watermelon, cantaloupe, honeydew, canary, galia, sugar kiss, snowball, or any other variety

Place the melon in a blender and blend until smooth, about 1 to 2 minutes.

Pour into a glass and serve immediately.

TIPS

- It's best to enjoy melon on an empty stomach or only after lemon or lime water and celery juice. Wait the customary 15 to 20 and ideally 30 minutes after finishing your celery juice before enjoying your Melon Smoothie.

- Feel free to double or triple this recipe according to your appetite.

- All ripe melons create truly delicious smoothies that hold an abundance of healing benefits, so feel free to use any melon variety you enjoy. Do make sure to stick to one melon variety per smoothie, though. Experiment with different varieties over time to see what you like.

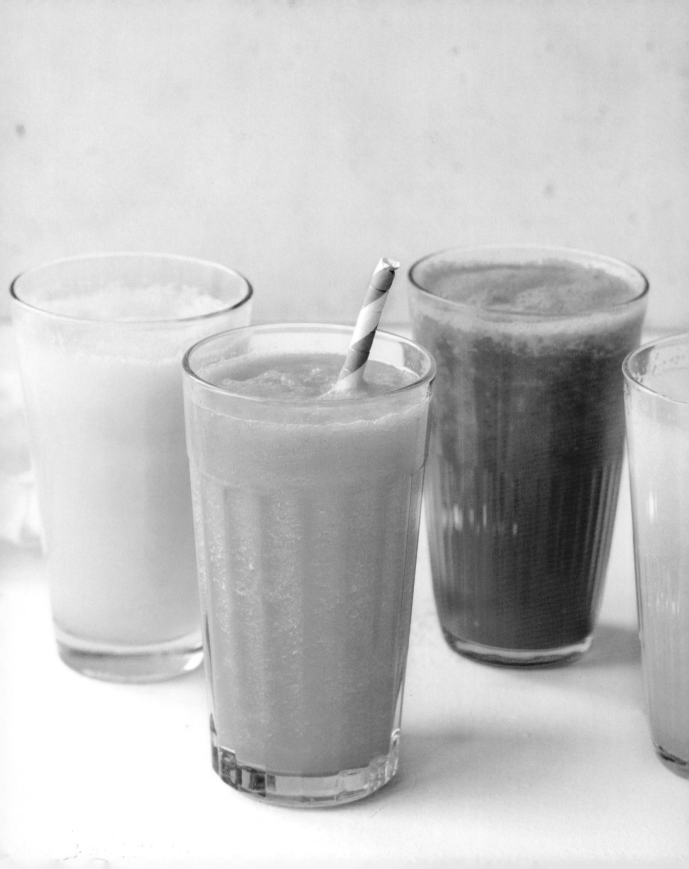

GREEN SMOOTHIE

Makes 1 serving

This simple smoothie is a quick and easy way to pack in plenty of leafy greens without having to chomp through a big salad. The banana or mango not only gives this smoothie its sweetness; it also provides critical glucose to drive the nutrients from the greens to where they need to go in the body.

3 medium-sized bananas, roughly chopped, or 3 cups diced mango

1 to 2 stalks celery, chopped

4 cups spinach, tightly packed, or 4 cups romaine lettuce, tightly packed

1 cup water, to blend

Place all the ingredients in a blender and blend until smooth. Serve immediately.

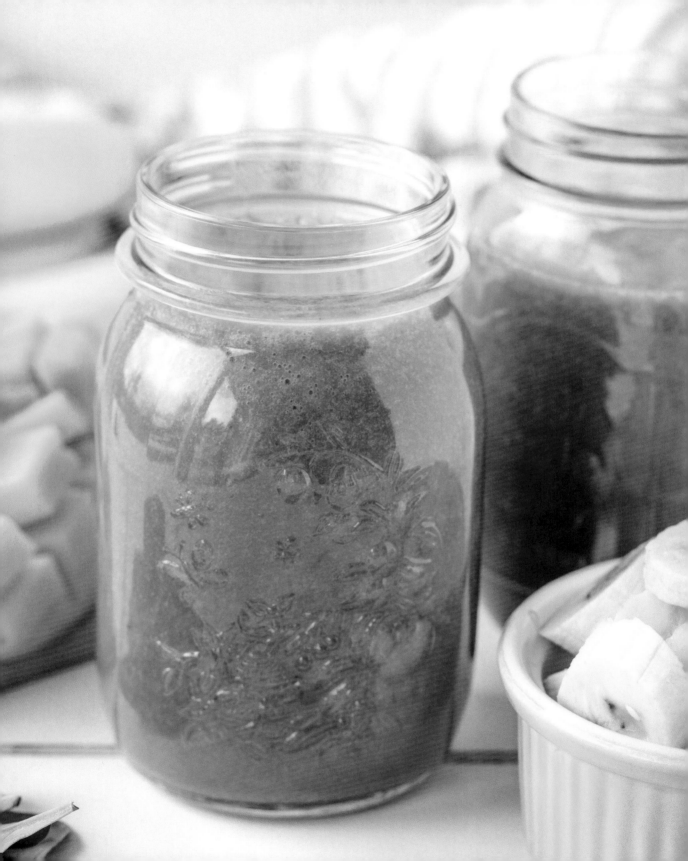

PAPAYA PUDDING

Makes 1 serving

The key to this vibrant healing pudding is to let your papaya properly ripen. When ripe, papaya is sweet and delicious and blends into a creamy, thick pudding you can savor.

½ large Maradol papaya, cubed

Place the papaya in a blender and blend until smooth. Serve immediately.

TIPS

- It's important to only use papayas that aren't genetically modified. Maradol papayas are a large variety that are not GMO.
- Make sure to use only ripe papaya—you want the flesh to be spoonable. You can usually judge ripeness from the outside, when the skin gets some orange or yellow and yields like a ripe avocado under pressure from your thumb.

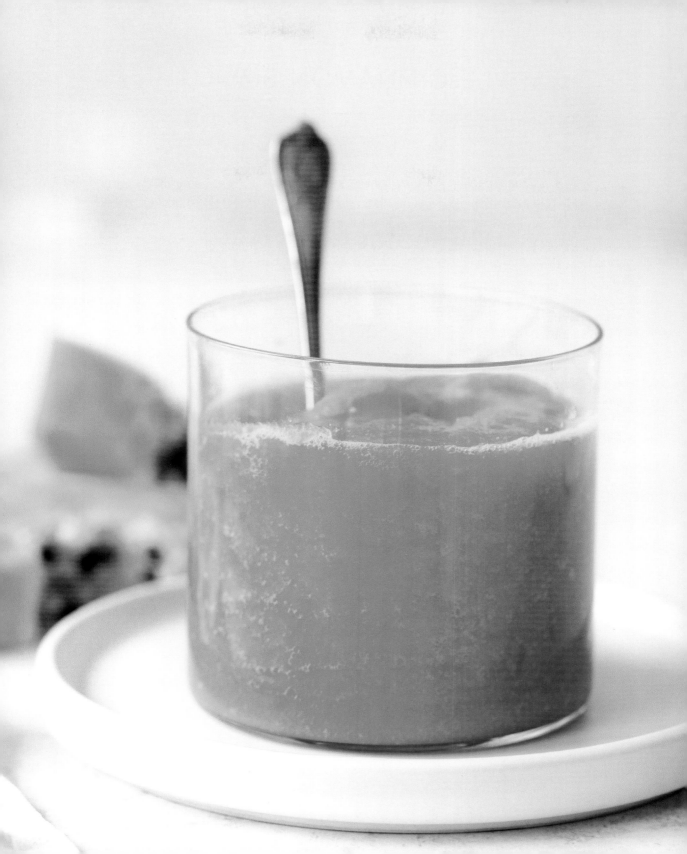

APPLE CINNAMON SMOOTHIE

Enjoy the delicious flavors of apple pie in this heavenly smoothie. It's so creamy, satisfying, and sweet, you will feel like you are indulging in a dessert, without any of the drawbacks that come with the wheat, eggs, butter, lard, and refined sugar of regular apple pie. This recipe is packed with only healing ingredients, so you can feel good about making it for yourself and your family over and over again.

2 medium-sized red apples, cored and cut into chunks

1½ frozen bananas

1 cup water

1 teaspoon pure maple syrup or 1 medjool date (optional)

¾ teaspoon ground cinnamon

¼ teaspoon ground ginger

Pinch of ground nutmeg

Place all the ingredients in a blender and blend until smooth. Serve immediately.

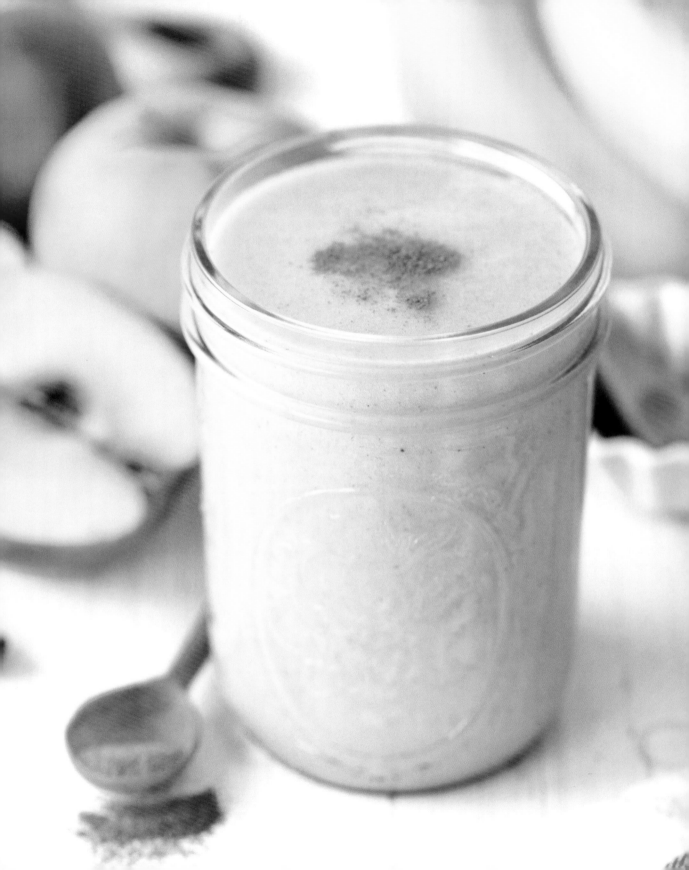

WATERMELON FRIES

Have the fun of eating fries with this perfect sweet replacement: watermelon! These Watermelon Fries are hydrating, healing, and delicious. Lime juice and zest plus chili powder give these fries a pop of flavor that will keep you coming back for more. Enjoy this breakfast all on your own or make enough to share with family or friends. This recipe is also easy to pack up and take with you for a picnic at a park or beach.

1 small watermelon, cut into fries

Zest from 1 lime

1 tablespoon lime juice

½ to 1 teaspoon chili powder

Arrange the watermelon fries on a plate or platter. Add the lime zest, juice, and chili powder. Serve immediately.

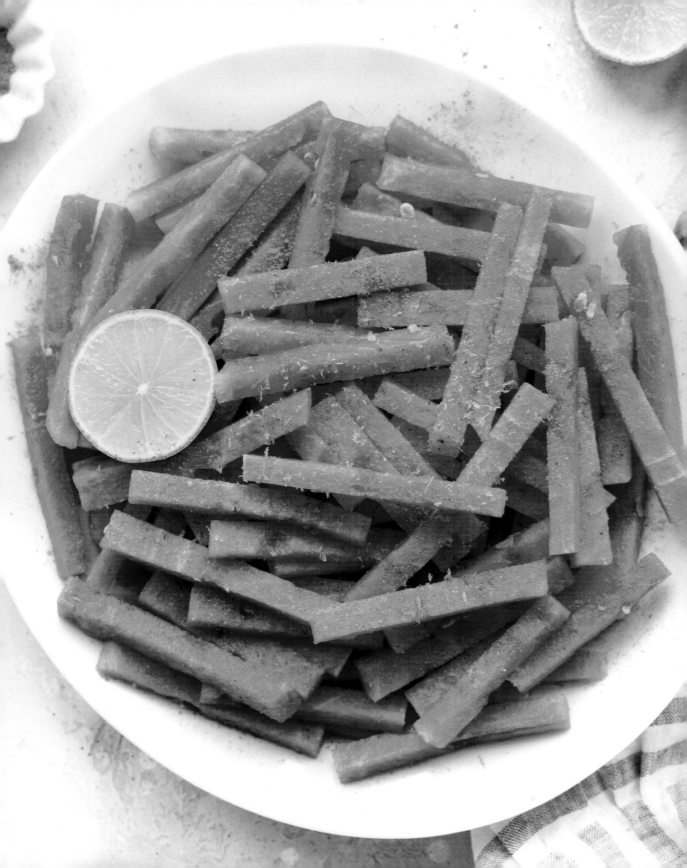

APPLESAUCE

Makes 1 serving

Don't be fooled by this recipe's simplicity—applesauce is one of the most profoundly rejuvenating, revitalizing foods for your liver cells, and that means wonders for the rest of your body. Plus it's sweet and delicious and easy to whip up anytime.

1 to 2 red apples, diced

1 to 3 medjool dates, pitted (optional)

1 stalk celery, chopped (optional)

¼ teaspoon cinnamon (optional)

Blend the diced red apple and other desired ingredients in a blender or food processor until a smooth, even applesauce forms.

Serve and enjoy immediately or squeeze some fresh lemon juice over the top and seal tightly if you'd like to save it for later.

TIPS

- If you're making this recipe to fill in for apples as part of the 3:6:9 Cleanse, be mindful about how many dates you add to your applesauce, if any. Pay attention to whether a given snack calls for them and adjust the amount of dates you include accordingly. As beneficial as dates are, you want to make sure you leave room for water-rich foods. With too many dates, you could fill up so much that you miss out on the other healing cleanse foods.

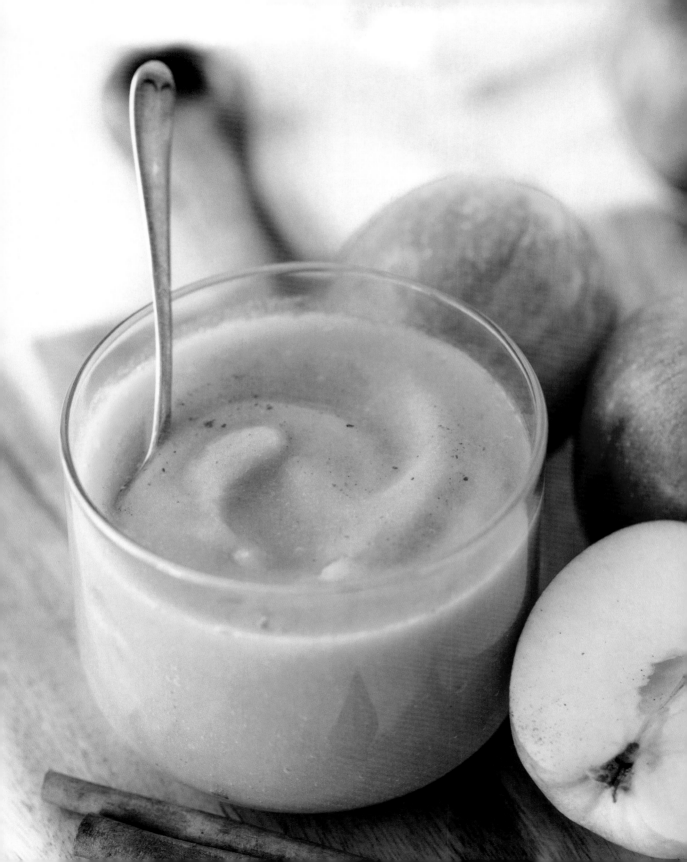

PEAR SAUCE

Makes 1 serving

Pear Sauce is a delicious variation on the Applesauce recipe for anyone who doesn't like apples or simply wants another option.

3 ripe pears, diced

Blend the diced pears in a blender or food processor until a smooth, even pear sauce forms.

Serve and enjoy immediately or store sealed tightly if you'd like to save it for later.

TIPS

- Waiting until your pears are soft and juicy will make it easier to blend them into sauce, and it will make the sauce gentler on your digestion.
- For Day 9 of the 3:6:9 Cleanse, it's important to make this recipe with pears alone; however, feel free to make it with additional ingredients such as dates, cinnamon, lemon juice, cardamom, or nutmeg after the Cleanse.

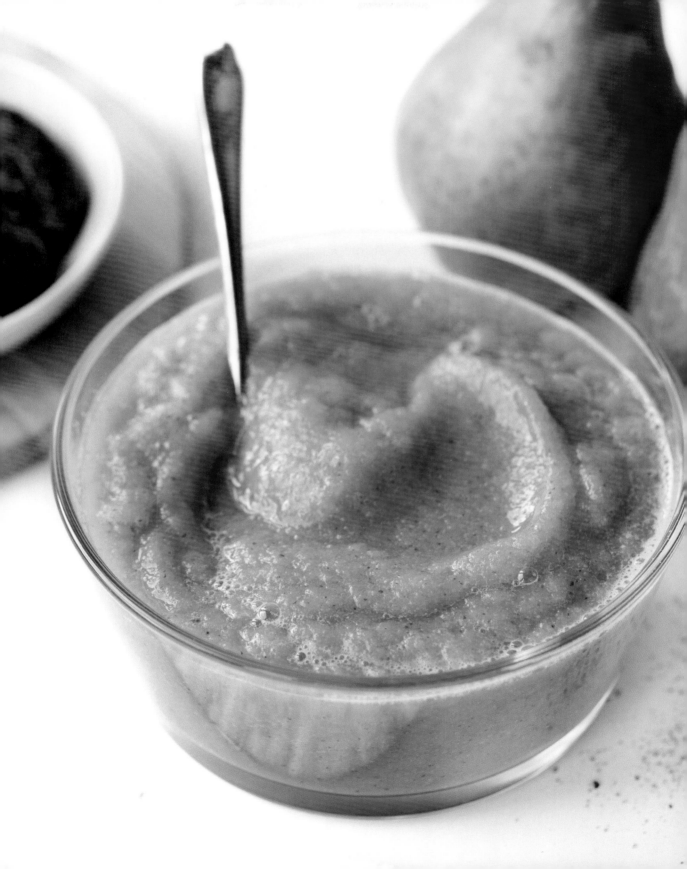

PITAYA SMOOTHIE BOWL

Let the color and nutrients in this smoothie bowl breathe light into your morning. The supercharged antioxidants—an undiscovered variety I call hyperantioxidants—in pitaya make it a standout ingredient in this recipe. It's certainly beautiful too!

2 frozen bananas or 2 cups frozen diced mango

1 cup fresh, 2 packets frozen, or 2 tablespoons powdered red pitaya (dragon fruit)

¼ to ½ cup fresh orange juice or water, to blend

TOPPINGS

2 to 3 fresh strawberries, chopped

2 tablespoons fresh blueberries and/or fresh raspberries

¼ cup sliced banana

¼ cup diced mango

Place all the ingredients for the smoothie in a high-speed blender and blend until smooth. Pour into a bowl and add toppings of your choice. Serve immediately.

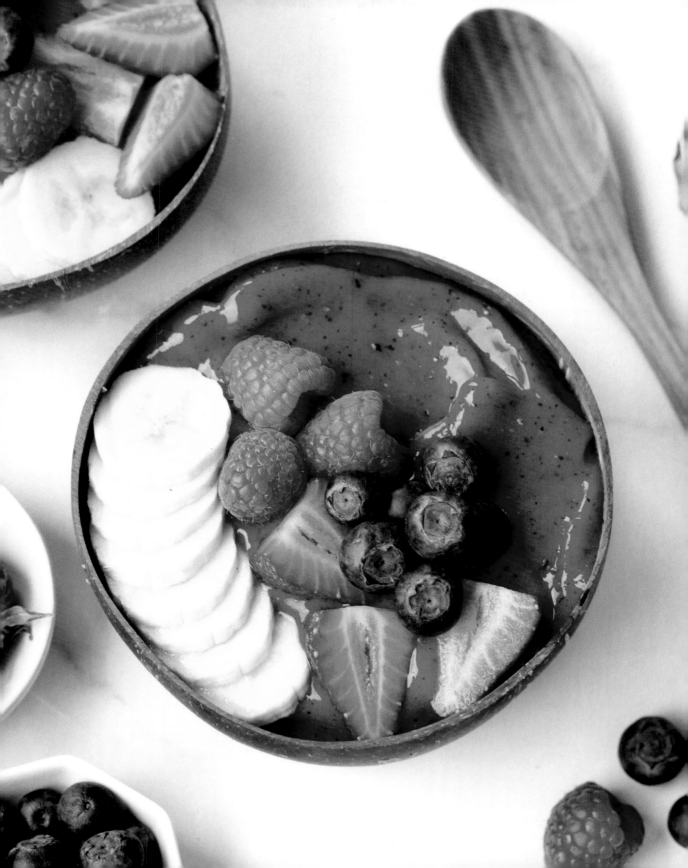

MELON PLATTER

Makes 1 serving

There's nothing quite like eating a big helping of your favorite melon for breakfast. Whether it's watermelon, cantaloupe, honeydew, or any specialty melons such as canary, galia, or Santa Claus, your body will thank you—as will your taste buds!

½ small or ¼ large watermelon, or ½ to 1 small melon of another variety

Eat straight up or arrange on a plate or in a bowl and enjoy!

TIPS

- It's best to eat melon alone, not with other fruit.
- Many of us are used to eating only a slice of watermelon here or a wedge of cantaloupe there. With melon as your main meal, make sure to serve yourself enough that you feel satisfied.

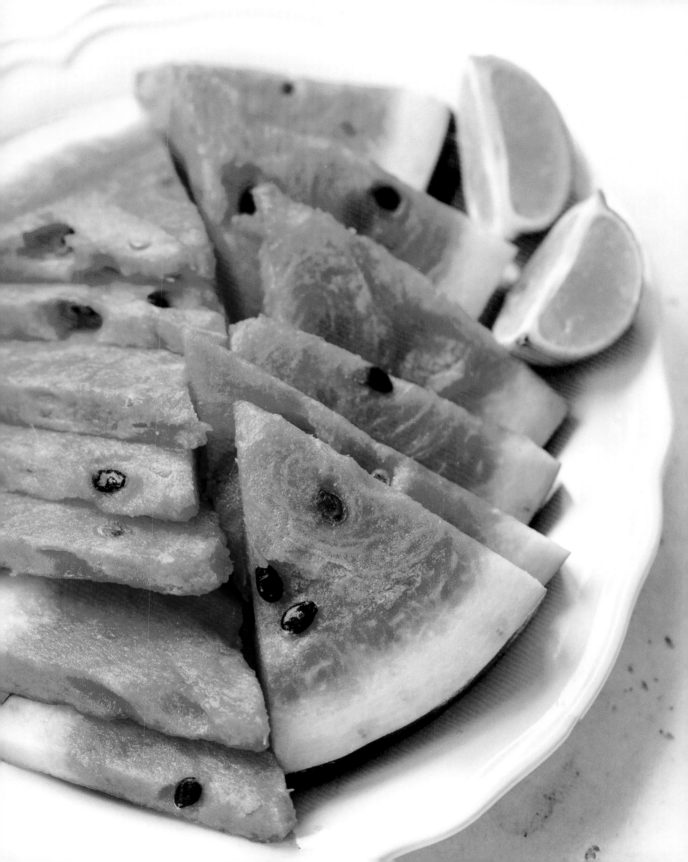

FRESH FRUIT BREAKFAST

Makes 1 serving

With so many fruits to choose from, this simple breakfast option can be as varied as you'd like. Simply pick your favorite fruits and enjoy. For optimal digestion, choose just one fruit, such as papaya or bananas, and eat enough to feel fully satisfied. Or choose just two or three fruits, such as berries with bananas, for a simple breakfast fruit bowl.

A hearty amount of any fresh fruits you like, such as papaya, berries, bananas, nectarines, grapes, oranges, peaches, figs, mangoes, apricots, apples, pears, or any other fresh fruit you love

Eat straight up or arrange on a plate or in a bowl and enjoy!

TIPS

- Make sure you serve yourself enough fruit for a whole meal. One or two apples, one banana, a cup of berries, or a couple of kiwifruit on their own is usually not enough breakfast for most people. If you prefer to eat small amounts, make sure you graze on more fresh fruit every hour to hour and a half throughout the morning.

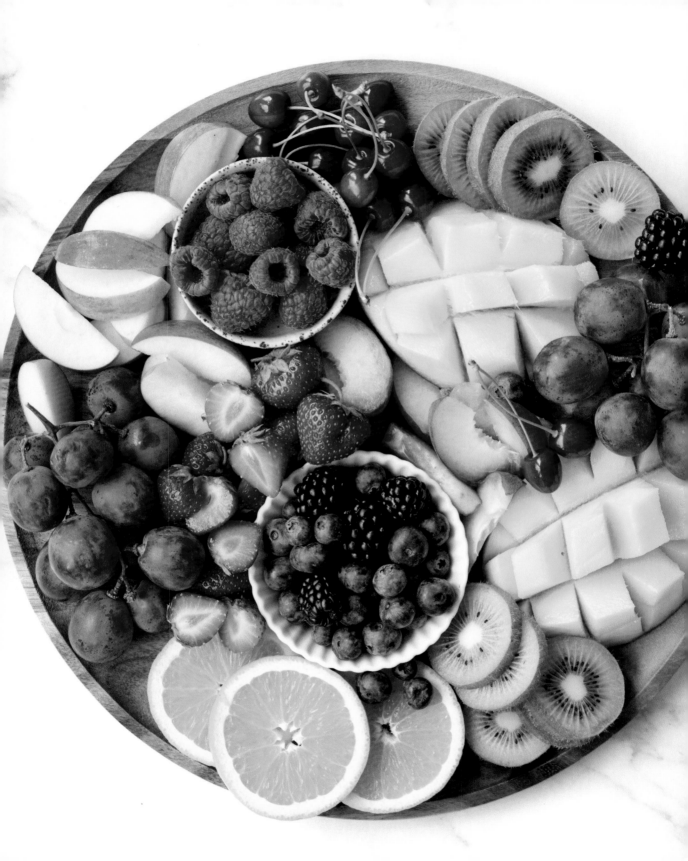

FRUIT CEREAL

Love cereal? This sweet, delicious fruit cereal is a wonderful alternative to the traditional version. Made with chopped mangoes and sweet berries and topped with a cold, creamy banana milk, this offers the same satisfying sensations with fresh, nutrient-dense ingredients.

1 cup mixed berries

1 mango, diced

1 fresh banana

1 frozen banana

1 tablespoon dried mulberries (optional)

Combine berries and mangoes in a bowl.

To make banana milk, blend 1 fresh banana and 1 frozen banana with 1 cup of water. Pour over the fruit bowl, top with optional dried mulberries, and enjoy!

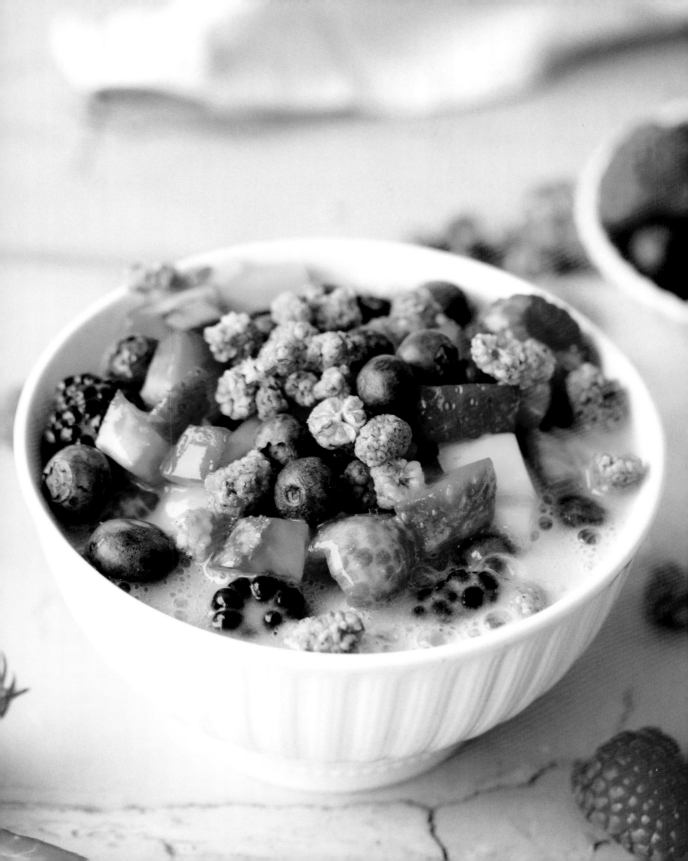

MANGO SMOOTHIE BERRY PARFAIT

Makes 1 serving

This gorgeous parfait is a feast for the eyes *and* the body. With its layers of bright orange smoothie topped with beautiful deep red and blue berries, you may find yourself serving this to family and friends long after the cleanse has finished.

2 cups frozen diced mango

2 to 3 tablespoons fresh orange juice or water, to blend

½ cup strawberries, raspberries, blueberries, and/or blackberries

Fresh mint, for garnish (optional)

Place the mango and orange juice (or water) in a blender and blend until smooth.

Pour a layer of mango-orange smoothie in a jar or bowl, scraping from the sides of the blender as needed. Top with half the berries. Repeat with another layer of the smoothie and berries.

Garnish with a few leaves of fresh mint, if desired, and serve.

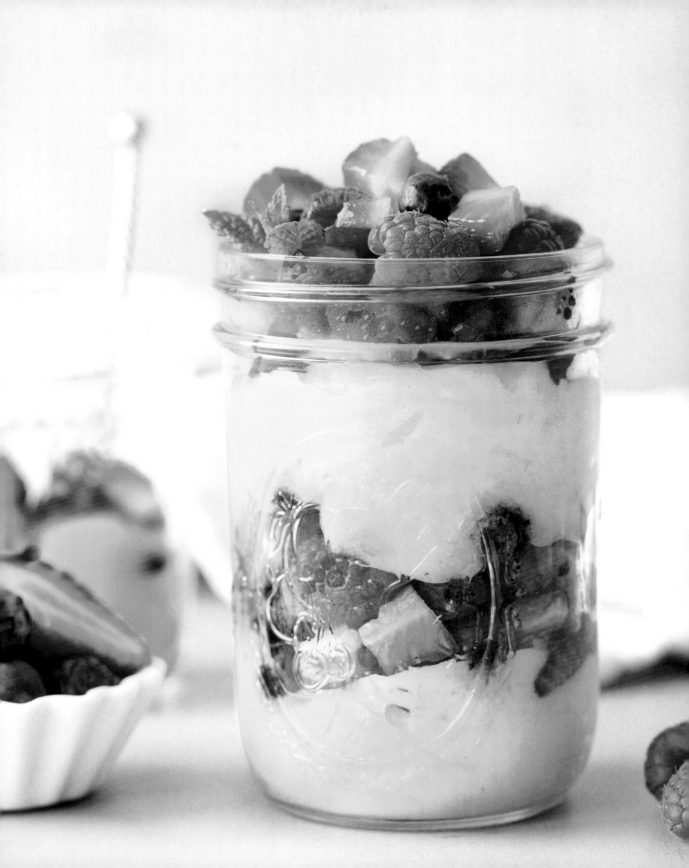

CARAMEL APPLE SOFT SERVE

Makes 1 serving

Trade dairy soft serve for this heavenly, creamy, fruit-based option. Made with banana, apple, and dates, this soft serve is a virus-fighting, liver-healing treat you can feel good about enjoying as often as you'd like!

1 apple, diced and frozen

1 frozen banana

2 to 3 medjool dates, pitted

1 teaspoon alcohol-free vanilla extract or ¼ teaspoon vanilla bean powder (optional)

2 to 3 tablespoons water, if needed to blend

Place all the ingredients in a high-speed blender or food processor and blend until smooth. Add as little water as possible and scrape down the sides as needed. Serve immediately.

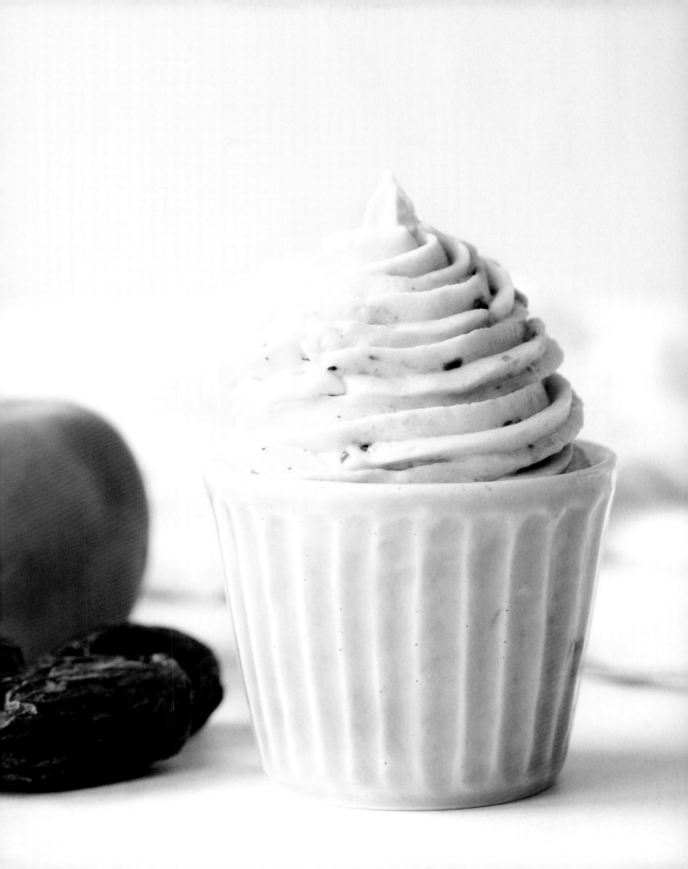

RAW APPLE BANANA "OATMEAL"
WITH BLACKBERRIES

A bowl of regular gluten-free oatmeal without dairy milk can be a healthy choice. For an even healthier version, try this "oatmeal" recipe made from apples, banana, and spices! It's creamy and satisfying and offers a wonderful alternative for anyone avoiding or limiting grains.

2 apples, diced

1 large ripe banana, roughly chopped

¼ teaspoon cinnamon

⅛ teaspoon cardamom

½ cup blackberries

OPTIONAL

raisins or dried cranberries

Place the apples, banana, cinnamon, and cardamom in a food processor and pulse until chunky and creamy.

Transfer the mixture to a bowl and top with blackberries and raisins or cranberries, if desired. Serve and enjoy.

TIPS

- If you'd prefer to use another berry, such as strawberries, raspberries, wild blueberries, or mulberries, go ahead. Any berry will be a healing food packed full of antioxidants and more.

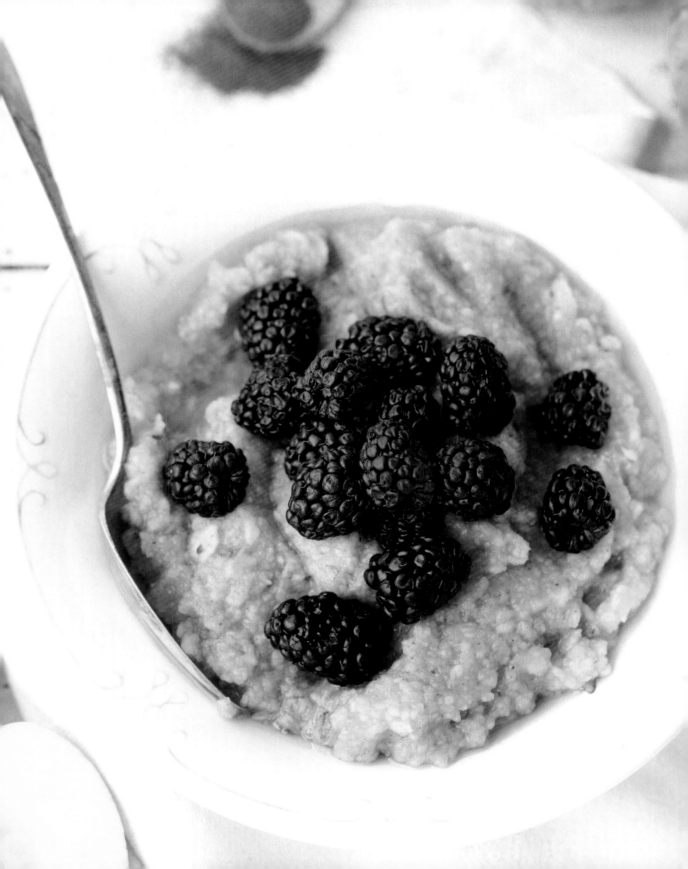

WILD BLUEBERRY PORRIDGE

A more traditional porridge than the Raw Apple Banana "Oatmeal," this recipe uses millet or gluten-free oatmeal with the addition of a secret weapon: wild blueberries. These little purple gems offer an explosion of delicious flavor, and their healing properties for the liver and the rest of the body are a true miracle.

1 cup millet or gluten-free oats

2 cups water; more if needed

½ teaspoon cinnamon

½ cup wild blueberries

2 tablespoons fresh wild or cultivated blueberries, or frozen wild blueberries, for garnish

Pure maple syrup or raw honey, to taste

Place the millet, water, and cinnamon in a small saucepan, stir, and bring it to a boil. Add more water if needed. Reduce to a simmer, cover, and cook until soft, about 10 to 15 minutes, stirring intermittently. Once it's cooked, remove the saucepan from the heat, cover it, and let it sit for a few minutes.

Alternatively, place the oats, water, and cinnamon in a small saucepan and bring to a simmer. Add more water if needed. Cover and cook until soft, about 5 to 10 minutes.

Stir in the wild blueberries and maple syrup to taste. Serve topped with the 2 tablespoons of blueberries.

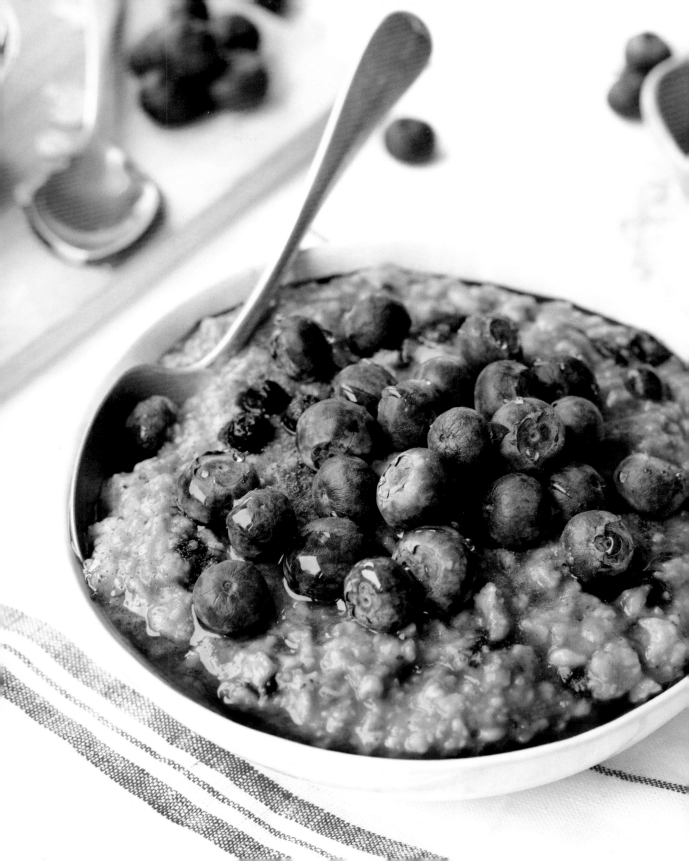

SPAGHETTI SQUASH HASH BROWNS

This unique spin on hash browns gives you a fun way to enjoy a childhood favorite while still allowing your liver and body to heal. You can serve these hash browns on their own or top with chopped tomato or a fresh tomato salsa.

½ large spaghetti squash (yields about 2 cups cooked)

1 teaspoon dried herbs, such as rosemary or thyme

Handful of chopped green onions or parsley, for garnish

Preheat oven to 400°F/200°C.

Scoop the seeds out of the spaghetti squash. Place it cut side down on a baking sheet lined with parchment paper and pierce the squash a few times with a fork. Roast it in the oven for 30 to 40 minutes, until soft. Cool the squash completely.

Once the squash is cooled, use a fork to scoop strands of "spaghetti" out of the squash and place them in a bowl. Add the herbs. Mix until combined. Form the mixture into patties, and then place the patties between pieces of kitchen towel and squeeze out the moisture.

Place a ceramic nonstick pan over medium-high heat and add the hash browns. Cook until browned, about 5 to 6 minutes on each side. Serve immediately with chopped green onions or parsley.

TIPS

- To save cooking time on busy mornings, you can cook the spaghetti squash in advance and then use it to make hash browns when you're ready.

- These hash browns can be served with any meal, not just breakfast. They are great paired with the Leafy Green Salad or a fresh tomato, basil, and spinach salad or salsa. A little drizzle of lemon juice and raw honey over your salad and squash is another nice option.

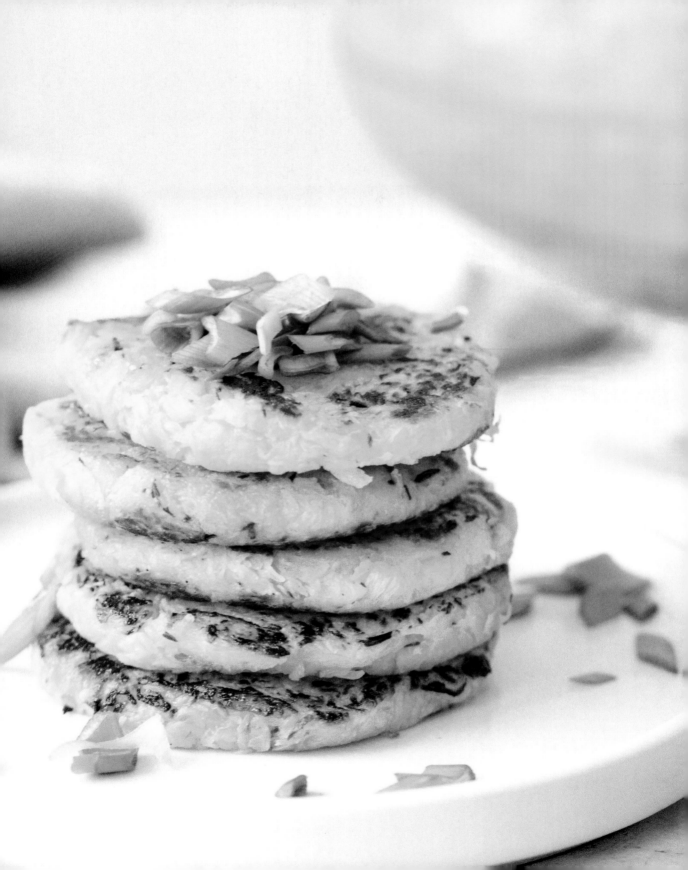

GLUTEN-FREE BANANA OAT BREAKFAST COOKIES

Makes 8 cookies

With just a few key ingredients, these Breakfast Cookies couldn't be simpler, with no flavor sacrificed. You can make them in advance for busy mornings or pack in lunch boxes for the whole family.

1 large ripe banana (about ½ cup mashed)

1 cup gluten-free oats

1 teaspoon cinnamon

¼ cup cranberries or raisins (optional)

Preheat oven to 350°F/180°C. Line a baking sheet with parchment paper.

Place the banana in a medium-sized mixing bowl and mash with a fork. Add the oats, cinnamon, and cranberries or raisins, if desired. Mix until uniform.

Scoop out the mixture using a heaping tablespoon measure—you should get about 8 cookies. Place them on the baking sheet and flatten them slightly to make discs.

Place the cookies in the oven and bake for 15 to 20 minutes, until browned on the sides. Cool completely before eating.

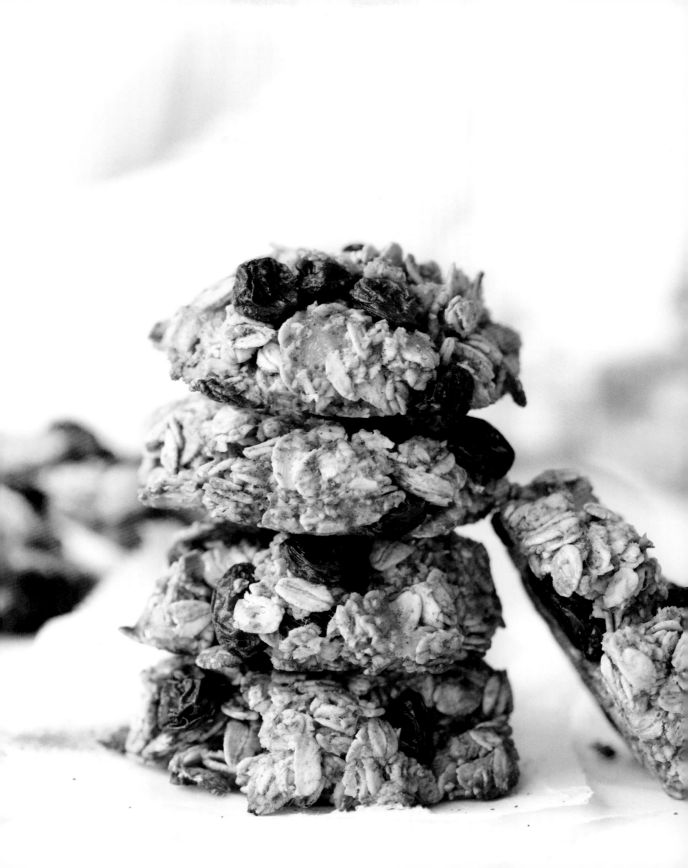

RAW MINI APPLE PIE TARTS

These pretty little tarts are a wonderful snack to fuel the liver and body with the glucose they need to heal and function. Enjoy them as a snack and store any leftovers in the fridge or freezer to share with friends and family another day.

CRUST

2 cups pitted medjool dates
1 cup mulberries

FILLING

3 apples, cored and diced
2 to 3 medjool dates, pitted
⅛ teaspoon cinnamon
Pinch of nutmeg
2 teaspoons fresh orange or lemon juice

TOPPING

½ apple, very thinly sliced
½ teaspoon cinnamon
1 to 2 teaspoons raw honey (optional)

To make the crust, combine the dates and mulberries in a food processor and process until well combined.

Line a muffin tin with pieces of parchment paper or plastic wrap large enough to hang over the edges for easy removal. Press the mixture to the bottom and up the sides, making 6 to 8 tart bases. Set aside.

Make the filling by blending together the apples, dates, cinnamon, nutmeg, and orange or lemon juice until smooth. Spoon into the tart shells and place in the freezer for 30 minutes.

Remove the tart bases from the muffin tin and pull away the parchment paper or plastic wrap. Place the tarts on a plate or platter and arrange the apple slices on top. Sprinkle with cinnamon and drizzle with raw honey, if desired.

Serve immediately or keep in the fridge or freezer for later.

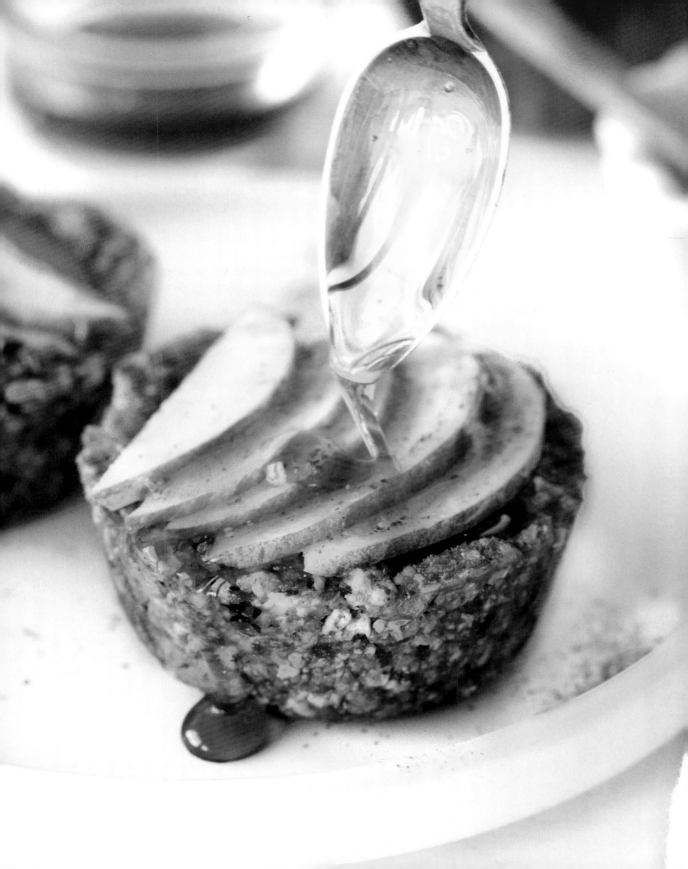

APPLE CINNAMON STUFFED DATES

Makes 2 servings

While dates are a perfect, easy snack on their own, these Apple Cinnamon Stuffed Dates take snacking to another level of deliciousness! Pair them with celery sticks and cucumber slices for a sweet, salty, and hydrating snack.

1 apple
½ teaspoon cinnamon
6 medjool dates

Cut the apple into thin wedges, removing the core and seeds. Lay the slices flat on a plate or platter and sprinkle with cinnamon.

Make an incision on one side of the date and remove the pit. Open the date and place a cinnamon apple wedge in the middle.

Repeat with the rest of the dates and serve.

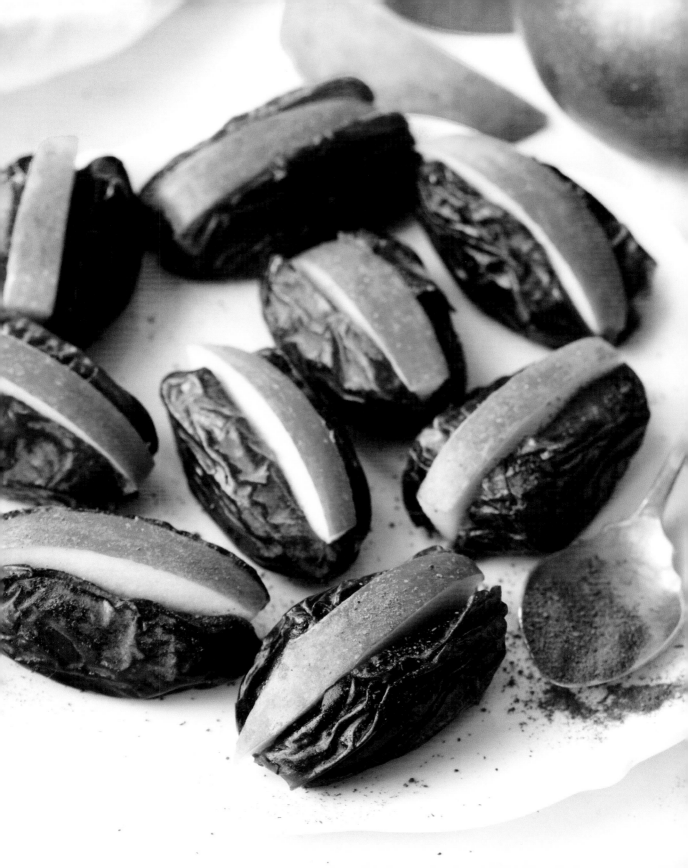

APPLE PIE FILLING

Enjoy this fun and cute way to savor the flavors of apple pie. With only a few ingredients, this recipe gives you plenty of taste bud satisfaction. It also keeps well for multiple days in the fridge, so consider making extra to reach for throughout the week.

½ cup pitted medjool dates

½ cup water

¼ teaspoon cinnamon

Pinch of nutmeg

3 medium-sized apples, diced

Blend together the dates, water, cinnamon, and nutmeg until smooth. Place in a bowl and add the diced apples. Mix until combined. Serve immediately or place in an airtight container in the fridge to keep for later.

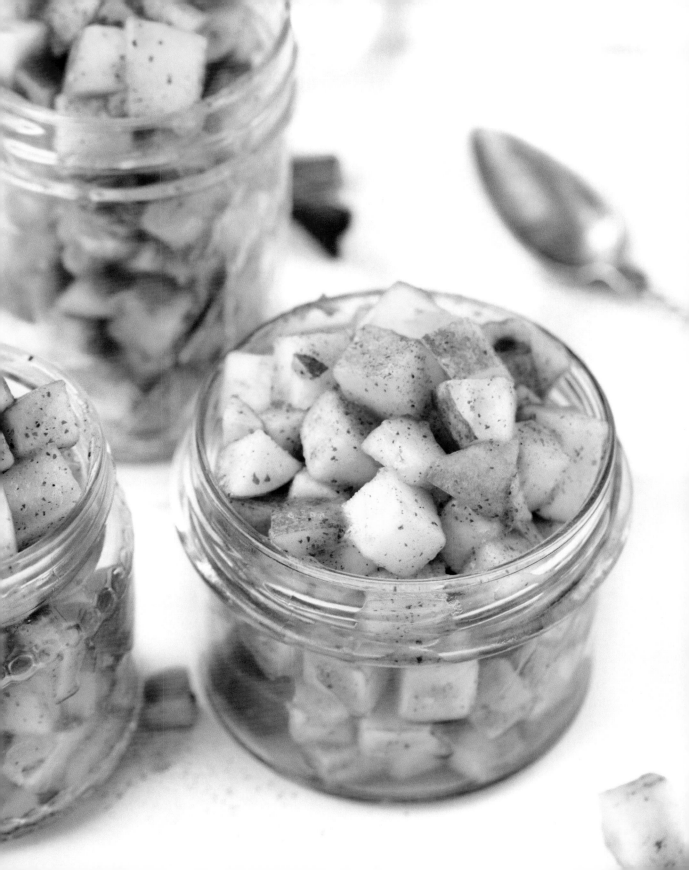

LIVER RESCUE SALAD

Makes 1 to 2 servings

These two salad options are brimming with healing properties for your liver. They're great for when you want a lighter meal, and they're also perfect additions to a cooked meal such as the steamed asparagus, brussels sprouts, zucchini, and summer squash in the 3:6:9 Cleanse. You can customize each salad with any of the healing foods listed below so that you never get bored. If you try the fat-free Orange "Vinaigrette" Dressing, it is sure to become a staple in your kitchen. It's flavorful, sweet, and satisfying for anyone to enjoy.

8 cups any variety of leafy greens (spinach, arugula, butter lettuce, romaine, kale, mâche, etc.), loosely packed

1 lemon, lime, or orange, juiced

OPTIONAL TOPPINGS

Apple	**Fresh herbs** (cilantro,
Grapes	parsley, basil, dill,
Mango	mint, oregano, thyme,
Papaya	rosemary, etc.)
Orange	**Atlantic dulse**
Tangerine	**Garlic**
Berries	**Onion** (any variety
Banana (only if the	you like—leeks,
salad doesn't include	red, sweet, yellow,
tomato, as banana	green, etc.)
and tomato don't	**Radish**
digest well together)	**Bell pepper** (ripe,
Fresh figs	not green)
Cucumber	**Sugar snap peas**
Celery	**Snow peas**
Tomato	**Raw cauliflower**
Asparagus	**Sundried tomatoes**
Cabbage (red or	(unsalted, oil-free,
green)	unsulfured)
Carrot	**Steamed green**
Sprouts	**beans**
Microgreens	

OPTIONAL ORANGE "VINAIGRETTE" DRESSING

1 cup orange juice

1 garlic clove

1 teaspoon raw honey

¼ cup water

⅛ teaspoon cayenne (optional)

Place the leafy greens of your choice and your desired toppings from the list in a bowl and mix together to form the base of the salad.

Drizzle the fresh lemon, lime, or orange juice over top to taste.

Alternatively, make the Orange "Vinaigrette" by blending all of its ingredients until smoothly combined. Toss with your salad until well mixed.

Serve and enjoy.

TIPS

- During the Original 3:6:9 Cleanse, it may be tempting to skip the Liver Rescue Salad if you enjoy the asparagus and/or brussels sprouts so much that you fill up on those at lunch and dinner. Try to be mindful so that this doesn't happen—unless it's dinner on Days 7 or 8, when the salad is optional.

- If you don't have room to eat the full salad with the other items called for in your cleanse meal, it is okay to cut this recipe by as much as half so you have an appetite for it all. That is, scale back how many toppings you include and cut the base from 8 cups of greens to 4 cups of greens.

- If you're really highly sensitive, you can even make the raw Liver Rescue Soup in place of this recipe. As a last resort on the Original 3:6:9 Cleanse, it's okay to opt for the Liver Rescue Juice recipe instead to get the nutrients in yourself that way. When your digestion is that compromised, you may prefer to start with the Mono Eating Cleanse from Chapter 18.

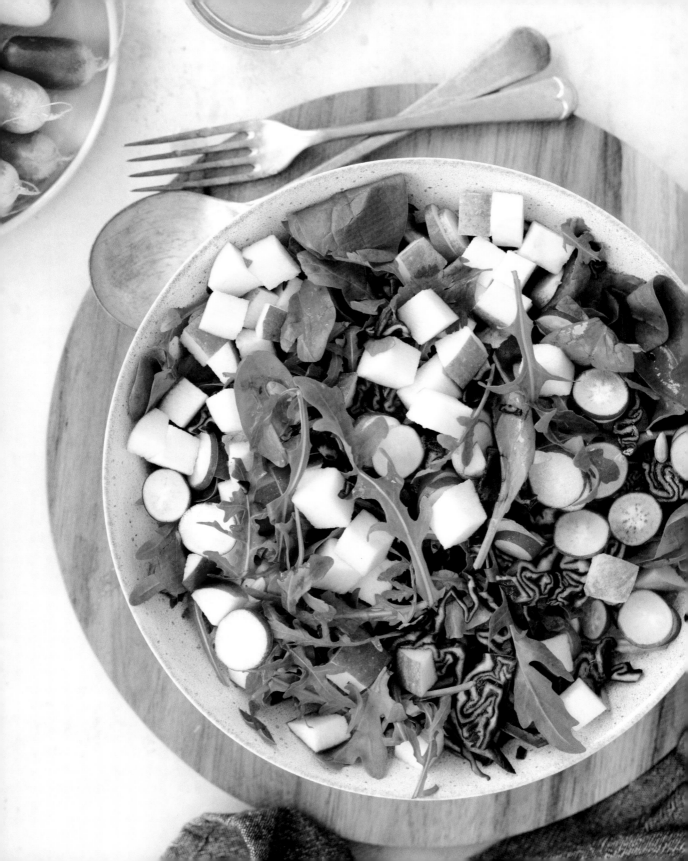

SPINACH SOUP

One of the amazing benefits of incorporating more fruits, vegetables, and leafy greens into our diet is the way our taste buds change and we begin to crave more and more of these fresh ingredients over time. When you find yourself yearning for leafy greens and the benefits they provide, this easy-to-make, richly flavored soup is a great way to incorporate them into your day in an easily digestible form. With all of the minerals the spinach provides, you'll also help curb any cravings for the foods you know don't serve your health right now.

1 pint grape tomatoes

1 stalk celery

1 garlic clove

1 orange, juiced

4 cups baby spinach, loosely packed

2 basil leaves or a few sprigs of fresh cilantro

½ to 1 cucumber (optional; leave out the cucumber noodles on Day 9 of the Simplified Cleanse)

Place the tomatoes, celery, garlic, and fresh orange juice in a high-speed blender and blend until smooth.

Add the spinach by the handful and blend until completely incorporated.

Add the basil or cilantro and blend until smooth.

If desired, make the cucumber into noodles using a spiralizer, julienne peeler, or vegetable peeler. (As noted at the beginning of this chapter, when using organic cucumber, you can leave the skin on or peel the cucumber first, depending on preference. With conventional cucumber, peel the cucumber if possible and discard skins.) Place the noodles in a serving bowl.

Pour the blended soup into the serving bowl and serve immediately.

TIPS

- If you can't use spinach, you can substitute butter leaf lettuce.

- If you can't use tomatoes, you can substitute ripe mango. If you can't get fresh, sweet mangoes, you can substitute thawed frozen mango.

- If neither tomato nor mango are options, you can blend up banana with greens instead. Be sure not to include both banana and tomato in the recipe, as they don't digest well together. Use banana only for this substitution.

- English cucumbers are a fun option when making cucumber noodles because of their small seeds.

- As was mentioned, if you are having Spinach Soup on Day 9 of the Simplified 3:6:9 Cleanse, leave out the cucumber noodles. You can blend cucumber into the soup if you'd like. You want to stick to juiced or blended foods only for that day.

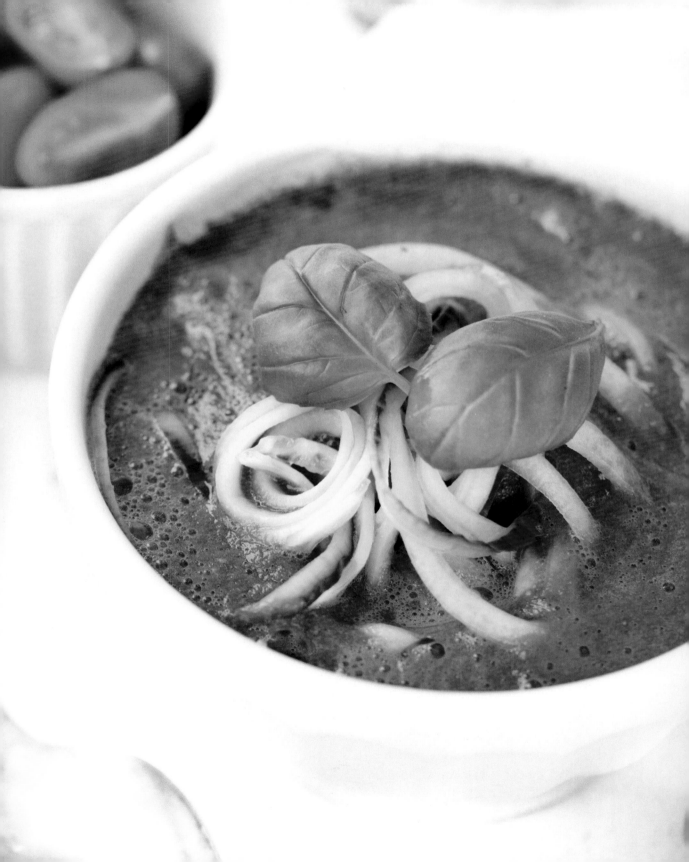

LIVER RESCUE SOUP

Makes 1 to 2 servings

If you're not into eating salads, Liver Rescue Soup is a fantastic healing alternative to Liver Rescue Salad so you can still get important cleansing and healing foods into your body. This raw soup is also a great choice for anyone who has difficulty chewing, has little time to eat, or suffers with sensitive digestion.

2 cups grape tomatoes

1 cup diced cucumber

2 celery stalks

¼ cup fresh cilantro, tightly packed

¼ cup parsley, tightly packed

4 cups leafy greens (spinach, arugula, butter lettuce, etc.), loosely packed

2 tablespoons fresh lemon, lime, or orange juice

1 cup chopped asparagus

1 to 2 medjool dates or 1 to 2 teaspoons raw honey (optional)

½ cup water

Place all the ingredients in a high-speed blender and blend until smooth. Serve immediately.

TIPS

- If Liver Rescue Soup is not to your taste, choose mild flavored leafy greens such as spinach instead of stronger-tasting greens such as arugula and kale.

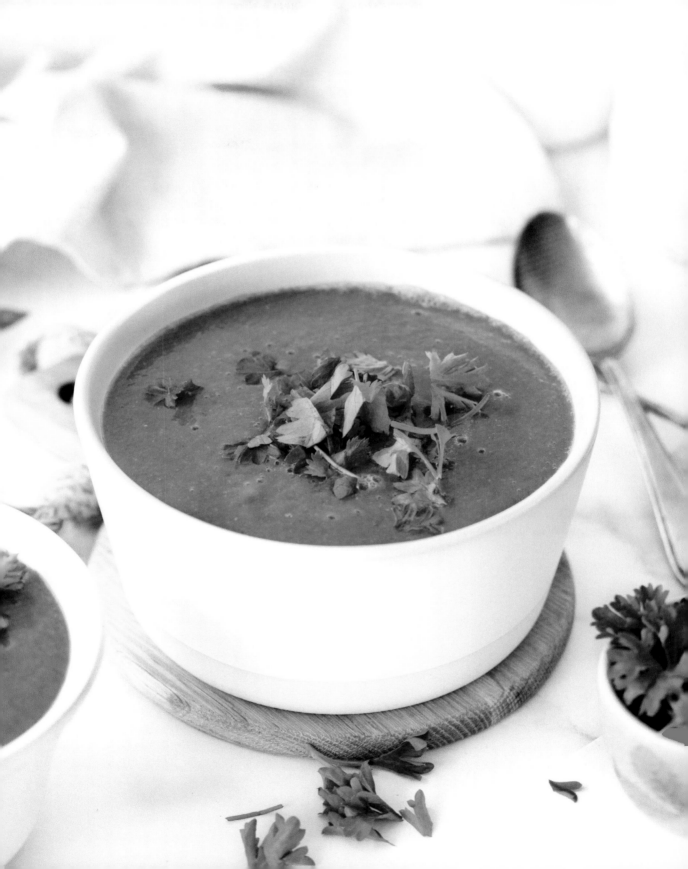

BRUSSELS SPROUT SLAW

Makes 1 to 2 servings

If you've never tried brussels sprouts raw, you might be surprised by how delicious they can be, especially when thinly sliced, grated, or shaved and served with a dressing. In this recipe, more traditional slaw components such as carrots and cabbage accompany the star ingredient of brussels sprouts, a gift for your cleansing and healing. Add fresh herbs and a delicious, simple dressing, and you may find yourself developing a new love for raw brussels sprouts! Enjoy the same day or make it in advance—both are delicious!

1½ cups thinly sliced brussels sprouts

1 cup shredded carrots (optional)

1 cup thinly sliced red cabbage

½ cup chopped fresh cilantro

¼ cup chopped green onions

1 garlic clove, finely grated

2 tablespoons lemon or lime juice

1 teaspoon raw honey or pure maple syrup (optional)

Place the brussels sprouts, shredded carrots (if using), red cabbage, cilantro, and green onions in a large mixing bowl. Toss until combined.

Add the grated garlic, lemon juice, and raw honey (if using) to the salad. Mix well.

Taste and adjust seasoning. Serve and enjoy.

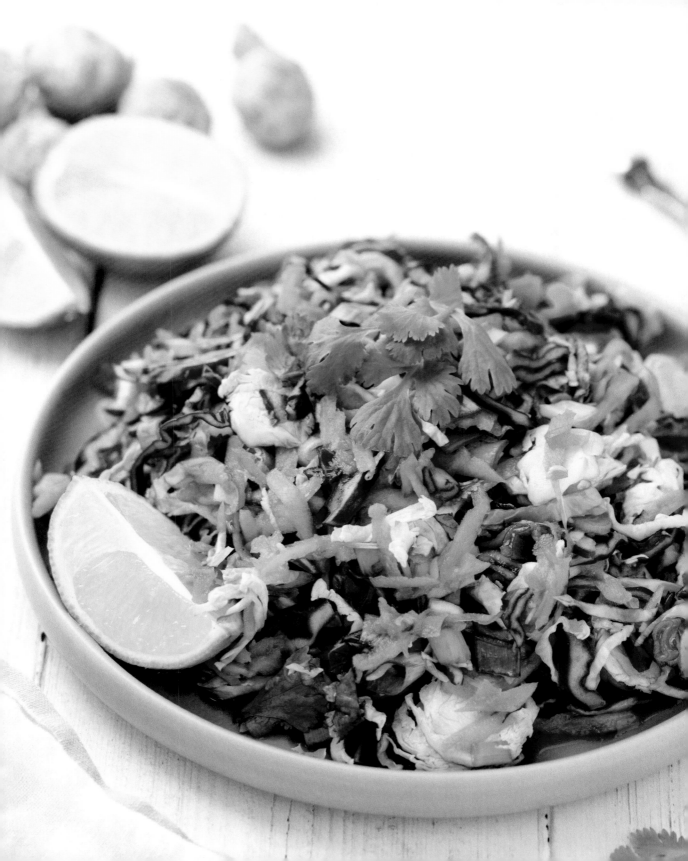

SHAVED BRUSSELS SPROUT, ASPARAGUS, RADISH, AND APPLE SALAD

Makes 1 to 2 servings

A little bit sweet and a little bit spicy, this salad is bright, clean, and flavorful. Its raw brussels sprouts, asparagus, apple, and radish are all powerhouse foods for your liver and other organs. This salad holds up well in the fridge as leftovers.

1 pound brussels sprouts, ends trimmed, shaved on a mandoline or thinly sliced

1 pound asparagus, ends trimmed, sliced into thin rounds

½ cup thinly sliced radish

1 medium-sized red apple, very thinly sliced

SAUCE

1 garlic clove, finely grated

1 teaspoon finely grated red onion

1½ teaspoons raw honey or pure maple syrup

3 tablespoons fresh lemon juice

Place the shaved brussels sprouts, asparagus, radish, and apple in a large mixing bowl. Mix well and set aside.

Make the sauce by whisking together the grated garlic, red onion, raw honey or maple syrup, and lemon juice in a small bowl or jar. Pour on top of the salad and toss to coat.

Divide between bowls and serve.

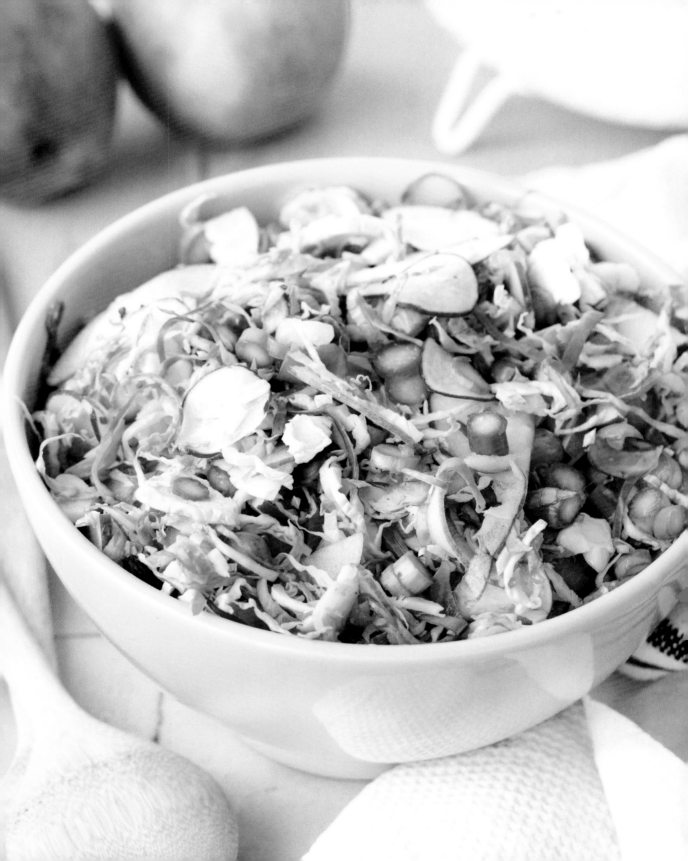

LEAFY GREEN SALAD

This salad can be as simple or varied as you'd like. In a pinch, throw some leafy greens in a bowl, add a squeeze of lemon or lime, and enjoy! Especially when serving it as a side salad, sometimes that's all you need. When you want to add other ingredients, consider tomatoes, cucumbers, onion, or any vegetables you prefer to make it your own.

4 cups leafy greens (such as spinach, arugula, butter lettuce, etc.), loosely packed

2 tablespoons lemon or lime juice

OPTIONAL ADDITIONS

¼ cup halved cherry tomatoes or chopped tomatoes

½ cup chopped cucumber

¼ cup thinly sliced red cabbage

¼ cup thinly sliced radish

¼ cup thinly sliced red onion

1 teaspoon raw honey or pure maple syrup

Add the leafy greens of your choice to a bowl and squeeze the lemon juice on top. Toss until coated.

Add any additions you like and serve.

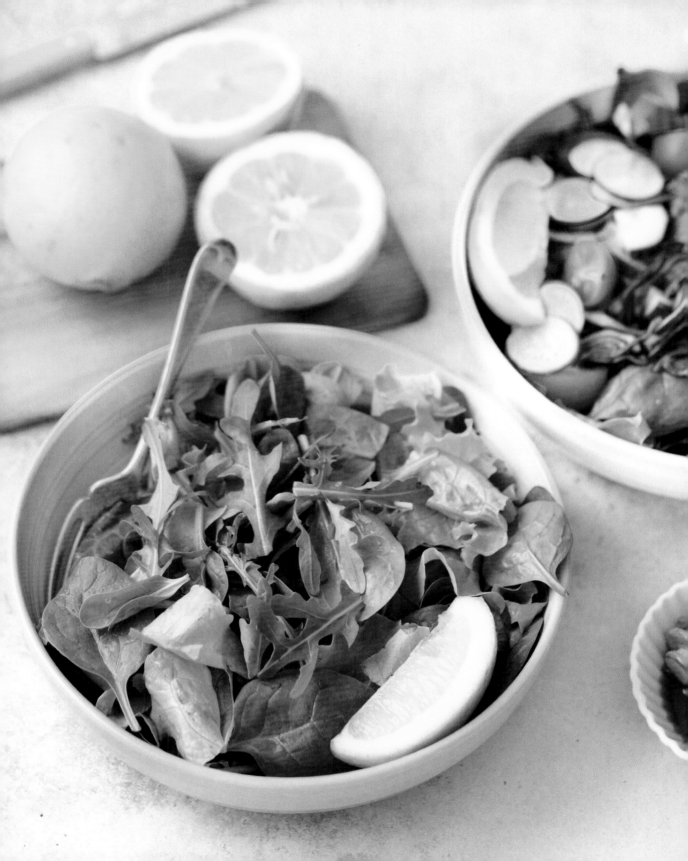

CAULIFLOWER SUSHI

Makes 2 servings

Raw cauliflower rice is a fun way to mimic the experience of white rice, with far more healing benefits. Pair the cauliflower rice with your vegetables, herbs, and fruits (such as mango, Maradol papaya, or orange) of choice—keeping the sushi fat-free—and roll them up in nori for a delicious and fun eating experience.

1 pound cauliflower florets

2 to 3 nori sheets

1 red pepper, thinly sliced

½ cucumber, cut into sticks

1 to 2 carrots, cut into sticks

1 cup thinly sliced red cabbage

1 to 2 tablespoons green onions, for garnish

Wasabi powder mixed with water, to serve (optional)

EXTRA DIPPING SAUCE

2 teaspoons pure maple syrup

2 tablespoons lime juice

¼ teaspoon cayenne

½ teaspoon grated ginger

Place the cauliflower florets into a food processor and pulse until a rice-like texture forms. Set aside.

Place one sheet of nori shiny side down on a cutting board. Scoop about 3/4 cup of cauliflower rice onto the end of the nori sheet closest to you and spread it into an even layer covering the bottom half of the nori. Arrange the desired vegetables and/or fruits in the middle of the cauliflower rice.

Carefully lift the nori from the bottom edge close to you and begin rolling it tightly toward the top. Just before finishing the roll, dip your finger in water and run it along the top edge of the sheet.

Using a sharp knife, slice each sushi roll into even pieces.

To make the dipping sauce, whisk together the maple syrup, lime juice, cayenne, and ginger.

Serve the sushi with the dipping sauce and wasabi if desired.

TIPS

- Instead of regular wasabi, look for a clean wasabi powder made of just wasabi powder or wasabi powder with horseradish. Mix the powder with a touch of water to create your own clean wasabi paste. If you're sensitive, keep in mind that wasabi is very spicy.

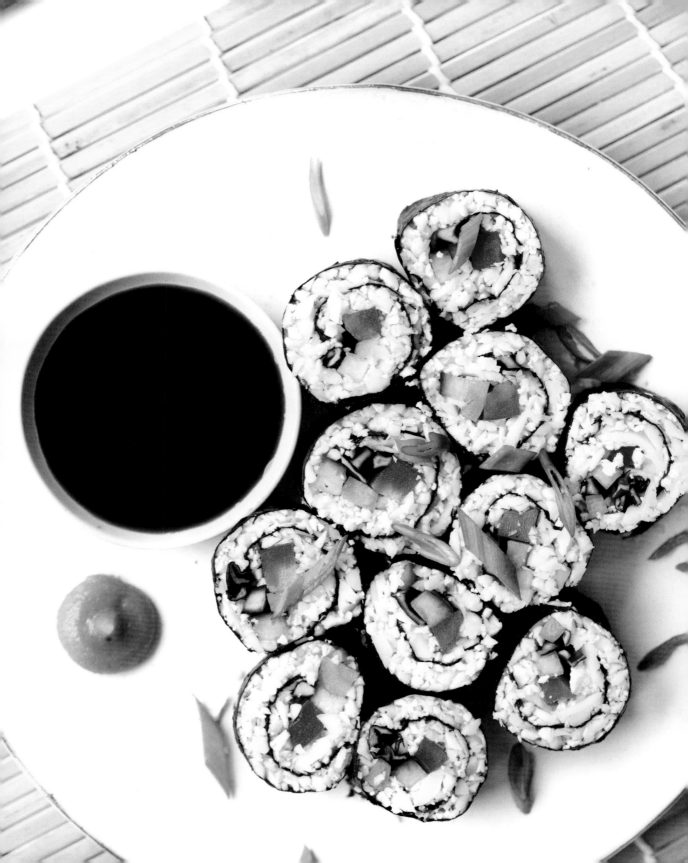

KALE SALAD

If you're used to eating kale salads with lots of avocado, oil, or dressings, you may be surprised at just how delicious this fat-free recipe is—it doesn't compromise on flavor, especially with the optional addition of garlic, chili pepper, and dates. If you normally avoid raw kale altogether because it seems fibrous, this is a fantastic recipe for you to try. Breaking up and mixing the ingredients in a food processor helps the flavors combine, and also makes the kale and other healing foods in this recipe easy to eat.

½ bunch kale, stems removed and roughly chopped

½ bunch green onions, roughly chopped

1 cucumber, roughly chopped

3 celery stalks, roughly chopped

2 large tomatoes, roughly chopped

¾ cup chopped asparagus

Juice of 1 to 2 oranges

1 garlic clove, finely minced (optional)

1 chili pepper, finely chopped (optional)

1 to 2 dates, finely chopped (optional)

Place the chopped kale and green onions in an even layer in the food processor and process at high speed until very finely chopped. Scrape down the sides as needed, and then remove and add to a large bowl.

Place the cucumber in the food processor and pulse until chopped, for about 3 seconds. Remove and add to the kale and green onions.

Place the celery in the food processor and pulse 1 to 2 times, until chopped. Add to the bowl.

Place the tomatoes in the food processor and pulse 1 to 2 times, until roughly chopped. Add to the bowl.

Add all the salad ingredients back to the food processor together with the chopped asparagus, orange juice, and additional options. Pulse 1 to 2 times, until evenly mixed.

Serve and enjoy.

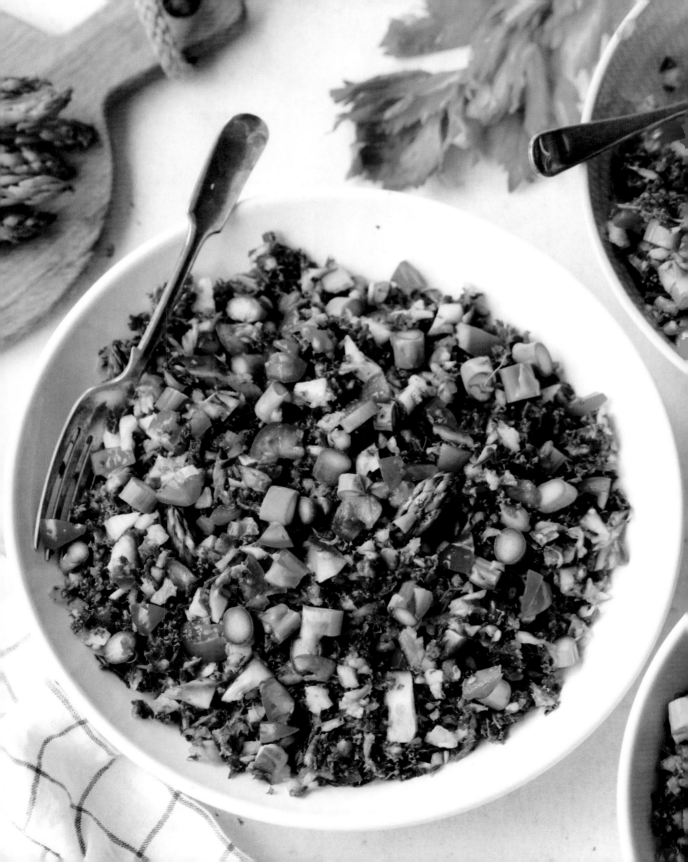

CAULIFLOWER AND GREENS BOWL

Makes 1 to 2 servings

This recipe only takes a few minutes to make and comes together easily. Enjoy it on its own in a bowl or scoop it into lettuce leaves and eat like tacos. Either way, it tastes delicious and is bursting with nutrients. Enjoy customizing the recipe to your tastes with the optional ingredients or other pure herbs and spices you love.

FOR THE CAULIFLOWER

1 medium-sized cauliflower, cut into florets

1 cup chopped green onions

1 cup chopped tomatoes

¼ cup tightly packed fresh cilantro, finely chopped

¾ cup chopped asparagus

½ teaspoon ginger powder (optional)

2 teaspoons dried basil (optional)

1 garlic clove, finely minced (optional)

½ to 1 teaspoon chili pepper flakes, to taste (optional)

1 teaspoon Atlantic dulse flakes, or more to taste (optional)

Juice from 2 medium-sized oranges or 2 dates, pitted

FOR THE SALAD BASE

8 cups loosely packed leafy greens of your choice (such as romaine, butter lettuce, spinach, and/or mâche, etc.), chopped

Juice from 1 orange or ½ lemon

Place the cauliflower florets in a food processor along with the dates (if using) and pulse until a rice-like texture forms. Place in a large bowl. Add the chopped green onions, tomatoes, cilantro, asparagus, and (if using) ginger powder, dried basil, garlic, chili pepper flakes, and dulse flakes plus the orange juice to the bowl. Mix well.

Divide the leafy greens between bowls and top with freshly squeezed orange juice. Top with the cauliflower mixture and serve.

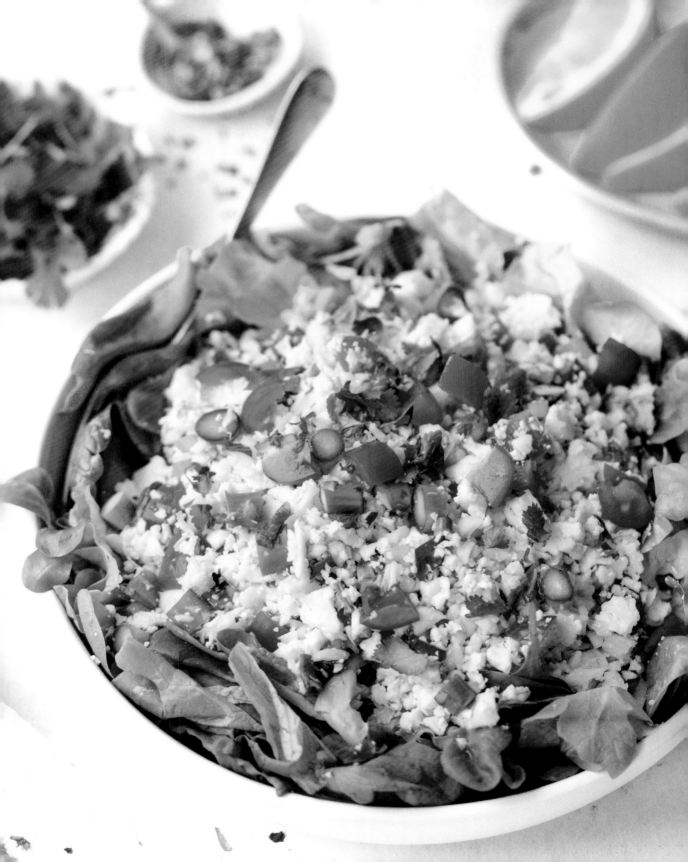

TOMATO, CUCUMBER, AND HERB SALAD

Makes 2 servings

Fresh herbs and thinly sliced cucumber and tomato make this simple recipe something special. Whether you use multicolored tomatoes or deep red varieties, the beauty of this recipe will come to life in front of you. While this salad is included as one of the dinner options for the Advanced Cleanse, you may just find yourself making it on a weekly basis long after the Cleanse is finished.

4 to 5 medium-sized tomatoes (any color), very thinly sliced

1 medium-sized cucumber, very thinly sliced

½ red onion, very thinly sliced

1 garlic clove, finely grated

1 cup chopped asparagus

1 cup loosely packed fresh basil, finely chopped

1 cup loosely packed fresh parsley, finely chopped

½ cup loosely packed fresh dill, finely chopped

1 tablespoon lemon juice

3 tablespoons orange juice

1 teaspoon Atlantic dulse flakes, more to taste (optional)

FOR THE SALAD BASE

6 cups loosely packed leafy greens (such as romaine, butter lettuce, spinach, and/or mâche)

2 tablespoons freshly squeezed orange or lemon juice

Place the tomatoes, cucumber, onion, garlic, asparagus, and herbs in a medium-sized bowl. Toss until evenly mixed. Add the lemon juice, orange juice, and dulse flakes. Toss again and set aside. Place the leafy greens of your choice in a large bowl and top with freshly squeezed orange or lemon juice. Top with the cucumber and tomato mixture. Serve immediately or keep in the fridge until needed.

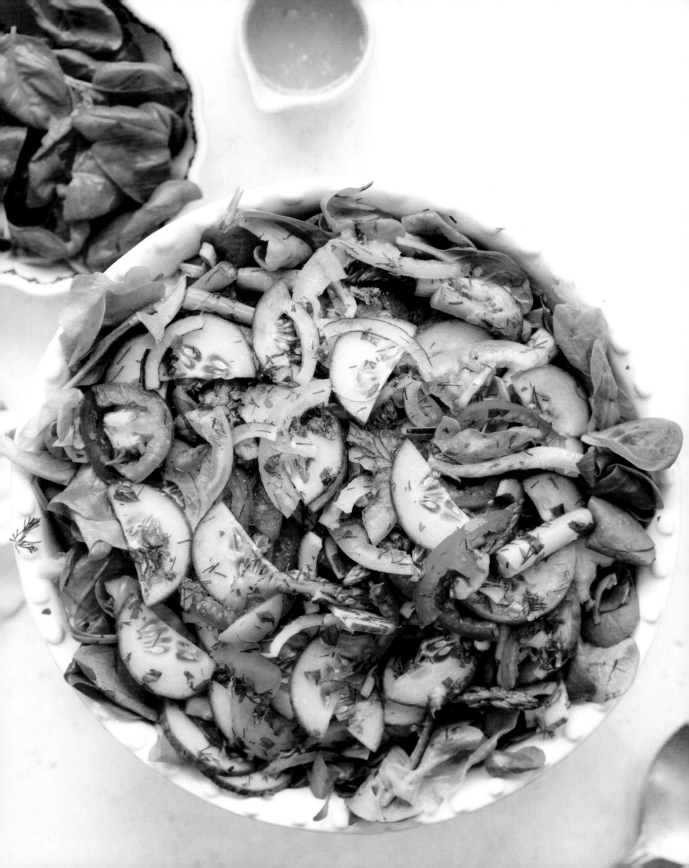

LEAFY GREEN NORI ROLLS

Makes 1 to 2 servings

These nori rolls give you a fun and easy way to consume a large volume of leafy greens without having to crunch through a big bowl of salad with a fork. The leafy greens are the focus of this recipe for a reason. While it's fun to add other ingredients into nori rolls, for the purpose of the Advanced Cleanse dinners, it's important to stick closely to the quantity of leafy greens indicated in the recipe.

4 sheets of nori

6 cups loosely packed leafy greens (such as romaine, butter lettuce, arugula, and spinach, etc.)

1 medium-sized tomato, cut into 4-inch strips

½ medium-sized cucumber, cut into 4-inch strips

8 spears asparagus (or 4 very large spears), ends trimmed

2 scallions, cut into 4-inch strips or ¼ sweet onion, thinly sliced (optional)

¼ cup sprouts

4 strips of Atlantic dulse or 2 to 3 teaspoons Atlantic dulse flakes (optional)

¼ cup fresh orange or lemon juice

Place a nori sheet shiny side down on a chopping board with the long edge close to you. Arrange the leafy greens, prepared vegetables, sprouts, and dulse (if using) on one end of the sheet. Brush orange or lemon juice across the other end of the sheet, and then roll up tightly. Cut in half and serve immediately.

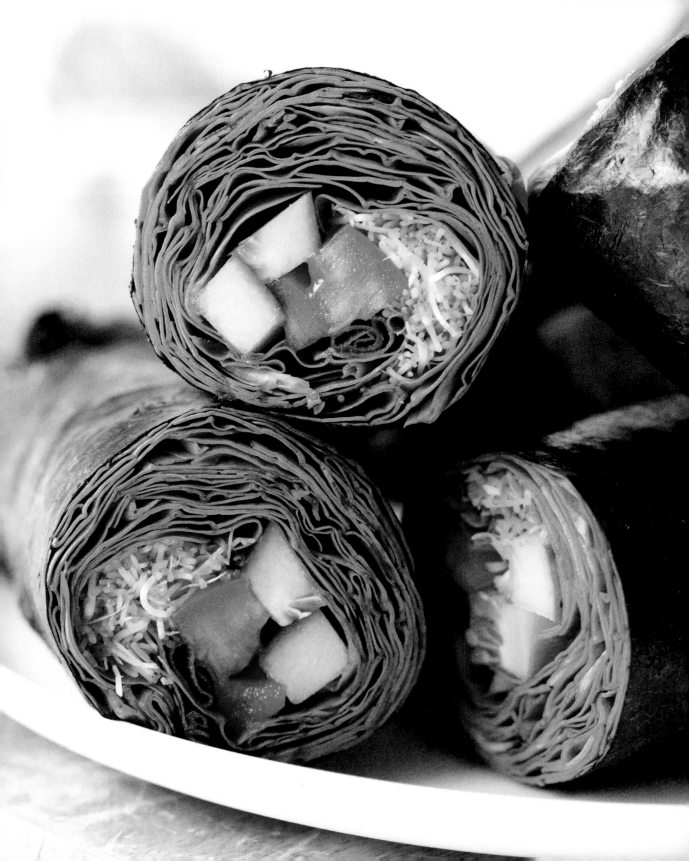

ROASTED EGGPLANT DIP WITH VEGETABLE CRUDITÉS

Makes 2 servings

This creamy, comforting dip is the perfect fat-free accompaniment to vegetable crudités. Serve yourself a platter of your favorite vegetables and dip to your heart's content! This recipe is also a wonderful choice for serving to friends and family at social gatherings.

2 medium-sized eggplants

4 whole garlic cloves

1 teaspoon paprika

½ teaspoon ground cumin

1½ tablespoons lemon juice

½ teaspoon onion powder

¼ medjool date

¼ cup fresh parsley or cilantro, tightly packed

VEGETABLE CRUDITÉS

2 carrots, cut into sticks

½ cucumber, cut into wedges

3 celery stalks, cut into sticks

1 red pepper, cut into wedges

Preheat oven to 400°F/200C°.

Slice the eggplants in half and pierce with a fork. Place them on a baking tray together with the garlic cloves and roast for 40 to 45 minutes, until the eggplant is very tender throughout. Remove from the oven and cool slightly.

Once the eggplant and garlic are cool enough to handle, scoop out the inside of the eggplant into a food processor or blender, and discard the skins. Peel the roasted garlic cloves and add them to the blender together with the paprika, ground cumin, lemon juice, onion powder, and date. Pulse the mixture a few times until the dip is smooth yet chunky.

Transfer to serving bowls and top with fresh parsley or cilantro. Serve with vegetable crudités.

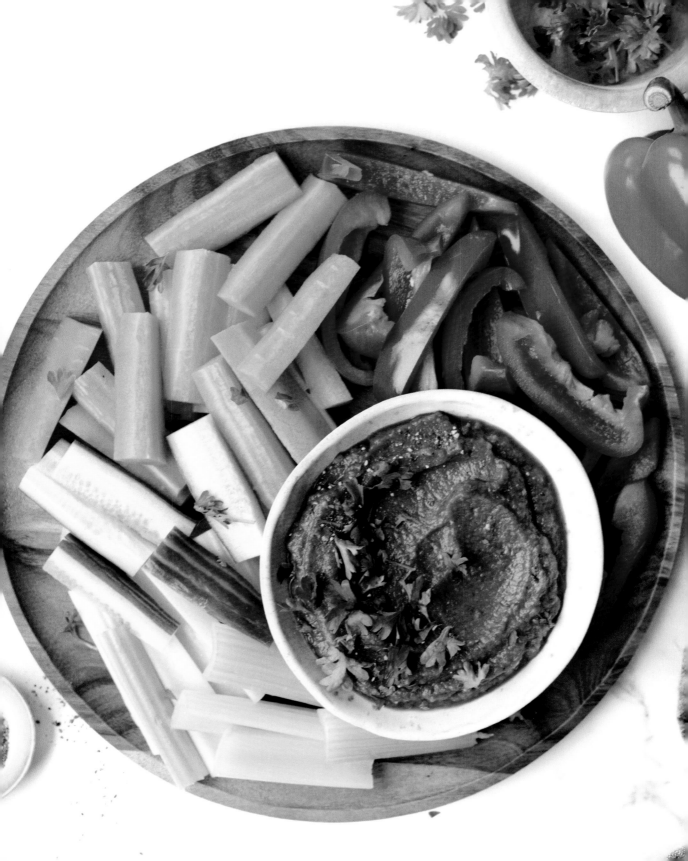

LEMON ASPARAGUS WITH ROASTED TOMATO AND SPINACH SALAD

Makes 1 to 2 servings

This recipe is a beautiful demonstration of how a simple selection of foods can come together to make a dish that's both healing and flavorful. Roasted cherry tomatoes, fragrant basil, subtly earthy asparagus, and bright lemon zest bring depth to the simplicity of this meal.

FOR THE SALAD

3 cups cherry or plum tomatoes

½ teaspoon dried thyme

4 cups spinach, loosely packed

1 cup loosely packed basil, roughly chopped

1 tablespoon fresh lemon juice

FOR THE ASPARAGUS

1 pound asparagus, ends trimmed

2 tablespoons lemon juice

½ teaspoon lemon zest

Preheat oven to 400°F/200°C. Line a baking dish with parchment paper.

Place the tomatoes in the baking dish and sprinkle with dried thyme. Roast in the oven for 15 to 20 minutes, until bursting. Set aside.

While the tomatoes are roasting, add 3 inches of water to a medium-sized pot, bring it to a boil, and add a steaming basket. Place the asparagus in the basket, cover, and steam for 6 to 9 minutes, depending on the thickness of the asparagus, until tender.

Remove and place in a bowl. Add the lemon juice and zest and toss to coat. Set aside.

To make the salad, combine the spinach and basil in a mixing bowl. Add the lemon juice. Toss to coat and divide between bowls.

Top the salad with the roasted cherry tomatoes and steamed asparagus. Serve immediately.

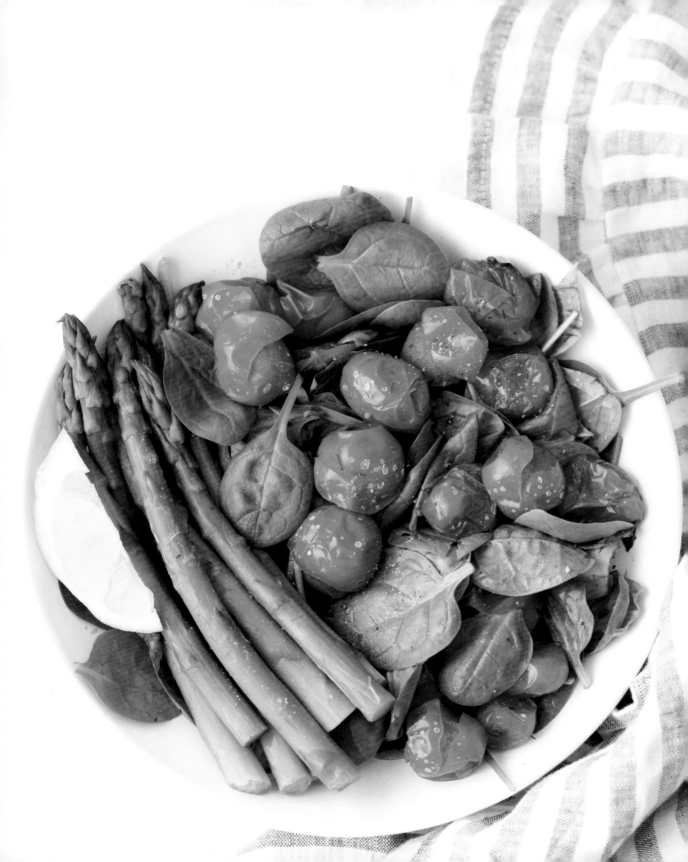

STEAMED ASPARAGUS

Makes 1 to 2 servings

The simple preparation for this healing food is one you can use over and over again. Steamed (or raw) asparagus is an incredible food for cleansing. Thanks to its ability to detoxify and support the liver's healing, asparagus is a key part of the Original 3:6:9 Cleanse. It brings order to a chaotic, sick liver and instantly strengthens the liver's immune system to help defend the rest of your body.

1 pound asparagus, ends trimmed

Add 3 inches of water to a medium-sized pot, bring it to a boil, and add a steaming basket. Place the asparagus in the basket, cover, and steam for 6 to 9 minutes, depending on the thickness of the asparagus, until tender.

Remove and serve.

TIPS

- If fresh asparagus isn't available, find it in the frozen food aisle and stock up so that you'll have plenty on hand. Don't worry if you can only find conventional; it's so beneficial to the liver that it outweighs any downsides to eating nonorganic asparagus. You can either steam it just before your meal or prepare it ahead of time and enjoy your asparagus cold or reheated (without butter or oil).

- Asparagus can also be eaten raw instead of steamed if you prefer. Simply wash, trim, and munch away. You may find that by the end of the 3:6:9 Cleanse, you have more appreciation for this rejuvenating, fountain-of-youth vegetable than ever before!

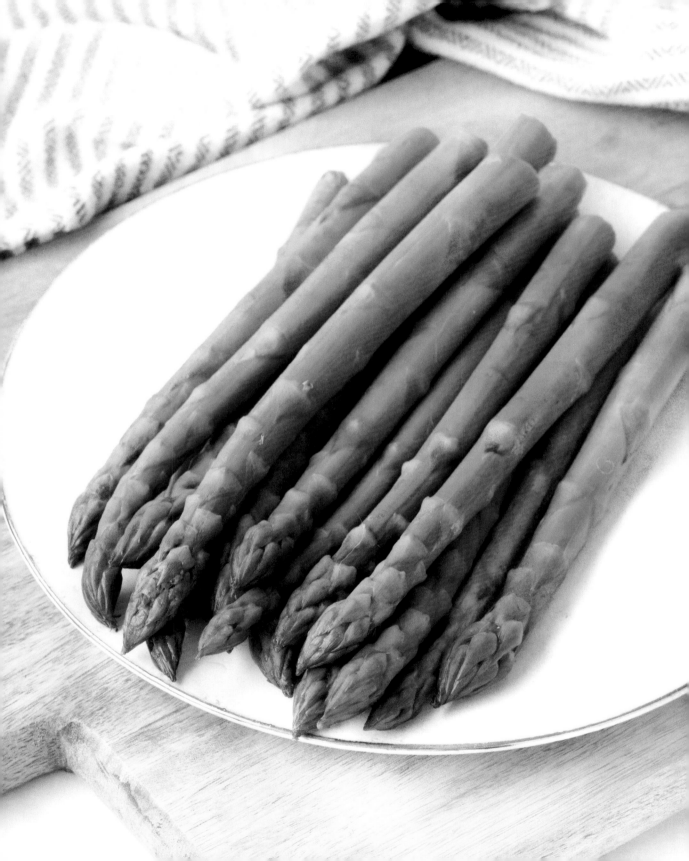

STEAMED BRUSSELS SPROUTS

Makes 1 to 2 servings

Like asparagus, brussels sprouts are key to the Original 3:6:9 Cleanse. Their unique sulfur has the ability to loosen hardened prison cells of inherited troublemaker toxins in the liver, cling to the poisons, and safely escort them out of the body so you can get relief from your symptoms and conditions. Whether or not simple steamed brussels sprouts are already a favorite food, over time you may find you develop more of a taste for these gems and start to seek them out for their incredible healing and satiating properties.

1 pound brussels sprouts, ends trimmed

Rinse the brussels sprouts in cold water. Remove any brown leaves and, with a sharp knife, cut away the end (just the tip) of each sprout and discard. Slice in half.

Add 3 inches of water to a medium-sized pot, bring it to a boil, and add a steaming basket. Place the brussels sprouts in the basket, cover, and steam for 6 to 8 minutes or more, depending on the size, until tender.

Remove and serve.

TIPS

- As with asparagus, if fresh brussels sprouts aren't available, find them in the frozen food aisle and stock up so that you'll have plenty on hand. Don't worry if you can only find conventional; they're so beneficial to the liver that it outweighs any downsides to eating nonorganic brussels sprouts. You can either steam the vegetable just before your meal or prepare it ahead of time and enjoy your brussels sprouts cold or reheated (without butter or oil).

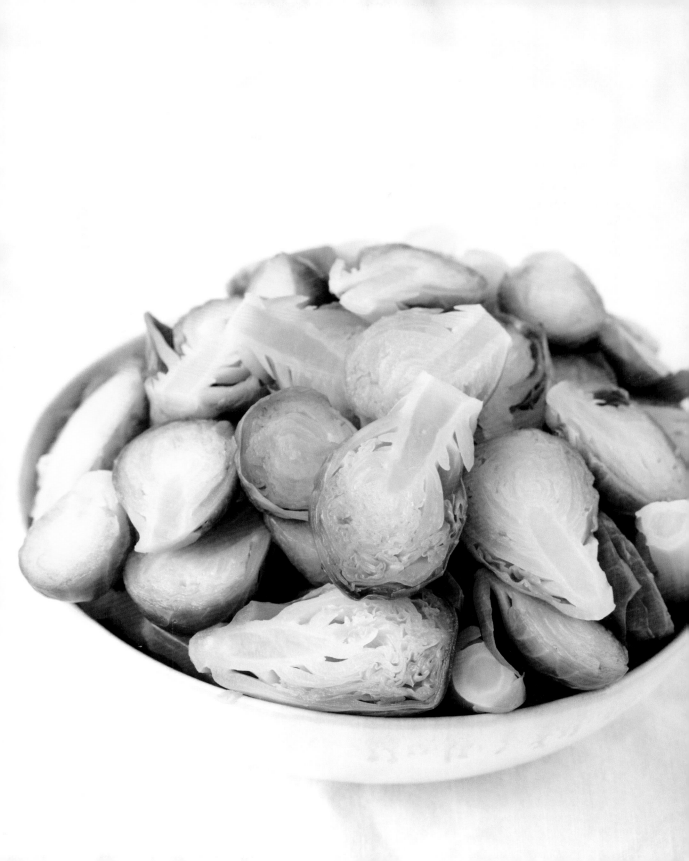

STEAMED ZUCCHINI/SUMMER SQUASH

Makes 1 to 2 servings

Simple steamed zucchini or summer squash is an important feature of the Original 3:6:9 Cleanse's initial three days. Plus, if you are unable to access or eat steamed asparagus or brussels sprouts when the cleanse calls for them, steamed zucchini and summer squash make wonderful substitutes. They gently purge the liver while also pushing pathogens out of the intestinal walls.

1 medium-sized zucchini, sliced

1 medium-sized summer squash, sliced

Add 3 inches of water to a medium-sized pot, bring it to a boil, and add a steaming basket. Place the sliced zucchini and summer squash in the basket, cover, and steam for 6 to 8 minutes, depending on the size, until tender. Remove and serve.

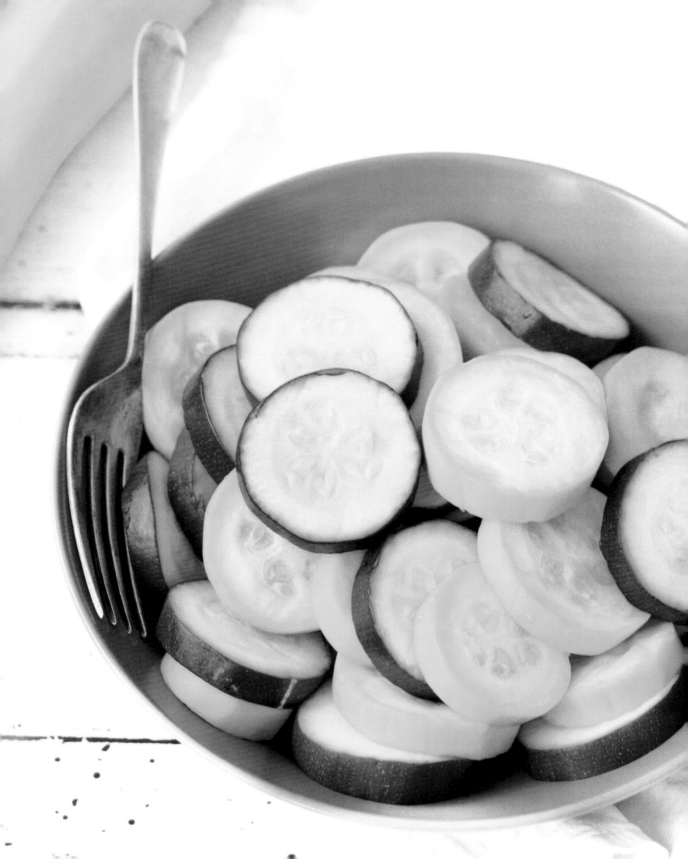

ROASTED RED PEPPER AND TOMATO SOUP

Makes 2 to 3 servings

This vibrant soup is as rich in flavor as it is in color, and it's very straightforward to make. Throw everything in to roast and then simply blend it into this inviting soup. This is a great recipe to make fresh or in advance for leftovers—it tastes fantastic either way.

1 pound roughly chopped red bell peppers

1 pound plum tomatoes

1 cup diced onion

3 garlic cloves, roughly chopped

½ cup chopped celery

1 teaspoon dried thyme

½ teaspoon red pepper flakes (optional)

1½ cups water or Liver Rescue Broth (recipe on page 394)

Fresh basil, to serve

Preheat oven to 400°F/200°C. Line a baking dish with parchment paper. Add the chopped peppers, tomatoes, diced onion, garlic, celery, thyme, and red pepper flakes (if desired) to the baking dish. Mix well. Place in the oven and roast for 20 to 25 minutes, until browned and tender.

Remove from the oven and add to a blender together with the water or Liver Rescue Broth. Blend until smooth. Pour into a pot and heat until simmering. Ladle into soup bowls and garnish with fresh basil. Serve immediately.

TIPS

- When choosing between water and Liver Rescue Broth for the ingredients, keep in mind that the broth will produce a richer flavor. Store-bought vegetable stock isn't called for because it's very difficult to find a variety that's free from oil, salt, natural flavors, and/or other additives. For convenience, make a batch of Liver Rescue Broth in advance and freeze it (consider ice cube trays for easy thawing) so you have it on hand for recipes like these.

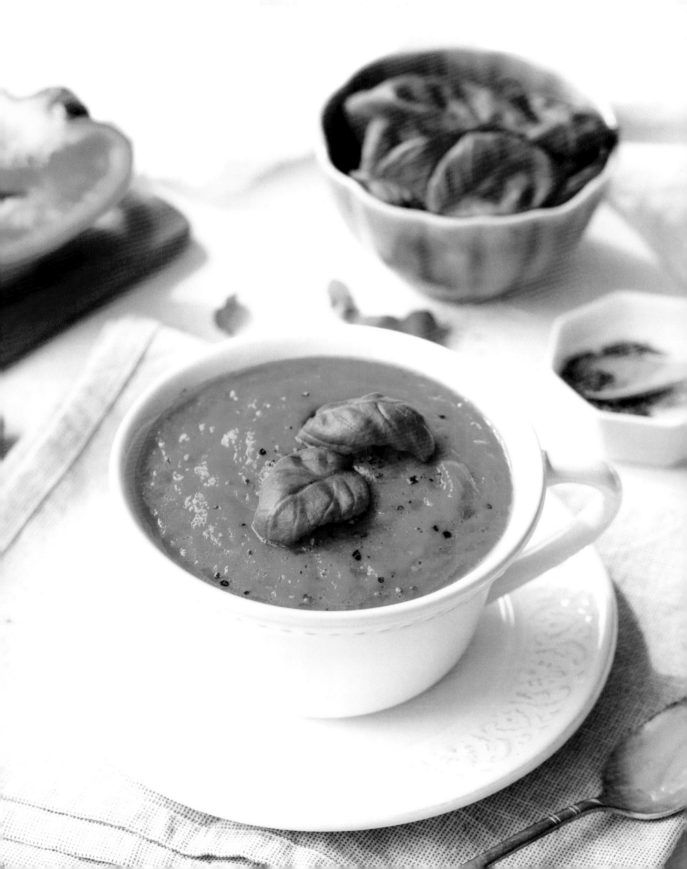

STEAMED BRUSSELS SPROUTS AND ASPARAGUS IN MAPLE CAYENNE SAUCE

Makes 1 to 2 servings

There are endless ways you can flavor and prepare brussels sprouts and asparagus, so you can enjoy variety while still getting enough of these incredible healing foods during the 3:6:9 Cleanse. Topping them with a delicious sauce is often all it takes to ignite a new love for these vegetables. This simple Maple Cayenne Sauce is a wonderful example of how regular steamed vegetables can be easily transformed into something quite special.

1 pound brussels sprouts, ends trimmed and halved

1 pound asparagus, ends trimmed and cut into 2-inch pieces

SAUCE

1 tablespoon pure maple syrup

½ to 1 teaspoon cayenne

1 garlic clove, finely grated

1 tablespoon fresh lemon juice (optional)

Add 3 inches of water to a medium-sized pot, bring it to a boil, and add a steaming basket. Place the brussels sprouts and asparagus in the basket, cover, and steam for 5 to 10 minutes, until tender. Remove and place in a bowl.

Make the sauce by whisking together the maple syrup, cayenne, grated garlic, and lemon juice, if desired. Pour on top of the steamed asparagus and brussels sprouts. Mix until coated. Divide between bowls and serve.

TIPS

- If fresh brussels sprouts and asparagus aren't available or you don't have time to prep them, substitute frozen in this recipe.

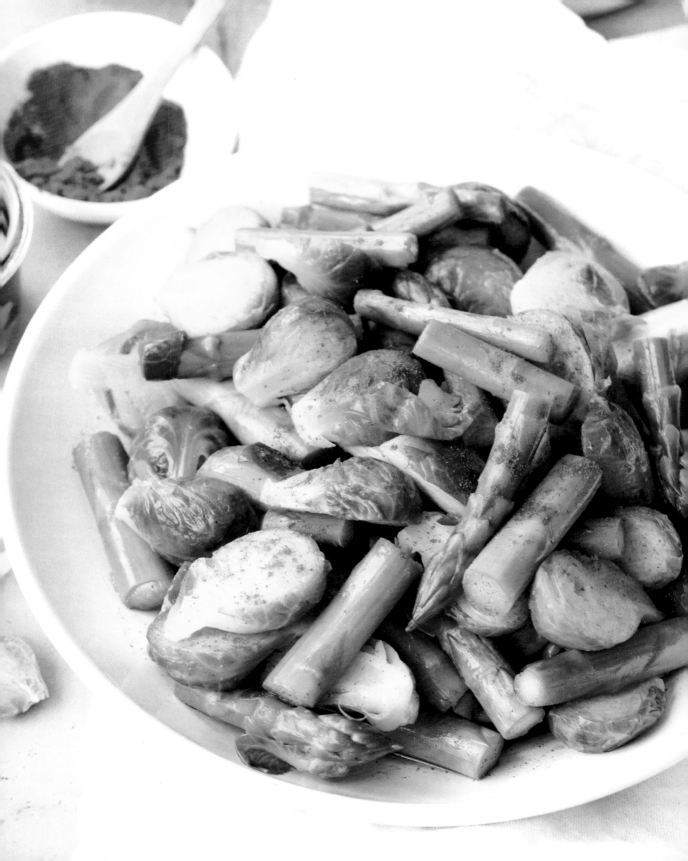

STEAMED BUTTERNUT SQUASH NOODLES

Makes 1 to 2 servings

This simple preparation of butternut squash gives you a fun way to enjoy this healing fruit that might be new to you—as noodles! Whether you serve them with simple additions and let their flavor speak for itself, or you top your noodles with a fresh tomato salsa, they are delicious and a delight to eat.

1 large butternut squash (about 4½ pounds), yields about 6 cups of noodles

2 tablespoons finely chopped parsley

1½ garlic cloves, finely grated

2 teaspoons fresh lemon juice

To prepare the noodles, chop off the top stem and the bulbous end of the squash, leaving just the straight part in the middle, which doesn't usually contain seeds. Peel off the skin using a sharp knife or vegetable peeler and chop the squash section into quarters, so it's easier to handle. Spiralize the squash to create thick noodles.

Add 3 inches of water to a medium-sized pot, bring it to a boil, and add a steaming basket. Place the butternut squash noodles in the basket, cover, and steam for 3 to 5 minutes until tender. Do not overcook, as they get soft very quickly.

Place in a bowl and add the parsley, garlic, and lemon juice. Mix well and serve immediately.

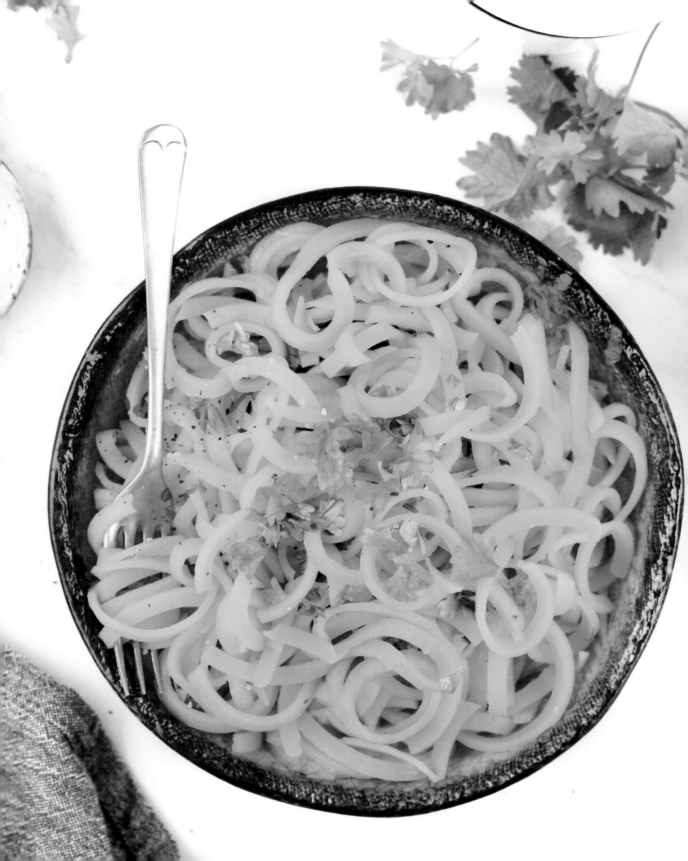

CHILI GARLIC BRUSSELS SPROUTS AND ASPARAGUS

If you're a lover of garlic, onion, and chili pepper, this might be your favorite way to enjoy brussels sprouts and asparagus. It only takes a few minutes to prepare this sauce that provides an explosion of flavor to a simple steamed dish. You'll also receive the many healing benefits of the raw garlic, onion, chili, lime juice, and honey.

1 pound brussels sprouts, ends trimmed and halved

1 pound asparagus, ends trimmed and chopped

1 tablespoon finely chopped fresh red chili pepper

1 tablespoon minced garlic

2 tablespoons finely chopped green onion

3 tablespoons lime juice

1½ teaspoons raw honey

Add 3 inches of water to a medium-sized pot, bring it to a boil, and add a steaming basket. Place the brussels sprouts and asparagus in the basket, cover, and steam for 5 to 10 minutes, until tender. Remove and place in a bowl.

Add the chopped chili, garlic, green onion, lime juice, and raw honey. Mix until coated. Divide between bowls and serve.

TIPS

- If fresh brussels sprouts and asparagus aren't available or you don't have time to prep them, substitute frozen in this recipe.

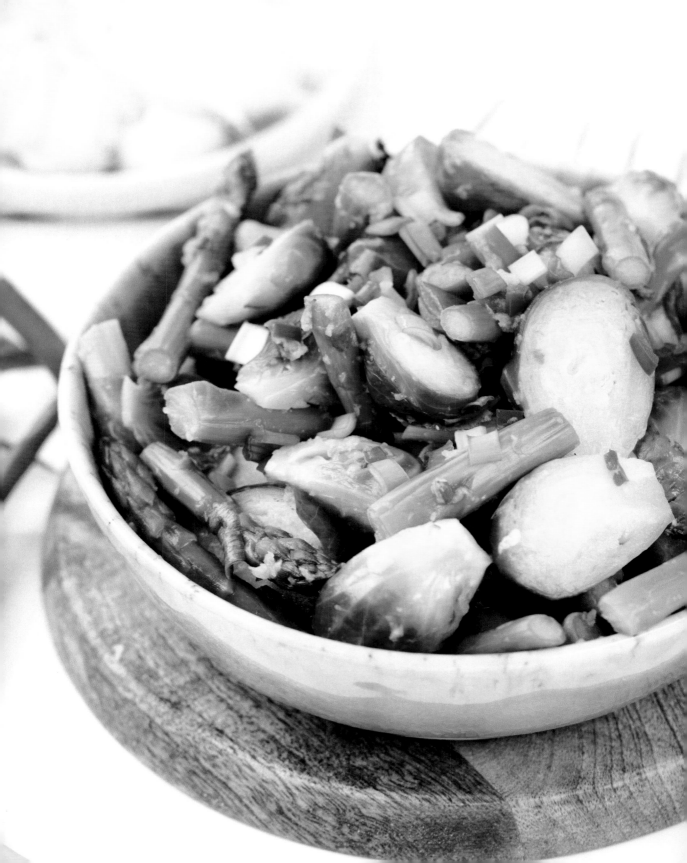

ZUCCHINI BASIL SOUP

Makes 2 servings

This pretty soup is one you may find yourself turning to over and over again. The zucchini lends a depth and creaminess, while the basil brings a brightness that makes it unique and special.

1 cup diced onion

3 garlic cloves, minced

3 medium-sized zucchini, chopped (about 2 pounds)

2½ cups water or Liver Rescue Broth (recipe on page 394)

1 teaspoon dried thyme

1 tablespoon lemon juice

1½ cups fresh basil, plus more to serve

Place a large ceramic nonstick pot on medium-high heat and add the onion and garlic. Cook for 3 to 5 minutes, until the onion is translucent, adding a spoonful of water if needed.

Add the chopped zucchini and cook for a further 5 minutes, until the zucchini begins to soften.

Add the water or Liver Rescue Broth, dried thyme, and lemon juice. Bring to a simmer and cook for 10 to 15 minutes, until the zucchini is very tender.

Ladle the soup into a blender, add the basil, and blend until smooth (you may need to do this in batches). Alternatively, you can use an immersion blender.

Pour the soup back in the pot and bring to a simmer. Taste and adjust seasoning. Divide between bowls and serve.

TIPS

- When choosing between water and Liver Rescue Broth for the ingredients, keep in mind that the broth will produce a richer flavor. Store-bought vegetable stock isn't called for because it's very difficult to find a variety that's free from oil, salt, natural flavors, and/or other additives. For convenience, make a batch of Liver Rescue Broth in advance and freeze it (consider ice cube trays for easy thawing) so you have it on hand for recipes like these.

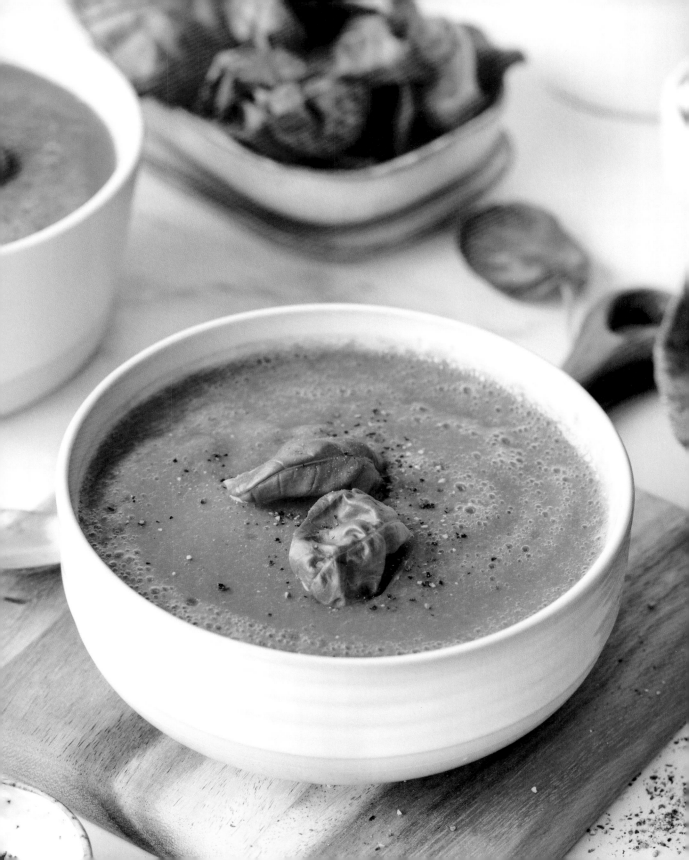

LEMON GARLIC STEAMED BRUSSELS SPROUTS

Makes 1 to 2 servings

Fresh garlic and lemon elevate the simple steamed brussels sprouts in this recipe. This is a wonderful dish to serve alongside a salad or other vegetable dish during or after the 3:6:9 Cleanse.

1 pound brussels sprouts, ends trimmed and cut in half
2 garlic cloves, finely grated
1 teaspoon lemon zest
2 tablespoons lemon juice

Add 3 inches of water to a medium-sized pot, bring it to a boil, and add a steaming basket. Place the brussels sprouts in the basket, cover, and steam for 6 to 8 minutes or more, depending on the size, until tender. Remove and place in a bowl.

Add the grated garlic, lemon zest, and lemon juice to the steamed brussels sprouts. Mix until coated. Divide between bowls and serve.

TIPS

- If fresh brussels sprouts aren't available or you don't have time to prep them, substitute frozen in this recipe.

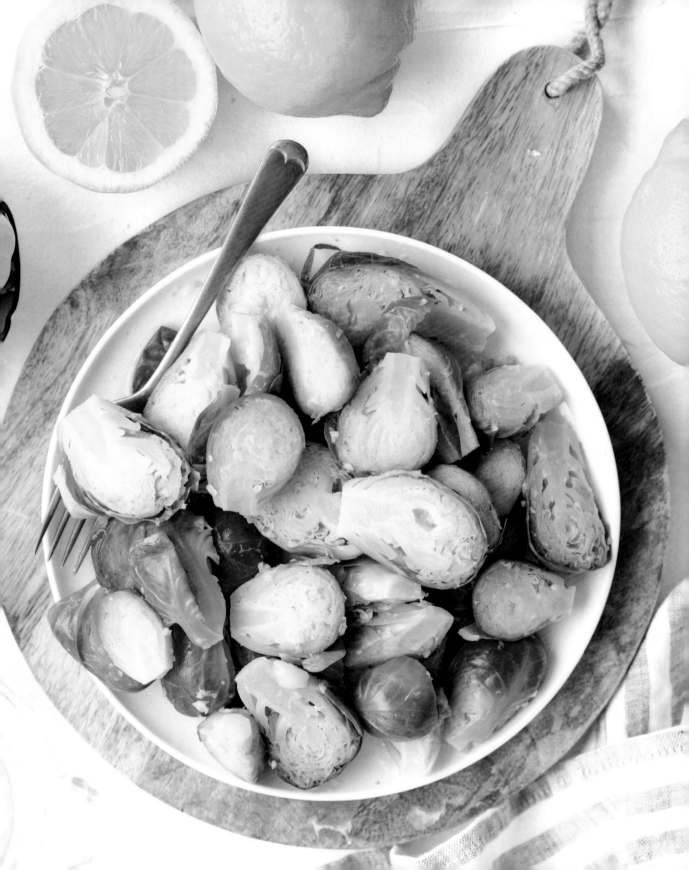

CURRIED CAULIFLOWER AND PEAS

The vibrant color, flavor, and fragrance of curry make this dish a standout. As a bonus, it comes together quickly and easily; you'll be sitting down to enjoy a beautiful meal in no time! Enjoy this wonderful Curried Cauliflower and Peas alone or with a salad such as Leafy Green Salad.

1 medium-sized head of cauliflower, cut into florets

¾ cup green peas, fresh or frozen

½ cup chopped green onions

2 garlic cloves, minced

1 teaspoon grated fresh ginger

3 teaspoons curry powder

½ teaspoon ground turmeric

½ teaspoon ground cumin

½ teaspoon ground coriander

¼ teaspoon chili powder (optional)

¼ cup tightly packed fresh cilantro, roughly chopped for garnish

Add 3 inches of water to a medium-sized pot, bring it to a boil, and add a steaming basket. Place the cauliflower and peas in the basket, cover, and steam for 3 to 4 minutes, until just tender. Remove from heat.

Place a large ceramic nonstick skillet on medium-high heat and add the green onions, garlic, and ginger. Cook for 2 to 3 minutes, adding a spoonful of water if needed, until the green onion begins to soften.

Lower the heat and add the curry powder, turmeric, ground cumin, ground coriander, and chili powder (if using). Cook for 2 to 3 minutes. If the mixture starts sticking to the pan or burning, add a bit of water.

Add the steamed cauliflower, peas, and ½ cup water. Stir until well mixed and coated. When all the water has evaporated and the peas are soft, remove from heat. Serve garnished with fresh cilantro.

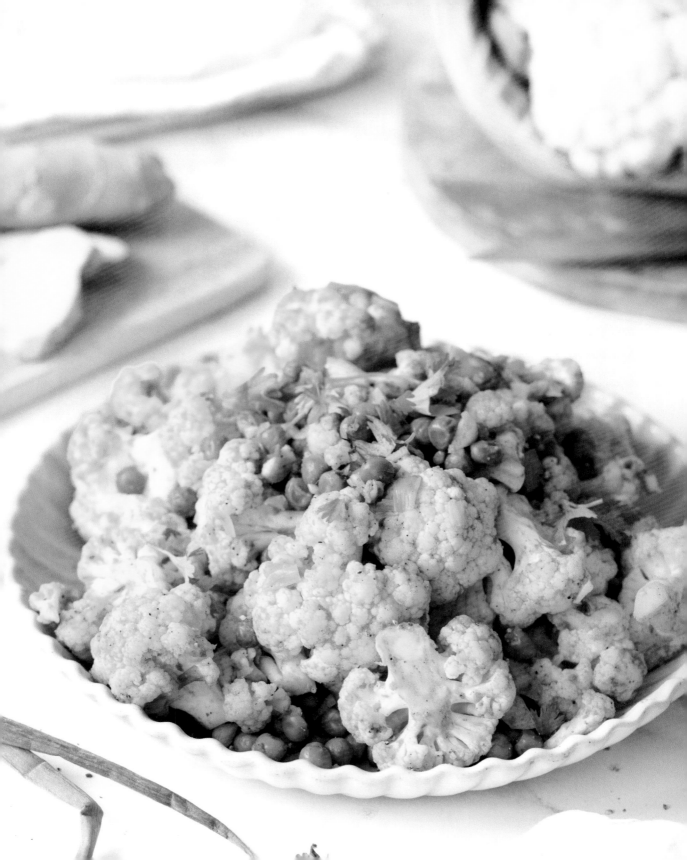

"CHEDDAR" BROCCOLI SOUP

Makes 2 to 3 servings

This soup is oh so creamy and dreamy. The potatoes add a natural creaminess to the soup without the use of cream, butter, or milk, and the broccoli adds some texture. Serve yourself up a big bowl of this soup when you're looking for a comforting, grounding meal. Pair it with Leafy Green Salad or Liver Rescue Salad if you wish.

3 cups diced potatoes

1 cup diced carrot

1½ teaspoons turmeric

2 teaspoons garlic powder

1 tablespoon onion powder

1 teaspoon paprika

2½ tablespoons fresh lemon juice

1 cup water or Liver Rescue Broth (recipe on page 394)

1 medium-sized head broccoli, chopped into bite-sized pieces (yields about 4 cups)

Add 3 inches of water to a medium-sized pot, bring it to a boil, and add a steaming basket. Place the potatoes and carrots in the basket, cover, and steam for 8 to 12 minutes, until soft.

When they're ready, remove the potatoes and carrots and place them in a blender together with the turmeric, garlic powder, onion powder, paprika, lemon juice, and water or Liver Rescue Broth. Blend until very smooth. Pour into a pot and bring to a simmer.

To make the broccoli, steam it for 5 to 10 minutes, until tender yet not mushy; you want the broccoli to hold up well in the soup. Stir it into the soup. Divide the soup between bowls and serve.

TIPS

- If you don't like broccoli, you can use cauliflower or asparagus.

- When choosing between water and Liver Rescue Broth for the ingredients, keep in mind that the broth will produce a richer flavor. Store-bought vegetable stock isn't called for because it's very difficult to find a variety that's free from oil, salt, natural flavors, and/or other additives. For convenience, make a batch of Liver Rescue Broth in advance and freeze it (consider ice cube trays for easy thawing) so you have it on hand for recipes like these.

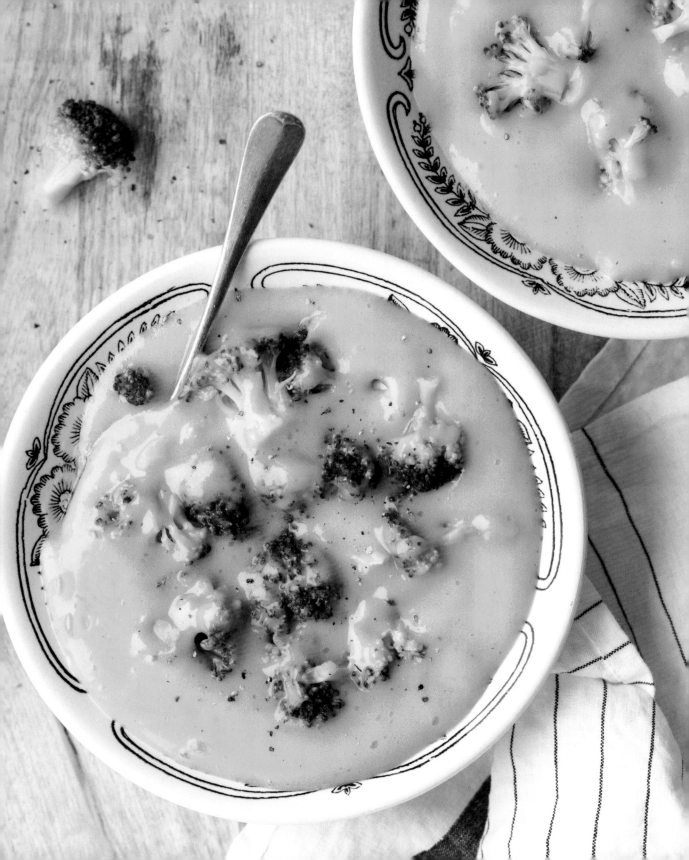

BRUSSELS SPROUT VEGETABLE SOUP

Makes 2 to 3 servings

If you like chunky vegetable soups in fragrant, delicate broth, this is the soup for you. It's light, delicious, and packed full of nutrients. Enjoy as much of this soup as you like and store the rest in the fridge or freezer for another day.

1 cup chopped onions

2 celery stalks, sliced

½ cup chopped carrot

4 garlic cloves, minced

1 teaspoon grated or minced ginger

1 cup chopped tomato

1 teaspoon dried thyme

1 teaspoon dried oregano

1 teaspoon lemon juice; more to taste

6 cups water or Liver Rescue Broth (recipe on page 394)

1 cup chopped cauliflower

3 cups thinly sliced brussels sprouts

1 tablespoon chopped fresh parsley

Place a large ceramic nonstick pot on medium-high heat. Add the onion and cook for 3 to 5 minutes, until soft, adding a spoonful of water if needed. Add the celery, carrots, garlic, and ginger and cook for another 2 to 3 minutes.

Add the tomato, thyme, oregano, lemon juice, and water or Liver Rescue Broth. Stir well and bring it to a boil. Lower the heat and simmer for 15 minutes, until the carrots and celery are almost done.

Stir in the cauliflower and brussels sprouts. Cook for a further 3 to 5 minutes, soft, adding a spoonful of water if needed. Ladle into serving bowls, top with fresh parsley, and serve.

TIPS

- You're also welcome to blend this soup using the final instructions from the next recipe, Asparagus Soup.

- When choosing between water and Liver Rescue Broth for the ingredients, keep in mind that the broth will produce a richer flavor. Store-bought vegetable stock isn't called for because it's very difficult to find a variety that's free from oil, salt, natural flavors, and/or other additives. For convenience, make a batch of Liver Rescue Broth in advance and freeze it (consider ice cube trays for easy thawing) so you have it on hand for recipes like these.

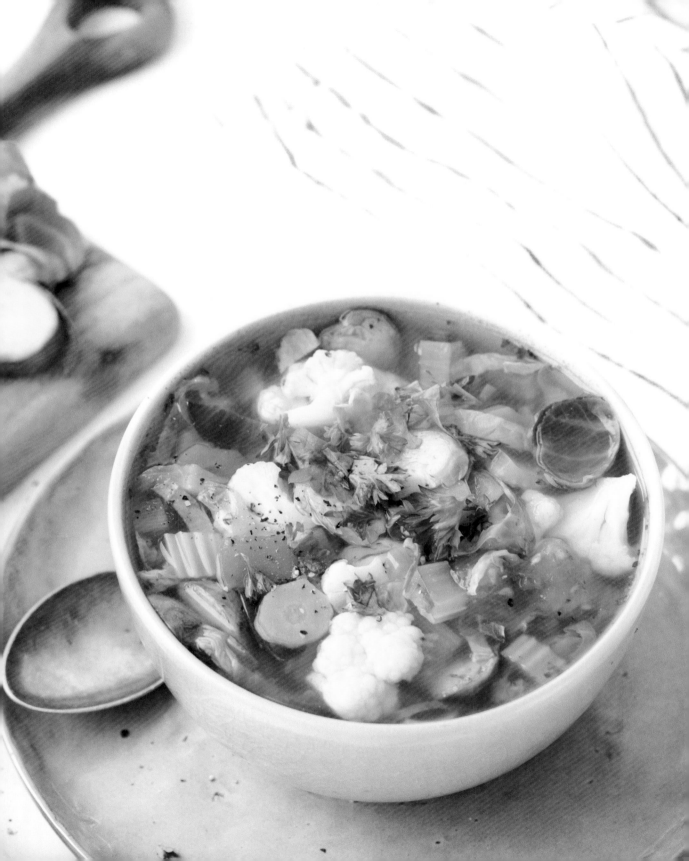

ASPARAGUS SOUP

Makes 2 servings

If you're looking for more ways to enjoy asparagus, try this nourishing Asparagus Soup. This recipe lets asparagus speak for itself, while offering accents of lemon and herbs to bring out its natural flavor. It's a lovely, light choice all on its own, served alongside a flavorful salad, or alongside another dish of your choice after the 3:6:9 Cleanse.

1 cup chopped onions
or leeks

3 garlic cloves, minced

2 pounds asparagus, ends
trimmed and chopped

3 cups water or Liver Rescue
Broth (recipe on page 394)

1 teaspoon dried thyme
or basil

1 tablespoon lemon juice

½ teaspoon lemon zest

Asparagus ribbons, for
garnish (optional)

Place a large ceramic nonstick pot on medium-high heat and add the onion and garlic. Cook for 3 to 5 minutes, until the onion is translucent, adding a spoonful of water if needed. Add the chopped asparagus and cook for a further 3 minutes, until the asparagus begins to soften.

Add the water or Liver Rescue Broth, dried thyme, lemon juice, and lemon zest. Bring to a simmer and cook for 10 to 15 minutes, until the asparagus is very tender.

Ladle the soup into a blender and blend until smooth, letting steam escape as needed (you might need to do this in batches). Alternatively, you can use an immersion blender for this.

Pour the soup back in the pot and bring to simmer. Taste and adjust seasoning. Divide between bowls. If desired, use a vegetable peeler to create asparagus ribbons as garnish. Serve immediately.

TIPS

- If you have this soup on Day 9 of the Simplified 3:6:9 Cleanse, skip the garnish of asparagus ribbons and just enjoy the blended soup.

- When choosing between water and Liver Rescue Broth for the ingredients, keep in mind that the broth will produce a richer flavor. Store-bought vegetable stock isn't called for because it's very difficult to find a variety that's free from oil, salt, natural flavors, and/or other additives. For convenience, make a batch of Liver Rescue Broth in advance and freeze it (consider ice cube trays for easy thawing) so you have it on hand for recipes like these.

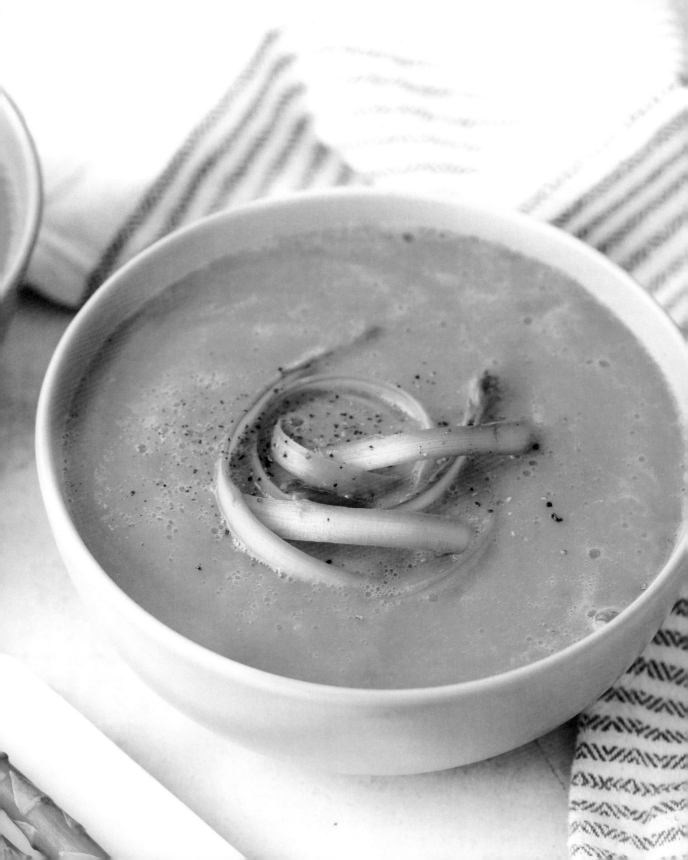

LIVER RESCUE BROTH

This broth is warming liquid gold. It's also ideal to make ahead and then freeze (try ice cube trays) so you always have bursts of flavor on hand to add to other recipes.

1 bunch celery, diced

6 carrots, diced

1 winter squash (such as butternut), cubed

2 yellow onions, diced

1 inch ginger root, peeled and minced

1 inch turmeric root, peeled and minced

1 cup peeled and sliced burdock root

1 cup cilantro, loosely packed

6 garlic cloves, peeled

12 cups water

Place all the ingredients in a large stock pot.

Cover the pot and bring the water to a boil over high heat, and then reduce the heat and simmer for at least 1 hour and up to 4 hours.

Strain and enjoy.

TIPS

- As an alternative, you can blend the broth with the vegetables for a pureed soup.
- This recipe may also be enjoyed as a chunky vegetable soup by leaving the vegetables whole within the broth.

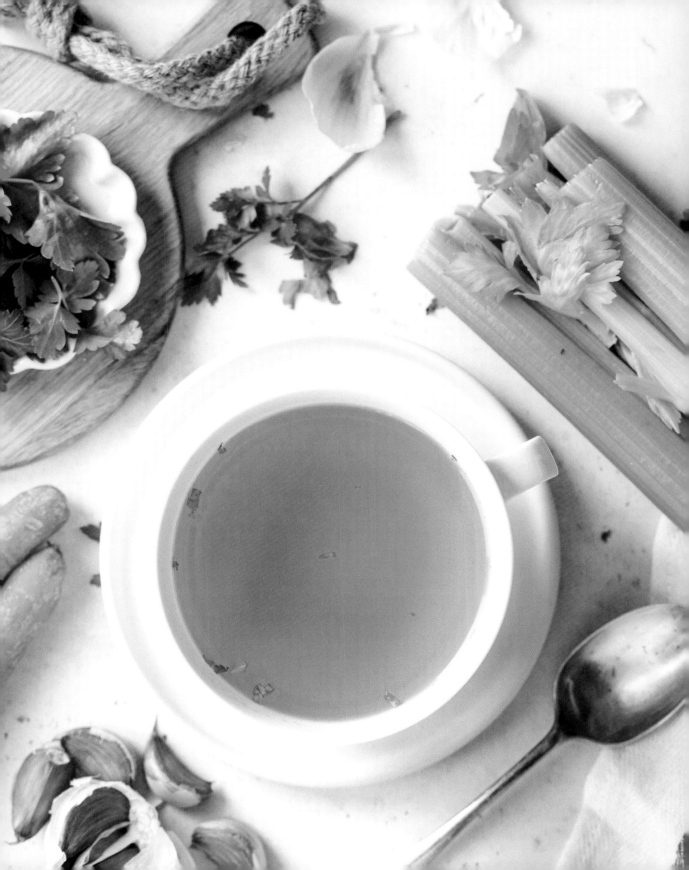

SWEET POTATO NOODLES WITH GARLIC, RED PEPPER, AND ASPARAGUS

Makes 1 to 2 servings

While you might have heard about or tried zucchini noodles, or even butternut squash noodles . . . have you tried sweet potato noodles? They're delicious and fun! In this recipe, they are combined with asparagus, garlic, and red pepper to make a beautiful meal that will delight your eyes and your body.

1½ pounds sweet potatoes (yields about 4 cups of noodles)

½ pound asparagus, ends trimmed and chopped

2 garlic cloves, minced

½ teaspoon red pepper flakes (optional)

1 medium-sized red pepper, cored and thinly sliced

1 tablespoon lemon juice

Peel the sweet potatoes, slice them in half, and spiralize them into thick noodles. Set aside.

Place a medium-sized pan over medium-high heat and add the noodles, asparagus, garlic, and red pepper flakes. Sauté for 3 to 5 minutes, adding a bit of water if desired and tossing and gently scraping down the sides as needed.

Add the sliced red pepper and 2 to 3 tablespoons of water. Place the lid on and cook for 3 to 5 minutes, until the noodles are tender. Be careful not to overcook—the noodles can turn mushy very quickly.

Season with lemon juice. Serve immediately.

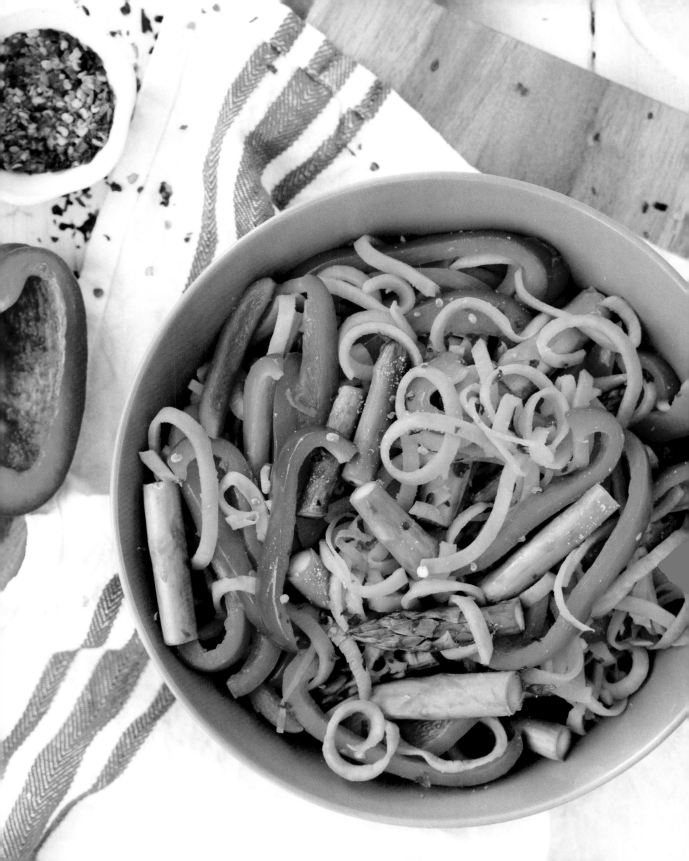

ZUCCHINI AND SUMMER SQUASH STIR-FRY OVER CAULIFLOWER RICE

Makes 2 servings

Fresh, light, and yet satisfying, this stir-fry lets the zucchini and summer squash shine. Enjoy it over cooked or raw cauliflower rice if you wish. Whichever way you choose to enjoy it, it's sure to be delicious.

CAULIFLOWER RICE

1 pound cauliflower florets
¼ cup water

STIR-FRY

1 medium-sized zucchini
1 medium-sized summer squash
2 garlic cloves, minced
¼ cup chopped green onion
1 teaspoon red pepper flakes
1 teaspoon pure maple syrup or raw honey
1 tablespoon lemon or lime juice

To make the cauliflower rice, place the cauliflower florets in a food processor and pulse until you get a coarse, rice-like texture.

Place a skillet on medium-high heat. When it is hot, add the water, followed by the cauliflower rice. Cover and cook until tender, about 2 to 3 minutes. Set aside.

To make the stir-fry, add the zucchini, summer squash, garlic, green onion, and red pepper flakes to a large ceramic nonstick pan or wok over medium-high heat. Cook for 5 to 6 minutes, until the squash starts to soften.

Add the maple syrup or raw honey and lemon juice. Cook until soft.

Serve with cauliflower rice.

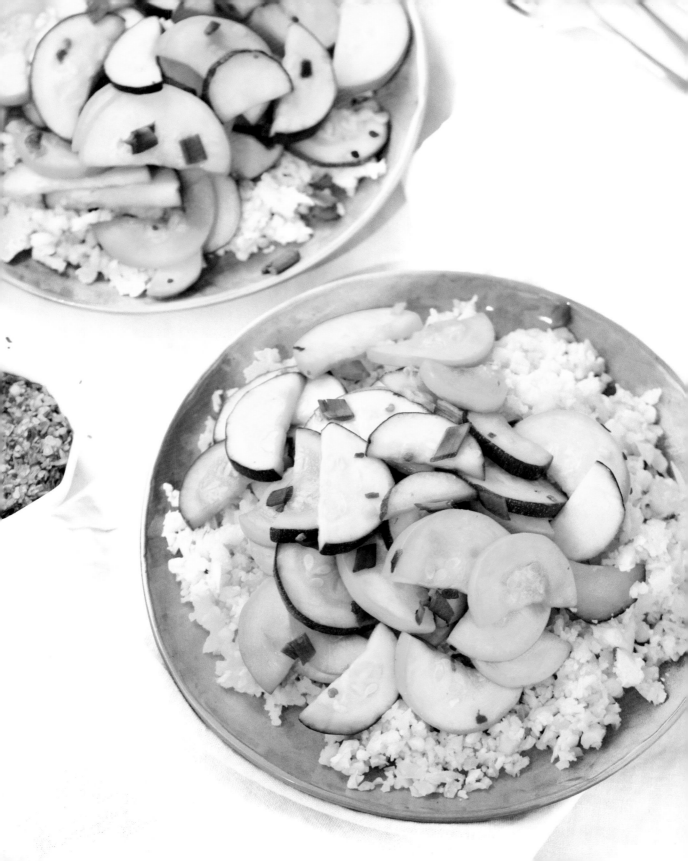

POTATO SALAD

Makes 2 servings

It's hard to beat a good potato salad. Whether you enjoy it during the 3:6:9 Cleanse or you make it a staple afterward, it's a meal that is always satisfying and comforting. The fresh herbs plus the cucumber and radish in the potato salad give it flavor and crunch while helping you digest the potatoes better. That's a win-win.

2 pounds potatoes, peeled and diced

1 garlic clove, minced

¼ cup roughly chopped fresh parsley

2 tablespoons finely chopped green onion

½ teaspoon mustard powder

2 teaspoons fresh lemon juice

OPTIONAL ADDITIONS

½ cup thinly sliced radish

½ cup thinly sliced cucumber

½ cup chopped asparagus, steamed or raw

Add 3 inches of water to a medium-sized pot, bring it to a boil, and add a steaming basket. Place the potatoes in the basket, cover, and steam for 5 to 10 minutes, until tender.

Remove and place in a bowl. Add the garlic, parsley, green onion, mustard powder, and lemon juice. Mix well. Add any additions you would like.

Divide between bowls and serve.

TIPS

- If you don't like parsley, you can replace it with another herb you do like, such as basil, dill, or cilantro.

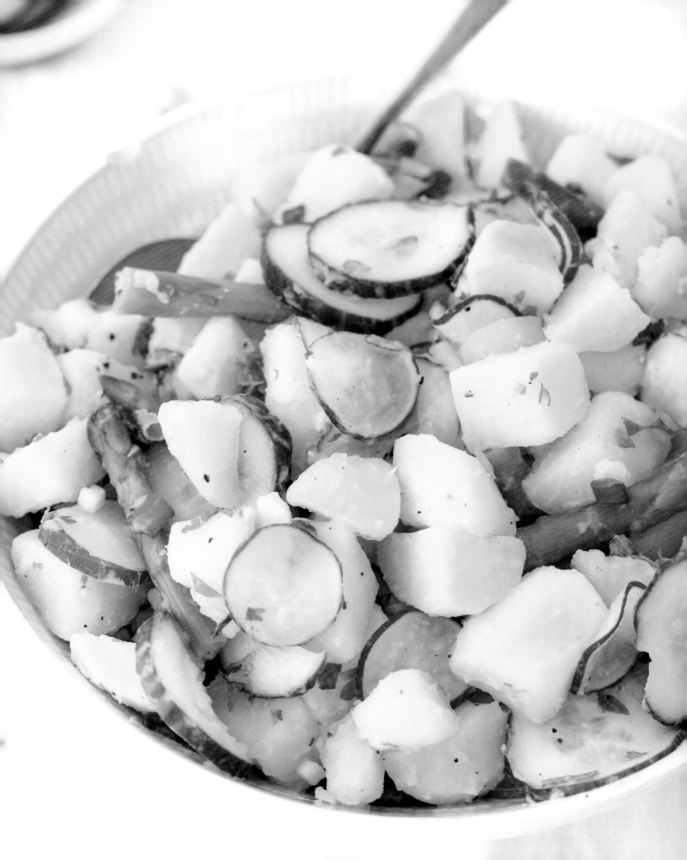

POTATO AND HERB STUFFED PEPPERS

Makes 2 to 3 servings

These stuffed bell peppers look beautiful and taste even better. If you're a mashed potato fan, you will likely enjoy this fun presentation of a family favorite. Serve with a fresh Leafy Green Salad for a perfect meal.

2 pounds potatoes, peeled and diced

1½ teaspoons onion powder

1 teaspoon garlic powder

½ teaspoon paprika

2 tablespoons finely chopped parsley; more for garnish

2 tablespoons finely chopped chives; more for garnish

1 tablespoon lemon juice

3 yellow, red, and/or orange bell peppers

Preheat oven to 400°F/200°C.

Add 3 inches of water to a medium-sized pot, bring it to a boil, and add a steaming basket. Place the potatoes in the basket, cover, and steam for 5 to 10 minutes, until tender. Remove and cool.

Place the potatoes in a large bowl or pot. Add the onion powder, garlic powder, paprika, chopped parsley, chopped chives, and lemon juice. Mash until smooth using a potato masher. You may need to add a few tablespoons of water if the potatoes are very dry.

Slice the bell peppers in half and remove the seeds and core. Place them in a baking dish. Divide the potato mash between the halves.

Cook in the oven for 20 to 25 minutes, until browned on top. Remove and serve. Garnish with chopped parsley and chives.

TIPS

- It's important to choose bell peppers that aren't green. If they are green, it means they are unripe and can cause some discomfort. Red, orange, yellow, and purple peppers are ripe and the best choices.

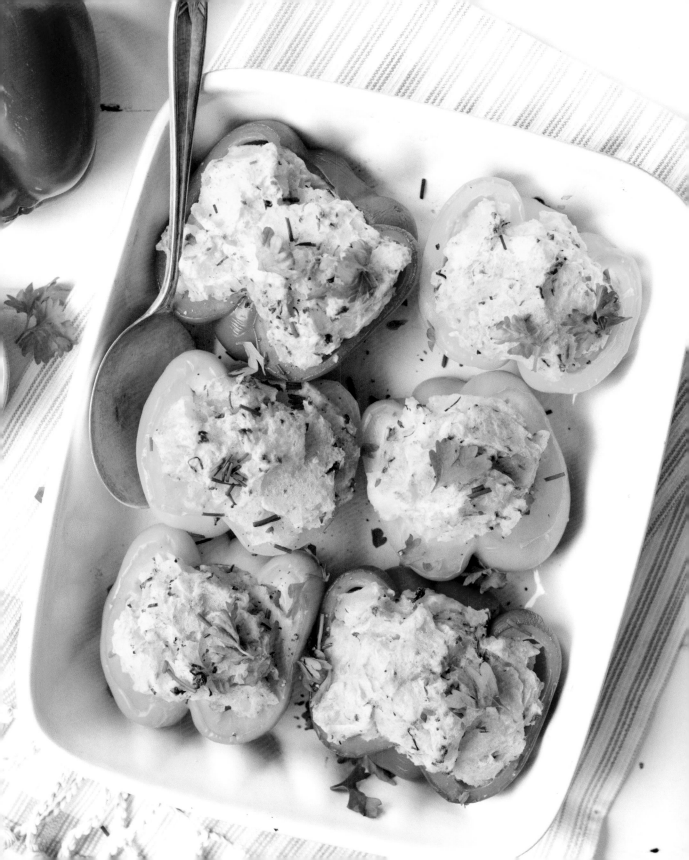

SWEET POTATO AND ZUCCHINI STEW

Makes 2 servings

Stews really are comfort in a bowl. Sweet potato and zucchini come together in this recipe to provide a delicious, liver-healing meal you can enjoy all for yourself or to share with loved ones. This stew is wonderful on its own or with a fresh salad by its side.

1 cup chopped onion

2½ cups diced sweet potato

3 garlic cloves, minced

2½ cups roughly chopped zucchini

1 teaspoon ground cumin

1 teaspoon ground coriander

½ teaspoon turmeric

1 teaspoon paprika

½ teaspoon red pepper flakes

1 cup diced tomato

2 tablespoons pure tomato paste (find one without additives)

1 cup hot water

¼ cup tightly packed fresh cilantro, roughly chopped, to serve

Place a saucepan on medium-high heat, and then add the onion, sweet potato, and garlic. Cook for 3 to 5 minutes, until the onion is soft. If the vegetables stick to the pan, add a bit of water.

Add the zucchini, together with the ground cumin, ground coriander, turmeric, paprika, red pepper flakes, tomato, tomato paste, and the cup of hot water. Stir well. Place the lid on, lower the heat, and simmer for 10 minutes.

Remove the lid and cook for another 10 minutes, until the sweet potato is cooked through and the stew has thickened.

Serve topped with fresh cilantro.

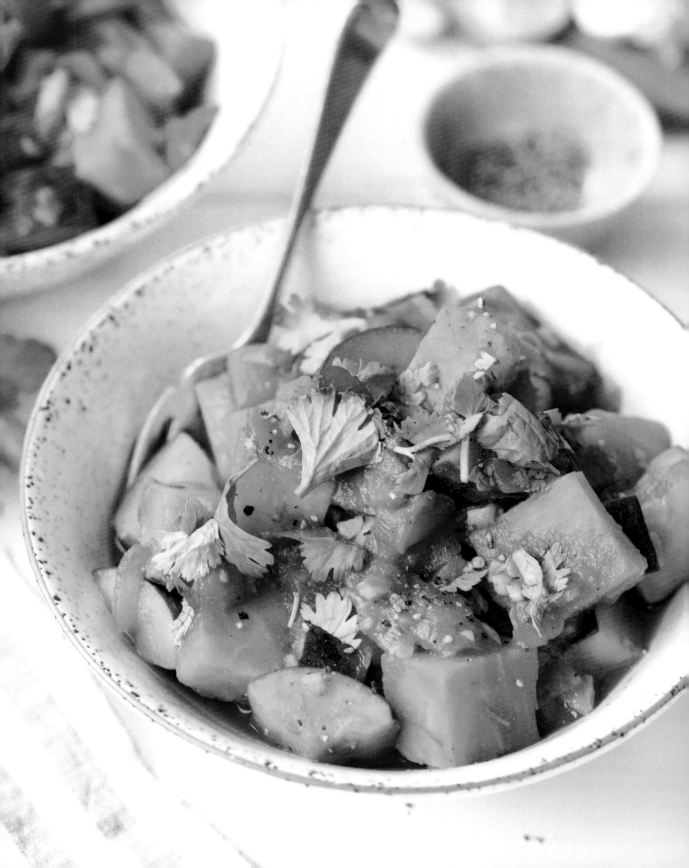

WARM SPICED ROASTED VEGETABLE SALAD

Makes 1 to 2 servings

Fresh arugula and spinach tossed with warm roasted vegetables makes for a heavenly pairing. This Warm Spiced Roasted Vegetable Salad is a great way to get all-important leafy greens in while also enjoying the comfort and satiation of roasted vegetables.

1 cup diced carrot

2 cups chopped butternut squash

½ cup diced red onion

2 cups roughly chopped zucchini

1 teaspoon ground coriander

½ teaspoon ground cumin

1 teaspoon paprika

1 teaspoon raw honey

2 cups spinach, loosely packed

2 cups arugula, loosely packed

¼ cup tightly packed fresh cilantro, chopped

FOR THE DRESSING

3 tablespoons freshly squeezed orange juice

¼ teaspoon finely grated orange zest

½ garlic clove, finely grated

1 teaspoon raw honey

1 tablespoon lemon juice

Preheat oven to 400°F/200°C. Line a large baking sheet with parchment paper.

Place the diced carrot, butternut squash, red onion, and zucchini on the baking sheet. Add the ground coriander, ground cumin, paprika, and raw honey. Mix until evenly coated.

Place in the oven and roast for 20 to 25 minutes, until tender and browned.

While the vegetables are roasting, make the dressing by whisking together the orange juice and zest, garlic, raw honey, and lemon juice.

Place the spinach, arugula, and cilantro in a serving bowl or divide between two. Top with roasted vegetables and drizzle the dressing on top. Serve immediately.

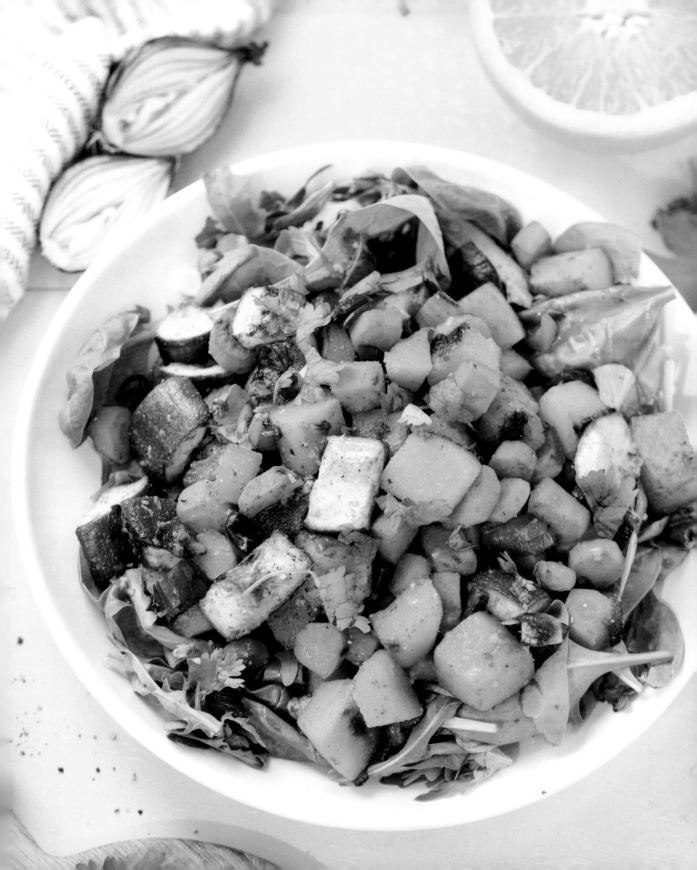

CARROT, ZUCCHINI, AND POTATO PATTIES

Makes 8 patties/3 to 4 servings

These veggie patties are so incredibly versatile that you can make them a regular lunch or dinner choice without getting bored. Try them over a salad, with steamed vegetables, topped with salsa, in a lettuce or cabbage leaf, dipped into the natural ketchup recipe on page 420, or any other way you can dream up.

2 potatoes
2 carrots
1 zucchini
1 teaspoon garlic powder
1 teaspoon onion powder
1 teaspoon dried oregano
1 teaspoon paprika

Add 3 inches of water to a medium-sized pot, bring it to a boil, and add a steaming basket. Place the potatoes and carrots in the basket, cover, and steam for 15 to 20 minutes, until tender. Remove from heat and cool completely.

Preheat oven to 350°F/180°C. Line a baking sheet with parchment paper.

Grate the zucchini and place it in a muslin cloth or nut milk bag to squeeze out all the water. Make sure that the zucchini is very dry; otherwise it will take the patties longer to crisp up in the oven. Add it to a mixing bowl. Grate the potatoes and carrots and place them in the bowl with the grated zucchini. Add the garlic powder, onion powder, dried oregano, and paprika and mix until combined.

Form the mixture into about 8 patties and place them on the baking sheet. Place in the oven and cook for 45 to 60 minutes, until browned and crispy, flipping them halfway through. Allow the patties to cool for 10 to 15 minutes before eating so they firm up.

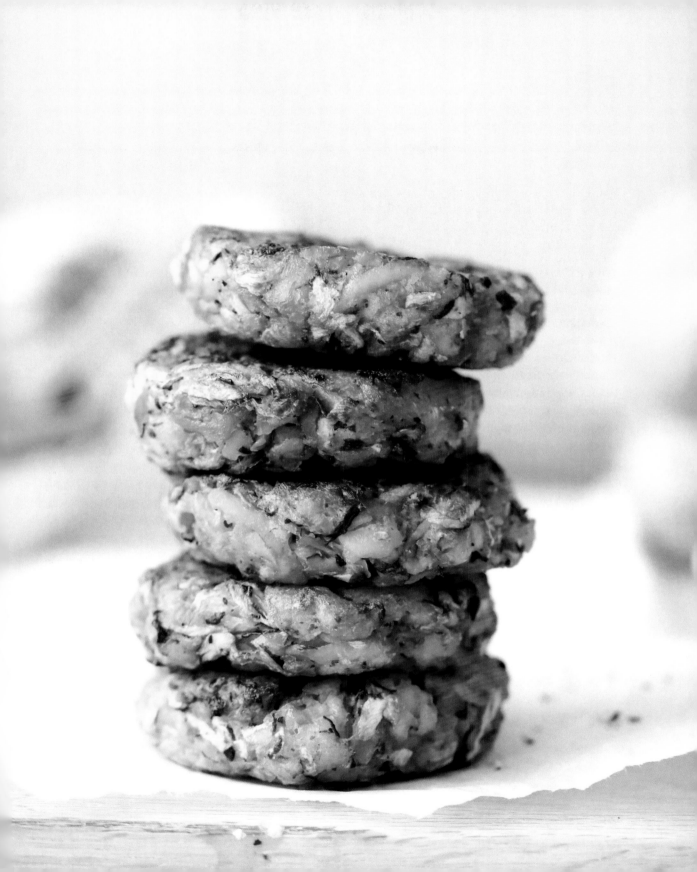

STUFFED BUTTERNUT SQUASH

Sweet and savory come together in this Stuffed Butternut Squash. Follow the recipe provided or choose your own favorite vegetables for the filling and experiment with your favorite pure spices, keeping the recipe fat-free. The Stuffed Butternut Squash halves stay well in the fridge for a few days; you can easily reheat them in the oven when you're ready and sprinkle them with fresh parsley.

1 large butternut squash, halved and seeds removed

2¼ cups cauliflower florets

½ cup diced onion

2 garlic cloves, minced

¼ cup finely diced carrot

1 cup chopped mushrooms

1 celery stalk, finely chopped

½ teaspoon dried thyme

½ tablespoon pure maple syrup

1 tablespoon chopped parsley; more for garnish

½ tablespoon lemon juice

Preheat oven to 400°F/200°C. Line a baking tray with parchment paper.

Place the squash halves on the baking tray. Roast in the oven for 40 to 50 minutes, depending on the size of the squash, until very tender when pierced with a fork.

Add the cauliflower florets in a food processor and pulse until you get a coarse, rice-like texture. Set aside.

Place a skillet on medium-high heat. Add the diced onion and cook for 3 to 5 minutes, until translucent, adding a bit of water if needed.

Add the garlic, carrots, mushrooms, and celery. Cook for 5 to 10 minutes, until the mushrooms and carrots are soft. Remove and place in a bowl.

Add the cauliflower rice to the vegetable and mushroom mixture together with the dried thyme, maple syrup, chopped parsley, and lemon juice. Mix well.

When the butternut halves are tender, fill them to the brim with the filling. Place them back in the oven to roast for 5 to 10 minutes.

To serve, arrange the halves on a platter or individual plates. Garnish with fresh parsley.

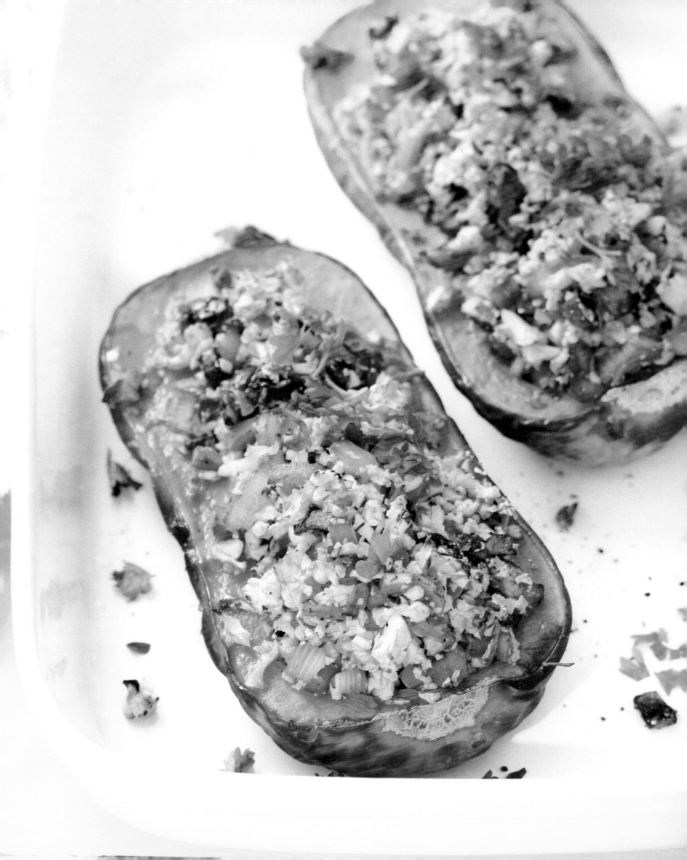

POTATO PIZZA BOATS

Makes 2 to 3 servings

The versatility of the humble potato is impressive. From steamed to baked to salads to pizzas to stuffed to mashed and more, there are endless ways to draw on its flexibility. Potatoes often get a bad rap because of the other ingredients that accompany them. When prepared without butter, cream, cheese, or bacon bits, the potato is an incredibly healing vegetable that can help knock down your viral load. These Pizza Boats show one more delicious way you can enjoy the potato.

4 large russet potatoes

SAUCE

½ cup pure tomato paste (find one without additives)
1 teaspoon dried oregano
½ teaspoon dried thyme
1 teaspoon raw honey
¼ cup water

TOPPING OPTIONS

¼ cup chopped zucchini
¼ cup chopped red pepper
¼ cup halved cherry tomatoes
¼ cup chopped red onion
Fresh basil, to serve

Preheat oven to 400°F/200°C. Line a baking sheet with parchment paper.

Pierce the potatoes with a fork and place them on the baking sheet. Bake them in the oven for 45 minutes to 1 hour, until tender. Remove and cool.

While the potatoes are roasting, make the tomato sauce by whisking together the tomato paste, dried oregano, dried thyme, raw honey, and ¼ cup water. Set aside.

When they are cool enough to handle, cut the potatoes in half lengthwise and scoop out the top of each potato half, creating a boat. Place a couple of tablespoons of tomato sauce in each and add toppings of your choice.

Place them back in the oven and roast for 15 to 20 minutes, until the toppings are cooked through. Serve immediately.

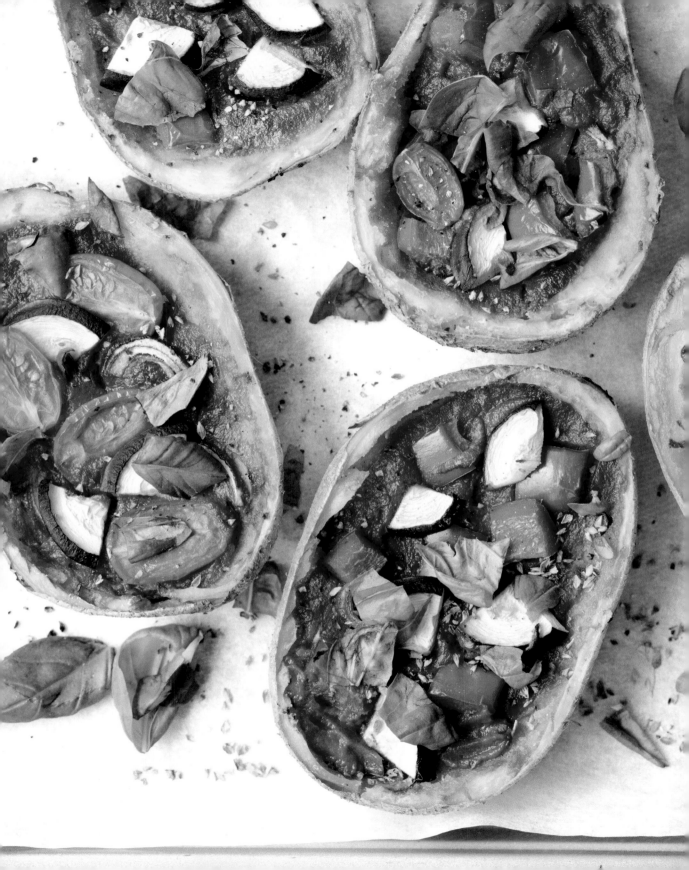

CHUNKY SWEET POTATO FRIES WITH SPINACH PESTO

Makes 2 servings

In this recipe, piping hot chunky sweet potato fries are served with a cooling and flavor-packed fat-free spinach and herb pesto. The spinach lends a touch of creaminess to the pesto while amplifying the nutrient value of this meal. You may want to make extra for any hungry bystanders in the house!

2½ pounds sweet potatoes (purple, Japanese, or orange), cut into thick fries

1 teaspoon dried oregano or thyme

SPINACH PESTO

3 cups baby spinach, loosely packed

1 cup fresh basil or parsley, loosely packed

2 to 3 tablespoons fresh lemon juice, to taste

1½ garlic cloves

3 tablespoons water or Liver Rescue Broth (recipe on page 394)

½ teaspoon raw honey

Preheat oven to 400°F/200°C. Line two large baking sheets with parchment paper.

Spread the sweet potato fries out into a single layer over the baking trays and sprinkle them with dried oregano or thyme.

Bake for 40 to 45 minutes, or until golden and cooked through.

While the fries are baking, place all the pesto ingredients in a blender or food processor and process until combined, leaving a little texture. Scrape down the sides as needed. Taste and adjust seasoning as desired.

When the fries are ready, remove them from the oven and serve with pesto.

TIPS

- When choosing between water and Liver Rescue Broth for the ingredients, keep in mind that the broth will produce a richer flavor. Store-bought vegetable stock isn't called for because it's very difficult to find a variety that's free from oil, salt, natural flavors, and/or other additives. For convenience, make a batch of Liver Rescue Broth in advance and freeze it (consider ice cube trays for easy thawing) so you have it on hand for recipes like these.

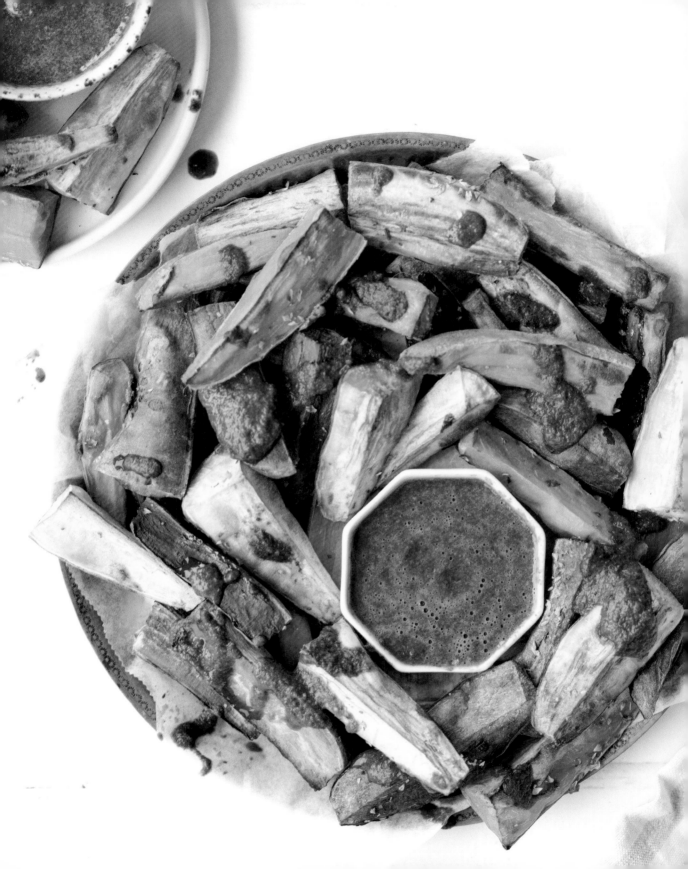

BUTTERNUT SQUASH FALAFELS WITH SALAD

Makes 2 servings

Golden falafel balls made with butternut squash instead of chickpeas are the star of this recipe. Served over tender greens and brightened with a squeeze of fresh lemon juice, this recipe is delicious, simple to pull together, and lets the ingredients speak for themselves.

3½ cups diced butternut squash

1 cup diced red onion

2 garlic cloves, peeled and roughly chopped

1 cup fresh cilantro or parsley, loosely packed

1 teaspoon ground coriander

1 teaspoon ground cumin

½ teaspoon ground ginger

1 tablespoon fresh lemon juice

GREEN SALAD

2 cups spinach, loosely packed

2 cups arugula, loosely packed

1 tablespoon fresh lemon juice

Preheat oven to 400°F/200°C. Line a baking sheet with parchment paper; don't skip this step, as the falafel mixture is very sticky. Place the diced butternut squash on the baking sheet and roast for 20 to 25 minutes until just tender.

Let it cool for 10 minutes, and then add it to a food processor along with the onion, garlic, fresh cilantro or parsley, ground cumin, ground coriander, ground ginger, and lemon juice. Blend the ingredients for 1 to 2 minutes, until the mixture is mostly smooth, with some bigger pieces.

Form the mixture into about 12 balls, roughly the size of golf balls, and then place them on the baking sheet and flatten them slightly. Bake the falafels for 30 minutes, or until lightly browned, and then flip and bake them for another 10 minutes.

Make the green salad by combining the spinach and arugula in a bowl. Add the lemon juice and toss to coat. Place the salad in a bowl and top with falafels. Serve immediately.

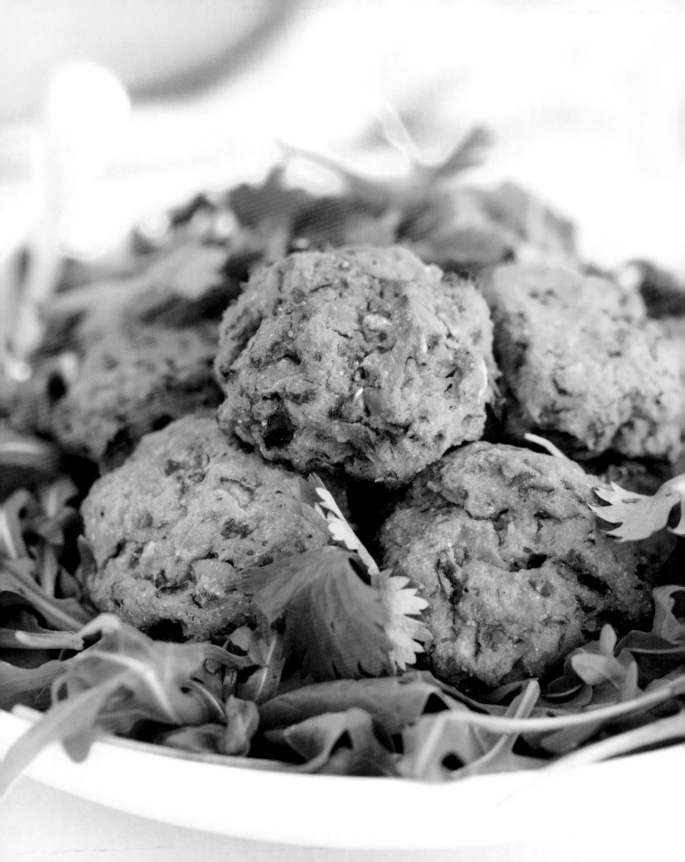

ZUCCHINI LASAGNA

A veggie lasagna without the dairy, grains, or fat? It's not only possible; it's delicious! Layers of flavorful tomato sauce, creamy potato béchamel, and baked zucchini make this recipe truly special and also healthy! This is a fun recipe to share with family and friends.

FOR THE LASAGNA

4 small to medium zucchini

5 to 6 fresh basil leaves, chopped (for garnish)

FOR THE POTATO BÉCHAMEL

6 medium-sized potatoes, peeled and diced (about 1½ pounds)

1 tablespoon onion powder

¼ cup arrowroot starch

1 tablespoon fresh lemon juice

¾ cup water

FOR THE MARINARA SAUCE

4 cups crushed or diced tomatoes

1 onion, diced

3 garlic cloves, minced

1 teaspoon dried oregano

1 teaspoon dried thyme

¼ cup tightly packed fresh basil, chopped

Preheat oven to 350°F/180°C.

Cut the ends off the zucchini, and then slice into about ¼-inch-thick ribbons, best done carefully with a mandoline. Arrange them on two or three large baking sheets covered with parchment paper and bake them in the oven for 20 to 25 minutes, until most of the moisture has evaporated. Remove from the oven and cool completely. If the slices still seem wet, dab them a few times with paper towels to remove excess moisture.

To make the potato béchamel, add 3 inches of water to a medium-sized pot, bring it to a boil, and add a steaming basket. Place the potatoes in the basket, cover, and steam for 15 to 25 minutes, until tender. Remove from the heat and place in a blender, along with the onion powder, arrowroot starch, lemon juice, and water. Blend until smooth. Set aside.

To make the marinara sauce, add the crushed or diced tomatoes, onion, garlic, oregano, and thyme to a medium-sized saucepan and cook on high heat for 15 to 20 minutes, until thick and reduced. Add the basil. Let cool for 10 minutes.

To assemble the lasagna, cover the base of the lasagna dish with a layer of baked zucchini. Next, add one-quarter of the marinara sauce, just enough to cover the zucchini. After that, add one-quarter of the potato béchamel, just enough to cover the tomato layer. Adding too much of either will result in a runny lasagna. Repeat, making layers with the zucchini, marinara, and potato béchamel, adding up to four layers in total.

Bake in the middle of the oven for 45 to 50 minutes, until browned on top and the zucchini is tender. Let cool for at least 20 minutes before slicing so the sauce can thicken. Serve with chopped fresh basil on top.

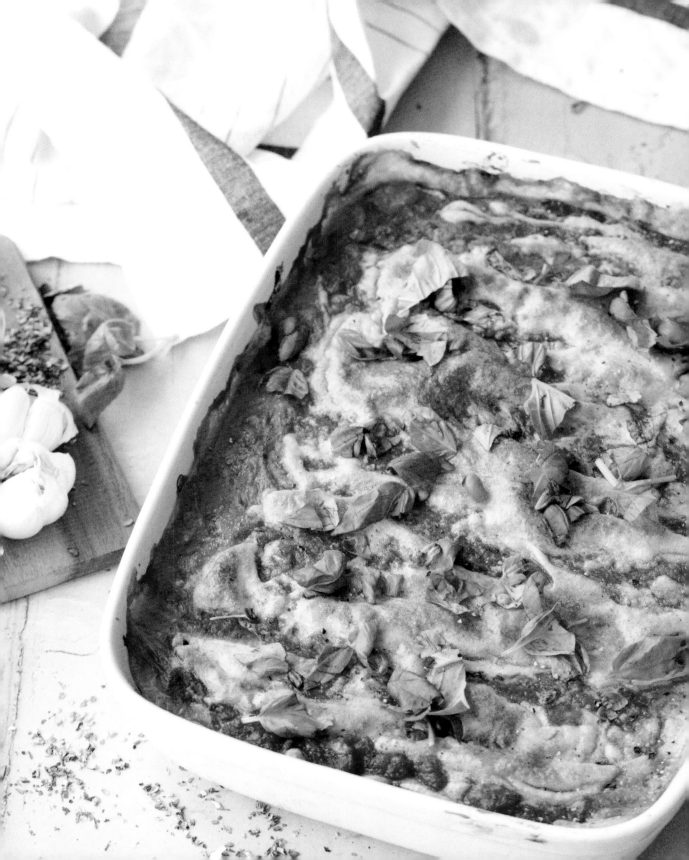

SWEET POTATO TOTS

Makes 2 servings

Enjoy this unique, healing spin on a childhood favorite. They're delicious served with salad or with the Spinach Pesto recipe (see page 414).

2 medium-sized sweet potatoes

1 teaspoon dried herbs such as oregano, thyme, or rosemary

OPTIONAL KETCHUP

6 ounces pure tomato paste (find one without additives)

⅓ cup apple juice

2 tablespoons fresh lemon juice

2 teaspoons raw honey

¼ teaspoon dried onion powder

¼ teaspoon garlic powder

¼ teaspoon dried oregano

¼ teaspoon cayenne pepper (optional)

Preheat oven to 375°F/190°C

Add 3 inches of water to a medium-sized pot, bring it to a boil, and add a steaming basket. Place the sweet potatoes in the basket, cover, and steam for 20 to 25 minutes, until tender on the outside yet firm in the middle. Remove from heat and cool completely.

Remove the skins from the sweet potatoes and grate them using the large side of a box grater. Place the grated sweet potato into a bowl and add the herbs. Mix until combined. Use a tablespoon to scoop the mixture, and then use your hands to form the tots into small cylinders.

Place the tots on a baking sheet lined with parchment paper and bake for 40 to 45 minutes, flipping them halfway through, until browned. For a crispier tot, turn the heat up to 400°F/200°C for the last 10 minutes of baking. Let the tots cool for 5 to 10 minutes before eating.

To make the ketchup, combine all the ingredients in a bowl and whisk until smooth. Serve with tots.

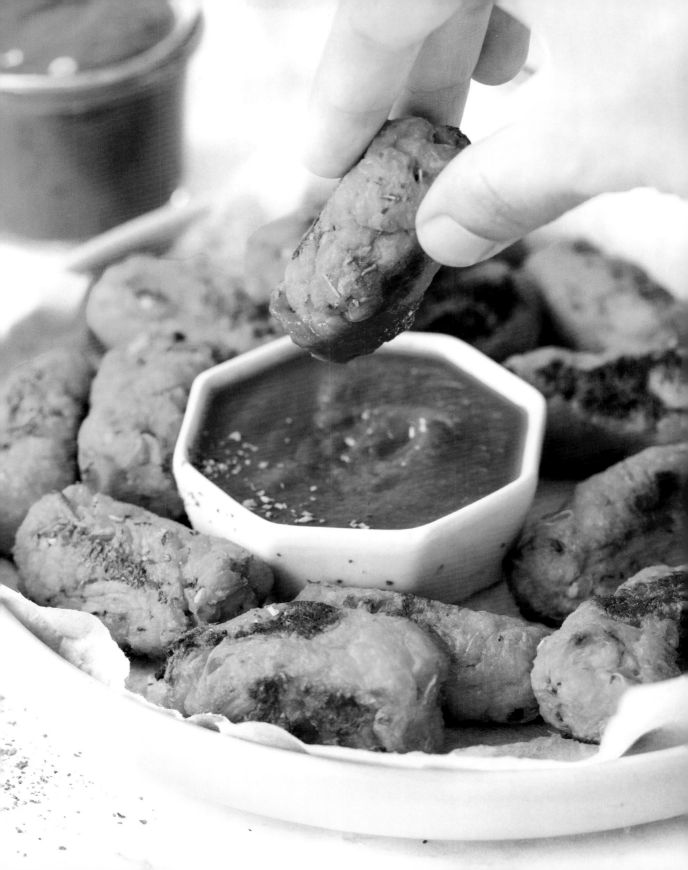

PORTOBELLO STEW

Makes 4 to 6 servings

This hearty stew is so satisfying and mouth-watering. Portobello mushrooms, carrots, potatoes, onions, and fresh herbs come together in a delicious gravy-style sauce. This is a great meal to serve to hungry friends and family or to keep in the fridge or freezer for leftovers. Enjoy with a fresh salad for a truly soul-comforting meal.

1 onion, roughly chopped

2 celery stalks, chopped

1 pound portobello or portobellini mushrooms, stems removed and chopped

4 cloves garlic, minced

2 carrots, roughly chopped

1½ pounds potatoes, quartered

2 tablespoons fresh thyme leaves

1 tablespoon chopped fresh rosemary

3 cups water or Liver Rescue Broth (recipe on page 394)

1 tablespoon pure tomato paste (find one without additives)

2 tablespoons arrowroot plus 3 tablespoons cold water, to thicken (optional)

2 tablespoons chopped fresh parsley, for garnish

Place a large ceramic nonstick pot on medium-high heat and add the onion. Cook for 3 to 5 minutes, until it starts to soften, adding a spoonful of water if needed. Add the celery and cook for another 2 minutes. Add the mushrooms and cook until softened and browned, about 5 to 7 minutes. Then add the garlic, carrots, potatoes, thyme, and rosemary. Stir well. Pour in the water and tomato paste and bring it to a boil. Cook uncovered for 15 to 20 minutes, until the potatoes and carrots are soft.

If desired, mix together the arrowroot and cold water in a small bowl to make a slurry. Pour the slurry into the stew and stir well. Cook for 2 to 3 minutes, until the stew has thickened.

Remove from heat and serve, topped with fresh parsley.

TIPS

- When choosing between water and Liver Rescue Broth for the ingredients, keep in mind that the broth will produce a richer flavor. Store-bought vegetable stock isn't called for because it's very difficult to find a variety that's free from oil, salt, natural flavors, and/or other additives. For convenience, make a batch of Liver Rescue Broth in advance and freeze it (consider ice cube trays for easy thawing) so you have it on hand for recipes like these.

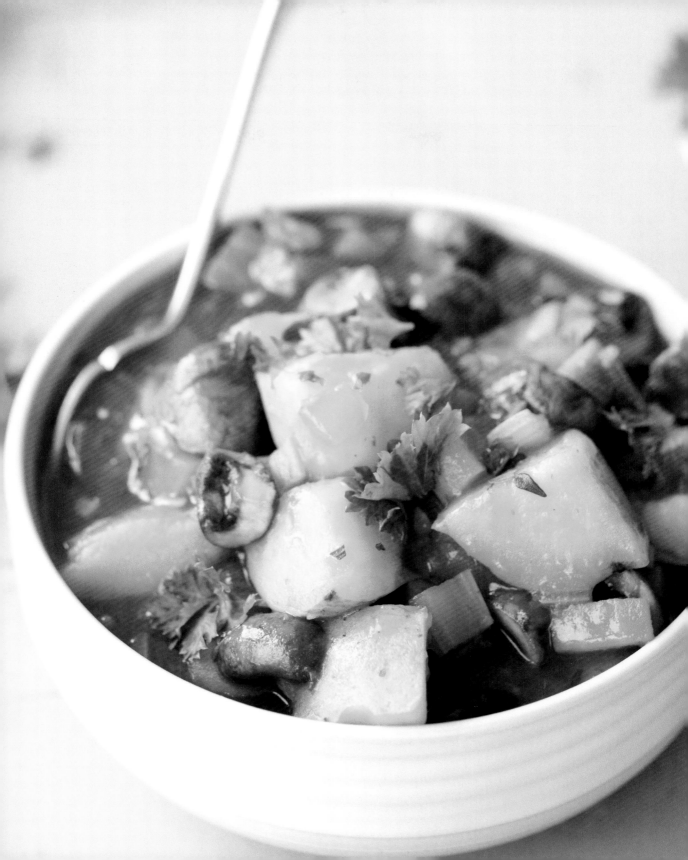

MINI POTATO CAKE PIZZAS

These delectable Mini Potato Cake Pizzas can satisfy a pizza craving without leaving you feeling sluggish. Pile the potato cake bases high with tomato sauce and your favorite vegetables and dig in with joy!

2 pounds potatoes, peeled and diced

1 teaspoon garlic powder

1 teaspoon onion powder

1 teaspoon dried oregano

SAUCE

¼ cup pure tomato paste (find one without additives)

½ teaspoon dried oregano

¼ teaspoon dried thyme

½ teaspoon raw honey

TOPPING OPTIONS

3 to 4 yellow and red cherry tomatoes

¼ small red onion, thinly sliced

2 to 3 mushrooms, thinly sliced

3 to 4 zucchini or summer squash slices

Small handful arugula

Small handful basil

Preheat oven to 400°F/200°C. Line a baking sheet with parchment paper.

To make the base, add 3 inches of water to a medium-sized pot, bring it to a boil, and add a steaming basket. Place the potatoes in the basket, cover, and steam for 5 to 10 minutes, until soft. Remove and cool completely.

Place the potatoes in a bowl together with the garlic powder, onion powder, and dried oregano. Mash with a fork or potato masher until smooth.

Using a ⅛ cup measure, form the mixture into 8 patties about ½ to ¾ inch thick and 3 to 4 inches in diameter. Place in the oven and bake for 20 minutes.

While the patties are baking, make the sauce by mixing together the tomato paste, dried oregano, dried thyme, raw honey, and 2 tablespoons water.

Remove the potato cakes from the oven and spread 1 to 2 tablespoons of tomato sauce on each. Arrange toppings on each of the mini potato cakes and place back in the oven for 15 to 20 minutes, until browned and firm.

Remove from the oven and add arugula and basil. Serve and enjoy.

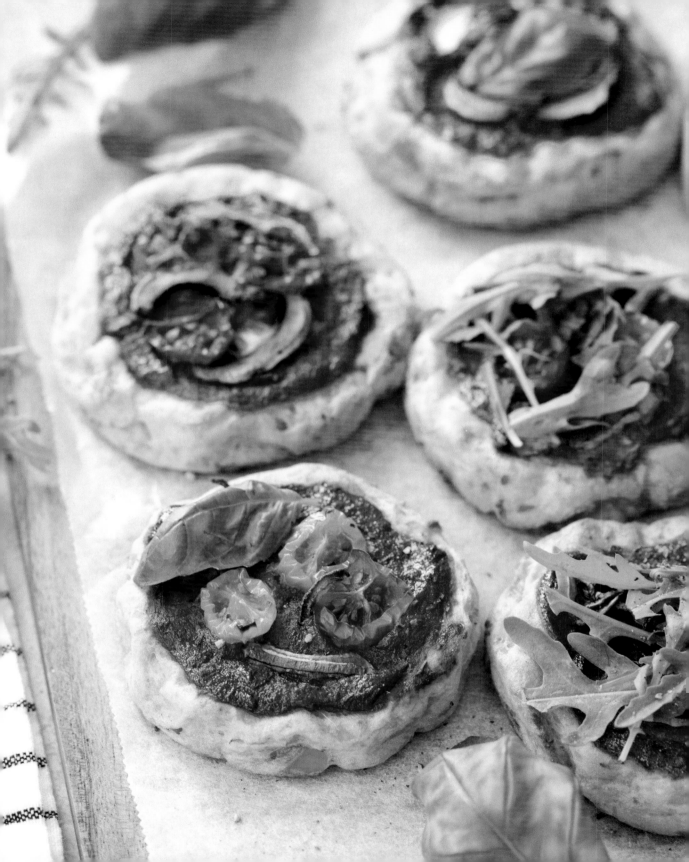

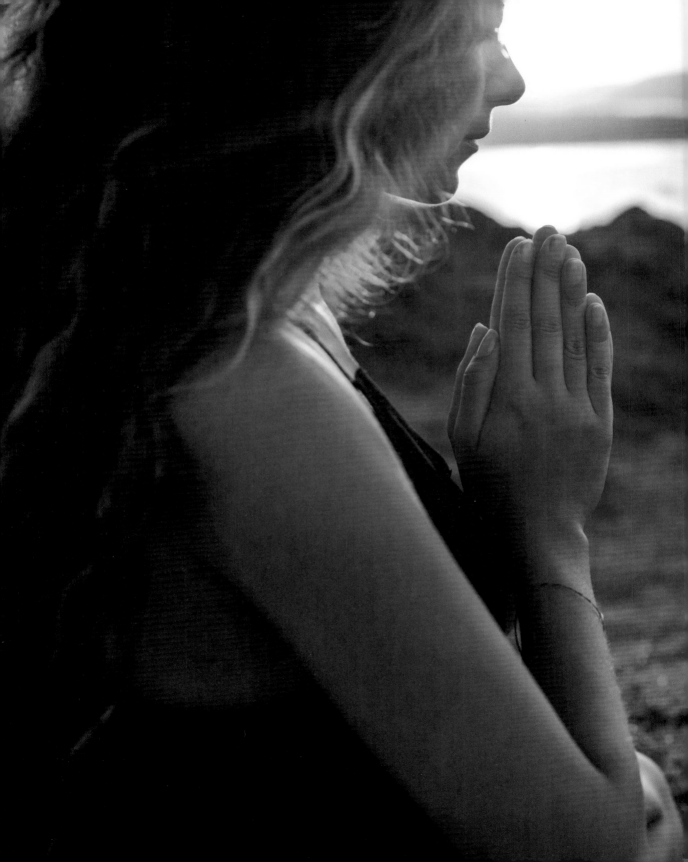

PART V

MORE SPIRITUAL & SOUL-HEALING SUPPORT

Living Words for Underdogs and a Note for Critics

Bullying: you don't deserve it. Whatever you've been through, whatever haters you've faced in life, whoever tried to hold you back from doing good: you did not deserve it. Maybe you had to suffer through it because it wasn't safe to speak up. Maybe you never got to say or do what you wished you could have. Maybe it was only years later that you got validation for calling out a situation that was not okay. Maybe you saved someone with your voice. Maybe you saved yourself. Somehow, you lived through it. You're still here. And with the life ahead of you, you can choose to be part of a powerful healing movement.

We all know that bullying doesn't stop when we grow up. The health realm is one area where that's abundantly clear. It can happen when someone spreads advanced information about healing, it can happen when someone sets out to heal using that information, and it can even happen when someone actually heals. Who would bully a person who has been through debilitating exhaustion and maddening pain, and has finally found a way to feel alive again? Plenty of people, I'm sorry to say. A long history of doubt and shame stretches behind us when it comes to suffering and well-being—especially when it comes to women's suffering and well-being. With the rise of social media, it has become easier to target those brave enough to share their stories. At the exact same time, mercifully, it's become easier for people who are struggling with chronic health issues to find resources and find each other.

Critical thinking: we need this in our confused world. Haters: we don't. Critics want to learn. They educate themselves on what they're critiquing and aim to leave personal opinion out of it, which creates room for them to change their minds. Haters cast their votes with no intention to change. The bullying this leads to is not the way it's supposed to be. Still, we must find a way to cope and stay grounded in its presence, to offer information in the face of hate and also offer compassion in the face of ill will. Above all, we must save ourselves.

Life can be so hard. When people are in pain emotionally, and sometimes even physically, because of the injuries they've experienced in life, a portion of them become haters. Out of their suffering, they adopt hatred. Yes, we have to have some compassion for these people. At the same time, we need to realize that there are a lot of other people out there in the world who have been injured by emotional or physical suffering, and they would never become hateful against others. They would never bully anyone or try to tear them down. We can't give forgiveness and allowance to every hater to the point of disrespecting the ones who would never be harmful or hurtful to others, even in the midst of their worst suffering. If we don't understand the distinction here between haters trapped in darkness and pain who want to pull others into their nightmare and people who are suffering who only wish for the alleviation of others' suffering, we're letting the haters off the hook.

Yes, we have to have compassion. We can't go so far with it that we injure ourselves. If we believe everybody is good, we're going to believe we're doing something wrong in the end. If we don't realize that there are haters who could hurt us in our healing process, then it will hit us in our core of self-worth and self-doubt when we're struggling and trying to heal. Darkness works in this way. Good people tend to give themselves their own lashings and punish themselves when they didn't even do anything wrong. If we don't come to the realization that there are certain people who dwell in hatred and keep light from entering their heart and soul, we could get hurt even more along the way, and that could be detrimental to the healing process.

You can protect yourself, knowing that you are a good person and it's not your fault and you didn't do anything wrong to deserve your pain.

We're taught that everyone is inherently good in this world. My job is to tell you the truth so you can protect yourself. If we believe naïvely that everyone is looking out for our best interest, then the haters can cause harm to our soul and physical body in many ways. That doesn't mean that all haters are hopeless. A miraculous event can change a person. There is always hope that a reversal can occur, where light and goodness can enter a person's heart and awaken them. Still, how much damage was caused along the way? How many people were emotionally harmed to get them to this awakening, and for how many years to come will those selfless individuals suffer for sacrificing their own well-being?

This is a message for the people who are struggling and trying to heal. This is not a message for the hater who doesn't like or believe in the information in this book or that it has helped so many. Critics are welcome here. If you're one of them, I know you're a good person. This is about taking the conversation to another level, opening your eyes so that you can see past your surroundings. My job is to look out for the underdogs who have been through hell and back. There are people who have been bullied and hurt very badly, and it has scarred them. If that's you, let these living words serve as a little lesson on haters so that you don't get hurt by the people trying to drag you into their own pain. Think of the living words here as your anti-bullying tool kit, your refuge when that old schoolyard feeling starts to surface.

THE SICK AND THE NOT-SO-SICK

The person who has never been down on their knees with health problems may be quick to judge the person who has. It's vastly different to experience a bit of bloating, mild acne, intermittent low energy, or slight weight gain than it is to be truly sick, to seek help from multiple doctors over several years for serious symptoms that impede the ability to function properly. To the sick person who has been on a long, grueling journey of trying to recover from severe fatigue, body pain, and brain fog and has tried both conventional and alternative approaches, who knows all too well what it is to be plagued by often invisible struggles, it would feel like a total blessing to experience occasional bloating or breakouts and nothing more. To the not-so-sick person who only visits the doctor for physicals, or perhaps a quick follow-up here or there, it can seem doubtful that chronic suffering is even real.

It's this distance that can make a not-so-sick person much more judgmental of answers to health and healing—for example, the need to cleanse. Toxic heavy metals causing harm inside our bodies? Pathogens such as viruses creating so many diseases and symptoms? Celery juice as a powerful medicinal for it all? It's easy to laugh off or brush aside these life-saving understandings if you haven't been humbled by suffering.

I call this the divide between the sick and the not-so-sick. Because let's face the reality: in today's world, most everyone is dealing with some sort of health challenge, even if it's one that they can live alongside without disruption . . . for now. At this moment, the not-so-sick may enjoy the privilege of their health issues not bringing their lives to a screeching halt.

That doesn't mean it will stay that way forever, especially if they go down the path of ridiculing the very answers that could one day save their lives.

Looking Out for All of Us

When someone is unwell and doesn't get over it quickly, it tends to get old fast to people in their life. Maybe not to a mom concerned about her child. And some of the not-so-sick hold enough humility to respect that just because they don't know what it is to suffer on a daily basis doesn't mean that what others go through isn't real. On the other hand, some not-so-sick can mistake the luck of their seemingly good health for superiority. They find a way not to think about their own vulnerability and instead think they simply know better and live better and that this gives them the right to invalidate people's stories of suffering and healing. There can be a complacence among the not-so-sick, a feeling that they understand life more fully than the sick. Over the past decades, as the rates of chronic illness have increased, a lack of compassion for the chronically ill has grown at the same time.

Some of the not-so-sick take what seems to be good health in the moment and make a living off flaunting it as "proof" that a certain lifestyle is the answer as their rank and popularity climb. It's even becoming popular to fib, for someone to say they have a symptom in order to make a splash on social media and become known so they can showcase a lifestyle as being the answer that saved them, meanwhile using the platform to promote their companies or sell products. This phenomenon of not-so-sick people who can't get movement on social media unless they pretend to have symptoms is becoming very popular, and it's an insult to the people who really do suffer with symptoms. It's manipulation to attract views. It's exploitation of the long fight of the chronically ill to be believed and taken seriously. When you're really sick and suffering and you hear that somebody else has gone through something similar, you may feel validated. Be cautious about what you buy into. Make sure it's not a lifestyle of the not-so-sick showcased in a pretty way to bait and hook sick people.

When a sick person is on the merry-go-round of seeking answers for chronic illness, that person comes to find that medical research and science do not yet have all the answers. Conventional, functional, integrative, holistic, alternative medicine: they all still come up short. While this can sound like sacrilege to the not-so-sick person who hasn't experienced the limits of even alternative medicine—and as well-meaning as the professionals who go into medicine are, and as advanced as so many areas of medicine can be—it is simply the truth that practitioners are not trained with the tools to heal chronic illness.

When someone who has been sick finds a solution such as celery juice and starts consuming it daily, they know the truth they have found. They know what a drop-off they feel on the days when they don't drink it. They respect that even as there are multiple facets that go into healing, this one tool has a special power to move you forward no matter where you are with your health. They are aware that Spirit of Compassion is looking out for us *all* if we don't let the industries, naysayers, disempowerers, or even our own selves stand in the way.

Finding the Gold

So many theories circulate about health remedies. The sick and the not-so-sick have two completely different takes on this. For the not-so-sick, it can be almost fun or lighthearted to try the latest trend. For the sick, it's about survival. Those with chronic illness know that whether it's supplementation with deer antler, kombucha, collagen, probiotics, colostrum, apple cider vinegar, or neem, it doesn't move the needle. These holistic approaches, like so many that have come before them and so many yet to come, do not move someone who is chronically suffering forward. Celery juice, on the other hand—a medicinal I've written a whole book about that's also part of every cleanse in these pages—has shown, through the millions drinking it, healing, and sharing their stories, that it operates on another level.

Here's a key distinction between the sick and the not-so-sick: far from the stereotype of "lazy," people who are sick put in the work on healing protocols. Someone who's not so sick may try a week of celery juice without paying attention to the guidelines, because they don't read the Medical Medium books and get the entire picture. They mistakenly add lemon, collagen, or ACV to their celery juice, purchase celery juice off the shelf that's gone through the HPP (high-pressure pasteurization) process, consume their celery juice at the same time as eating other food, or only drink celery juice for five to seven days to film a video for social media at the same time they play with a new supplement or cut out gluten on the days it doesn't feel too hard. Because of half-hearted adherence to key understandings, they may miss out on the real benefits and walk away feeling like they tried yet one more cute trend that didn't deliver. On top of this, not-so-sick people aren't being held back by a symptom or illness, so they don't experience just how quickly some freshly juiced celery with nothing added to it that's sipped on an empty stomach can make a difference when you've been suffering, how it can move your health forward when nothing else has. Someone who's sick will pay meticulous attention to what it takes to get a protocol right. They'll study the Medical Medium information, become expert in it, put in the work to apply it correctly—and because of this, see their lives change.

To hear them both tell it, it would be easy to think that the not-so-sick person and the sick person put in the same work; it would be easy to believe the not-so-sick person who said they gave it a real go. With a true look, though, you'd see two entirely different situations: one where a person barely scratched the surface, and another where somebody dug in and found the gold. With attention and dedication, this health information can heal some of the most difficult health compromises.

CHRONIC AND MYSTERY ILLNESS: AN EPIDEMIC

One critical tool to defend yourself from bullying is knowledge that's founded in truth from above. With this knowledge, you won't doubt yourself in the face of bullies who threaten to weaken your stance and conviction. So let's look more closely at *why* having Medical Medium healing information that's different from both mainstream alternative and conventional medicine is necessary: because chronic illness is at an all-time high. In America alone, more than 250 million people are sick or dealing with mystery

symptoms, and that number is growing. These are people leading diminished lives with no explanation from either conventional or alternative medical research or science, or living with explanations that don't sit right or that make them feel even worse, such as the autoimmune theory (which says that your body's own immune system is destroying your glands and organs and that you have to live without answers) or the gene theory (which says that your genes are faulty and mutated, and the very essence of your physicality and who you are is in question) or the hormone theory (where every symptom you experience is blamed on your hormones). You may be one of these people. If so, you can attest that medical science is still puzzling through what's behind the epidemic of mystery symptoms and suffering.

Why are we letting the system tell us false answers based on theories that were never proven to begin with? Because medical research and science in the area of chronic illness have created a bully system that breaks our spirit and can even injure our soul by telling us lies about our body that were never true. I'm not talking about the good people who go into medicine and the study of chronic illness with the highest intentions. I'm talking about the system that breaks their spirits too. You can use this anti-bullying tool kit against that system, and against the not-so-sick people who have bought into medical research's and science's body-shaming lies. Now you have a way to defend yourself against the falsehoods that say that your body is faulty or attacking itself.

A Field Held Back by Funding

Let me be clear, as always, that I revere good medical science. There are incredibly gifted and talented doctors, surgeons, nurses, nurse practitioners, physician assistants, technicians, researchers, chemists, and more doing profound work in both conventional and alternative medicine. I've had the privilege of working with many of them. Thank God for these compassionate healers. Learning how to understand our world through rigorous, systematic inquiry is one of the highest pursuits imaginable.

Most doctors have an innate wisdom and intuition that tell them that the medical establishment doesn't give them what they need in order to offer the best diagnosis and treatment plan when it comes to chronic illness. How many times have you heard, "There is no known cure for [fill-in-the-blank disease]"? You could fill in eczema, psoriasis, lupus, MS, ALS, Alzheimer's disease, Hashimoto's thyroiditis, PCOS, endometriosis, fibromyalgia, every autoimmune disease, now even Lyme disease, and the list could go on and on and on. Even at the best, most elite medical schools, there are doctors who graduated at the top of the class who are honest about the fact that they finished school unprepared to work with chronic-illness patients. They had to learn to fly on their own. Then there are doctors who believe that they *are* given all the answers in school and for some reason think that their training supersedes the mysteries of chronic illness; they think everything else is nonsense and hocus-pocus, which is unfortunate, since they live in denial of the millions of people who are suffering with no real answers.

Either way, it's not doctors' or researchers' fault that the medical industry hasn't been able to solve the mysteries of chronic illness. Every day, amazing, brilliant minds in science stumble upon discoveries that require a green light from investors and decision makers at the top in order to move forward. Thousands of discoveries that could really change people's lives for the better are kept from going anywhere, and individuals in the field of science are held back.

The Ideal versus the Reality

We sometimes treat medical science like pure mathematics, governed solely by logic and reason. Though at times intertwined, math and medical science aren't the same. Math is definitive; science isn't. True science applies to an outcome, a result of applying theory. You can use math in medical science; you can use it to make a drug, for example, though the drug shouldn't be deemed a viable scientific option until there's a proven result and the numbers make sense in the end. Science labs are often play shops of highly intelligent people methodically slapping together different materials to test out different hypotheses and theories while investors apply pressure to rush a favorable outcome. Too often, theories are treated as fact before they ever get a chance to be proven—or disproven. That's especially the case with chronic illness. It's extremely rare in the medicine of chronic illness that you ever get a straight answer that's correct.

Wouldn't it be nice if science were the ideal we sometimes make it out to be? If it were a pursuit where money never mattered and only the truth won out? Like any human pursuit, medical science is still a work in progress. Think about the recent recognition of the mesentery as an organ. Here this active, mesh-like connective tissue has been hiding in plain sight in the gut all along and even acknowledged along the way, and only now is it beginning to get its full due. There's more to come;

new breakthroughs occur every day. Science is constantly evolving, and so theories that one day seem like they're heading to a huge discovery can be revealed the next day to be obsolete or even harmful. Ideas that one day seem laughable can be proven the next to be life-saving. What this translates to is: science doesn't have every answer yet.

We've already waited 100-plus years for real insights from medical communities into how people who live with chronic health problems can get better—and they haven't come. You shouldn't have to wait another 50 or more years for scientific research to let the right people in the door to find the real answers. You shouldn't have to wait a lifetime for medical research and science to stop ignoring the truth that they don't have the answers for chronic illness yet, and to stop pushing unfounded theories and dressing them up to look like answers while keeping people disempowered and in the dark. If you're stuck in bed, dragging through your days, or feeling lost about your health, you shouldn't have to go through one more day of it, let alone another decade. You shouldn't have to watch your children go through it either—and yet millions do.

A HIGHER SOURCE

That's why Spirit of the Most High, God's expression of compassion whom I call Spirit of Compassion, came into my life when I was four years old: to teach me how to see the true causes of people's suffering and to get that information out into the world. If you'd like to know more about my origins, you'll find my story in *Medical Medium: Secrets Behind Chronic and Mystery Illness and How to Finally*

Heal. The short version is that Spirit of Compassion constantly speaks into my ear with clarity and precision, as if a friend were standing beside me, filling me in on the symptoms of everyone around me. Plus, Spirit of Compassion taught me from an early age to see physical scans of people, like supercharged MRI scans that reveal all blockages, illnesses, infections, trouble areas, and past problems.

We see you. We know what you're up against. And we don't want you to go through it a moment longer. My life's work is to deliver this information to you so that you can be elevated above the sea of confusion—the noise and rhetoric of today's health fads and trends—in order to regain your health and navigate life on your own terms.

The material in this book is authentic, the real deal, all for your healing benefit. This book is not like other health books. There is so much packed in here that you may want to come back and read it again and again to make sure you get all the information to heal and protect yourself and your loved ones. Sometimes this information has surely seemed to be the opposite of what you've heard before, and sometimes it's probably sounded closer to other sources, with subtle and critical differences.

The reason it could sound similar to health information already out there is that before I started to publish the Medical Medium books, I spent the previous 30-plus years spreading this advanced medical and spiritual information to tens of thousands of individuals, many of them professionals in the field of health who needed help with their most difficult cases. Throughout the years, the chronically ill, along with doctors, nurses, and health coaches, have learned information from my lectures and my personal guidance using Spirit of Compassion, and they've spread it to other sources. You'll notice that because these other sources have mixed this information with misdirected ideas along the way, when you hear versions of this health information out in the world, it has holes in it. In this book and its companion books in the series, you've finally found the origin, the real source. The whole truth is here. It's not repackaged or recycled theory made to sound like a new understanding of chronic symptoms and illness. The information here doesn't come from broken science, interest groups, medical funding with strings attached, botched research, lobbyists, internal kickbacks, persuaded belief systems, private panels of influencers, health-field payoffs, or trendy traps.

In Search of Truth

Those hurdles—from interest groups to trends to payoffs—get in the way of medical research and science making the leaps and bounds it's meant to in understanding chronic illness and what heals it. Think about this: If you're a scientist with a theory, once you've conjured that theory, you need to get investors. That means you need to pitch to them. If investors like your pitch, it's usually because they want to see a certain outcome, and so they fund your endeavor. This comes with incalculable pressure to produce favorable, tangible results and proof that justify the amount of money the investors poured into it. Scientists in this position are afraid that if they blow it, they'll never get another investor to back another theory again, and their name won't hold any merit within the profession.

That doesn't leave much space for scientists or lab technicians to follow what's supposed to be the natural path of inquiry: to have ideas not pan out sometimes, go in unexpected directions, or reveal that certain foundational beliefs that started an endeavor to begin with are faulty. This constriction calls into question whether the reportedly breakthrough study results we read about are always quite as favorable as they appear. When outside sources have a vested interest in obscuring certain truths for their own gain, then precious research time and money get spent in unproductive areas. Certain discoveries that would truly advance the treatment of chronic illness get ignored and lose funding, which closes the door for virology to advance and find critical life-saving discoveries to prevent autoimmune disease. The scientific data we think of as absolute can, instead, be skewed—contaminated and manipulated—and then treated by other health experts as law, even though it's inherently flawed. That's why trying to keep up with health information is so confusing and conflicting. Most of it is not truth.

Medical Medium cleanses have already proven themselves to be effective, tested in people's hands and people's homes with no agenda or funding to force a certain outcome. The documentation is only growing that the 3:6:9 Cleanse and other Medical Medium cleanse techniques and Medical Medium information are helping people. They are becoming more and more validated by the day. The millions of people getting better from celery juice, many of whom are changing nothing in their lives other than adding celery juice, take it out of the realm of the theoretical and into the domain of medical truth. In its original meaning, science is knowledge. I've seen no more certain knowledge than that in the eyes of someone who, after trying everything, has seen Medical Medium information such as celery juice, the Heavy Metal Detox Smoothie, and the 3:6:9 Cleanse take them from bedridden to alive again.

Where Are the Citations?

To go with the facts and figures about cleansing and chronic illness throughout this book, you'll notice you haven't seen citations or mentions of scientific studies spawned from unproductive sources. You don't need to worry that the information here will be proven wrong or superseded, as you do with other health books, because all of the health information I share here comes from a pure, untampered-with, advanced, clean source—a higher source: Spirit of Compassion. There's nothing more healing than compassion.

If you're someone who only believes in what science has to say, know that I like science too. When it comes to chronic illness, though, the industries using science for conventional and "natural" medical treatments are mostly selling drugs and nutraceuticals and are often corrupt. While we're in a great time, where it seems like advancements, from heart surgery to cancer imaging, are raining out of the sky everywhere, we're also sicker and more tired than ever before in history. If medical professionals had any idea what really causes people's suffering, there would be a revolution in the way we think about nearly every aspect of our health.

Unlike many other areas of science, which are strongly founded on weights and measures and math, scientific thinking about chronic illness is all still theoretical—and today's theories hold very little truth, which is why so many people are still dealing with chronic symptoms and conditions. If it keeps going like this, we'll reach a point where there won't be any studies at all in which agendas and interests aren't driving the outcomes against your favor. This trend is why the scientific establishment has let chronic illness communities down since the beginning, letting doctors down too, and leaving hundreds of millions to suffer. You don't need to be one of them.

QUESTION EVERYTHING

Once upon a time, we lived by the rule of authority. We were told that the earth was flat, and then that the sun revolved around the earth, so we believed it. Those theories weren't fact, and yet people treated them like they were. People living back then didn't feel like life was backward; it was just the way life was. Anyone who spoke out against the status quo seemed like a fool. Then came the paradigm shift of science. The questioners—the committed researchers and thinkers—the ones who all along hadn't been content to take a "fact" at face value finally proved that analysis could open the door to a much deeper, truer understanding of our world.

Now science has become the new authority. In some cases, this saves lives. Surgeons now use sterile tools, for example, because they understand the risk of contamination that surgeons of old didn't realize. Just because we've benefited from certain advancements, though, we can't stop actively questioning. It's time for that next paradigm shift. "Because science" isn't enough of an answer when it comes to chronic illness. Is it *good* science? What was the funding behind it? Was the sample size diverse enough? Big enough? Were the controls handled ethically? Were enough factors considered? Were the measurement tools advanced enough? Does the analysis stamped on the results tell a different story from the numbers themselves? Was the study rushed? Was there bias? Did an influencer with establishment power put a thumb on the scale? Some science will hold up brilliantly under this questioning. Some will reveal holes: payoffs, kickbacks, small sample sizes, poor controls. We're handed the word *science* as though we're meant to bow down to it without question—because we haven't shifted out of the authoritative belief system as much as we think. Progress doesn't happen without the very framework being questioned—and in our society today, we're not allowed to question the scientific framework.

Trends don't always look like trends. They often disguise themselves as sound medical advice. So much of the health information out there is repetition or, worse, garbled and distorted whisper-down-the-lane. We must be wary of someone sending out a message with an agenda so that when it reaches us, it's twisted. Good primary sources used to be the gold standard. Now, in an enormous push for content, some research for health literature gets rushed, published based on one okay-enough-sounding source. We must look at the special interests of those who are interpreting and posting. Even the research results themselves—can they be trusted?

Then there are the articles written by health hobbyists that get published on the Internet with no scientific studies behind them—which doesn't stop other health hobbyists from citing these articles as though they were based on science. Seeing these headlines, you may never realize there was no scientific study performed. Another tactic to look out for: articles that are backdated or changed as it's convenient. For example, an article could be written today with information that was stolen recently, and then the piece could be published online with an older date to make it look like the information was known years ago. Old articles get quietly manipulated too. We're in a place where integrity and fairness are not the norm anymore.

Food Wars

Science is so often used as an attack mechanism. That label can be used to put a spin on everything possible. Take the food wars, for example. Vegan and plant-based folks are battling paleo and animal-product keto folks with science as their sword and shield. Paleo and animal-product keto folks are battling vegan and plant-based folks with science as *their* sword and shield. They're both using studies to justify their sides—because you can find a study to justify practically anything. Never mind if the study was authentic or if other researchers even stand behind its methodologies. Never mind if the study only looked at 10 to 20 people of the same age and background who were paid for their participation, and if that's leading to gross generalizations and misinformation.

We're supposed to sit up and listen to anything that comes after the word *science* because conventional thinking would have you believe that science offers clear answers. People on all sides of any debate have learned to use that to their advantage. Are you willing to trust your life to debate tactics? It should tell you something when science plays both offense and defense for two warring camps; it should tell you that some of that science can't be real.

Some of it is flawed science, some of it is fake science, and some of it is underdeveloped science. Each side uses science specifically geared to its cause. Animal-product science doesn't believe in plant-based science. Plant-based science doesn't believe in animal-product science. These science entities are against each other. Meanwhile, the conventional mainstream medical science entity does not even treat food as medicine yet. Conventional medical science doesn't support either of these food science entities. So whose science is real and legitimate and whose isn't?

When even science isn't enough, food war participants go for the emotional aspect of the other's belief system. Vegan and plant-based folks tell paleo and animal-product keto folks they're killing animals. Paleo and animal-product keto folks tell vegan and plant-based folks they're starving themselves and their children.

Meanwhile, they all still get sick. *Regardless of the studies or beliefs they cite to try to disprove each other, they all encounter health challenges that neither they nor science understand.* Perhaps an illness comes and then goes . . . and then comes back three months or years later. It can be easier to brush off the first time. When someone falls victim to health trouble again—for example with an autoimmune issue such as eczema, psoriasis, ME/CFS, MS, celiac, Lyme disease, or Hashimoto's thyroiditis, or with PCOS, endometriosis, fibroids, anxiety, depression, brain fog, bloating, Crohn's, colitis, or vertigo—it can bring up doubt. Whatever belief system previously fit their agenda falls under scrutiny. If they'd been skittish about veganism to begin with and ran into trouble on a high-protein or high-fat, plant-based diet, plant foods seem like an easy reason to

blame for why they're sick. When someone from the animal-protein camp gets sick, sometimes they'll blame the food. More often, since animal protein holds such a heralded, god-like place in today's society, it doesn't get the blame. Instead, that person searches for other problems, cross-examining themselves about their attitude and whether they think positively enough, sometimes heading off on a spiritual retreat because they think they've caused their health decline with their thoughts. Or maybe they blame it on a piece of fruit they ate, or they look for mold, or they blame it on stress.

People from both camps find themselves on wild goose chases as they seek out doctors of alternative medicine and keep busy worrying about the microbiome, bacterial overgrowth in the gut, metabolism issues, or nutrient deficiencies. It's very easy to convince the plant-based camp that their symptoms are caused by deficiencies of vitamins, minerals, or especially protein, *Candida*, or leaky gut. Meanwhile, those in the animal-protein camp are just as nutrient deficient, although their diets are far less likely to get the blame at the doctor's office. Instead, they'll hear that it's from gene mutations or autoimmune. Sure, some slight improvements can come when either camp goes on assorted supplements and starts changing their routine a little and altering their foods. For most everyone, improvements will only be temporary because everyone is still lost. It's all still a guessing game.

Getting better is not about choosing sides or what you've adopted as a belief system in that moment—even if it's a belief system based on reports you've read of scientific studies. It's about understanding that we've been tricked along the way and that we also need to understand the true causes of why we're really sick.

An Open Heart

We won't get anywhere by treating science as God and treating those who question theories and findings as fools. Medical science looks out for medical science. While individual health-care providers can have the best of intentions, the greater industry is not about looking out for a person; it's about looking out for itself, since it has its authority to uphold. It's self-involvement in the most chronic way.

Let's be honest. Even today's science in those areas we think of as concrete sometimes shows cracks. If you've heard about recalls of hip replacement parts or hernia mesh, you know what I'm talking about. These are tangible items that were designed with exacting scientific standards, then went through rigorous scientific testing before being put to use, and even that highly scientific process wasn't guaranteed. Certain products developed unforeseen problems, and an area of science that seemed indisputable turned out to be fallible. Think, then, what kind of uncertainty remains in scientific understanding of chronic illness and how cleansing can alleviate it. The 3:6:9 Cleanse isn't a device that can be held in your hand, measured, and analyzed as solely independent from the rest of you. It's a protocol that taps into the body's undiscovered rhythms, and we all know the human body to be one of the greatest miracles and mysteries of life. If a protocol works with detoxification abilities of the liver that science doesn't even know exist yet, to go after problems in our bodies that science doesn't know exist yet, how can we trust any source that says

cleansing is bogus? Again, science is a human pursuit and a work in progress, especially when that work involves decoding the human body. It takes constant vigilance, receptiveness, humility, and adaptability to keep that work truly progressing.

If you've never struggled with your health, suffering for years with no answers for your condition, or if you feel cemented within a certain medical, scientific, or nutritional belief system, I hope that you read these words with curiosity and an open heart. The meaning behind today's widespread chronic symptoms and suffering is so much bigger than anyone has yet discovered. What you'll read here is unlike any information about chronic health issues or healing you've seen before. It's information that has helped millions of people heal over the past decades.

BATTLING MISINFORMATION

When you're feeling strong, it may seem inconceivable that bathing or brushing your teeth could feel as exhausting as running a marathon for those who are struggling with their health. That's one reason why the chronically ill often face so much discrimination: because from the outside looking in, they may look "fine" or "normal." Until it happens to you, you'd never think that hearing "But you look great!" could feel so demoralizing when you're feeling just the opposite. It's a natural human drive to want validation for our suffering—and for our healing. And yet, when it comes to chronic illness, and when it comes to *healing* from chronic illness, that validation can be sorely lacking.

The Intimidation Factor

Healthy skepticism is one thing, if it's also accompanied by curiosity and openness. Instead, what we see all too often are bullies—because again, the chronically ill have always been bullied. Bullying is not something everyone left behind decades ago on the school playground. It's alive and well on social media, at workplaces—if someone with chronic illness can still work—and even in people's homes.

In larger numbers, people who've been hiding their suffering from the world are using social media to express themselves. The world can have a surprising reaction to this. When a person shares her story of illness, she'll often find acceptance on the Internet, or at least she'll be left alone to express herself. While there may be some doubters in the comments, the noise will be at a tolerable level—until she begins to heal.

Once she starts voicing a story of getting better, that's when the bullying can really arise. It's a sad truth of today that when the army of the chronically ill rises up and starts finding relief, that's when people really start to receive flak and flagellations, sometimes even direct antagonism. When someone finds an answer such as celery juice, they may get picked on, as if they have no right to heal or to share about it. That's when the hate parade can begin.

It's almost as if some people want the chronically ill to stay down, hidden, quiet, and meek. They don't want these brave, forgotten souls to express the truth of their suffering, or worse, the truth of what's finally healing them. Keeping the chronically ill down grants power to the people who have no compassion. It makes them feel better than the chronically ill,

better about their selfish selves and their lack of caring for others. It's a way to control the chronically ill.

Because the chronically ill usually have confidence problems from suffering for so long, a feeding frenzy of antagonism can instantly stymie them, which is exactly the intended result of the coldhearted souls who don't want the chronically ill to get their bearings back or rise out of the ashes—who don't want the chronically ill to sing joy. They want them feeling inadequate, useless, and hopeless so that they can manipulate them energetically, systematically, and corruptively to their liking.

I know this sounds drastic. I wish it weren't true. As new as this intimidation factor seems today, though, and as specific as it seems to the Internet and social media, it's a tactic that's been around for centuries. People with leprosy (once known as lepers) went through it. People with HIV in the 1980s and '90s went through it. Now the chronically ill on the whole are going through it.

So when you tell the truth about the struggles happening in someone's life, whether a loved one's or your own, and when you point out that this should not be the norm, you can draw scrutiny. When you go beyond that and share advanced information that's ahead of medical research and science about how to get better, you can experience blowback. Where does the blowback often come from? From the not-so-sick or the very few who aren't dealing with symptoms (who are usually men, by the way). Always remember that any scrutiny, naysayers, or negativity you ever face in life about the powerful, good actions you take means you're doing the right thing. It means you're making a difference—because it stimulates jealousy out there in the world of disapproval.

Remember too that the work you put into your healing is profound and powerful. It speaks to others who need that healing truth, that healing information, that inspiration to be hopeful and not want to give up. Your healing tells others that there is a way out from suffering and that they can heal too when they offer the body what it really needs. When you inspire people to get out of bed and fight for their health freedom and recover—those are the ones you're speaking to. There's no greater work on a spiritual level than changing people's lives so they see the light and realize that their bodies aren't faulty, that they're not bad people, and that they deserve to feel better, get better, and heal like you have. So the work you're doing by spreading your story of healing overrides the noise and scrutiny from others who have no compassion or care about people's struggles, hardships, and suffering. You're a world changer now. You have to remember that there are silent, reserved viewers and listeners who found you when they were in the midst of struggle and are taking your words to heart. They want to take your advice and information seriously and apply it to rise out of the ashes and heal. We're all in this together. We have to remember this.

All in This Together

Since I first started to share Spirit of Compassion's information, I've been so blessed to see it make a difference for the people who have found it. With the publication of the Medical Medium book series, I've been incredibly moved to see this information reach the wider world and help thousands more.

I've also noticed that some of these messages have been manipulated as certain career-driven individuals try to climb the ladder of acclaim and notoriety. This approach touches the raw nerve of suffering at people's core and takes advantage of it.

This is not how the gift I was given was ever meant to be used. Spirit of Compassion is a voice for the ones in need of answers, a source independent from any system filled with traps that have wasted so many lives along the way. We love it when people become experts on the health information I share and cite this original source, and when they spread the compassionate message far and wide in the name of truly helping others. I am so thankful for this. It gets dangerous when that information is tampered with—intermixed and twisted with trendy misinformation, changed just enough so that it sounds original, or blatantly poached and attributed to seemingly credible sources that are anemic of the truth. This leads to people who are suffering with chronic illness trusting the sources that hijacked and altered this information, which in turn means that people in need of healing can't find their way back to the original source. I say this because I want you to know to protect yourself and your loved ones from the misguidance out there.

This book is not repetition of everything you've already read. It is not about a belief system that blames your genes or says your body is faulty, nor is it about putting a spin on a trendy high-fat or high-protein diet to keep symptoms at bay. Because it comes from a higher source, it's not human-based theory. It's information, and it's being applied and studied as people bring it into their lives. This information is fresh—an entirely new perspective on the symptoms holding back so many people in life, and an entirely new perspective on how to heal.

As I mentioned earlier, I respect critics. If you're one of those critics, I respect you. Critics want to learn. Critics put in the work. They'll read the material here and *then* decide its value, not write it off without taking time to understand it. I get it if you're wary as you approach these pages. We react, we judge; that's what we do. It can be an instinct that protects us in certain circumstances; sometimes, it gets us through life. In this case, I hope you'll reconsider. You may judge yourself out of learning the truth. You could lose the opportunity to help yourself or somebody else.

I want you to become the new expert on protecting yourself and your family from the pathogens and toxins of this world. We are all in this together with getting people better.

FAR FROM ALONE

Long after we're gone, this information will still be here for those who come next. In that sense, it is timeless. This planet will continue to present challenges, often in the form of pathogens and other toxic troublemakers, to the people living on it. The human body will continue to hold the capacity for healing—if the coming generations know how to tap into its cleansing rhythms.

Many people who have discovered the Medical Medium information make it a part of their family. They hope that this will be part of their legacy, that their loved ones will continue to use this healing knowledge to protect themselves when they can no longer do that job. While we're still here, sometimes we'll need to fight for this information and fend off the bullying. We can do that with a greater sense of purpose. We can even do it with a sense of humor.

When you find yourself challenged to defend yourself, remember that you are far from alone. You are part of an empowering movement. By standing up for yourself, you are standing up for the crowd of people with hopes and dreams for their lives who do not deserve to be held back by chronic suffering.

Thank you for coming with me on this healing journey and taking the time to read this book. Bringing the truths you read here into your life will change everything for you and the ones around you.

"Always remember that any scrutiny, naysayers, or negativity you ever face in life about the powerful, good actions you take means you're doing the right thing. It means your light is changing the world."

— Anthony William, Medical Medium

CHAPTER 25

The Emotional Side of Cleansing

Cleansing is an emotional venture all on its own. Just the thought of changing our foods from the norm we're used to can stimulate emotion. Many of us don't like change, and we're afraid of embarking on something new. Even if you're someone who loves to try new things, including new foods, you may still find that the idea of cleansing brings up emotions.

It's a challenging endeavor to change up what we're used to eating every day. So many of us like to eat what we want, even if we keep that within relatively healthy guidelines. A cleanse, by definition, is restrictive. The 3:6:9 Cleanse is no different. Its restrictions are in place to protect us: to make sure that the pathogens that reside inside of us do not get fed, that they starve, that the toxic fuel that feeds them gets cleaned out too, and that at the same time *we're* not starving.

So many of us have emotional injuries around food, whether from being told what to eat as a child, being forced to eat something at school, being told we're not eating right, being reprimanded or challenged by our family for eating differently, or not being able to afford enough food growing up. We all

sustain little or big emotional injuries around food. Many families think their teen or young adult has an eating disorder if they start eating like a friend who's making healthier choices. A lot of "Where's your protein?" concern comes into play, or "Science says you need more fat in your diet to be healthy." They may be peer pressured by family and friends because they're leaving the pack.

When you embark on a cleanse, similar concern may be directed your way. Others may make you feel like you're not normal—if "normal" is everyone getting a pizza and enjoying a slice (or three) together, going out to dinner and ordering barbecue, or digging into macaroni and cheese. When we try to eat for our health, it can spark insecurity in everyone else because it makes them question their own food choices, and having that insecurity directed at and projected onto us can stir up our old emotional experiences around eating. If you have a history of disordered eating, you've since stabilized from that and reached a healthier place, and now you're trying one of the cleanses in this book, you can feel a sense of sadness if people around you start to fear you're back in eating disorder territory. It may bring up a bit of what you went through in your darkest hour.

Keep in mind that everyone has issues around eating. There's no one who doesn't, because there's never been a perfect situation with our food, ever. Our forebears waited in line during the Depression for a loaf of bread, and they never forgot that; they passed the stories along. Or maybe you were alive at the time and experienced the rationing yourself, on top of the times of struggle you heard about from your own ancestors about failed crops or earlier wartime food shortages. All the way back to the beginning, worry has been part of our relationship with food because food is part of our survival. Generation to generation, that's been instilled in us.

Many siblings at the dinner table, not enough food to go around, and everyone leaving the table hungry night after night—this can lead to strong particularities around food as an adult, even if the preferences are ones so deeply instilled in us as survival techniques that we're unaware of them, or if they're not what anyone would label an eating disorder. Survival techniques around food can also repeat themselves generation after generation, with so many different varieties of particularities reoccurring, whether because we learned them from our parents or grandparents or because difficult circumstances repeated themselves. Relatives don't necessarily believe there are eating disorders within their family network; it becomes part of the norm. Misinformation and mistaken theories about food also get passed along from family before us. Brainwashing about protein from decades ago gets perpetuated. Availability and affordability of fresh food resources, the need to rely on canned food or fast food—it's different for everyone and creates imbalances for us all.

That's right: everybody's eating is imbalanced. When a health professional says, "Oh, you need to eat a balanced diet," who's to say their "balanced" diet is correct or even balanced? It's not. It's a decision by some man out in the world about what we should or should not eat, an opinion that he then schooled a group of health professionals into believing. Beliefs and interpretations about what's balanced are rampant, inherited, everywhere.

At the same time, so many people have so many things going wrong with their health. So many people have pathogens active inside them causing their symptoms and conditions, and no one understands that—not the doctors, not the dieticians. If we're going to change that and heal, we need to change our food. The Medical Medium information that I share from Spirit of Compassion centers around specifics on what to eat and what not to eat for personal, individual situations because throwing around the term "balanced" isn't an answer. Balanced for whom? Balanced for what health issue? Who really knows what to eat or not if they don't know the real reasons why people are sick? It's all guesswork.

So don't be intimidated when you hear the term *balanced diet*. Those who promote the idea are confused and misled. Everyone has issues around food, even those who say they don't govern their lives around food, that they just live their lives. "I don't think about food" or "I'm not trapped by rules around food"—that whole game is really a sign that someone is a prisoner to their food. We're all wrapped up in food, from different tastes to dislikes to emotional issues. An experience as simple as a babysitter striking a child's hand for reaching in the cookie jar could leave a lasting impression, and that's without even eating. It's endless. An endless—well, brainscrew. And it's not all negative, not remotely. Food is life. We *have* to think about food. It's reality, and no one is above reality. It's part of the human condition on earth.

Keep this in mind as you embark on your cleanse. If emotions come up, that's perfectly natural—and we'll get to exactly why in a moment. If cravings come up, those too have explanations. We live with a lot stored up inside of us—emotions, toxins, viruses, unproductive bacteria—and they're more tied up with each other than anyone realizes. The 3:6:9 Cleanse and the other Medical Medium cleanses are ways to release them safely. If every moment of cleansing isn't happy and shiny and social media–ready, don't let it worry you. You are steering your own ship now, and the ups and downs as waves of emotion come and go are part of a greater rhythm. Keep your eye on the horizon and know that all of it is beneficial, setting you up to reap rewards long after the cleanse while carrying you to a better and healthier place in life.

DECODING CRAVINGS

You won't necessarily experience cravings while on the cleanses in this book. Cravings vary person by person and day by day and even minute by minute. If you do experience cravings, they're very natural—and to ride them out, it helps to understand why they're happening.

Pathogenic Die-Off

First, let's be clear that a craving for a bacon cheeseburger or a sausage, egg, and cheese sandwich while on a cleanse is not your body telling you that you need fat or protein. It *is* a signal coming from within your body . . . only it's not originating *from* your body itself, and it doesn't want to help you. When we withhold our standard comfort foods, emotions start to surface. One reason cravings occur is that when we withhold troublemaker foods, viruses and unproductive bacteria begin to starve. Because they're not getting the foods they want (such as eggs, gluten, and dairy), these pathogens start to excrete signal chemicals. The chemicals can then enter our brain and stimulate hunger messaging receptors, triggering us to want those very foods.

When you understand this, it can be a lot easier to feel some distance from a craving and let it pass by—because you don't want to be at the beck and call of a viral or bacterial strain, do you? You want to be the one in control, taking away its fuel source and ushering the pathogen out of your body. You can even take cravings as a good sign, one that the viruses and bacteria in your body are losing strength—and doing a little whining on the way out.

As you read in Chapter 20, "Your Body's Healing Power," some of us also feel a little sicker when we start to cleanse. That can have an emotional effect too; it can stir up fear and doubt that cleansing is the right thing to do and make us question whether we should go back to eating our normal foods. At the very least, it can make us crave those comfort foods. It helps to know what's really happening: that we're often viral without realizing it, and that viruses as well as viral neurotoxins and dermatoxins have filled up our fat cells. Those fat cells protect us in a way in everyday life, making us feel less sick because they act as a buffer. When we start cleansing fat cells, which means that the viruses and viral waste they've absorbed get released, that's when we can feel a little under the weather for a little while. You don't have to have weight on you to experience this; I'm not just talking about the fat cells that may be visible as extra weight. We all have fat cells within our organs that can suspend viruses and viral waste, and so any of us can experience these effects of cleansing them. While it can make us worry that we're temporarily moving backward, it's really a sign of release that will move us forward.

If someone feels sicker during a cleanse and they're dealing with more pronounced fatigue, it's a sign that they've been viral for a very long time. It means that neurotoxins—whether from one of the over 30 varieties of shingles, one of the over 60 varieties of EBV, herpes simplex, HHV-6, CMV, or the many other varieties of undiscovered herpetic family viruses—are already saturating their body and making them sick. When they cleanse, it's bringing out even more neurotoxins. Tricky as this is, it's what we need to do to heal. We need the viruses to die, and when they die, they're going to release neurotoxins and dermatoxins. It wouldn't help us to keep the neurotoxin buildup, nor would it help us to keep the viruses alive and active. Starving viruses and boosting your immune system with a cleanse is only going to help you in the long run, so that you can get out of your illness completely. You can protect yourself through the ups and downs of the healing process with this knowledge that underneath it all, you're making incredible progress.

For special insights into the emotional side of cleansing viral neurotoxins, see "More Secrets of Viral Cleansing" later in this chapter.

Adrenaline Release

Pathogens aren't always behind our cravings when we avoid certain foods. Cravings also have an emotional component. People tend to belong to one of two schools when it comes to eating and emotions. In the one school are folks who eat to take their mind off their pain. When we're in this school and we take away certain comfort foods, sometimes we start to experience a few feelings we were trying to use food to suppress. That old, familiar sadness, loneliness, fear, shame, guilt, or anger starts to cast a shadow over our thoughts, or even creeps in as a sinking in the stomach or tightness in the chest, and in that moment, the pleasures of pizza or mac and cheese or ice cream seem like the perfect antidote.

I say "trying" to suppress because does eating really suppress emotions? Only temporarily. And is suppression the real goal? Probably not—healing is. True emotional suppression can happen sometimes, when you've been harmed and the adrenaline that harbors the pain of that trauma gets stored deep in the neurons of the emotional centers of the brain. That's usually not a bad thing; emotional walls exist to protect us. Other than this truly suppressed trauma, though, pain tends to resurface. When we start thinking about it again, we feel that urge to eat certain foods again, and that can keep happening over and over again if we don't know which foods can actually help our brains and bodies heal.

One of the reasons we consume comfort foods in the first place is to sop up the adrenaline that comes with emotional disturbances or conflicts. Traditional comfort foods (think tacos, nachos, pizza, mac and cheese, ice cream, spaghetti with meatballs, pancakes, French fries, lobster with butter, chicken wings, pulled pork sandwiches, grilled cheese, fried eggs) are usually high in fat; that fat is what's doing the sopping up. Once fat has soaked up adrenaline, the stress hormone becomes trapped in our fat cells—fat cells that then become part of us as they take up residence in our organs. Here's the key point: adrenaline holds information. In the case of adrenaline that was released at highly emotional times, it holds information about the fear, hurt, betrayal, injury, or stress overload we were experiencing in that moment.

The minute we start taking away these comfort foods, such as when we're on one of the cleanses in this book, the old fat cells start to dissolve, and that releases the adrenaline that had been trapped away. Past emotions tied to the adrenaline can surface, and that can make us want to reach for the foods we ate last time around to tamp them back down. Rationally, we know that picking up the pizza (whether regular or even vegan), ice cream (dairy-free or not), or pastry (regular or gluten-free) can lead to cycles of sadness and depression. The gratification of traditional comfort foods only lasts so long, and we can only eat so much of them. Cravings aren't about rationality, though. So how do you handle the magnetic pull of temptation? By connecting to this new knowledge about the physiological reasons why cravings arise. Knowledge puts the power in your hands. The cleanses in this book are about eating foods that help you cleanse adrenaline rather than store it and can comfort you at the same time on a spiritual and soul level.

Let's also not forget about the other school of emotions and eating. In this school are folks who prefer to avoid food when they're in pain. Often triggered because their emotions have taken away their appetite or made them feel sick, this approach can turn into an addiction to having no appetite, where they become afraid to eat because it feels like a loss of control. They already feel that they don't have control over their environment or situations happening around them or people in their life, and so, whether consciously or subconsciously, they try to exert extreme control over what they put into their mouths. (People from the other school, those who overeat, often struggle with loss of control too; they happen to have a different way of dealing with the sensation.) For those who withhold food, while food cravings may still surface, and surface intensely, their even stronger craving is *not* to eat, or to eat very little. One doesn't always stay in this pattern forever. Sometimes hunger can become overpowering—because the body can only function for so long with adrenaline filling in for critically needed blood sugar—to the point that somebody ends up switching over to the other school. Our organs, especially our brain, require the natural sugar of glucose to feed cells so we can stay strong and function. Suddenly, someone who withheld food may find themselves reaching for those foods they tried to avoid for so long—again, unless they know which foods can actually help the brain and body heal.

Toxin Release

Adrenaline isn't all that gets stored away in our organs and fat cells. Along with the adrenaline are environmental and pathogenic toxins as well as toxins from troublemaker foods themselves. When we start to cleanse, these toxins can start to surface as they travel through the bloodstream on the way out of the body, and with that can come cravings for the same foods that trapped the toxins. Take, for example, pizza. As you embark on a cleanse that takes pizza away, your body can finally start to rid itself of any buried remainders of that food. And along with the food's fat cells and residues will surface whatever toxins your body was trying to process and expel at the time you ate that food—or whatever gluten in the crust, pharmaceuticals such as antibiotics in the dairy products, toxic hormones, heavy metals, or other toxins the food contained and had to bury because processing the troublemaker food itself took priority.

When cravings arise as a result of this toxin release, it's another instance of detox cravings as good signs that mean your system is cleaning itself out. Back to that idea that an intense, specific craving for a food does not mean your body is experiencing a deficiency: if you're overcome by the need for a bacon cheeseburger while cleansing, there's a good chance that it means your body is letting go of pathogenic fuel that was inside of a bacon cheeseburger or similar food you ate in the past. That's exactly why you're cleansing in the first place: to let go. If you interrupt that process by actually reaching for the cheeseburger, you'll work against your very intention. You don't need to waste mental energy deciphering what the craving is telling you, because now you know:

pathogenic die-off, fat cell dissolution, and adrenaline and toxin release. You'll serve your healing process best by reaching for one of the flavor-rich cleanse foods instead and reminding yourself exactly why you're doing that.

Fluid Retention Release

When we're detoxing, it's not only about fat cell release. We're also cleansing toxic fluid from our lymphatic system. When our bodies are overloaded with troublemakers, our lymph glands fill with a thick and stagnant yellow sludge that's loaded with poisons and toxins, ranging from viral and bacterial byproduct to adrenaline released during intense situations to poisons and toxins that have overflowed from our liver and become trapped in our lymphatic system. As polluted as that fluid has become, it's a protector; it's there in the lymphatic system to keep toxins diluted slightly, so their concentrations are less aggressive.

As the fluid becomes more and more polluted with troublemakers, we start to retain water. That can add pounds to the scale and contribute to a weight problem that we may misconstrue as solely fat buildup. Most of the time, a significant proportion of weight gain is, in truth, water retention. Someone could be carrying around 5, 10, 15, or 20 pounds of retained fluid as their lymphatic system fights to keep toxins suspended. You could be 40 pounds overweight, for example, and 15 to 20 pounds of it could be this sludgy fluid retention. There are even situations where someone is 100 pounds overweight and 30 to 40 pounds of it could be water retention. While not everyone has that much, many people do have a lot.

When people start to change their diet and detox with one of these cleanses, they may experience rapid weight loss at first as this polluted sludge leaves the lymphatic system and heads to the kidneys and sweat glands to be eliminated. That's a healthful, positive process. It can also come with some emotions, since the fluid buildup can contain adrenaline from past emotional situations, a lot of pathogenic byproduct (both bacterial and viral), and other toxins. As that's released, waves of sorrow, fear, guilt, shame, or feelings of being lost and confused can surface. As you saw above, toxins are really intense emotionally. Some waves will be bigger and some will be smaller, and they may bring cravings with them. It's all about riding out these short, temporary storms as everything is being released so you can come out unburdened and stronger for it when the waves calm and the sky clears.

HOW TO COPE

If you've experienced even the mildest emotions around food—and everyone has—you could feel some of them come up when you do the 3:6:9 Cleanse or any other cleanse. Without your standby comfort foods to distract from the daily pain and sorrow of whatever you've dealt with in life, you could start to miss your usual fancy coffee drink, matcha latte, bagel with cream cheese, or even comfort foods you haven't leaned on in a while for the reasons we just explored.

These cravings won't unmoor you, though, because here's what sets Medical Medium cleanses apart from whatever else you've heard about or tried before: They're designed to feed you. They're designed to nourish you. They're designed to offer you emotional and even spiritual support at the same time that they're helping you heal on a deeper physical level than ever before—which in the long term helps cravings start to lose their grip on your life.

While you're cleansing, can it be tough to miss the foods that usually bring you comfort? Sure. There's not much chance to dwell on the cravings, though, because throughout the day, you're reaching for a beverage or a meal or a snack that gives your brain fuel for repair and makes your liver happy and is easy on digestion. This combination can come as an enormous relief; we have no idea how much an overheated, overloaded liver and a taxed digestive tract can affect our state of mind.

And brain support—real brain support—can come as a revelation. We're so used to starving our brain (and the rest of our body) of glucose; too much fat in the bloodstream keeps cells from being able to access and absorb this critical fuel. When we lower our dietary fat and our brain cells actually start receiving high-quality glucose, not to mention rich mineral salts from living sources such as celery juice, our brain can heal and function at a new level, changing our entire relationship with cravings and challenging emotions.

Some cleanses out there are reckless. It's right to be wary of how they may affect you emotionally. Even water fasting, which does have its uses when done right, can create a flood of emotional processing and be far too intense for someone with a history of trauma.

The cleanses in this book, on the other hand, are designed to feed you and safeguard you. They can completely change your relationship with food. The 3:6:9 Cleanse is not designed to unleash horrible past experiences and torture you into a bad episode. The whole point of the 3:6:9 Cleanse is to offer healing. As long as you're following the cleanse instructions and not eating too little and putting yourself into starvation mode because you believe that's what a cleanse should be, then when emotions are released, they can't do damage because of that vital glucose that the 3:6:9 Cleanse—and the other Medical Medium cleanses—provide to the brain.

I'll say it again: glucose protects your emotional stability. It helps protect you from post-traumatic stress symptoms and emotional trauma. It's when we go into glucose deprivation on cleanses of other kinds, not to mention every-day diets that are devoid of natural sugar from fresh fruit and similar sources, that we get into harmful territory. If we're not keeping our brain cool with glucose, protecting the emotional centers of the brain, we can go into glucose deficit, and that's when we're susceptible to a relapse of trauma. The 3:6:9 Cleanse is created to do the opposite. Even with the Mono Eating Cleanse, you get enough glucose. That's part of the very purpose of any Medical Medium cleanse. Glucose is that critical.

Be Kind to Yourself

The idea of cutting out foods from your diet, even for the short space of a mini cleanse, can be loaded. For women especially, societal messaging has attached shame to food choices for far too long. I've always said that I'm not the food police, and that will always be true. Remember this: when you see a Medical Medium recommendation to limit or temporarily cut out a certain food, that is never attached to judgment. A Medical Medium cleanse is never about virtuousness versus shame. It's about healing. And from a medical perspective, shame is not healing. Instead, shame releases

a harsh adrenaline blend that's corrosive and abrasive to our nervous system and can weaken our immune system.

If you set out with the very best intentions for your health and then have a terrible, stressful day where appointment after appointment ends up on your calendar and you get over-hungry and reach for a food that's outside the cleanse because it's sitting right there in the break room, does that mean that you should feel guilty? No, never. Whatever food choice you make at whatever time, it's not "bad" or shameful. It's only that—a choice you made—and next time, you can make another choice. In the case of the 3:6:9 Cleanse, it does mean that you'll need to go back to Day 1, because food choices outside the guidelines break the cleanse. In those moments of intense craving, it may help to ask yourself, "Do I have it in me to start all over again? Or would I rather ride out this craving?"

(With the cleanses from Part III, add three days to the end of the cleanse if you break the cleanse partway through. For example, if you're doing 30 days of the Morning Cleanse and in the second week, you have a milky coffee drink, get yourself back on track and then add a 31st, 32nd, and 33rd day to the cleanse.)

When you eat a food that you know doesn't take you closer to feeling relief from your symptoms, self-punishment shouldn't come into the picture. Rather than enter that headspace, try to remind yourself gently that physically, the best choice you can make is to be kind to yourself. What does that kindness look like? It would seem like the ultimate triumph over food shame would be to eat anything you want at any time. I wish that were true. You *can* do that. It's certainly an option, if your resources allow. That will take you down a route where you end up sicker, though. Self-compassion looks more like a pause whenever you get the impulse to reach for a food that isn't part of the cleanse. It looks more like that big-picture question: "Do I have it in me to start all over again?" And it looks like respect for yourself if the answer is that this time, you made a choice you wish you hadn't. Chances are, if you do eat a troublemaker food mid-cleanse, you're going to feel enough of a difference in your gut, mood, or otherwise to encourage you to select a healing food next time.

Don't Be a Hero

Another way to show compassion for yourself is to think ahead, taking into account the fundamental truth that you get to have an appetite. Hunger is a sign of life. You have nothing to prove by going all morning without breakfast or skipping lunch. So don't try to be a hero by undereating on a cleanse! It doesn't save anyone, least of all yourself. All it does is set you up to run on adrenaline and get tired, irritable, and over-hungry (a common theme with people who are intermittent fasting)—to the point where you're far too tempted to reach for a food that makes you break the cleanse and have to start all over again.

Whenever you can, plan ahead. Prep your snacks and meals ahead of time on days you'll be away from home or when you know you'll get too busy to stop and spend time in the kitchen midday. Think about ordering cases of produce, if that's what you need to have enough ingredients on hand and make them more affordable. Take a cooler bag with food along to work or on errands or other obligations. The extra thought on the front end will save you mightily when you're in the middle of a stressful day, realize suddenly that you need to eat, and all you want is to grab a tuna fish sandwich off a tray at that lunch function you're required to attend.

Preparing for our needs instead of pretending we don't have them is far more effective in the long run. It helps us stay steady in the face of food cravings—which are often only surface cravings, in a way. Our deeper craving is to feel well. No matter what you may hear otherwise, nobody wants to stay sick. We all have an innate impulse to be well. We simply haven't been handed the tools to do that before now. With healing options at our fingertips, we're far better positioned to listen to that deeper craving and make the choice that's going to keep us on the cleanse so our body can continue its process of letting go and repairing.

As you heal, you're likely to find that the surface food cravings start to alleviate. Some will lift because your liver and brain aren't as burdened as they were before and have started getting proper glucose replenishment, giving you relief from some of the emotions that had sent you to certain comfort foods. Some will lift because enough time off troublemaker foods will give you distance to feel the difference without them—you'll realize how certain foods were directly interfering with the digestive system, neural function, and other body processes. And some will lift because the healing foods in Medical Medium cleanses in this book give you direct emotional and spiritual support. (You can read more about just how that works in *Life-Changing Foods*.)

Food is here to nourish us, and we get to enjoy it.

FATS AND FEELINGS

After an extended period of cleansing during which you've been off radical fats, it can be an adjustment to return to eating fats. The major reason that we lower or eliminate radical fats in the first place is to ease up the load on the liver. Essentially, we're eating for the liver in order to serve the brain and the rest of the body, and as we've well established, food and eating hit the emotional core in all of us. We have so many issues around foods, both growing up and living life in this hard world, and having to hold back from certain comfort foods translates to the set of experiences that we just explored. Now let's explore the feelings that come up specifically around radical fats.

Back to Life

What happens after the cleanse, when we start to diversify what we eat again? Emotions can come up then too. That's because at the end of a cleanse, we often have a sense of accomplishment and feel emotionally strong. Sometimes we're on such a high that we're not even sure we're ready to go back to regular life. So post-cleanse, if we're up against a little bit of stress or an emotional trigger and a food calls out to us at the store and we decide to eat it, even if it's a healthy food such as tahini or avocado, we might feel a little guilty. Maybe feelings of defeat or failure will come up. Maybe we'll feel that we've broken down or reversed or slowed down our healing process. Even if that's

how it feels initially, we can't look at it that way. Instead, we need to see that we succeeded. Whether we were off radical fats entirely or simply went low-fat, the fact that we did it at all is a great accomplishment for the liver and moved our healing process forward.

Sure, there's a distinction here. Grabbing some lard-filled cupcakes, frying up some bacon, or popping a frozen pizza in the oven is different from reintroducing tahini and avocado. Even in those cases, where we get triggered and eat the chocolate cake or pizza or other item that's not ideal, we still have to see our accomplishments. We can't punish ourselves for being triggered into a vice.

If we want to feel our best, then yes, it's wonderful to keep fats minimal after a cleanse such as the 3:6:9. Following the Morning Cleanse as a matter of course in your everyday life is very beneficial. And your body will love you for it if you limit radical fats to only higher-quality fats, consumed only two to three days a week (and only at lunchtime or after). That means four to five days a week where you avoid radical fats altogether. You can even stay fat-free, keeping radical fats out of your diet for as long as you'd like. Not that you deserve any judgment if this is not doable for you. It's simply knowledge for someone who's seriously focused and wants this as an option.

Any step we take to cleanse is a great accomplishment. We have to look at what we've achieved, because we have achieved some level of healing no matter how long we were on the 3:6:9 Cleanse, even if we stopped after three days. We get to recognize and celebrate that. If, after the cleanse, you need to go back and live in whatever world you're living in, the goal is to see if you can continue to avoid eggs, milk, cheese, butter, gluten, and some of the other top troublemaker foods from Chapter 7. If that's not workable and you need to go back to eggs, milk, cheese, butter, and the works, your body's going to love you for what you did on the nine-day cleanse. You succeeded majorly with it. You accomplished the greatest body cleanse you can do, one that tapped into your liver's hidden cycle of release and repair, and your liver is so critical to your well-being. This is to say that we can't punish ourselves for not being able to keep up 3:6:9 protocols in our everyday lives. There's a good chance that eventually, you will naturally get off the eggs, milk, cheese, butter, gluten, and more because you'll feel enough of a difference that it motivates you to take your health to the next level.

Physical Feelings

Going back on radical fats after a cleanse can affect how you feel physically as well as emotionally. You just went fat-free for what was most likely the first time in your life. Aside from all the other work you did to support your cleansing with special foods and drinks at special times, that on its own is incredible. If you go straight back to your normal level of fats afterward, whether that's a bunch of tahini or chicken, it's easy to feel uncomfortable. One reason it can hit you is because you're forcing your body to produce a lot of bile right after that vacation from radical fat. The other reason is that it can make you realize how hard on your body high levels of fat actually were all along.

When you eat fat-free for long enough, such as when you do the 3:6:9 Cleanse, you're just getting used to sending straight glucose to your brain for what could be the first time in your life. That experience of your neurons being fed more glucose, your neurotransmitters receiving more electrolytes, and your brain building up more glycogen storage can be life-changing. So when you switch from that freedom to having thick blood again due to too much fat in the bloodstream, it can have a mental and emotional effect, because fats in the bloodstream stop glucose from getting to your brain properly. If you're eating radical fats all day long, that means there's never a window where your brain can get what it really wants. Electrolytes drop in the brain, neurotransmitter chemicals are weakened, and you lose that full glucose supply, the very resource that allows you to think clearly and be mentally strong. That takes a toll on how you feel—especially when you just came off getting exactly what you need.

Sometimes you also get tired when going back on radical fats—again, because you notice how they were affecting you all along. Digesting radical fats is a larger undertaking for the digestive system. When you free your body of such a burden, of constantly having to process fats every single day, you finally experience a reprieve from this strain on your system. When you start back on fats again, you may feel a little down because you've become attuned to how different it feels when your brain and body don't have to do so much extra work. Some people are sensitive enough that the second they bring radical fats back in, they wake up to how they used to feel. You may find yourself realizing, *Was I always a little sad, confused, unfocused, ungrounded?*

The restoration process you accomplished during the 3:6:9 Cleanse upgraded your neurons, neurotransmitters, brain function, and immune system, which means that after the 3:6:9 Cleanse, you have the potential to be a healthier, more viable, mentally stronger you. When you go back to tahini, avocado, nuts, seeds, or olive oil, or other radical fats that may not be as healthy, you have the potential now to make better choices about how much of them you eat and what time of day, because now you can detect the subtle differences in how what you eat affects you. You're not as likely to slop down a food that previously you thought of as a worthwhile indulgence and now you see more as poisonous. With your guard up a little, your antennae up, you can protect yourself and your family to a greater degree, wise now to what your body's true needs are.

There are key subtleties here, differences between what your body really needs and *thinking* you're in touch with what your body wants. A prime example of how we lose the subtle connections to knowing what our bodies need is when we say, "My body needs eggs. It feels good on eggs," when in truth, eggs feed every pathogen known to man (and not known to man) inside our bodies. Given some time off eggs and other troublemaker foods, our intuitive skills enhance greatly. Post-cleanse, as we go back to a life that incorporates radical fats (if we want to), we're more inclined to choose a little tahini or avocado to go with our salad versus two boiled eggs or worse.

MORE SECRETS OF VIRAL CLEANSING

If someone has been viral over the years—for example, with EBV or herpes simplex—they've built up a substantial amount of neurotoxins too, most likely resulting in frustrating symptoms. So as fat cells drain, neurotoxins and even dermatoxins also drain back into the

bloodstream, floating throughout the body—with information inside them—on their way out. The information attached to neurotoxins and dermatoxins can be extremely distant and also vast. It can be very hard to put your finger on it as it stirs sensations. Nevertheless, someone can still experience those sensations, even if only mildly.

Neurotoxins' and dermatoxins' information depends on the story of the viral strain that produced them. How were you first exposed to EBV? Did you catch mono kissing a classmate as a teenager? Did you get a virus from your dad and mom, passed down in utero or via sperm at conception? Did the virus come from the public bathroom you used on a night out? From a restaurant you ate in? From a relationship? Before a virus was in you, it was in someone else, and in someone else before that, and in someone else before that. And as any viral strain moves through a person, it collects data along the way. Viruses have to vibe with their host. When you got infected with it, the virus already contained multiple levels of information, both emotional and physical, about the experiences of people the virus had inhabited. As the virus moved through you, it collected information about when you were first infected with it, how you became sick with it, and so on. Any neurotoxins and dermatoxins the virus then produced held this information.

When you're cleansing by removing foods, such as eggs, that viruses love, you're essentially starving the virus. The 3:6:9 Cleanse and all other Medical Medium cleanses are antiviral. Foods aren't removed from the diet during these cleanses because of a belief system about "good" and "bad" foods. One of the main reasons the troublemaker foods such as eggs from

Chapter 7 are kept out of these cleanses is that people are sick with chronic illnesses due to viruses and other pathogens, and these pathogens require certain food to stay alive inside of us. Cleansing not only removes toxins from our body; it starves viruses, helping kill them off and usher out the viruses' waste matter, which includes neurotoxins, dermatoxins, and other viral byproduct. With that cleansing can come some emotional sensations particularly keyed to the release of viral waste matter.

If you were having a positive experience when you picked up a virus, if you picked it up at a restaurant when you were having a night to remember, then as you clean out the neurotoxins from the virus, you may actually experience positive sensations as they leave. Or if you picked up a virus while in a bad relationship, then as its neurotoxins and dermatoxins leave your body during these antiviral cleanses, you may experience sadness. Then there's the whole history of a virus and its previous hosts to consider. Say you first received a mutation of one of the over 60 varieties of EBV from a chef who cut his finger in the kitchen of the restaurant where you dined. That particular viral strain could have come to you containing information about the ebbs and flows of his life, how he lives, and how he thinks. As you go through the 3:6:9 Cleanse or the Anti-Bug Cleanse and the virus starts to die and viral toxins are released (both from inside the virus cells themselves and from old "storage bins" in your body), the coping mechanisms that the previous host used in life could surface. You may suddenly get the sensation of how a chef you never even met handled hardship, without having any idea that's what you're feeling or why you're feeling it. Thankfully, it's all on its way out of you.

Try not to be hard upon yourself when you're experiencing unsettled emotions. Realize there could be much, much more at hand than anyone realizes, and that it's not your fault and you didn't create it. At times like this, it's important to rise through these emotional states without blaming yourself for how you're feeling. Instead, harness the truth: that these emotions shall pass and that you're not supposed to self-punish for what resides in these emotions as they pass through you. It would be unfair to judge yourself for these sensations that are difficult to decipher and understand. Know that you're only getting better and healthier and to a place where you will experience less emotional pain as you heal. As the neurotoxins and dermatoxins from these viruses leave the body, symptoms such as depression and anxiety start to subside over time.

MORE SECRETS OF ADRENALINE

Adrenaline deserves a closer look when we're talking about cleansing. First, let's establish that with each of your life experiences, your adrenal glands release a specific blend of hormones keyed to that event. When it's an intense experience, the adrenaline blend required is more potent, and that both protects you—by powering you through it—and can be injurious because of its strength. The hormone blend that your adrenal glands pump out also has information in it that associates itself to the experience in the moment. This adrenaline then gets stored in tissue and organs in the body. And as we touched on, when it's released out of your cells, tissue, and stored fat as you cleanse, you can re-experience the sensation of what you went through before.

Sometimes that can take the form of nostalgia. Intense experiences aren't always challenging ones—sometimes they're very happy times, or times of great excitement. Take, for example, the adrenaline keyed to a 16th birthday party where everything went perfectly and it ended with a car topped with a bow in the driveway. When we cleanse that adrenaline however many years later, finally allowing it to come out of storage from the cells that it saturated, we could feel nostalgic sensations.

What we call déjà vu could also come up as we cleanse old adrenaline from past experiences, where we can't put our finger on why we're feeling a certain way. We could also feel sensations of peace if we went through extremely peaceful times in the past that required adrenaline that's now releasing. Maybe, for example, we succeeded in a goal, with one adrenaline blend that propelled us through it, and then tremendous peace and tranquility from our success in that moment released another adrenaline blend associated to that experience through our body. Now that we're giving our cells the chance to let go, the adrenaline is flowing out, and we're feeling familiar sensations.

Cleansing adrenaline can be a mixed bag like this. As old hormones from your past experiences are being released from the storage pockets throughout the body that you're cleansing, memories of the difficult struggles and hard times can be accompanied by memories of some of the most joyous, happy times.

It helps to have a handle on why harder emotions can come up on a cleanse. Here's some perspective: if someone cheats on you in a relationship and you find out, the adrenaline that your adrenal glands pump out will be appropriate to the injustice that's happening in your life in that moment. Your body doesn't do this on purpose to hurt you. It's to give you strength to be able to process the harm done as information comes through the neurons to your brain's emotional centers and communicates that you've been betrayed.

Betrayal is something we all experience at least one time in our life. It could be anything, whether from a broken relationship of any kind, a school project where a classmate changes the whole topic without your permission, a coach telling you to sit out the most important sports game of your life for reasons you don't understand, or being let down by medical research and science when you're searching for answers to your chronic illness. As the accompanying adrenaline surges through your body, it has the uncanny ability to carry information within itself such as fear, hurt, and anger, and also to collect data. It can actually absorb the emotions that you're processing from the crime that was committed against you.

Whatever toxic experience (or even exciting experience) your adrenaline is there to power you through, and in that sense safeguard you, there's that other side to it: the high levels of adrenaline can be pretty harsh on the body. Technically, the adrenaline is supposed to leave the body when the experience is over; its presence is meant to be brief. These experiences don't always end in one day, though. When you find out your boyfriend has cheated on you or become disinterested, you're not over it in 24 hours. When you lose a loved one to an illness or tragedy, you may carry it for a lifetime; there could be moments through the years when the pain surfaces again in between your times of resolve.

These types of ongoing adrenaline overload can be a little tricky for your health, if the adrenaline doesn't leave the body easily—and one reason adrenaline wouldn't leave the body easily is if we're eating foods that aren't good for us or are toxic all on their own. Particularly at issue here are high-fat foods, which, if we're eating them without any breaks, can lead to fat cells collecting in our liver and other places in the body. Even if someone doesn't look like they have fat on them, they could have this stored body fat in the liver and elsewhere, and it could end up collecting to the point that it makes itself known down the road. Here's the point: these fat cells get saturated with adrenaline. Fat aside, our *organ* cells get saturated with adrenaline; deep in your liver, for example, you could have adrenaline stored without fat.

A lot of times, the foods we eat in times of crisis don't allow adrenaline to leave the body. We often eat food to push down the hurt. Not that we're supposed to feel guilt or shame about that—it's natural to reach for food at difficult times as our brains and bodies ask for fuel to cope. We're not taught which foods can actually help us, so instead we reach for foods that aren't the best for us, ones that can get saturated with the adrenaline coursing through us at the same time, meaning that the adrenaline can get stored more easily and deeply inside the body instead of leaving naturally as it's meant to do. When we have the opposite reaction and don't eat in times of crisis, adrenaline does tend to leave more quickly, although this doesn't mean it's productive to starve ourselves! Adrenaline still goes to the liver and other parts of the body and gets stored there if we don't take active steps to cleanse.

When a crisis subsides and life goes back to something like normalcy, the adrenaline from that and other past tough times is still stored in various places in the body. As the years go on, we absorb more and more liver

and body troublemakers into our system too. We breathe in pollutants and other environmental toxins, they enter our body through our skin, or we ingest them, all of it giving viruses and unproductive bacteria the chance to thrive and proliferate inside our liver and other organs—and so we start to develop symptoms and conditions.

If we start cleansing using one of the 3:6:9 Cleanse plans or even one of the cleanses from Part III, toxins and old debris from organs and tissue start to loosen up and enter the bloodstream. Fat cells actually explode, and what comes out as they drain is old adrenaline, along with many different toxins and poisons. That old adrenaline carries with it information about old hurt (or, as you read, old excitement or old joy). Everybody is different. Some people haven't experienced a lot of hurt in life. Many people have. Not everybody who has experienced hurt has had to live in it every day; maybe they feel they've processed it or moved on. If it's still in you, though, when that old adrenaline from a breakup or other heartbreak or injustice or emotional injury or physical injury is released as part of cleansing and starts floating through the bloodstream, you may start to feel some emotions and not know what's causing them—which can be puzzling as other aspects of the cleanse are giving you so much relief.

Now, the cleanse is not the *cause* of these feelings. The cleanse is a tool that you're using in this moment so the process of healing can occur. Healing may not feel perfectly straightforward as old adrenaline reenters the bloodstream and the past harm or fear you've experienced that was packed into your cells finally gets a chance to leave. This can lead to some sadness when cleansing, some nervousness, or a vague unsettled feeling. It could also lead to some mild depression or a bit of anxiousness, or it could ignite emotional dreams that may or may not make total sense. You may remember some experiences you've forgotten, or you may remember a feeling that you can't quite put your finger on and yet is familiar.

Everyone's emotional cleanse experience is different because everyone is packed with different toxins and poisons. Many people have recreational drugs in their system from the past, or prescription drugs they became addicted to and overused. When that's the case, it usually means the drugs were consumed during emotional and/or physical hardship—times when the body was pumping out adrenaline to cope. At the same time, the drugs themselves triggered adrenaline release. All of this adrenaline harbored emotional information about our struggle, adrenaline that got stored in the liver along with the drugs. For example, if we go through an emotional crisis and we take a benzodiazepine, other anti-anxiety medication, or any other type of prescription or recreational drug to get us through, we don't realize that both the drug and the divorce, breakup, betrayal, or other difficult time trigger adrenaline that contains information about the experience, and that this adrenaline gets packed into our liver cells with the medication. When we cleanse, then, we've got those old drugs, whether recreational or prescribed, coming out of our cells and releasing into our bloodstream along with the old adrenaline that can trigger hurt, pain, fear, or sadness.

A SISTERHOOD AND BROTHERHOOD OF HEALING

Everybody has a different set of experiences. The betrayal one person went through might have been substantially different from someone else's, and yet maybe the negative impact it had on their lives could in some sense be equal. Sometimes people experience much more hardship, more losses, more breakups as they look for love in life, more business relationships that are hurtful rather than fruitful. And as people find their way, find their true calling, crawl out of the depths of a hardship they thought was their fault and in reality was the depths of darkness (some people see darkness for what it is; many don't), they have different ways of handling difficult memories and experiences, releasing as much as they safely can while some memories become buried in the subconscious. While we're all different in our experiences, there is still a sisterhood and a brotherhood to what we go through in this life.

The chronically ill often find power in numbers when they connect over their shared suffering. Even if their physical symptoms vary, with one person experiencing migraines, anxiety, or depression and another going through back pain, neck pain, or insomnia, there's still a resonance that unites them. Similarly, it's hard to find an emotional experience that is so unique that not a single other soul has ever been faced with even a fraction of it before. Everyone knows what broken trust feels like. We've all experienced relationships, whether with friends, family members, spouses, or others, that became difficult or even harmful in some way. Many of us have experienced physical injury that went along with emotional injury. We've all been let down.

Either way, physically or emotionally, even when the details are different, we can find enough similarities to one another's hurt to identify with each other. That is, if we're not isolated from those who have gone through similar situations. Sometimes we feel completely alone, especially when the experts we consult or the people in our lives imply or outright tell us that we've imagined or created our illness. Because there's still stigma around chronic suffering—a result of how little it's understood—it can be hard to find true help from someone who gets it. Rest assured: even if you believe that you are the only one to know the particular pain of fighting for your life while those around you look at you with skepticism that your muscle stiffness or brain fog or fatigue is really that bad, others who've been through nearly the exact same struggle are out there. You're not alone. The sisterhood and brotherhood with these people, once you find them, is strong.

The emotions that went along with fighting to be heard are some of what we release when we cleanse. Those struggles also led to emotion-based adrenaline that flowed through our veins and got stored in our cells. As we detox, then, these are some of the feelings that can come back up in different ways. One person may find themselves with nostalgia that's almost uncomfortable in a way. Another may go through intense dreams. Yet another may feel a little sadness, with tears coming up periodically without knowing exactly why. Not that everybody goes through this with cleansing, not at all. These are the more pronounced cases, where someone has gone through substantial hurt. Whatever you've gone through and whatever comes up, on any level, is important.

Medical Medium cleanses are designed to support throughout. This means that even as cells release old adrenaline that carries difficulties from our past, it's not a reckless process. Your brain is getting critical glucose and mineral salts to give you grounding as this all happens in the background. You don't need to engage or process the emotions and feelings that come up on a cleanse. It's usually not the time or space to deal with them. It could happen—everyone is different in how or when they need to process life. Sometimes miracle states of emotional healing can happen naturally during one of these cleanses. A great lifting of energy could occur, a sensation of weight off our back, and we may be able to identify it and we may not be able to identify it, and that's okay. There's no rule about how our emotional processing is supposed to happen. Usually, the shift occurs after the cleanse is over, when we've had enough time to gain insight into what surfaced during the cleanse. After a cleanse, we become wiser in the emotional arena in so many ways.

As we release poisons and toxins that were deeply embedded into cells of all kinds, including fat cells that are now bursting and draining while we cleanse, those poisons and toxins that are now flowing through our bloodstream on their way out of the body can affect our senses of taste and smell. Sometimes while cleansing, someone will taste a manufactured food they ate when they were a child—a cheeseburger, for example, from a chain fast food restaurant. Sometimes they'll taste smoke from cigarettes. Sometimes it's a type of ice cream or cheese or doughnut or cookie they used to consume. Sometimes it's a familiar flavor they can't quite pin down. Sometimes it's a chemical essence. Sometimes it's pungent and rotten, ammonia- or sulfur-like, and makes the breath smell like aging cheese or rotting flesh. That can all connect to feelings. The smells and tastes can change over the course of the cleanse too, and after you've released a certain amount of toxins, your senses can even become more fine-tuned. You'll notice that what won't come up on the cleanse is the taste of a grape or apple or celery stick or strawberry. These are foods that fight toxins; they aren't toxic foods themselves. You'll notice that it's only the toxic food that surfaces during a cleanse.

Your emotional well-being can become more fine-tuned as well. This doesn't mean that you become more emotional after cleansing—rather, that you can become more emotionally protected and emotionally sound. Old hurt can create such a fog, allowing us to make the same mistake over and over again, just as when we're in pain from burning our hand on the stove, we may turn away in fear, and in our haste, accidentally back into the fireplace. When we aren't filled with poisons and fear-based, betrayal-based, harm-based adrenaline—when leftover hurt that was stored deep in our cells leaves our system—we're going to know we burned our hand on the stove, and yet it's not going to send us reeling. We're going to be able to see the momentary pain clearly rather than find ourselves in a fog of old percolating hurt, and that's going to let us take care of ourselves properly rather than hurt ourselves even more by making mistakes out of fear or desperation.

After cleansing the right way, you often become wiser beyond your years. You may find yourself a little more guarded, in a good way. You're more cautious about when to be vulnerable, make better decisions about whom to involve yourself with and whom to confide in, and you're more intuitive about when to drop your guard and open the door for healthier friendships and relationships. You become more keen, less reactive, more mindful—because when you've rid your cells of enough toxins and poisons and viruses and unproductive bacteria and enough old adrenaline that harbored past emotions, you become better able to avoid repeating mistakes. Once you've released old hurts and fears from broken relationships, your adrenaline passageways become clearer. Your own deep understanding of what you're truly feeling, and who you truly are, can surface. In the end, what this all amounts to is freedom from the old chains of toxins, bugs, and hurt that have been holding you back throughout a lifetime.

"Empowerment is more than a word. It's more than an understanding of confidence. It's the mortar between the bricks of a person's sense of value here in life on earth. When it's used for good, when it's healthy and positive, it's crucial to shaping goals, aspirations, and human life and sending us in a direction that only betters humanity."

— Anthony William, Medical Medium

CHAPTER 26

Empowered Souls

Empowerment. When we are allowed to understand ourselves after we've been purposely held back from doing so, it's one of the most sensible, higher-minded, spiritually conscious, critical aspects of elevating confidence, and even more so, of feeding the soul with something larger. When times are challenging, confidence wanes. Empowerment is there to catch you. It should be considered a spiritual word—because when it's used in a positive light and not in an unfair way, when it's used for protecting and helping people, it can absolutely be spiritual. True spiritual, not imaginary spiritual.

The word *empower*—that is, the granting of power—can imply that power was once taken away. Not everybody knows they're disempowered when they're disempowered. When it comes to women's health, power has been taken away. Health is a gender issue. While there's no denying that men suffer too, chronic illness affects women in disproportionate numbers, and not because women are weak. A woman struggling with chronic illness should never be blamed for a "victim mentality." Women bear chronic illness with immense strength and courage.

We're supposed to be living in the most empowering time for womankind. Can we be, when young women in their teens, 20s, and 30s are being sidelined by symptoms at record rates? When unexplainable pain and fatigue have women in their 40s, 50s, and 60s at a loss about how to care for their families and careers? When women in retirement aren't able to enjoy that time because they're trying to solve their health mysteries?

Women are being kept in the dark about why they're sick and how to get better. Not that medical research and science have all the answers and they're simply keeping them quiet. Rather, conventional world powers that be within the larger system are trying to distract from the truth that they *don't* have all the answers. Chronic illness remains a great mystery to the medical establishment, and so they point the finger at women's bodies, at women's own selves, as the problem. They point at faulty genes, for example, as if after all these thousands of years, women's genes have suddenly hit an expiration date just in the last two decades. They discredit healing tools such as celery juice and cleansing that are saving women's lives. That's disempowerment.

It doesn't have to be this way.

MORE THAN A WORD

If a woman is sick with symptoms that are holding her back, or keep coming back, or a diagnosis from which she's not getting better because she doesn't know the true cause of her suffering, is that woman truly empowered?

And why, in this time of modern technology, with seemingly advanced pharmaceuticals and medical research, do women not have answers to over 90 percent of the illnesses, symptoms, and diseases from which they suffer? Why are women experiencing an all-time high in reproductive system conditions?

In daily life, we don't hear about how many women have to give up precious time going to multiple doctors searching for answers. We don't hear about the great hope they lose when they find that the "answers" they are given aren't the true causes of their pain and suffering and don't provide relief. This is not talked about. Women have to bear this alone.

Empowerment is more than a word. It's more than an understanding of confidence. It's the mortar between the bricks of a person's sense of value here in life on earth. Empowerment can also be used in a negative light. It can be misdirected, used to empower someone to inflict emotional or other harm on someone else. Yet when it's used for good, when it's healthy and positive, it's crucial to shaping goals, aspirations, and human life and sending us in a direction that only betters humanity.

No one wants to be disempowered. No one wants to be told to be quiet, for their voice to be stifled, for their thoughts and feelings to go unheard. No one wants their purpose suppressed or their qualities, creativity, and value to be oppressed on any level.

Womankind has had some trying times in history. Women have been held down in the past, kept from achieving their dreams because that didn't fit into the world that was. Today, in many places, women's rights have come a long way. Empowerment is being taken seriously as a force that allows an individual to grow, achieve, and become oneself on a more equitable level, with the opportunity and right to survive, and even more than that, to strive for the best quality of life. We're at a place now, here, when you don't have to look far to see empowerment woven into the fabric of society. It's in words written in articles and in books; it's in stories told person to person and across media outlets, from social media to news sites to talk shows. Empowerment is a miracle for womankind, evolving every day in a land where it was never allowed to be not so long ago.

Because of these positive changes and headlines, it's easy to walk around with the belief instilled that in this modern, present moment, women are protected. Because it is true that women are being taken more seriously than ever before, it's easy to get comfortable thinking that women really are fully empowered. That women really are valued as being as important as men. That time has caught up, and women really do get an equal playing field. As true as this is in some areas of life with all the undeniable advances, there is still this area where women are disempowered and even held back deliberately, and it's the most important area for a woman to have power: her health.

We often say that health is paramount. We say that women's well-being is a number-one focus, medically and institutionally. We say that giving a woman a right to choose any direction she needs for her personal health should be part of this, that having options for women's health is critical. All this talk should mean women are empowered, right? The truth is that when it comes to chronic illness, women were disempowered many decades ago, and women are disempowered still.

Everything changes when a woman becomes sick. Every day, women become ill with chronic issues such as fatigue, thyroid disease, PCOS, fibroids, endometriosis, migraines, hair loss, anxiety, depression, eczema, and psoriasis—and lose their rights with their health. The first part of the journey is learning about the medical system. Women find out rather quickly that the system isn't set up to give the proper direction that so many need to heal from chronic illness. When you're not dealing with a problem, it's easy to accept that this is how it is. Yet when you're the one going from doctor to doctor, sitting on the exam table hearing about your diagnosis and hearing "no known cure"— or not even receiving a diagnosis for your health struggles—getting the message that you need to accept a lack of answers about your health as your life, the limits of how we address chronic illness suddenly come into focus. This is the reality millions of women are facing every day.

As more and more women become doctors every day, it translates into more women patients being heard about their symptoms and conditions than years ago. Since that's the case, why would disempowerment still exist in the medical system, holding back women

in the area where they should be most protected? Because doctors of all genders aren't being given the training and tools they need to move the needle on chronic illness.

Disempowerment can happen in a very dark way, a very secretively hidden way. You could be disempowered—held back, suppressed, harmed—and not realize at first that's what it is. The nuts and bolts of the medical system are geared to keep women in the dark about their bodies, allowing them to stay disempowered. Let's be clear: It's not doctors who are disempowering women. It's the system within which doctors operate. In the 1940s and '50s, many doctors joined in with the system that disempowered women, saying chronic illness was not real and that women were either making it up, bored, just tired, lazy, or even crazy. Those days are mostly behind us. Today, doctors are boxed into new viewpoints about chronic illness: that it's a woman's own immune system attacking her body, for example, or that her genes or hormones are to blame for her suffering. What's different today versus decades ago is that now, most doctors are compassionate and caring enough to realize that the patient is struggling with a real condition.

Still, this progress with the physicians themselves and how they treat patients doesn't free a woman of disempowerment when it comes to her health, because the "answers" she's being given aren't answers. It leads to a sort of whiplash, with the genuine, caring physician (Dr. Jekyll) making you feel safe while the medical establishment (Mr. Hyde) tells you something is wrong with who you are. Hearing that your body is disgusting, faulty, and broken explained to you in the most kind, compassionate way creates an almost abusive relationship with the medical system, where you get a pat on the head just before you're thrown aside. Even though these theoretical belief systems about the body attacking itself or faulty genes causing chronic illness do not have scientific proof behind them, these are the explanations that medical systems hand doctors, and they're what doctors offer patients. This Jekyll and Hyde dynamic undermines everything that today's compassionate doctors are trying to do to help patients with chronic illness.

A DESIGN FLAW THAT DIVIDES US

We're facing some critical problems in this current age we live in together. One is that when a woman falls ill and it becomes more than just a headache once in a while or some temporary back pain or a small bout of anxiety, she isn't truly heard as much as we would like to think she is. Classes divide between those who feel well and those who feel sick, and those who are well usually don't want to hang around or hear too much from people who are really sick. It's not a simple matter of men not wanting to listen to women about their problems. When someone from the unwell class has a few too many complaints because they can't get the help they need and they can't get their symptoms to subside as they're traveling from doctor to doctor for answers, in many cases they will quickly learn who their friends truly are. Because the chronically ill class is often made up of women, this can lead to a divide among women.

There's some irony here. As much energy as healthy people put into keeping their distance from those who suffer chronically, in this day and age, many of those healthy people become sick later. No one is immune from the varying levels of chronic illness. Nearly everyone, no matter their gender, is developing symptoms over time, whether those symptoms are labeled "chronic illness" or whether they're the type of symptoms that we all seem to accept as a normal part of life—such as sinus problems, acne, UTIs, migraines, painful periods, anxiety, and depression—symptoms that become more serious over time and start to impede how someone lives, even affecting what they can do in their leisure time.

In the past, before social media, women struggling with their health were rarely heard in the wider world. There was no platform for them. If a chronic illness was serious enough, then the hope was that a very wealthy person or group of wealthy people would create a charity and a board in hopes that once or twice a year, there would be a gala or other benefit to raise money for this disease affecting women. With online platforms now, women who are sick are able to voice themselves about their different illnesses and conditions and symptoms. Even though it's improving on that level, women are still suppressed. When it comes to feeling unwell, not feeling strong, it's not always detectable to the outside eye, which makes it even harder to be taken seriously.

It takes a lot of compassion, deep understanding, and the ability to not be completely self-absorbed for someone who's healthy now to at least acknowledge the friends and family and other people in this world who are struggling with real illnesses and real symptoms, people who are in need and not allowed to project their concerns, issues, and opinions so easily. It takes someone with a caring, loving heart to acknowledge someone they know who struggles and to give them the time and energy they need.

Life is difficult as it is. Everyone has so much going on; it's not always easy to have that compassion or set aside that time for a friend. The responsibility shouldn't all be on individuals who are healthy to look out for those struggling with illness. It should be the duty of something larger, the system of medical research and science and top health authorities, to take responsibility and change the misinformed, grandfathered laws and theories that are holding back womankind. That greater framework should be designed so that women can take measures to prevent and heal illness based on what's really happening inside their bodies, and so that women can discover the empowering truth about who they are as beings.

THE OTHER KIND OF BODY SHAMING

One of the most important fights for womankind, if not the most important, is the fight for her health. We all know that on some level. To understand it better, we need to look at some of the beliefs that seem to be set in stone to keep women from understanding the truth about chronic illness and moving forward: there are forms of body shaming that go beyond shape, size, and appearance (which are already bad enough). I'm talking about theories of chronic illness that say a person's genes are faulty, that their body is attacking itself, that the problem is their mind, that they have a slow metabolism, or that their hormones are "off." These are forms of control from a system that doesn't have answers—and

that last one, hormone blame, is a particular strike against gender.

In the 1950s, the body-attacking-itself theory of "autoimmune" gained traction, positing that the immune system can get confused and start going after your own organs and glands. Imbalanced hormones were another popular theory of the day, blaming practically anything that went amiss with a woman's health, such as moods and issues categorized as "appearance," on hormones. So was the idea that someone with symptoms such as heart palpitations, hot flashes, and headaches that couldn't be easily explained was really just bored, lazy, or crazy—that they were malingering, and it was all in their head. This thinking placed the blame for illness on someone's own body and mind, creating the ultimate shame about who someone was inside at a cellular level.

While hormone blame is alive and well—just think how many times you've heard someone say, "Oh, she's just hormonal"—the old "it's all in your head" model did start to shift and diminish through the decades. Now the more popular notion when someone asks, "How come I'm sick?" is to answer that they created their own illness by not generating a positive flow to attract health like someone else did. It's another form of disempowerment for women, sending them the message that if they don't feel well, it's their fault because they don't understand how the universe works and they're not thinking positively enough to create abundance. So on top of body and mind shaming, we have spirit shaming. Young women are becoming convinced that their unhappiness is why they're sick, not that they have real issues that medical research and science haven't discovered yet that are the actual, physical problems plaguing women's health.

And we can't forget about the gene blame game. This one names certain chronic diseases as genetic, leaving someone to feel faulty and trapped as it shames the very fiber of their being. When you actually dig into this, you see that the *theory* is faulty, not people's bodies. The BRCA gene mutation, for example, is said to spell doom and gloom for developing breast cancer, which isn't true. Just as many cases of breast cancer occur where a BRCA mutation is not present, and the real reason they place the blame on inherited gene mutations is that they haven't yet discovered the cause of breast cancer that I revealed in my book *Thyroid Healing*. Gene blame is becoming entangled with other theories too—for example, that the body attacks itself *because* it's genetically flawed. It is yet more shaming and disempowerment.

If we step back for perspective, we can understand why the shaming happens: because the system of medical research and science needs to protect itself. It has credibility to uphold—among patients and also among the doctors and other health professionals who work within it. And so the system offers what seem like answers for practitioners to offer, in turn, to patients and their family members. These "answers" may seem like they're protecting women's best interests. In truth, they're protecting the medical establishment at women's expense.

Women who have tried alternative therapies and healing have faced so much scrutiny over the years. From roughly the 1940s up until the early 2010s, women took so much flak and even hatred from family and friends for leaving conventional pathways and searching for other ways to heal from their illnesses. If you were a woman in the 1970s who wanted to seek out an alternative therapy or a healthier way of eating, you were mocked or ridiculed. Young women—and men too—were not accepted by their families, or they were even cut off, because they wanted to eat better or go plant based. In the 1980s and '90s, it was seen as bizarre, outlandish, or dangerous to choose an alternative way of thinking with health. Imagine, or maybe you can remember, what it was like to go an herbal route for an illness rather than choosing medication. The judgment you'd receive was a whole other form of suppression and oppression because it limited people's freedom of choice about how to help themselves through their symptoms and conditions.

Some of this still exists today. You see both conventional-minded and alternative-minded diet professionals, for example, trying to stop women from drinking celery juice. If only they knew that in their attempts to guard women from the unfamiliar and outside-the-box, they were doing the opposite and keeping women from the very solutions that can *protect* their health.

Have you ever wondered *why* millions of people have searched outside the box for answers for their health? Could it be because the medical industry as a whole hasn't offered the answers to their chronic struggles, suffering, symptoms, and conditions? When people can't find the relief they need for their chronic health issues from the existing medical system and then are doubted or ridiculed for going outside that system to find relief, shouldn't it be obvious that the system is broken? By the way, you can be alternative-minded and offer alternative theories when trying to help people out there and at the same time still be attached to or working for a broken medical system that's behind the disempowerment of women's health. Alternative health professionals believe in the same grandfathered laws as do conventional professionals, like that someone's body is attacking itself and that's the reason they're sick. The difference is that these practitioners have a different wheelhouse of treatments.

TAKE THE BLAME OFF YOUR SOUL

Do we ever think about what happens to a person when they're physically hurt in some way and told they're to blame? Do we even realize what kind of soul harm is done when that occurs? If we're so concerned about building women up—and that seems to be what we're trying to do in today's world, with support groups to overcome the scars of being made to feel inadequate, less-than, and worthless; with conversations about women's advancement in the workplace; and with tools to raise children with enlightened thought—then how come we miss this most critical aspect of all? If we care about womankind, wouldn't we care enough to find out about the soul injury that's sustained?

When you experience a symptom that you can't figure out how to control and you lean on the medical system for support, it's not uncommon to find that what we think of as one of the most important parts of our world—the medical system—is not as stable, reliable, and all-knowing as we believed. We can't blame medical research and science for not having answers about chronic suffering yet. We do need to be aware of what little children, and especially young women, are raised to believe: That science makes us safe and has all the

answers. That when we're sick, it's because of something wrong with a facet of who we are. Long after they're grown up, women keep hearing this. So again, when that happens, where does the inevitable injury go? It settles itself within the soul. Over time, it breaks a person's spirit too.

This means, then, that discovering the truth behind chronic and mystery illness is about keeping the soul strong within a woman, child, or any other person, for that matter. It's about protecting your soul. One of the most important foundations to hold on to is that *no matter what, in the end, it's not your fault.* You can't be empowered if self-hatred is dominating you, self-hatred controlled by negligence from the medical establishment that operates above doctors. From their very work, medical research and science know it is human nature to blame ourselves the moment we fall ill. Once you take the blame off your own soul and realize your symptom, condition, illness, or disease is not your fault—and not your body's fault—you can become truly empowered. This kind of empowerment is more important than we know. It rises above false empowerment that's based on entitlement and ego. You are not the reason you have unknown symptoms and conditions. *You* are not why you're sick.

HEALING IS POSSIBLE

There are heroes within the health community. Doctors are some of those heroes. It's not always within their power, though, to talk about what it's like to have a woman walk into their office and tell her story of visiting neurologists and other specialists, of trying treatment upon treatment, and what it's like to see despair in her eyes because none of it got her out of pain. Doctors don't always have a platform or safety net to express what they're seeing, or the bewilderment they're feeling themselves because they don't have the literature or tools to offer new insights for the people who are struggling. There are other heroes, too, within the healing community, in mainstream, alternative, and social media outlets, including the heroes who tell their own stories of getting better. Even with all this, it's a very small percentage of people sending out the message that women are in trouble with their health, that they're not getting the answers they need, and that *healing is possible*.

We can find comfort in the knowledge that it doesn't have to be this way. There are true freedom and empowerment in having control over your health and well-being, and not only over one aspect or decision—control over the big picture. That control comes from having answers: Answers about what could cause future illness and how you can help prevent that now. Answers about what's causing your current illness and what to do about it, with information and a plan to move yourself forward and heal.

I'll say it again: empowerment is having answers. It's knowing that your body is not attacking itself. It's knowing that your genes or hormones are not responsible for your sickness, that you are not a faulty person. It's knowing that you're not a bad person either, and that you didn't create your illness with your mind-set and emotions. Empowerment is knowing there are real problems that can happen inside the body with real causes that simply haven't been seen yet by medical research and science, or haven't been realized or understood by professionals in all realms of healing. There's a growing practice of telling women that they're creating their illness with how they think, or that they haven't learned the correct meditation tools or forms of positive thinking or attraction methods for getting positive results in life, or that they're carrying around negative energy, or that their frequency and vibration are off. These are the theories that perpetuate when people walk around struggling with no answers. Once again, they're theories that put the blame on our existence. This can be very disempowering when you're sick, or when you're battling real physical issues.

If we want life to be best for women and their children, is it best for everyone to be in the dark about what causes chronic suffering, for us to blame it on emotions and genes and fate? Or is it best to reveal that these illnesses that are sidelining more and more women are caused by troublemakers such as toxic heavy metals and pathogens such as the over 60 varieties of Epstein-Barr virus? These are causes that are not your fault, that can be worked on. In this book, you have found the answers to cleansing the very toxins, poisons, and pathogens responsible for chronic symptoms and conditions, so that you can take control of your health and make the choices that are best for you to protect you and your family. You didn't create your symptoms, you are a good person, and now that you hold control, you can move forward on a path of healing.

As you've seen, we're in a time when we think women are the most empowered they've ever been, and this isn't entirely true. The reality? We're in a time when women are being held back more than ever in areas of critical meaning: health, safety, and vitality. Women are being trained to think and believe that their physical bodies are weak and faulty. The reason this is happening is that when a woman is strong and healthy, she is a world changer. Not on a small scale. On a level that battles darkness. Those who are in power behind the scenes and run the world know this: that the stronger women are, the more good will occur, the more positive change will come. That's not in the best interests of darkness. The ones in power behind the scenes, the ones who threaten the planet, fear the strength and uprising of womankind, because women's strength and uprising truly are the greatest threat to the age of industries and fortune that bank on women's suffering. When women are strong, it only works for the good of humanity.

"The work you put into your healing is profound and powerful. It speaks to others who need that healing truth, that healing information, that inspiration to be hopeful and not want to give up. Your healing tells others that there is a way out from suffering and that they can heal too when they offer the body what it really needs. When you inspire people to get out of bed and fight for their health freedom and recover—those are the ones you're speaking to. There's no greater work on a spiritual level than changing people's lives so they see the light and realize that their bodies aren't faulty, that they're not bad people, and that they deserve to feel better, get better, and heal like you have."

— Anthony William, Medical Medium

PART VI

KNOWING THE CAUSE & THE PROTOCOL

CHAPTER 27

What You Need to Know about Supplements

Why is the world of nutraceuticals exploding? Why has it crossed over from alternative to mainstream medicine, becoming almost as big an industry as pharmaceuticals? It's not because anyone likes to wake up and gobble down a bunch of pills. It's not like taking medication is such a fun pastime that everyone decided it would also be a pleasure to take multivitamins, probiotics, amino acids, fish oil, and the like—no one enjoys filling prescriptions and facing down a tray of pink, blue, yellow, and orange capsules. No one really wants to spend their time swallowing dozens of pills a day, even if they're natural ones.

Adopting a regimen of capsules and pills does not come with the satisfaction of caring for ourselves in other ways. There's a difference, for example, between brushing your teeth to keep plaque and tartar away versus swallowing a painkiller because your jaw hurts with no answers. There's a difference between getting up and washing your face in the morning versus taking antibiotics for stubborn acne, and between doing a few stretches and a short meditation to center yourself for the day versus starting your morning at the medicine cabinet to take your acid reflux, high blood pressure, and high cholesterol medications.

Helpful as they can be, it's true for nutraceuticals too. Taking a refreshing shower at the beginning of the day is very different from staring down your lineup of supplement bottles as you prepare to take 15 to 20 capsules. And there's a distinction between deciding to walk or ride your bike to work or school versus having to plan your day around getting to the store before noon to replace the used-up bottle of tablets that your doctor recommended.

Which isn't to say pharmaceuticals and nutraceuticals don't have their place. Medications and supplements are necessary in many cases. That's why Part VI, "Knowing the Cause and the Protocol," is here. Relying on them hasn't become popular because it's fun, though. Someone could have a positive attitude about it; they could be optimistic, bright, and cheery about opening their pillbox. At the same time, they only started taking them because they had to, because they were told or felt they needed them for a specific symptom or condition, or they wanted to improve a health aspect such as hair, skin, and nails. Both pharmaceuticals and nutraceuticals are costly, and most everyone would prefer to put that money toward something they love. Even the person who starts out as an enthusiast, happy to go above and beyond with a regimen because it makes them feel better, may start to tire of the routine of taking supplements in six months or a couple of years.

Taking pills, no matter how motivated someone is about it, is a chore. That refreshing shower, that small bout of meditation, washing your face, cleaning your teeth, taking a walk—simple tasks like these can have an enjoyable side to them when we're feeling well. For the chronically ill, those who struggle to get out of bed and get through the day, they can be like mountains to climb. A daily pill regimen, on top of a basic self-care routine, can feel like a nightmare. People do it because they're soldiers in the trenches fighting the battles of symptoms and illnesses that won't go away, and those medications or supplements are their rations. Whether in the form of pharmaceuticals or nutraceuticals, people turn to them because they need help. They do it because something's not right.

These final chapters are here for you. Throughout this book, we've explored cleansing as a way to bring your body back to its rightful state of health. Sometimes you need more help, and that's where the proper herbs and supplements can be critical to rebuild your immune system, reverse deficiencies, fight off and kill pathogens, and protect yourself from stress. After important tips about how to navigate supplementation while cleansing,

we'll get to lists of supplements for over 100 specific symptoms, conditions, illnesses, and diseases. If you're coming to this book from *Liver Rescue*, don't skip this section. Many of the lists offer upgrades to the supplement lists you found there, not to mention that there are dozens more health issues covered here.

One important feature is that each list will include insights into the true cause of the health problem, because in order to understand what the proper herbs and supplements even are for a health problem, we need to discover what the underlying issue is. Chronic illnesses and chronic symptoms such as acne, UTIs, fatigue, bloating, and eczema are largely a mystery to current medical research and science, so science can't offer those answers—and when something's not right, you deserve answers.

SUPPLEMENTATION WHILE CLEANSING

It's an important question: How do you integrate supplements with a cleanse? We'll get to a few key tips to guide you in a moment. First, let's address the most important aspect of supplementation while cleansing: which supplements to *avoid*.

Supplements to Avoid while Cleansing

If you are on supplements that are not Medical Medium–recommended—for instance, whey protein powder, plant protein powders, fish oil, collagen, chlorella, multivitamins, hair-nail-skin supplements, glandular supplements, and gut powder blends—hold off on taking those while on any Medical Medium cleanse. You may also want to reevaluate whether you want them in your life at all, because supplements other than what I recommend may be contributing to your problems in the first place. Remember, because medical research and science don't know why people are sick with chronic illness, supplementation is a guessing game for them. If you stay on a non-recommended supplement while cleansing, you may not see the benefits you want to see.

Whey protein powder, for example, feeds viruses and other pathogens—so instead of starving the bugs that are keeping you sick, which a Medical Medium cleanse is meant to do, consuming whey protein powder during a cleanse actively feeds the pathogens that make you sick to begin with. You have to look out for plant protein powders too, because they have hidden MSG in their flavorings, which may feed pathogens in your body as well.

Same with fish oil, which has traces of mercury—because all fish oil, no matter how clean, has traces of this toxic heavy metal. I've talked before about how eating a piece of fish is vastly different from taking fish oil. The fish oil extraction process destabilizes the mercury present in the fish. No matter what advanced technology is used, fish oil still contains homeopathic traces of mercury. Mercury feeds the pathogens that cause your inflammation and chronic illness, so if you take fish oil regularly and you continue that routine while on a cleanse, it's hard to see the cleanse benefits as well as you could; you're keeping the bugs alive with the fish oil. For more on fish oil, revisit Chapter 7, "Troublemaker Foods."

That's not to mention that fish oil is a radical fat. Say you're on the ninth day of the 3:6:9 Cleanse and you decide to take a couple of fish oil capsules with your celery juice. Not only does that interfere with the celery juice, and not only does it introduce mercury into your system at the precise time you're trying to remove it—it also breaks the cleanse with oil. It's a common mistake and a prime example of why it's best to hold off on supplements that are not Medical Medium–recommended during the cleanses in this book.

Tips and Guidelines for Medical Medium–Recommended Supplements on a Cleanse

- If you're already on some of the supplements in Chapter 29's Medical Medium–recommended lists and you want to stay on them while cleansing (whether with the 3:6:9 Cleanse, the Anti-Bug Cleanse, the Morning Cleanse, the Heavy Metal Detox Cleanse, or the Mono Eating Cleanse), you're welcome to do so.

- If you aren't already taking Medical Medium–recommended supplements and you're looking for relief from a symptom or condition, you're welcome to start supplementation at the same time you start one of the cleanses in this book. You don't need to start supplements with the 3:6:9 Cleanse, the Anti-Bug Cleanse, the Morning Cleanse, the Heavy Metal Detox Cleanse, or the Mono Eating Cleanse, although you have the option to do so.

- Celery juice is a part of every cleanse and every supplement list in this book, and the recommended celery juice amounts will sometimes differ between a cleanse and a supplement list. If you're following one of these cleanses while following one of these supplement lists, go with the recommended amount of celery juice from the cleanse.

Keep in mind that when you go full steam ahead with new supplements while cleansing, it can amplify their power. Supplements will be stronger while you're on a cleanse because there are no fats in the way of the glucose that's binding itself to the supplementation and delivering it into your cells. High-fat/high-protein diets get in the way of your receiving nutrients from your supplementation. Medical Medium cleanses allow all the nutrients from supplementation to enter into your cells.

Balance also plays a role. When you start taking new supplements, it takes your body a few days or a week to find balance with them. So if you're starting supplements at the same time as a cleanse, your body is just beginning to acclimate to the new supplements. You may not get relief quite yet. Any supplements that you're already on, your body had to take time to adjust to and develop a relationship with, while at the same time it was developing a relationship between those new supplements you were taking and the foods you were used to eating. The minute you change your foods, even for the better, that balance is disrupted. Not in a negative way—it simply shifts the balance.

What if you want to take your Medical Medium–recommended supplements while cleansing? You can. Because they will be more potent, you may want to consider at first cutting your dosage in half for every supplement you take while on one of these cleanses. Supplements are almost diluted by our everyday way of eating. When we minimize or get rid of troublemaker foods while on a Medical Medium cleanse, half dosages of supplements will basically have the potency that a full dosage would have on our regular diet. While on a longer-term Medical Medium cleanse, you're welcome to start working your way up from supplement half dosages after nine days of cleansing.

INDIVIDUAL SUPPORT FOR YOUR SYMPTOMS AND CONDITIONS

Before you leap into the supplement lists in the coming chapters, be sure to read through this guidance.

To Cleanse or to Supplement?

As we've covered, trying these supplements is an optional step beyond cleansing. If you prefer to focus on foods for healing, you're more than welcome to do that. You don't have to play in Supplement Land yet if you don't want to. Do stay open to supplements for the future if you're struggling with symptoms and conditions. Any of the cleanses that you've read about here are powerful; they lower fats, avoid troublemaker foods, and add in healing foods to help with all your problems. For extra power afterward, these supplements are here for you.

This supplement guide is for people looking for something more, looking for options because their situations are perplexing to them. If that's you, then keep reading for a treasure trove of options in the form of specialized supplement lists for the individual symptoms and conditions in this book. It's important to know that our deficiencies are a big part of why we're sick. Zinc, for example, is practically nonexistent in food today, and a zinc deficiency lowers the immune system, so we're always in need of it. We also have a lot of toxic heavy metals in us, and spirulina is critical for removing those metals.

Where to Start?

If you're dealing with more than one symptom or condition at the same time, pick the one that looms largest in your life. For example, if you're plagued by fatigue, focus on taking care of that and don't worry about bloating. Over time, you may find that working on one issue takes care of another, or you can switch off after a little while and focus on a different supplements list in these pages.

Once you've found your symptom or condition here, you don't need to take every supplement listed for it. If you're sensitive, you can try one supplement a day. If not, you can put them all together as your daily regimen. Or as a middle ground, you can choose a couple to start off with, and then take it from there. Celery juice is always a good place to begin. Beyond that, if vitamin B_{12}, zinc, vitamin C, and/or lemon balm are in your list, bring in those. Then, if you're ready to move forward and your list contains spirulina, curcumin, cat's claw, and/or L-lysine, add those as your next step. Later on, if you're not experiencing what you want from these supplements, you can add a few more from your list. And you can always take smaller amounts than the listed dosages if you feel you're sensitive.

Further, any supplement from this chapter that's not in your specific symptom or condition list is still an option to use, if your expert sense of what your body needs or your physician's recommendation tells you to do so. They're all helpful supplements for chronic health issues.

You may already be taking other supplements. Again, be very discerning about supplements not recommended in the next chapters. A lot of supplements have ingredients that work against you—as you read a few pages ago in "Supplements to Avoid while Cleansing," some supplements such as fish oil and whey protein powder can work against your healing by feeding pathogens that create the symptoms and conditions that you'll be reading about in the pages to come.

How Long?

The length of time to stay on these supplements depends on factors such as how deficient you are (in areas that bloodwork cannot even determine) and how viral you are (meaning what kind of low-grade, undetected, undiagnosed viral infections you're dealing with), as well as how many toxic heavy metals you may have in your brain and liver, how depleted your organs are of glucose and mineral salts, how much mystery inflammation you're experiencing from undiagnosed, low-grade viral and bacterial infections, and how weakened your overall body systems may be—all of it occurring beyond detection at the doctor's office. You may be someone who says, "My doctor checked me. I'm not deficient. They didn't say anything about heavy metals. Why should I be on supplements?" The point is that a doctor isn't given the training or tools to see all the factors behind chronic illness. Even if you checked out at the doctor's office, are your symptoms and conditions still persisting? That's a sign to stick with supplementation to address the underlying issues.

The other measures you're taking to care for yourself—that is, regularly turning to options such as the Morning Cleanse, the 3:6:9 Cleanse, and the Heavy Metal Detox Cleanse and supporting yourself at other times by incorporating healing foods, lowering fats, and avoiding toxic troublemakers and troublemaker foods—will make a big difference to your healing timeline. How much your body was struggling and how long you'd been suffering when you started on your healing path will make a big difference too. Everyone has a different healing process and time frame. You may have been ill for a long time, in which case supplements are great for maintaining critical progress after you heal. Even as you're feeling better and recovering, with your specific symptoms fading away, continuing with supplements is important.

Singles for a Reason

You'll notice that almost every one of the items to come is a single herb or supplement. What you won't find here are bottles and bottles of supplement with dozens of ingredients each—dozens of herbs, vitamins, amino acids, and more. There's a reason for this. When you fill a capsule with anywhere from 10 to 40 nutrients, it's only going to contain a speck of each one, and that's not going to help you heal. This is a practice some supplement companies employ so that they don't have to use up their cheap, low-grade ingredients in large amounts in each capsule. And if one of those ingredients is a high-quality ingredient, they're saving money by only using a speck of it. Either way, whether the

product is of quality or not of any quality at all, you end up getting ripped off. When your digestive system is weakened, you may get virtually no absorption of those specks.

At the same time, most people with chronic illness of any kind are highly sensitive. If you have a reaction to a pill, powder, or tincture filled with that many ingredients, you'll never know what's causing the reaction, so you'll never get to learn from it. Plus, a supplement with dozens of ingredients is a concoction thrown together according to what a so-called expert in the field of nutraceuticals believes, not what your liver needs or what addresses the true cause of why you're sick and suffering to begin with.

Each one of the supplements in these lists holds God-given powers to help your body heal. Your liver, a processing center of your body, can understand each one of these and knows how to use it. So if you see in Chapter 29, "The True Cause of Your Symptoms and Conditions with Dosages to Heal," a list of 10 to 15 different single supplements to take for an illness or symptom, the healing benefits far surpass taking 10 to 15 different bottles of gimmicky supplements, even if they're supposedly high quality. What they really are is filled with dozens and dozens and dozens of guesses at what's good for you that end up disrupting and overburdening your liver and other areas of your immune system.

What it boils down to is that chronic symptoms and conditions like the ones in Chapter 29 remain mysteries to medical communities. How can an expert recommendation of a blended supplement help if no one knows what's really causing your ailment or disease? Only by knowing what really causes your health issue, as you can discover in these lists and throughout the Medical Medium book series, can you know what to take for it specifically. With the herbs and supplements here, the power is in your hands to take care of your specific symptoms and conditions.

Quality Matters

I'm continually asked, what is the most effective form of a given supplement, and does it really matter? Yes, it matters greatly. There are subtle and sometimes critical differences among the different supplement types available that can affect how quickly your viral or bacterial load dies off, if at all; whether your central nervous system repairs itself and how fast; how quickly your inflammation reduces; how long it takes for your symptoms and conditions to heal; and if you can safely remove toxic heavy metals or not. The supplement variety you choose can make or break your progress. To speed up healing, you need the right kinds of supplements. For these very important reasons, I offer a directory on my website (www.medicalmedium.com) of the best forms of each supplement listed in Chapters 28 and 29.

Dosages

In the pages to come, you'll find lists of supplements that can offer specific support for you. You're welcome to start at a much lower dose with anything. Even with a smaller dose of one of these high-quality supplements, you will get more health benefits than a large amount of ingredients in a lower-quality supplement. If you're sensitive, use your own experience or healing intuition or talk to your physician about what dosage your body can handle.

Teas and Tinctures

When it comes to herbal tinctures, actively seek out alcohol-free versions (avoid the word *ethanol* too). The alcohol in tinctures is normally corn grain alcohol, and therefore GMO-contaminated, even if it's organic, which (1) cancels out the herb's benefits and (2) soaks into the herb anyway and alters it, not to mention that (3) alcohol hurts your liver and lowers your immune system. Corn grain alcohol feeds the pathogens responsible for chronic symptoms and conditions. Grape alcohol in a tincture, while it may not feed pathogens, still soaks into the herb, cancels the herb's benefits, and affects your liver and immune system.

If more than one herbal tincture is recommended for your symptom or condition, you're welcome to mix them—that is, take them all at once in a small amount of water. The same is true if more than one herbal tea is recommended for your symptom or condition. For example, if your situation calls for rose hip tea, peppermint tea, and nettle leaf tea, that doesn't mean you need to drink three separate mugs of tea—that could feel especially overwhelming if you're meant to drink the tea twice a day. You can instead put a rose hip tea bag plus a peppermint tea bag plus a nettle leaf tea bag into one mug together, or create a loose-leaf blend with all three herbs.

When preparing your teas and tinctures, you're welcome to add fresh lemon juice or raw honey.

Celery Juice as a Medicinal

In every supplement list to come, you'll find a recommended amount of fresh celery juice. As you can read about in my book *Celery Juice*, celery juice is a powerful medicinal that elevates whatever you're doing right in your life. That's why it was part of every cleanse in this book too.

The same guidelines apply for celery juice as always:

- Fresh, plain, unadulterated, straight celery juice. No added ice, lemon juice, apple cider vinegar, collagen, or other mix-ins. Also, as beneficial as green juice blends can be, they're not a substitute for pure celery juice.

- Juice means juice. Drinking blended celery without straining the pulp doesn't yield the same benefits—turn back to Chapter 6, "The Juicing versus Fiber Debate," for more on why.

- Fresh means fresh. Making a drink from reconstituted celery powder won't deliver the right benefits, nor will drinking pasteurized or HPP (high-pressure pasteurization) celery juice. Any kind of juicer is okay for celery juice, and you can also choose to purchase your fresh celery juice from a juice bar rather than making your own. For best results, drink it freshly made. If you can't drink it immediately after juicing—for example, if you're having a second serving in the day—that's okay. Store it chilled in an airtight container for up to 24 hours. After 24 hours, it loses its potency.

- Drink your fresh celery juice on an empty stomach. If you drank some water or lemon water beforehand, wait at least 15 to 20 and ideally 30 minutes before drinking your celery juice. After finishing your celery juice, wait at least 15 to 20 minutes and ideally 30 minutes before consuming anything else.

- If you're drinking celery juice later in the day, give any food you've eaten plenty of time to digest first. If your last snack or meal was high in fat/protein, it's best to wait a minimum of two hours and ideally three hours before having your celery juice. If you last ate something lighter such as fruit, vegetables, potatoes, or a fruit smoothie, you can drink your celery juice 60 minutes after eating.

- If you are on a doctor-prescribed medication, it's okay to take it either before or after your celery juice, depending on whether it's supposed to be taken on an empty stomach or with food. (Please note that if your medication is supposed to be taken with food, celery juice does not count as a food.) If you take the medication first, try to wait at least 15 to 20 minutes and ideally 30 minutes before you drink your celery juice. If you drink your celery juice first, try to wait at least 15 to 20 minutes and ideally 30 minutes before you take your medication. For any further questions or concerns, consult your physician.

- When it comes to the other supplements in these lists, please hold off on taking them *with* your celery juice. While the supplements will do fine with the celery juice, the celery juice is better without most supplements. It's best to wait to take your supplements until at least 15 to 20 minutes and ideally 30 minutes after you've finished your celery juice.

- If you have any further questions about bringing celery juice into your life, *Medical Medium Celery Juice* is an entire book of answers waiting for you.

Children

With the exception of a few instances where noted, the dosages listed are for adults. If you're considering supplements for a child, consult with her or his physician about what's safe and appropriate.

When selecting celery juice amounts for children, you can refer to this table. These are recommended daily minimums. It can be less if that feels right for your child, or more. You don't need to worry that going over these minimums is harmful.

——— CELERY JUICE AMOUNTS FOR CHILDREN ———

AGE	AMOUNT
6 months old	1 ounce or more
1 year old	2 ounces or more
18 months old	3 ounces or more
2 years old	4 ounces or more
3 years old	5 ounces or more
4 to 6 years old	6 to 7 ounces or more
7 to 10 years old	8 to 10 ounces or more
11 years old and up	12 to 16 ounces

Pregnancy and Breastfeeding

Every woman who is pregnant should check with her doctor about any type of supplements she's considering.

If you're a mom struggling with symptoms or conditions while breastfeeding, you're welcome to partake in any of the supplementation listed here. If you have any questions about using supplements in your particular situation, talk to your doctor.

Secrets of Supplements

The supplements to come are listed in alphabetical order, not necessarily order of importance. An exception is celery juice, which you'll see at the top of each list. As you read through these pages, keep in mind that the extent of what these supplements do for your body and brain remains undiscovered by medical research and science. While a few are on their radar, many of them are completely unknown as health rescuers, and the benefits go far beyond what anyone realizes.

One powerful undiscovered tip is to consider taking your supplements with a piece of fruit such as a banana or even some potato, sweet potato, winter squash, raw honey, pure maple syrup, or coconut water (as long as it's the right kind of coconut water—see Chapter 19, "Critical Cleanse Dos and Don'ts"). Natural sugar is what carries vitamins, minerals, and other nutrients through the bloodstream to help them find their way to where they need to go, and an organ won't accept vitamins, minerals, and other nutrients without sugar to assist it. This is one reason why low-carb, high-fat/high-protein diets long term can cause serious deficiencies in vitamins, minerals, trace minerals, antivirals, antibacterials, antioxidants, and healing phytochemical compounds—because it takes natural sugar to deliver these nutrients into a cell. Taking your supplements with natural sugars ensures that the liver (your processing center) and other parts of your body can actually use them.

"You have the right to heal.
You deserve to feel strong and productive
and to experience your body as a precious vehicle
that can carry you through life with ease."

— Anthony William, Medical Medium

CHAPTER 28

Medical Medium Shock Therapies

Medical Medium Zinc Shock Therapy and Medical Medium Vitamin C Shock Therapy are powerful healing tools you'll find referenced in some of the supplement lists to come. These are tools to rebuild your immune system quickly by fueling it with what it needs to fight an infection, whether you're dealing with a condition that's occurring for the first time or you're experiencing a relapse.

Zinc feeds the immune system, providing it with one of the most critical trace minerals for the immune system to function optimally. Everyone is zinc deficient, which is one reason why we end up with immune systems that viruses and unproductive bacteria can take advantage of to cause us harm. Zinc makes pathogens docile, slow, and less active, which helps stop them from proliferating quickly, in turn allowing your immune system to get ahead of the viruses and unproductive bacteria.

Vitamin C is an antioxidant that feeds your immune system. On top of which, the viruses and unproductive bacteria that are responsible for symptoms and conditions are highly allergic and sensitive to vitamin C. While protecting your own cells from oxidation, vitamin C has the ability to oxidize a pathogen, causing it to become injured, break down, and disperse.

Try these Medical Medium therapies if you have any of these conditions: cold and flu, UTIs, sties, cold sores (herpes simplex 1), herpes simplex 2, shingles, rash, cough, sore throat, sinus infection, lung infection, canker sores, or mono.

MEDICAL MEDIUM ZINC SHOCK THERAPY

Medical Medium Zinc Shock Therapy is a useful technique because most everyone is zinc deficient. It's a mineral that left our soils long ago due to a reaction that occurs when toxic heavy metals enter our soils, including our organic farm soils, and create dead soil over time by destroying the soil's immune system. Trace mineral zinc in foods at this point is minuscule and only becoming rarer as passing-by pollutants (such as pesticides, herbicides, car exhaust, old asbestos from car brakes in decades past, and DDT and toxic heavy metals falling from the sky) continue to enter our soil and deplete the soil's immune system. Zinc is supposed to be our own immune system's number-one defense, and because we're deficient, we're in dire need of it.

If we don't have enough zinc in the body, our immune system may overreact to an invader such as a flu strain or underreact to a chronic viral infection such as Epstein-Barr. Overreaction could mean higher fever and other more advanced, severe symptoms. Underreaction could mean prolonged low-grade symptoms that become chronic over time. When our immune system is well supplied with an abundant amount of zinc, this overreaction or underreaction doesn't take place. Zinc also slows down viruses and unproductive, aggressive bacteria on its own merit. Viruses and unproductive bacteria are allergic to zinc; the mineral repels and weakens them, even making pathogens docile, which allows the immune system to kill off and eliminate the pathogens more quickly.

Medical Medium Zinc Shock Therapy Directions

- If you think you're coming down with a bug, you're already sick with the flu, or you have one of the infections listed above, then for an adult, squirt 2 dropperfuls of high-quality liquid zinc sulfate into your throat every three hours. Let it sit for one minute before swallowing. If the flu isn't making you nauseated and you can palate the zinc, you can do this up to five or six times a day (that is, two squirts of zinc every three hours for a total of 10 to 12 dropperfuls a day) for two days.

- If your palate is more sensitive, you're welcome to try a milder Medical Medium Zinc Shock Therapy: 1 dropperful every three hours up to five times a day or 2 dropperfuls three times a day. In any version of Medical Medium Zinc Shock Therapy, after the two days, bring the zinc dosage down to what your supplement list says.

For children, here are the adjusted amounts of liquid zinc sulfate for this supplement therapy:

- **Ages 1 to 2:** 2 tiny drops (not dropperfuls) in juice, water, or directly in the mouth every three hours during waking hours

- **Ages 3 to 4:** 3 tiny drops (not dropperfuls) in juice, water, or directly in the mouth every three hours during waking hours

- **Ages 5 to 8:** 4 small drops (not dropperfuls) in juice, water, or directly in the mouth every three hours during waking hours

- **Ages 9 to 12:** 10 small drops (not dropperfuls) in juice, water, or directly in the mouth every three hours during waking hours

- **Ages 13 and up:** 1 dropperful directly in the mouth every four hours during waking hours

Because of children's special sensitive nature, it's especially important to get the right kind of liquid zinc sulfate, which you can find on my directory online at www.medicalmedium.com. Almost all companies make zinc that's aggressive in taste and hard to palate, often with harsh additives too.

MEDICAL MEDIUM VITAMIN C SHOCK THERAPY

Why does Medical Medium Vitamin C Shock Therapy bring healing to a new level? Because it takes a specific type of glucose that you'll find mainly in raw honey, pure maple syrup, and fresh-squeezed citrus to bind onto the right type of vitamin C to drive it into cells and organs. The raw honey and the squeezed orange combined attach themselves directly to the vitamin C, allowing this powerful delivery of antiviral, antibacterial healing nutrients to occur within the body.

Medical Medium Vitamin C Shock Therapy Directions

- **For Medical Medium Vitamin C Shock Therapy for adults, the ingredients are 2 500-milligram capsules of Micro-C, 1 cup of water (preferably warm), 2 teaspoons of raw honey, and the freshly squeezed juice from one orange.**

- **Here's how to prepare it: Open the Micro-C capsules and pour their powder into the warm water. Stir until dissolved. Add the raw honey and orange juice and stir well. Starting at the first sign of cold, flu, or any of the infections listed, drink this tonic every two hours during waking hours. You can do this for two days and then switch to the dosage in an individual supplement list, or you can use this technique throughout the duration of a cold or flu.**

- If you feel you need more vitamin C per drink, you can add more than 2 capsules of Micro-C to each. If you don't want to use raw honey, you can use 100 percent pure maple syrup (not maple-flavored syrup) in its place. If you don't like orange, you can substitute the juice of one lemon.

For children, here are the adjusted amounts of vitamin C for this supplement therapy:

- **Ages 1 to 2:** 1 500-milligram capsule Micro-C emptied and mixed with ½ cup water, 1 teaspoon raw honey, and the freshly squeezed juice from half an orange, every six hours during waking hours

- **Ages 3 to 4:** 1 500-milligram capsule Micro-C emptied and mixed with ½ cup water, 1 teaspoon raw honey, and the freshly squeezed juice from 1 orange, every five hours during waking hours

- **Ages 5 to 8:** 1 500-milligram capsule Micro-C emptied and mixed with 1 cup water, 2 teaspoons raw honey, and the freshly squeezed juice from 1 orange, every four hours during waking hours

- **Ages 9 to 12:** 1 500-milligram capsule Micro-C emptied and mixed with 1 cup water, 2 teaspoons raw honey, and the freshly squeezed juice from 1 orange, every two hours during waking hours

- **Ages 13 and up:** 2 500-milligram capsules Micro-C emptied and mixed with 1 cup water, 2 teaspoons raw honey, and the freshly squeezed juice from 1 orange, every three hours during waking hours

CHAPTER 29

The True Cause of Your Symptoms and Conditions with Dosages to Heal

Spirit of Compassion has always said to me throughout the years of helping so many people heal that knowing the true cause of why you're sick is half the battle won. Knowing what to do, what to take, and how to apply those tools is the other half the battle won. In this chapter, you will learn why you're struggling with symptoms and conditions and how to address that "why" with supplements that you can add to your life. Supplementation is not a replacement for cleansing. Make sure to go back and read Chapter 27, "What You Need to Know about Supplements," for guidance on how to integrate supplementation and cleansing.

CRITICAL TIPS—READ THIS FIRST

Before you leap into the supplement lists to come, first make sure you read Chapter 27 fully so you can interpret these lists correctly. Then make sure to read these critical tips.

- When you see the term *dropperful*, that means as much liquid supplement as fills the bottle's eye dropper when you squeeze its rubber top. It may only fill up halfway; that's still considered a dropperful.

- There are also some supplements where dosages are given in drops. Make sure to check carefully whether it says *drops* or *dropperfuls*.

- Most of the liquid and powder supplements below are meant to be taken in water. Check the directions on the supplement's label.

- When you see multiple herbal tinctures in a list, you're welcome to combine them into one ounce or more of water and take them together.

- Again, the same goes for teas. If multiple teas are listed for your symptom or condition, feel free to combine the herbs to make yourself a special tea blend or use a few different tea bags together.

- One cup of tea translates to either 1 tea bag or 1 to 2 teaspoons of loose leaf tea.

- Some of the dosages are listed in milligrams. If you can't find capsules that line up with the exact suggestions, try to get ones that are close.

- Remember: almost all of these are adult dosages. Talk to a physician about what's right for a child.

- When you see the term *daily*, that means to take the given dosage of the supplement over the course of the day, and it's your choice how you do that. You're welcome to take the whole dose once a day. If you're sensitive, you may want to break it up into multiple servings. For example, if it says to take 2 teaspoons of barley grass juice powder daily, you may decide either to put both teaspoons together into a smoothie or have 1 teaspoon in a morning smoothie and 1 teaspoon in some water at night.

- When you see *twice a day,* that means two installments taken at any time of day, as long as they're at least four hours apart. If you miss one of the installments on any given day, try to start fresh the next day.

REAL REASONS FOR YOUR SUFFERING

Before each list, you'll find the true cause of each symptom and condition. What's listed are the *main* causes. While multiple factors can contribute to a given health issue, and those factors can be different from person to person, you'll find only the leading causes that fit here, due to space. To explore further and find much more detail about chronic health issues, you can look into the rest of the Medical Medium book series.

Often, these true causes will challenge both conventional and alternative wisdom, so prepare yourself to see the unexpected. Only with real understanding of what's behind chronic suffering can we conceptualize what's needed to heal. Almost all of these symptoms and conditions are still misunderstood by medical research and science. The root problems that cause the majority of these health problems are mysteries to medical communities, much as it may seem otherwise when you hear labels and theories circulating as facts.

The explanation behind autoimmune disease, for example—that the body attacks itself—seems like a verified medical fact. It's not. It's simply a theory that gained popularity in the 1950s when no one could explain why symptoms and chronic illness started taking hold of the population. Your body never turns on itself. Your body never turns on *you.*

You'll see many mentions of common pathogens such as the Epstein-Barr virus, shingles virus, and *Streptococcus* bacteria. Many more strains of these pathogens exist than have yet been discovered, and they're at the root of many more health problems than anyone yet realizes. Often, they're burrowed so deeply in the body that they're beyond detection, at least as far as current medical testing goes. Because there are dozens of mutations of each, they can cause diverse symptoms—you'll see just how diverse in a moment.

If you want a refresher on where I get my information, my mission to protect you, and what to say to those who don't understand the steps you're taking to heal, turn back to

Chapter 24, "Living Words for Underdogs and a Note for Critics." You deserve to know the truth about your health.

DOSAGES TO HEAL

Everyday Liver and Health Maintenance

If you're not experiencing any of the symptoms or conditions in this chapter, here's a list of herbs and supplements to help maintain your general health.

- **Fresh celery juice:** work up to at least 16 ounces daily
- **Celeryforce:** 1 capsule twice a day
- **5-MTHF:** 1 capsule daily
- **Aloe vera:** 2 or more inches of fresh gel (skin removed) daily
- **Barley grass juice powder:** 2 teaspoons or 6 capsules daily
- **Chaga mushroom:** 2 teaspoons or 6 capsules daily
- **Curcumin:** 2 capsules daily
- **Lemon balm:** 3 dropperfuls daily
- **L-lysine:** 3 500-milligram capsules daily
- **Magnesium glycinate:** 2 capsules daily
- **Nettle leaf:** 2 cups of tea or 3 dropperfuls daily
- **Spirulina:** 2 teaspoons or 6 capsules daily
- **Turmeric:** 2 capsules daily
- **Vitamin B$_{12}$ (as adenosylcobalamin with methylcobalamin):** 1 dropperful daily
- **Vitamin C (as Micro-C):** 4 capsules twice a day
- **Zinc (as liquid zinc sulfate):** up to 1 dropperful daily

Abscesses

True cause: Acute or chronic viral or bacterial infections mostly residing within the lymph and more rarely inside an organ.

- **Fresh celery juice:** work up to 32 ounces daily, then work up to 64 ounces if possible
- **Barley grass juice powder:** 2 teaspoons or 6 capsules daily
- **Cat's claw:** 2 dropperfuls twice a day
- **Curcumin:** 2 capsules twice a day
- **Goldenseal:** 3 dropperfuls twice a day (two weeks on, two weeks off)
- **Lemon balm:** 4 dropperfuls twice a day
- **Mullein leaf:** 3 dropperfuls twice a day
- **Olive leaf:** 2 dropperfuls twice a day
- **Oregon grape root:** 2 dropperfuls twice a day (two weeks on, two weeks off)
- **Raw honey:** 1 tablespoon daily
- **Spirulina:** 2 teaspoons or 6 capsules daily
- **Vitamin B$_{12}$ (as adenosylcobalamin with methylcobalamin):** 1 dropperful twice a day
- **Vitamin C (as Micro-C):** 6 capsules twice a day
- **Wild blueberry powder:** 2 tablespoons daily
- **Zinc (as liquid zinc sulfate):** up to 2 dropperfuls twice a day

Acne

True cause: One or more strains from the over 50 groups of *Streptococcus* bacteria residing both in your liver and your lymphatic system. Having acne doesn't necessarily mean having a strep infection such as strep throat. Acne develops when strep has made a long-term home inside the body after (sometimes long after) a strep-related infection.

- **Fresh celery juice:** for teenagers, work up to 16 ounces daily; for adults, work up to 32 ounces daily

- **Barley grass juice powder:** 1 teaspoon or 3 capsules twice a day
- **Cat's claw:** 1 dropperful twice a day
- **Chaga mushroom:** 1 teaspoon or 3 capsules twice a day
- **Curcumin:** 2 capsules twice a day
- **GABA:** 1 250-milligram capsule daily
- **Goldenseal:** 2 dropperfuls twice a day (two weeks on, two weeks off)
- **Lemon balm:** 2 dropperfuls twice a day
- **Mullein leaf:** 2 dropperfuls twice a day
- **Nascent iodine:** 3 small drops (not dropperfuls) twice a day
- **Nettle leaf:** 2 dropperfuls twice a day
- **Oregano oil:** 1 capsule daily
- **Raw honey:** 1 tablespoon daily
- **Spirulina:** 1 teaspoon or 3 capsules daily
- **Thyme:** 2 sprigs of fresh thyme in hot water as tea or 4 sprigs in room temperature water daily
- **Vitamin B$_{12}$ (as adenosylcobalamin with methylcobalamin):** 1 dropperful daily
- **Vitamin C (as Micro-C):** 4 capsules twice a day
- **Zinc (as liquid zinc sulfate):** up to 1 dropperful twice a day

Addiction

True cause: A deficiency of glycogen and mineral salts in the brain from a lack of glucose entering the brain, partly due to years of high-fat/high-protein diet, and a lack of mineral salts from sources such as celery juice and leafy greens in the diet to feed neurotransmitters. Elevated levels of toxic heavy metals such as mercury, aluminum, and copper inside the brain can contribute to or cause addiction on their own. Emotional duress can amplify or further deplete someone, triggering addictive impulses.

- **Fresh celery juice:** work up to at least 16 ounces daily
- **Celeryforce:** 2 capsules three times a day
- **5-MTHF:** 1 capsule daily
- **Ashwagandha:** 1 dropperful twice a day
- **Barley grass juice powder:** 1 tablespoon or 9 capsules daily
- **Chaga mushroom:** 2 teaspoons or 6 capsules daily
- **Curcumin:** 2 capsules twice a day
- **EPA and DHA (fish-free):** 2 capsules daily (taken with dinner)
- **GABA:** 1 250-milligram capsule daily
- **Lemon balm:** 4 dropperfuls three times a day
- **L-glutamine:** 2 capsules twice a day
- **Licorice root:** 1 dropperful daily (two weeks on, two weeks off)
- **Melatonin:** 5 milligrams twice a day
- **Spirulina:** 1 tablespoon or 9 capsules daily
- **Vitamin B$_{12}$ (as adenosylcobalamin with methylcobalamin):** 3 dropperfuls twice a day
- **Vitamin C (as Micro-C):** 4 capsules daily
- **Wild blueberry powder:** 2 tablespoons daily
- **Zinc (as liquid zinc sulfate):** 1 dropperful twice a day

Adrenal Problems

True cause: Chronic fight-or-flight syndrome, a low-grade viral infection (such as from one of the over 60 varieties of EBV), too many years on a high-fat/high-protein diet, or regularly going too many hours without eating. In many cases, all four of these causes can contribute at the same time.

- **Fresh celery juice:** work up to 16 ounces twice a day or 32 ounces every morning
- **Celeryforce:** 3 capsules twice a day

- **Amla berry:** 1 teaspoon twice a day
- **Ashwagandha:** 1 dropperful twice a day
- **B-complex:** 1 capsule daily
- **Chicory root:** 1 cup of tea daily
- **Hibiscus:** 1 cup of tea daily
- **Lemon balm:** 2 dropperfuls twice a day
- **Licorice root:** 10 small drops (not dropperfuls) twice a day (two weeks on, two weeks off)
- **Magnesium glycinate:** 2 capsules twice a day
- **Nettle leaf:** 1 dropperful twice a day
- **Schisandra berry:** 1 cup of tea daily
- **Spirulina:** 2 teaspoons or 6 capsules daily
- **Vitamin B$_{12}$ (as adenosylcobalamin with methylcobalamin):** 1 dropperful twice a day
- **Vitamin C (as Micro-C):** 4 capsules twice a day
- **Zinc (as liquid zinc sulfate):** up to 1 dropperful twice a day

Aging

True cause: A long-term high-fat/high-protein diet (whether healthy or unhealthy fats) causing depletion of critically needed glycogen inside the liver, weakening the organ and allowing it to become overburdened with a variety of toxins (including from petrochemical byproducts, toxic heavy metals, old pharmaceuticals, air fresheners, scented candles, colognes, perfumes, viruses, and bacteria), in turn causing the skin and body in general to age more quickly than normal.

All the supplements in this chapter help prevent aging. If it's a particular concern for you, consider these hand-picked ones:

- **Fresh celery juice:** work up to 32 ounces daily
- **Celeryforce:** 2 capsules twice a day

- **Barley grass juice powder:** 2 teaspoons or 6 capsules daily
- **Chaga mushroom:** 1 teaspoon or 3 capsules twice a day
- **Curcumin:** 2 capsules twice a day
- **Glutathione:** 1 capsule daily
- **Nettle leaf:** 1 dropperful twice a day
- **Spirulina:** 2 teaspoons or 6 capsules daily
- **Vitamin B$_{12}$ (as adenosylcobalamin with methylcobalamin):** 2 dropperfuls twice a day
- **Vitamin C (as Micro-C):** 2 capsules twice a day
- **Wild blueberry powder:** 2 tablespoons daily
- **Zinc (as liquid zinc sulfate):** up to 1 dropperful twice a day

Alzheimer's Disease, Dementia, and Memory Issues

True cause: Toxic heavy metals (predominantly mercury and aluminum) oxidizing in the brain.

- **Fresh celery juice:** work up to at least 16 ounces daily
- **Celeryforce:** 3 capsules three times a day
- **5-MTHF:** 1 capsule twice a day
- **Barley grass juice powder:** 4 teaspoons or 12 capsules daily
- **B-complex:** 1 capsule daily
- **Cat's claw:** 1 dropperful twice a day
- **CoQ10:** 1 capsule twice a day
- **Curcumin:** 3 capsules twice a day
- **EPA and DHA (fish-free):** 2 capsules daily (taken with dinner)
- **Glutathione:** 1 capsule daily
- **Lemon balm:** 3 dropperfuls twice a day
- **L-glutamine:** 2 capsules twice a day
- **L-lysine:** 1 capsule twice a day

- **Magnesium glycinate:** 1 capsule twice a day
- **Melatonin:** 5 milligrams up to six times a day
- **Nettle leaf:** 3 dropperfuls twice a day
- **Spirulina:** 1 tablespoon or 3 capsules daily
- **Vitamin B$_{12}$ (as adenosylcobalamin with methylcobalamin):** 3 dropperfuls twice a day
- **Vitamin C (as Micro-C):** 2 capsules twice a day
- **Zinc (as liquid zinc sulfate):** 1 dropperful daily

Anorexia and Bulimia

True cause: Different cases of these eating disorders have different causes. Emotional distress, emotional injury, toxic heavy metal exposure, extreme stress, posttraumatic stress symptoms (PTSS), societal expectations, and body shaming about how we're "supposed" to look are some of the factors that can contribute, often in combination with each other. When purging is part of someone's struggle, extra adrenal support is needed, which is reflected in the list below.

- **Fresh celery juice:** work up to at least 16 ounces daily
- **Celeryforce:** 3 capsules twice a day
- **5-MTHF:** 1 capsule daily
- **Aloe vera:** 2 or more inches of fresh gel (skin removed) daily
- **Ashwagandha:** 1 dropperful daily (**note:** if purging is involved, 1 dropperful twice a day)
- **Barley grass juice powder:** 2 teaspoons or 6 capsules daily
- **Cat's claw:** 1 dropperful daily
- **Curcumin:** 1 capsule twice a day

- **D-mannose:** 1 tablespoon in water daily
- **EPA and DHA (fish-free):** 2 capsules daily (taken with dinner)
- **GABA:** 1 250-milligram capsule daily
- **Lemon balm:** 4 dropperfuls twice a day
- **Licorice root (only for cases of purging):** 1 dropperful daily (two weeks on, two weeks off)
- **Magnesium glycinate:** 1 capsule twice a day
- **Nascent iodine:** 6 small drops (not dropperfuls) daily
- **Nettle leaf:** 2 dropperfuls daily
- **Raspberry leaf:** 1 cup of tea with 2 bags daily
- **Spirulina:** 1 teaspoon or 3 capsules daily
- **Vitamin B$_{12}$ (as adenosylcobalamin with methylcobalamin):** 1 dropperful twice a day
- **Zinc (as liquid zinc sulfate):** 1 dropperful daily

Anxiety and Anxiousness

True cause of anxiety: When anxiety interferes with your life, it's caused by toxic heavy metals (such as mercury, aluminum, and copper), viruses (such as one of the over 60 varieties of Epstein-Barr virus or one of the over 30 varieties of shingles virus), or a combination of both toxic heavy metals and viruses. Most of the time, it's both at once, with one cause more dominant depending on the individual case. Anxiety can also be triggered, accelerated, or heightened by emotional conflict, although toxic heavy metals and/or a virus must be present for the anxiety to become sustained, chronic, and longer term.

True cause of anxiousness: Anxiousness that comes and goes in a milder form can have the same toxic heavy metal and/or viral causes, or it can result from mild emotional injury or prolonged stress on their own.

Supplements for Anxiety

- **Fresh celery juice:** work up to 32 ounces daily
- **Celeryforce:** 3 capsules three times a day
- **5-MTHF:** 1 capsule daily
- **Aloe vera:** 2 or more inches of fresh gel (skin removed) daily
- **Ashwagandha:** 1 dropperful twice a day
- **Barley grass juice powder:** 2 teaspoons or 6 capsules daily
- **B-complex:** 1 capsule daily
- **Curcumin:** 2 capsules daily
- **EPA and DHA (fish-free):** 1 capsule daily (taken with dinner)
- **GABA:** 1 250-milligram capsule daily
- **Ginger:** 2 cups of tea or freshly grated to taste daily
- **Lemon balm:** 4 dropperfuls four times a day
- **L-lysine:** 2 500-milligram capsules daily
- **Magnesium glycinate:** 3 capsules daily
- **Melatonin:** 5 milligrams at bedtime daily
- **Spirulina:** 2 teaspoons or 6 capsules daily
- **Vitamin C (as Micro-C):** 4 capsules twice a day
- **Vitamin B$_{12}$ (as adenosylcobalamin with methylcobalamin):** 3 dropperfuls twice a day
- **Vitamin D$_3$:** 1,000 IU daily
- **Wild blueberry powder:** 2 teaspoons daily
- **Zinc (as liquid zinc sulfate):** 1 dropperful daily

Supplements for Anxiousness

- **Fresh celery juice:** work up to at least 16 ounces daily
- **Celeryforce:** 2 capsules twice a day
- **Ashwagandha:** 1 dropperful daily
- **Barley grass juice powder:** 2 teaspoons or 6 capsules daily
- **B-complex:** 1 capsule daily
- **Chaga mushroom:** 2 teaspoons or 6 capsules daily
- **Curcumin:** 1 capsule twice a day
- **EPA and DHA (fish-free):** 1 capsule daily (taken with dinner)
- **GABA:** 1 250-milligram capsule daily
- **Hibiscus:** 1 cup of tea twice a day
- **Lemon balm:** 3 dropperfuls twice a day
- **L-lysine:** 2 500-milligram capsules twice a day
- **Magnesium glycinate:** 1 capsule twice a day
- **Melatonin:** 5 milligrams at bedtime daily
- **Spirulina:** 2 teaspoons or 6 capsules daily
- **Vitamin B$_{12}$ (as adenosylcobalamin with methylcobalamin):** 2 dropperfuls twice a day
- **Vitamin C (as Micro-C):** 4 capsules twice a day
- **Vitamin D$_3$:** 1,000 IU daily
- **Wild blueberry powder:** 2 teaspoons daily
- **Zinc (as liquid zinc sulfate):** 1 dropperful daily

Autoimmune Disorders and Diseases

If your individual autoimmune issue does not appear with its own supplement list in the coming pages, turn back to this list for support.

True cause: Unknown to medical research and science, health problems that are labeled "autoimmune" are, in truth, viral infections. Viruses that cause autoimmune conditions can be one or more of the over 60 varieties of Epstein-Barr virus, the over 30 varieties of shingles virus, many varieties of HHV-6 and HHV-7, varieties of the undiscovered HHV-10 through HHV-16, multiple varieties of herpes simplex 1 and herpes simplex 2, and many more. The cause of autoimmune disorders and diseases is *not* the body's immune system attacking its own organs and glands, a theory that gained popularity in the 1950s and unfortunately still persists today. Often, people who are dealing with the viruses responsible for these illnesses are living with that viral activity in combination with toxic heavy metals such as mercury, aluminum, and copper. These viruses also feed on foods such as eggs, dairy products, and gluten, which can worsen a person's condition.

- **Fresh celery juice:** work up to 32 ounces twice a day if possible; if not, work up to 32 ounces every morning
- **Celeryforce:** 3 capsules twice a day
- **5-MTHF:** 1 capsule twice a day
- **ALA (alpha lipoic acid):** 1 500-milligram capsule twice a week
- **Aloe vera:** 2 or more inches of fresh gel (skin removed) daily
- **Barley grass juice powder:** 2 teaspoons or 6 capsules twice a day
- **Cat's claw:** 2 dropperfuls twice a day
- **Chaga mushroom:** 2 teaspoons or 6 capsules twice a day
- **Curcumin:** 2 capsules twice a day
- **Glutathione:** 1 capsule daily
- **Hibiscus:** 1 cup of tea daily
- **Lemon balm:** 2 dropperfuls twice a day
- **Licorice root:** 1 dropperful daily (two weeks on, two weeks off)
- **L-lysine:** 4 500-milligram capsules twice a day
- **Lomatium root:** 1 dropperful daily
- **MSM:** 1 capsule twice a day
- **Mullein leaf:** 2 dropperfuls twice a day
- **Nascent iodine:** 3 small drops (not dropperfuls) twice a day
- **Nettle leaf:** 2 dropperfuls twice a day
- **Oregon grape root:** 1 dropperful twice a day (two weeks on, two weeks off)
- **Raw honey:** 1 to 3 teaspoons daily

- **Selenium:** 1 capsule daily
- **Spirulina:** 2 teaspoons or 6 capsules daily
- **Thyme:** 2 sprigs of fresh thyme in hot water as tea or 4 sprigs in room temperature water daily
- **Turmeric:** 1 capsule twice a day
- **Vitamin B$_{12}$ (as adenosylcobalamin with methylcobalamin):** 2 dropperfuls twice a day
- **Vitamin C (as Micro-C):** 6 capsules twice a day
- **Wild blueberry powder:** 1 tablespoon daily
- **Zinc (as liquid zinc sulfate):** up to 2 dropperfuls twice a day

Bloating

True cause: Most commonly, a diet too high in fat/protein (whether unhealthy or healthy fats) causing liver burnout. When an overworked liver must constantly overproduce bile to accommodate a chronic, long-term high-fat/high-protein diet, the stomach must in turn produce more hydrochloric acid to compensate for the reduction in bile reserves over time. Eventually, this causes the stomach glands to become depleted and produce less hydrochloric acid to break down and digest proteins, all while the liver is becoming more sluggish and stagnant.

As this happens, one or more strains from the over 50 groups of *Streptococcus* bacteria can begin irritating the intestinal wall linings and causing mild gastritis as well. At times, overabundant stress can also account for bloating, with the adrenals becoming overworked from either constant low-grade stress or extreme stress conditions. Excess adrenaline tends to affect the intestinal linings, causing irritation there, while tiring out the liver and contributing to its sluggishness and stagnation.

- **Fresh celery juice:** work up to 32 ounces every morning
- **Celeryforce:** 1 capsule twice a day
- **5-MTHF:** 1 capsule daily
- **Aloe vera:** 2 or more inches of fresh gel (skin removed) daily
- **Barley grass juice powder:** 1 teaspoon or 3 capsules daily
- **Burdock root:** 1 cup of tea or 1 root freshly juiced daily
- **Cat's claw:** 1 dropperful daily
- **Chaga mushroom:** 1 teaspoon or 3 capsules daily
- **Curcumin:** 1 capsule daily
- **Ginger:** 1 cup of tea twice a day or freshly grated or juiced to taste daily
- **Hibiscus:** 1 cup of tea daily
- **Lemon balm:** 1 dropperful daily
- **Licorice root:** 1 dropperful daily (two weeks on, two weeks off)
- **Magnesium glycinate:** 1 capsule daily
- **Milk thistle:** 1 dropperful daily
- **Peppermint:** 1 cup of tea daily
- **Raspberry leaf:** 1 cup of tea with 2 bags daily
- **Spirulina:** 1 teaspoon or 3 capsules daily
- **Vitamin B$_{12}$ (as adenosylcobalamin with methylcobalamin):** 1 dropperful daily

Brain Fog

True cause: Low-grade chronic viral infection (most commonly caused by one of the over 60 varieties of Epstein-Barr virus); toxic heavy metals such as mercury, aluminum, and copper; or both a viral load and toxic heavy metals in combination. For example, someone could have a low-grade viral infection with very low toxic heavy metals, or they could have no viral inflammation and elevated toxic heavy metal exposure. Metals often age over time, oxidizing as the years go by, accelerated by a high-fat/high-protein diet, and as a result the metals create discharge that spreads to adjacent brain tissue and causes neurotransmitters to weaken and diminish, electrical impulses to overreact, and neurons to become saturated with the toxic heavy metal oxidation runoff. The majority of brain fog cases have a little of both: a longstanding viral infection such as EBV plus an honest amount of toxic heavy metals, with mercury being the leading heavy metal in this case.

- **Fresh celery juice:** work up to 32 ounces every morning
- **Celeryforce:** 3 capsules three times a day
- **5-MTHF:** 1 capsule twice a day
- **Ashwagandha:** 1 dropperful twice a day
- **Barley grass juice powder:** 2 teaspoons or 6 capsules twice a day
- **B-complex:** 1 capsule daily
- **Cat's claw:** 1 dropperful twice a day
- **Chaga mushroom:** 1 teaspoon or 3 capsules twice a day
- **Lemon balm:** 1 dropperful twice a day
- **Licorice root:** 1 dropperful daily (two weeks on, two weeks off)
- **L-lysine:** 2 500-milligram capsules twice a day
- **Nettle leaf:** 1 dropperful twice a day
- **Spirulina:** 2 teaspoons or 6 capsules twice a day
- **Vitamin B$_{12}$ (as adenosylcobalamin with methylcobalamin):** 1 dropperful twice a day
- **Vitamin C (as Micro-C):** 2 500-milligram capsules twice a day
- **Wild blueberry powder:** 1 tablespoon daily
- **Zinc (as liquid zinc sulfate):** up to 1 dropperful twice a day

Breast Density

True cause: A stagnant, sluggish liver that's toxic and overburdened by a variety of toxins, including from low-grade pathogenic infections such as one of the over 60 varieties of Epstein-Barr virus or one of the over 30 varieties of shingles virus. Pathogens create byproduct and debris, which further burden a liver already tired from toxic heavy metals, pesticides, herbicides, colognes, perfumes, scented candles, air fresheners, petrochemicals, plastics, old pharmaceuticals, and other troublemakers, and that affects the lymphatic system directly connected to the breast tissue.

- **Fresh celery juice:** work up to 32 ounces daily
- **ALA (alpha lipoic acid):** 1 capsule daily
- **Aloe vera:** 2 or more inches of fresh gel (skin removed) daily
- **Ashwagandha:** 1 dropperful daily
- **Barley grass juice powder:** 1 tablespoon or 9 capsules daily
- **Burdock root:** 1 cup of tea or 1 root freshly juiced daily
- **Cardamom:** a pinch in food once a week
- **Chaga mushroom:** 2 teaspoons or 6 capsules daily
- **CoQ10:** 1 capsule daily
- **Curcumin:** 2 capsules twice a day
- **Dandelion root:** 1 cup of tea daily
- **Lemon balm:** 2 dropperfuls twice a day
- **Milk thistle:** 1 dropperful daily
- **MSM:** 1 capsule daily
- **Nettle leaf:** 4 dropperfuls daily
- **Oregano oil:** 1 capsule daily
- **Raspberry leaf:** 1 cup of tea with 2 bags twice a day
- **Spirulina:** 2 teaspoons or 6 capsules daily
- **Vitamin B$_{12}$ (as adenosylcobalamin with methylcobalamin):** 1 dropperful daily
- **Vitamin C (as Micro-C):** 4 capsules twice a day
- **Wild blueberry powder:** 1 tablespoon daily
- **Zinc (as liquid zinc sulfate):** 1 dropperful daily

Brittle, Ridged Nails

True cause: A stagnant, sluggish liver filled with toxins leading to a zinc deficiency.

- **Fresh celery juice:** work up to 16 ounces daily, then work up to 32 ounces if possible
- **5-MTHF:** 1 capsule daily
- **Barley grass juice powder:** 2 teaspoons or 6 capsules daily
- **B-complex:** 1 capsule daily
- **Burdock root:** 1 cup of tea or 1 root freshly juiced daily
- **Chaga mushroom:** 2 teaspoons or 6 capsules daily
- **CoQ10:** 1 capsule daily
- **Curcumin:** 1 capsule daily
- **Lemon balm:** 2 dropperfuls daily
- **Milk thistle:** 1 dropperful daily
- **Nettle leaf:** 1 dropperful daily
- **Spirulina:** 2 teaspoons or 6 capsules daily
- **Vitamin C (as Micro-C):** 4 capsules daily
- **Zinc (as liquid zinc sulfate):** 1 dropperful twice a day

Burnout

True cause: Burnout is often blamed on our inability to handle stress, when in truth, that's another way to blame us for our health problems. The toxic troublemakers and bugs we encounter in our daily world are what set us up to be susceptible to burnout. See Chapter 2, "What's Causing Burnout," for more.

- Fresh celery juice: work up to 32 ounces daily
- Celeryforce: 4 capsules three times a day
- 5-MTHF: 1 capsule twice a day
- Aloe vera: 2 or more inches of fresh gel (skin removed) daily
- Ashwagandha: 3 dropperfuls twice a day
- Barley grass juice powder: 1 tablespoon or 9 capsules daily
- B-complex: 1 capsule daily
- California poppy: 1 dropperful or 1 capsule twice a day
- Cat's claw: 1 dropperful daily
- Chaga mushroom: 1 tablespoon or 9 capsules daily
- CoQ10: 1 capsule daily
- Curcumin: 2 capsules twice a day
- EPA and DHA (fish-free): 1 capsule daily (taken with dinner)
- Goldenseal: 1 dropperful daily (two weeks on/two weeks off)
- Lemon balm: 3 dropperfuls four times a day
- Licorice root: 1 dropperful daily (two weeks on, two weeks off)
- L-lysine: 4 500-milligram capsules twice a day
- Magnesium glycinate: 2 capsules twice a day
- Melatonin: 5 milligrams at bedtime daily
- Nettle leaf: 2 dropperfuls twice a day
- Selenium: 1 capsule once a week
- Spirulina: 2 teaspoons or 6 capsules daily
- Vitamin B_{12} (as adenosylcobalamin with methylcobalamin): 4 dropperfuls twice a day
- Vitamin C (as Micro-C): 5 capsules twice a day
- Wild blueberry powder: 2 tablespoons daily
- Zinc (as liquid zinc sulfate): 2 dropperfuls twice a day

Cancer

True cause: The majority of cancers are caused by specific, aggressive strains of viruses from the herpetic family that take advantage of a weakened immune system and feed on toxins (such as mercury, aluminum, copper, other toxic heavy metals, pesticides, herbicides, fungicides, solvents, petrochemicals, scented candles, colognes, perfumes, and air fresheners), in turn releasing stronger toxins that denature, hinder, and destroy healthy cells. A small minority of cancers are caused by extreme toxic exposure, such as to asbestos or radiation, with a weakened immune system from general viral activity in the body creating greater susceptibility.

If you've been diagnosed with cancer, consult with your physician about whether supplements are appropriate with whatever treatment you're already undergoing.

- Fresh celery juice: work up to 32 ounces twice a day
- Celeryforce: 2 capsules twice a day
- ALA (alpha lipoic acid): 1 capsule daily
- Aloe vera: 2 or more inches of fresh gel (skin removed) daily
- Amla berry: 2 teaspoons daily
- Barley grass juice powder: 1 tablespoon or 9 capsules daily
- Cat's claw: 4 dropperfuls twice a day
- Chaga mushroom: 1 tablespoon or 9 capsules daily
- CoQ10: 1 capsule twice a day
- Curcumin: 3 capsules twice a day
- Glutathione: 1 capsule daily
- Lemon balm: 4 dropperfuls twice a day
- L-lysine: 2 500-milligram capsules daily
- Melatonin: work up to 20 milligrams twice a day
- Milk thistle: 1 dropperful twice a day

- **Nascent iodine:** 6 small drops (not dropperfuls) twice a day
- **Nettle leaf:** 3 dropperfuls twice a day
- **Oregon grape root:** 1 dropperful twice a day (two weeks on, two weeks off)
- **Raw honey:** 1 tablespoon daily
- **Rose hips:** 1 cup of tea twice a day
- **Selenium:** 1 capsule daily
- **Spirulina:** 1 tablespoon or 9 capsules daily
- **Turmeric:** 3 capsules twice a day
- **Vitamin B$_{12}$ (as adenosylcobalamin with methylcobalamin):** 2 dropperfuls daily
- **Vitamin C (as Micro-C):** 8 capsules twice a day
- **Wild blueberry powder:** 1 tablespoon daily
- **Zinc (as liquid zinc sulfate):** up to 2 dropperfuls twice a day

Canker Sores

True cause: A virus in the herpetic family that creates mouth and throat ulcers. Causes symptoms such as mouth pain, throat pain, tingling sensations in the gums and teeth, and pain on the tongue.

- **Fresh celery juice:** work up to 32 ounces daily
- **Cat's claw:** 2 dropperfuls daily
- **Curcumin:** 2 capsules daily
- **Goldenseal:** 3 dropperfuls twice a day (two weeks on, two weeks off)
- **Lemon balm:** 3 dropperfuls twice a day
- **Licorice root:** 2 dropperfuls daily (two weeks on, two weeks off)
- **L-lysine:** 4 capsules twice a day
- **Propolis:** 3 dropperfuls twice a day; also try to dry off the canker sore with a paper towel, then dab straight propolis drops onto the sore periodically throughout the day

- **Raw honey:** 1 tablespoon daily
- **Spirulina:** 2 teaspoons or 6 capsules daily
- **Vitamin B$_{12}$ (as adenosylcobalamin with methylcobalamin):** 2 dropperfuls daily
- **Vitamin C (as Micro-C):** 6 capsules twice a day
- **Zinc (as liquid zinc sulfate):** 2 dropperfuls daily

Cataracts

True cause: Long-term vitamin C deficiency from an overburdened, stagnant, sluggish liver filled with toxic heavy metals, pesticides, herbicides, and fungicides, including traces of DDT passed down from earlier generations or encountered through direct exposure. Accelerated by a high-fat/high-protein diet.

- **Fresh celery juice:** work up to at least 16 ounces daily
- **Celeryforce:** 1 capsule daily
- **5-MTHF:** 1 capsule daily
- **Barley grass juice powder:** 2 teaspoons or 6 capsules daily
- **B-complex:** 1 capsule daily
- **Chaga mushroom:** 2 teaspoons or 6 capsules daily
- **Curcumin:** 2 capsules twice a day
- **EPA and DHA (fish-free):** 1 capsule daily (taken with dinner)
- **Eyebright:** 1 dropperful daily
- **Lemon balm:** 2 dropperfuls daily
- **Nettle leaf:** 2 dropperfuls twice a day
- **Spirulina:** 2 teaspoons or 6 capsules daily
- **Vitamin B$_{12}$ (as adenosylcobalamin with methylcobalamin):** 1 dropperful twice a day
- **Vitamin C (as Micro-C):** 4 to 6 capsules twice a day
- **Wild blueberry powder:** 1 tablespoon daily

Chemical and Food Sensitivities

True cause: A combination of a sluggish, stagnant liver filled with toxic troublemakers (such as mercury, aluminum, copper, lead, nickel, cadmium, arsenic, solvents, conventional detergents, conventional cleaning supplies, air fresheners, pesticides, herbicides, fungicides, scented candles, perfumes, and colognes) plus viruses (such as one of the over 60 varieties of Epstein-Barr virus, one of the over 30 varieties of shingles, or one of the multiple strains of HHV-6) or bacteria (such as one or more strains from the over 50 groups of *Streptococcus* bacteria), all creating byproduct and other debris. When the liver becomes too burdened to handle this chemical, viral, and bacterial waste matter, the bloodstream becomes overloaded with it, since the person is not able to detox it properly, most likely due to a high-fat/high-protein diet, which is not helpful to the detox process. As a result, the central nervous system becomes mildly inflamed from the viral load, and the individual begins to react in the form of chemical and/or food sensitivities.

Everyone with chemical and food sensitivities is different. You're welcome to explore any of the supplements in this chapter. The list here is simply a starting point for some sensitive people. The fresh celery juice, Celeryforce, and raw honey can become part of your daily routine. For the other herbs and supplements, take only one supplement one day, another the next, and so on, cycling through the full list of what you want to try over the course of several days instead of taking them all in one day. If you decide to take all of the supplements in this list, it means you'll be on an eight-day cycle. A sensitivity is yet another reason to stay away from supplements with 50 ingredients in one bottle, which you will not find advised here.

Daily

- **Fresh celery juice:** try to work up to 16 ounces daily
- **Celeryforce:** 1 capsule daily
- **Raw honey:** 1 teaspoon or more daily

Cycle through, with one per day:

- **5-MTHF:** 1 capsule
- **Barley grass juice powder:** ½ teaspoon or 1 capsule
- **Lemon balm:** 1 dropperful
- **L-lysine:** 500 milligrams
- **Peppermint:** 1 cup of tea
- **Vitamin B$_{12}$ (as adenosylcobalamin with methylcobalamin):** 1 dropperful
- **Vitamin C (as Micro-C):** 2 capsules
- **Vitamin D$_3$:** 1,000 IU

Child Liver

True cause: Exposure to mercury, aluminum, copper, and other toxins (most commonly pesticides, herbicides, and fungicides) early on in a child's life, or even passed down via egg, sperm, or in utero, can lead to a sluggish, stagnant liver from the start. So can an early low-grade viral or bacterial infection (most commonly from one of the over 60 varieties of Epstein-Barr virus, one of the numerous strains of HHV-6, or a strain from the over 50 groups of *Streptococcus* bacteria). As I cover in more length in *Liver Rescue*, this condition that I call *child liver* determines more of children's health and well-being than we know.

- **Fresh celery juice:** refer to table on page 480 for children's amounts
- **Amla berry:** ½ teaspoon daily (mix powder with a liquid such as juice, smoothie, or water)

- **Barley grass juice powder:** ½ teaspoon daily (mix powder with a liquid such as juice, smoothie, or water)
- **Ginger:** 1 cup of tea twice a day or freshly grated or juiced to taste daily
- **Lemon balm:** 1 dropperful daily
- **Magnesium glycinate:** ¼ to ½ teaspoon daily (open capsule, then mix powder with liquid such as juice, smoothie, or water)
- **Milk thistle:** 6 small drops (not dropperfuls) daily
- **Spirulina:** ½ teaspoon daily (mix powder with a liquid such as juice, smoothie, or water)
- **Vitamin B$_{12}$ (as adenosylcobalamin with methylcobalamin):** 10 small drops (not dropperfuls) daily
- **Vitamin C (as Micro-C):** 1 capsule daily (if desired, open capsule, then mix powder with liquid such as juice, smoothie, or water)
- **Zinc (as liquid zinc sulfate):** up to 6 small drops (not dropperfuls) in juice, water, or directly in mouth daily

- **Fresh celery juice:** if possible, work up to 32 ounces twice a day; if not, 32 ounces daily
- **Amla berry:** 2 teaspoons twice a day
- **Barley grass juice powder:** 2 teaspoons or 6 capsules twice a day
- **Burdock root:** 1 cup of tea or 1 root freshly juiced twice a day
- **Chaga mushroom:** 1 teaspoon or 3 capsules twice a day
- **Chicory root:** 1 cup of tea twice a day
- **CoQ10:** 1 capsule twice a day
- **Glutathione:** 1 capsule daily
- **Hibiscus:** 1 cup of tea twice a day
- **Lemon balm:** 1 dropperful twice a day
- **MSM:** 1 capsule twice a day
- **NAC:** 1 capsule daily
- **Vitamin B$_{12}$ (as adenosylcobalamin with methylcobalamin):** 1 dropperful daily
- **Vitamin C (as Micro-C):** 5 capsules twice a day
- **Wild blueberry powder:** 1 tablespoon daily

Cirrhosis and Pericirrhosis

True cause: Low-grade infections from multiple pathogens (such as one or more of the over 60 varieties of Epstein-Barr virus and one or more of the over 30 varieties of shingles virus) plus buildup of old pharmaceuticals (recreational or prescribed), a long-term chronically high-fat diet, and toxins such as the toxic heavy metals mercury, aluminum, and copper. Alcohol use can contribute, although alcohol is not always involved. A high-fat/high-protein diet can accelerate the condition.

Taking supplements for cirrhosis depends on the severity of your case. Especially if you're in late-stage cirrhosis, consult with a physician before applying supplements.

Cold and Flu

True cause: What we call "colds" these days are actually mild versions of the flu. Many, many years ago, there were different varieties of common cold viruses that could give you the sniffles, a scratchy throat, and sometimes a fever under 100 degrees. In order for this to happen, you would really need to have a lowered immune system, which most often occurred due to not being clothed right for damp weather and experiencing temperature shock from being exposed to the elements. These cold viruses never created what we're up against in the present. Today, if we experience those symptoms and they're mild, we're really dealing with a mild influenza strain. When the symptoms are worse, we're still dealing with influenza. Colds are no longer—flus have dominated over any strain of cold virus. Even the stomach bugs that go around are particular strains of the flu.

The flu can enter a family of five and each individual can experience different symptoms as the strain leaves one family member and moves on to the next; the strain mutates from person to person, plus everyone's immune system reacts differently, so the last family member's flu may be very different from the first family member's. For example, one person may get a sore throat, runny nose, and cough for three days while the next gets a 103-degree temperature and a very long-lasting cough and sinus drainage.

Medical Medium Zinc Shock Therapy and Medical Medium Vitamin C Shock Therapy (see pages 482–484) can be very helpful techniques to apply at the first sign of contracting a bug. Because the flu often starts in the lungs, throat, and sinus cavities, Medical Medium Zinc Shock Therapy is geared to this region to try to head it off at the pass.

Supplements for Colds and Flus in Adults

- **Fresh celery juice:** work up to at least 16 ounces daily
- **Cat's claw:** 2 dropperfuls three times a day
- **Elderberry syrup:** 1 tablespoon three times a day
- **Eyebright:** 3 dropperfuls three times a day
- **Ginger:** 1 cup of tea or freshly grated in water twice a day
- **Goldenseal:** 4 dropperfuls three times a day
- **Lemon balm:** 4 dropperfuls three times a day
- **Lomatium root:** 3 dropperfuls three times a day
- **Mullein leaf:** 4 dropperfuls three times a day
- **Olive leaf:** 1 dropperful twice a day

- **Oregano oil:** 1 capsule twice a day
- **Osha:** 3 dropperfuls three times a day
- **Thyme:** 2 sprigs of fresh thyme in hot water as tea or 4 sprigs in room temperature water twice a day
- **Vitamin B$_{12}$ (as adenosylcobalamin with methylcobalamin):** 2 dropperfuls twice a day
- **Vitamin C (as Micro-C):** after optional Medical Medium Vitamin C Shock Therapy, 4 capsules three times a day
- **Zinc (as liquid zinc sulfate):** after optional Medical Medium Zinc Shock Therapy for two days, 2 dropperfuls twice a day

Supplements for Colds and Flus in Children Ages 1 to 2

- **Fresh celery juice:** refer to table on page 480 for children's amounts
- **Elderberry syrup:** 1 teaspoon three times a day
- **Goldenseal:** 4 tiny drops (not dropperfuls) three times a day
- **Lemon balm:** 6 tiny drops (not dropperfuls) three times a day
- **Lomatium root:** 3 tiny drops (not dropperfuls) three times a day
- **Mullein leaf:** 6 tiny drops (not dropperfuls) three times a day
- **Vitamin B$_{12}$ (as adenosylcobalamin with methylcobalamin):** 4 tiny drops (not dropperfuls) twice a day
- **Vitamin C (as Micro-C):** after optional Medical Medium Vitamin C Shock Therapy, open 1 500-milligram capsule and mix half (250 milligrams) into juice or smoothie twice a day
- **Zinc (as liquid zinc sulfate):** after optional Medical Medium Zinc Shock Therapy for two days, 3 tiny drops (not dropperfuls) in juice, water, or directly in mouth twice a day

Supplements for Colds and Flus in Children Ages 3 to 4

- **Fresh celery juice:** refer to table on page 480 for children's amounts
- **Elderberry syrup:** 2 teaspoons three times a day
- **Eyebright:** 4 tiny drops (not dropperfuls) three times a day
- **Ginger:** freshly grated to taste in juice daily
- **Goldenseal:** 6 tiny drops (not dropperfuls) three times a day
- **Lemon balm:** 6 tiny drops (not dropperfuls) three times a day
- **Lomatium root:** 3 tiny drops (not dropperfuls) three times a day
- **Mullein leaf:** 6 tiny drops (not dropperfuls) three times a day
- **Vitamin B$_{12}$ (as adenosylcobalamin with methylcobalamin):** 4 tiny drops (not dropperfuls) twice a day
- **Vitamin C (as Micro-C):** after optional Medical Medium Vitamin C Shock Therapy, open 1 500-milligram capsule and mix half (250 milligrams) into juice or smoothie three times a day
- **Zinc (as liquid zinc sulfate):** after optional Medical Medium Zinc Shock Therapy for two days, 4 tiny drops (not dropperfuls) in juice, water, or directly in mouth three times a day

Supplements for Colds and Flus in Children Ages 5 to 8

- **Fresh celery juice:** refer to table on page 480 for children's amounts
- **Elderberry syrup:** 1 tablespoon three times a day
- **Eyebright:** 10 small drops (not dropperfuls) three times a day

- **Ginger:** freshly grated to taste in juice daily
- **Goldenseal:** 15 small drops (not dropperfuls) three times a day
- **Lemon balm:** 1 dropperful three times a day
- **Lomatium root:** 6 small drops (not dropperfuls) three times a day
- **Mullein leaf:** 1 dropperful three times a day
- **Vitamin B$_{12}$ (as adenosylcobalamin with methylcobalamin):** 6 small drops (not dropperfuls) three times a day
- **Vitamin C (as Micro-C):** after optional Medical Medium Vitamin C Shock Therapy, 1 500-milligram capsule three times a day (optional: open capsule and mix into juice or smoothie)
- **Zinc (as liquid zinc sulfate):** after optional Medical Medium Zinc Shock Therapy for two days, 6 small drops (not dropperfuls) in juice, water, or directly in mouth three times a day

Supplements for Colds and Flus in Children Ages 9 to 12

- **Fresh celery juice:** refer to table on page 480 for children's amounts
- **Elderberry syrup:** 1 tablespoon four times a day
- **Eyebright:** 1 dropperful three times a day
- **Ginger:** freshly grated to taste in juice daily
- **Goldenseal:** 2 dropperfuls three times a day
- **Lemon balm:** 2 dropperfuls three times a day
- **Lomatium root:** 1 dropperful three times a day
- **Mullein leaf:** 2 dropperfuls three times a day
- **Osha:** 1 dropperful three times a day

- **Vitamin B$_{12}$ (as adenosylcobalamin with methylcobalamin):** 1 dropperful twice a day
- **Vitamin C (as Micro-C):** after optional Medical Medium Vitamin C Shock Therapy, 2 500-milligram capsules three times a day (optional: open capsules and mix into juice or smoothie)
- **Zinc (as liquid zinc sulfate):** after optional Medical Medium Zinc Shock Therapy for two days, 10 small drops (not dropperfuls) in juice, water, or directly in mouth three times a day

Supplements for Colds and Flus in Children Ages 13 and Up

- **Fresh celery juice:** refer to table on page 480 for children's amounts
- **Elderberry syrup:** 1 to 2 tablespoons four times a day
- **Eyebright:** 3 dropperfuls three times a day
- **Ginger:** freshly grated to taste in juice daily
- **Goldenseal:** 3 dropperfuls three times a day
- **Lemon balm:** 3 dropperfuls three times a day
- **Lomatium root:** 3 dropperfuls three times a day
- **Mullein leaf:** 4 dropperfuls three times a day
- **Osha:** 2 dropperfuls three times a day
- **Vitamin B$_{12}$ (as adenosylcobalamin with methylcobalamin):** 1 dropperful twice a day
- **Vitamin C (as Micro-C):** after optional Medical Medium Vitamin C Shock Therapy, 3 500-milligram capsules three times a day (optional: open capsules and mix into juice or smoothie)

- **Zinc (as liquid zinc sulfate):** after optional Medical Medium Zinc Shock Therapy for two days, 1 dropperful directly in mouth twice a day

Colorblindness

True cause: Exposure to aluminum toxicity at the beginning of eye tissue cell development or passed down via egg, sperm, or in utero from parents (who could have received it from your grandparents, who could have received it from even earlier ancestors) who carried toxic aluminum. Usually people who are colorblind end up experiencing degenerative eye problems earlier in life than others because the aluminum in their eyes can oxidize over time and create susceptibilities. For example, individuals who are colorblind tend to develop cataracts faster. Removing aluminum from the system may not repair the colorblindness factor; it can help prevent these other degenerative eye issues that would have been accelerated by aluminum toxicity.

As usual, these are adult dosages. If you're worried about colorblindness in your child, talk to your pediatrician about reducing these supplements to quarter dosages.

- **Fresh celery juice:** work up to at least 16 ounces daily
- **5-MTHF:** 1 capsule daily
- **ALA (alpha lipoic acid):** 1 capsule twice a week
- **Amla berry:** 1 teaspoon daily
- **Barley grass juice powder:** 2 teaspoons or 6 capsules daily
- **B-complex:** 1 capsule daily
- **Chaga mushroom:** 2 teaspoons or 6 capsules daily
- **CoQ10:** 1 capsule daily
- **EPA and DHA (fish-free):** 1 capsule daily (taken with dinner)

- Eyebright: 1 dropperful daily
- Lemon balm: 2 dropperfuls daily
- NAC: 1 capsule daily
- Nascent iodine: 3 small drops (not dropperfuls) daily
- Nettle leaf: 2 dropperfuls daily
- Spirulina: 2 teaspoons or 6 capsules daily
- Vitamin B$_{12}$ (as adenosylcobalamin with methylcobalamin): 1 dropperful twice a day
- Vitamin C (as Micro-C): 4 capsules twice a day
- Wild blueberry powder: 1 tablespoon daily

Congenital Eye Defects

True cause: Toxic heavy metals from generations past, with mercury the leading metal behind these issues. As a reminder, these are adult dosages.

- Fresh celery juice: work up to at least 16 ounces daily
- 5-MTHF: 1 capsule daily
- Barley grass juice powder: 2 teaspoons or 6 capsules daily
- Chaga mushroom: 2 teaspoons or 6 capsules daily
- CoQ10: 1 capsule daily
- Curcumin: 2 capsules daily
- EPA and DHA (fish-free): 1 capsule daily (taken with dinner)
- Eyebright: 1 dropperful daily
- Hibiscus: 1 cup of tea daily
- Lemon balm: 2 dropperfuls daily
- L-lysine: 2 500-milligram capsules daily
- Magnesium glycinate: 1 capsule daily
- Nettle leaf: 2 dropperfuls daily
- Rose hips: 1 cup of tea daily
- Spirulina: 2 teaspoons or 6 capsules daily

- Vitamin B$_{12}$ (as adenosylcobalamin with methylcobalamin): 2 dropperfuls daily
- Vitamin C (as Micro-C): 2 capsules twice a day
- Wild blueberry powder: 1 tablespoon daily
- Zinc (as liquid zinc sulfate): 1 dropperful daily

Conjunctivitis (Pink Eye)

True cause: Infection in the eye of a bacterial strain from one of the over 50 groups of *Streptoccocus*. As usual, these are adult dosages.

- Fresh celery juice: work up to 32 ounces daily
- Amla berry: 1 teaspoon daily
- Cat's claw: 1 dropperful twice a day
- Chaga mushroom: 1 teaspoon or 3 capsules daily
- Curcumin: 1 capsule twice a day
- Eyebright: 3 dropperfuls twice a day
- Goldenseal: 3 dropperfuls twice a day (two weeks on, two weeks off)
- Lemon balm: 4 dropperfuls twice a day
- Lomatium root: 3 dropperfuls twice a day
- Monolaurin: 1 capsule twice a day
- Mullein leaf: 3 dropperfuls twice a day
- Olive leaf: 2 dropperfuls twice a day
- Oregon grape root: 1 dropperful twice a day (two weeks on, two weeks off)
- Vitamin B$_{12}$ (as adenosylcobalamin with methylcobalamin): 1 dropperful daily
- Vitamin C (as Micro-C): 4 capsules twice a day
- Zinc (as liquid zinc sulfate): 2 dropperfuls twice a day

Constant, Mystery Hunger and Overeating

True cause: A lack of stored glycogen in the liver and brain due to a deficiency of critical clean carbohydrates in the diet and, in most cases, a low-grade viral infection, as well as insulin resistance from a high-fat/high-protein diet.

- **Fresh celery juice:** work up to 32 ounces daily
- **Celeryforce:** 2 capsules twice a day
- **5-MTHF:** 1 capsule daily
- **Barley grass juice powder:** 2 teaspoons or 6 capsules daily
- **Cardamom:** sprinkle on food to taste daily
- **Chaga mushroom:** 2 teaspoons or 6 capsules daily
- **Chicory root:** 1 cup of tea daily
- **Curcumin:** 2 capsules daily
- **Ginger:** 1 cup of tea or freshly grated or juiced to taste daily
- **Lemon balm:** 2 dropperfuls twice a day
- **Licorice root:** 1 dropperful daily (two weeks on, two weeks off)
- **Magnesium glycinate:** 2 capsules daily
- **Spirulina:** 1 tablespoon or 9 capsules daily
- **Vitamin B$_{12}$ (as adenosylcobalamin with methylcobalamin):** 1 dropperful daily

Constipation

True cause: A chronically sluggish, stagnant liver from a range of factors such as toxic heavy metals, various other toxins, and low-grade viral or bacterial infection in both the liver and the intestinal tract. When present in the gut, pathogenic infection can cause narrowing and/or expanding in both the small intestine and colon. Viral neurotoxins can also cause inflammation of the nerve endings around the intestinal tract, resulting in peristaltic slowdown and even gastroparesis. (For more on gastroparesis, see Chapter 18, "Mono Eating Cleanse.")

Another cause of chronic constipation is food that feeds viruses and unproductive bacteria in the small intestinal tract and colon, creating inflammation there—most commonly milk, cheese, butter, eggs, and gluten. The condition can progress due to a high-fat/high-protein diet.

Causes of acute constipation include emotional stress or nervousness creating overtightening or spasming in the abdominal muscles around the small intestine and colon. Long car rides and long plane flights coupled with foods that are not friendly to regularity can also lead to short-term constipation.

- **Fresh celery juice:** work up to 32 ounces every morning
- **Celeryforce:** 2 capsules twice a day
- **Amla berry:** 2 teaspoons twice a day
- **Barley grass juice powder:** 2 teaspoons or 6 capsules daily
- **Cat's claw:** 1 dropperful twice a day
- **Dandelion root tea:** 1 cup of tea twice a day
- **EPA and DHA (fish-free):** 1 capsule twice a day (taken with dinner)
- **Licorice root:** 1 dropperful daily or 1 cup of tea twice a day (two weeks on, two weeks off)
- **Magnesium glycinate:** 1 teaspoon of powder twice a day
- **Milk thistle:** 1 dropperful twice a day
- **Nettle leaf:** 1 dropperful or 1 cup of tea twice a day
- **Peppermint:** 1 cup of tea twice a day
- **Rose hips:** 1 cup of tea twice a day
- **Vitamin C (as Micro-C):** 4 capsules twice a day
- **Wild blueberry powder:** 1 tablespoon daily

Corneal Disease

True cause: Chronic, long-term viral infection, most commonly from one of the over 60 varieties of Epstein-Barr virus. Accelerated by deficiencies in antioxidants and trace minerals.

- **Fresh celery juice:** work up to 32 ounces daily
- **5-MTHF:** 1 capsule daily
- **ALA (alpha lipoic acid):** 1 capsule every other day
- **Barley grass juice powder:** 2 teaspoons or 6 capsules daily
- **B-complex:** 1 capsule daily
- **Cat's claw:** 1 dropperful twice a day
- **Chaga mushroom:** 2 teaspoons or 6 capsules daily
- **CoQ10:** 1 capsule daily
- **Curcumin:** 2 capsules twice a day
- **EPA and DHA (fish-free):** 1 capsule daily (taken with dinner)
- **Eyebright:** 1 dropperful twice a day
- **Lemon balm:** 2 dropperfuls twice a day
- **L-lysine:** 3 500-milligram capsules twice a day
- **Monolaurin:** 1 capsule daily
- **MSM:** 1 capsule daily
- **Nettle leaf:** 2 dropperfuls daily
- **Rose hips:** 1 cup of tea daily
- **Selenium:** 1 capsule daily
- **Spirulina:** 2 teaspoons or 6 capsules daily
- **Vitamin B$_{12}$ (as adenosylcobalamin with methylcobalamin):** 1 dropperful twice a day
- **Vitamin C (as Micro-C):** 4 capsules twice a day
- **Wild blueberry powder:** 1 tablespoon daily
- **Zinc (as liquid zinc sulfate):** 1 dropperful twice a day

Dark Under-Eye Circles

True cause: If not from a lack of sleep, this symptom is a sign of a liver struggling with an abundance of toxins such as toxic heavy metals; viruses and bacteria and their byproduct and debris; plastics and other petroleum-based byproducts; and pesticides, herbicides, and fungicides. This can lead to the blood getting thick because it can't detoxify properly due to a high-fat/high-protein diet. High blood fat also causes lower levels of oxygen in the blood, which can lead to chronic low-grade dehydration and blood thickening. Thick blood suspends toxins in the bloodstream, which can create this shadow under the thin layer of skin beneath the eyes.

- **Fresh celery juice:** work up to 32 ounces daily
- **Celeryforce:** 1 capsule twice a day
- **ALA (alpha lipoic acid):** 1 capsule daily
- **Barley grass juice powder:** 1 teaspoon or 3 capsules twice a day
- **B-complex:** 2 capsules daily
- **Burdock root:** 1 cup of tea or 1 root freshly juiced daily
- **Dandelion root:** 1 cup of tea twice a day
- **Hibiscus:** 1 cup of tea twice a day
- **Licorice root:** 1 dropperful daily or 1 cup of tea twice a day (two weeks on, two weeks off)
- **Red clover:** 1 cup of tea or 1 dropperful twice a day
- **Spirulina:** 2 teaspoons or 6 capsules daily
- **Turmeric:** 2 capsules twice a day
- **Vitamin B$_{12}$ (as adenosylcobalamin with methylcobalamin):** 1 dropperful twice a day
- **Vitamin C (as Micro-C):** 4 capsules twice a day
- **Wild blueberry powder:** 2 tablespoons daily
- **Zinc (as liquid zinc sulfate):** up to 1 dropperful twice a day

Depression

True cause: Traumatic loss, traumatic stress, and emotional injury are common, identifiable causes of depression. These traumas can create a lasting neurotransmitter deficiency, leading to depression that sometimes continues past the time of hardship. In other cases, we can point to identifiable daily challenges as the source of depression. And then there's unexplained depression, which is caused by toxic heavy metals such as mercury, aluminum, and copper, often with a low-grade viral infection of one or more of the over 60 varieties of Epstein-Barr virus, one or more of the over 30 varieties of shingles virus, or one or more strains of the multiple varieties of herpes simplex 1, herpes simplex 2, or cytomegalovirus. A brew of all of these factors at once could also create someone's depression, particularly if they experienced toxic exposure at the same time they suffered trauma.

- **Fresh celery juice:** work up to 32 ounces daily
- **Celeryforce:** 2 capsules three times a day
- **5-MTHF:** 1 capsule daily
- **Ashwagandha:** 1 dropperful daily
- **Barley grass juice powder:** 2 teaspoons or 6 capsules daily
- **B-complex:** 1 capsule daily
- **Curcumin:** 2 capsules daily
- **EPA and DHA (fish-free):** 1 capsule daily (taken with dinner)
- **GABA:** 1 250-milligram capsule daily
- **Hibiscus:** 1 cup of tea twice a day
- **Lemon balm:** 4 dropperfuls twice a day
- **Licorice root:** 1 dropperful daily (two weeks on, two weeks off)
- **L-lysine:** 2 500-milligram capsules daily
- **Magnesium glycinate:** 2 capsules daily
- **Melatonin:** 5 milligrams at bedtime daily
- **Nascent iodine:** 3 small drops (not dropperfuls) daily

- **Spirulina:** 2 teaspoons or 6 capsules daily
- **Vitamin B$_{12}$ (as adenosylcobalamin with methylcobalamin):** 2 dropperfuls twice a day
- **Vitamin C (as Micro-C):** 4 capsules twice a day
- **Vitamin D$_3$:** 1,000 IU daily
- **Wild blueberry powder:** 2 teaspoons daily
- **Zinc (as liquid zinc sulfate):** 1 dropperful daily

Diabetes (Type 1, Type 1.5 [LADA], and Type 2), Prediabetes, and Blood Sugar Imbalance

True cause: Type 1 and type 1.5 diabetes (the second of which is also known as latent autoimmune diabetes in adults, or LADA) is caused by injury to the pancreas, usually from a pathogen such as a virus or bacterium, and sometimes even a physical blow. The severity of the pathogen and the condition of the pancreas determine the severity of the individual case of diabetes. Sometimes the pathogenic injury is slow or happens later in life, which is what leads to type 1.5/LADA. At the same time as either types 1 or 1.5 diabetes, you can have a sluggish, stagnant liver and a diet too high in fat creating insulin resistance issues.

Type 2 diabetes comes from a sluggish, stagnant liver filled with various toxins, including viral toxins from a virus such as one of the over 60 varieties of Epstein-Barr. At the same time, the liver has lost its glycogen reserves so that the pancreas has to work harder, overextending itself due to the constant insulin resistance issues that come up from a long-term high-fat/high-protein diet.

- **Fresh celery juice:** work up to 32 ounces daily
- **5-MTHF:** 1 capsule twice a day
- **Amla berry:** 2 teaspoons twice a day

- Ashwagandha: 1 dropperful twice a day
- Barley grass juice powder: 2 teaspoons or 6 capsules daily
- Chaga mushroom: 2 teaspoons or 6 capsules daily
- Glutathione: 1 capsule daily
- Hibiscus: 1 cup of tea twice a day
- Lemon balm: 2 dropperfuls or 1 cup of tea twice a day
- L-lysine: 2 500-milligram capsules twice a day
- Nascent iodine: 6 small drops (not dropperfuls) daily
- Nettle leaf: 2 dropperfuls or 1 cup of tea twice a day
- Rose hips: 1 cup of tea twice a day
- Schisandra berry: 1 cup of tea twice a day
- Turmeric: 2 capsules twice a day
- Spirulina: 2 teaspoons or 6 capsules daily
- Vitamin C (as Micro-C): 4 capsules twice a day
- Vitamin B$_{12}$ (as adenosylcobalamin with methylcobalamin): 1 dropperful twice a day
- Wild blueberry powder: 1 tablespoon daily
- Zinc (as liquid zinc sulfate): up to 1 dropperful twice a day

Diarrhea (Chronic, Intermittent, Long Term)

True cause: A gut filled with unproductive bacteria such as strains from the over 50 groups of *Streptococcus* and one or more of the several common *E. coli* varieties; and/or viruses; and/or yeast, mold, or other unproductive fungus causing inflammation in various parts of the small or large intestinal tract. This can lead to a variety of gastrointestinal diagnoses.

- Fresh celery juice: work up to 16 ounces daily
- Aloe vera: 2 or more inches of fresh gel (skin removed) daily
- Barley grass juice powder: ½ teaspoon or 1 capsule daily
- Burdock root: 1 cup of tea or 1 root freshly juiced daily
- Cat's claw: 2 dropperfuls twice a day
- Curcumin: 1 capsule twice a day
- D-mannose: 2 teaspoons in water daily
- Ginger: 1 cup of tea or freshly grated or juiced to taste daily
- Goldenseal: 3 dropperfuls twice a day (two weeks on, two weeks off)
- Hibiscus: 1 cup of tea daily
- Lemon balm: 3 dropperfuls twice a day
- Licorice root: 1 dropperful twice a day (two weeks on, two weeks off)
- Lomatium root: 1 dropperful daily
- Magnesium glycinate: 1 capsule daily
- Monolaurin: 1 capsule twice a day
- Mullein leaf: 2 dropperfuls twice a day
- Nettle leaf: 2 dropperfuls twice a day
- Oregano oil: 2 capsules daily
- Vitamin B$_{12}$ (as adenosylcobalamin with methylcobalamin): 1 dropperful twice a day
- Vitamin C (as Micro-C): 1 capsule twice a day
- Zinc (as liquid zinc sulfate): 1 dropperful daily

Dirty Blood Syndrome

True cause: A lack of proper daily hydration from the right liquids combined with a diet too high in fat/protein over the years and a toxic, stagnant, sluggish liver leading to chronic dehydration that causes blood to thicken.

- Fresh celery juice: work up to 32 ounces daily

- **Amla berry:** 1 teaspoon twice a day
- **Barley grass juice powder:** 2 teaspoons or 6 capsules daily
- **Burdock root:** 1 cup of tea or 1 root freshly juiced twice a day
- **Chicory root:** 1 cup of tea twice a day
- **Dandelion root:** 1 cup of tea twice a day
- **Milk thistle:** 1 dropperful twice a day
- **Nettle leaf:** 1 dropperful or 1 cup of tea twice a day
- **Red clover:** 1 cup of tea or 1 dropperful twice a day
- **Spirulina:** 2 teaspoons or 6 capsules daily
- **Turmeric:** 2 capsules twice a day
- **Vitamin C (as Micro-C):** 4 capsules twice a day
- **Yellow dock:** 1 cup of tea twice a day

Diverticulitis

True cause: One or more strains from the over 50 groups of *Streptococcus* bacteria and/or one or more of the several common *E. coli* varieties. These bacteria tend to colonize the lining of the colon, creating divots and pockets there by feeding on troublemaker foods and repopulating themselves, widening the diverticula as the bacteria breed. Strep is the leading cause and *E. coli* the runner-up, with many people having pockets of both. When *Streptococcus* and *E. coli* are present at the same time, they feed on different foods—like two families panning for gold on the same riverbank, staking different claims.

- **Fresh celery juice:** work up to 16 ounces daily
- **Aloe vera:** 2 or more inches of fresh gel (skin removed) twice a day
- **Barley grass juice powder:** 1 teaspoon or 3 capsules daily
- **Cat's claw:** 2 dropperfuls twice a day
- **Curcumin:** 1 capsule twice a day

- **Ginger:** 1 cup of tea or freshly grated to taste daily
- **Goldenseal:** 4 dropperfuls twice a day (two weeks on, two weeks off)
- **Lemon balm:** 4 dropperfuls twice a day
- **Licorice root:** 1 dropperful twice a day (two weeks on, two weeks off)
- **Lomatium root:** 2 dropperfuls twice a day
- **Magnesium glycinate:** 1 capsule daily
- **Mullein leaf:** 4 dropperfuls twice a day
- **Nettle leaf:** 2 dropperfuls twice a day
- **Olive leaf:** 2 dropperfuls twice a day
- **Oregano oil:** 2 capsules twice a day
- **Peppermint tea:** 1 cup twice a day
- **Rosemary:** 2 sprigs of fresh rosemary in hot water as tea or 4 sprigs in room temperature water daily
- **Thyme:** 2 sprigs of fresh thyme in hot water as tea or 4 sprigs in room temperature water twice a day
- **Vitamin B$_{12}$ (as adenosylcobalamin with methylcobalamin):** 1 dropperful twice a day
- **Vitamin C (as Micro-C):** 2 capsules twice a day
- **Zinc (as liquid zinc sulfate):** 1 dropperful twice a day

Dry, Cracked Skin

True cause: An overburdened, stagnant, sluggish liver filled with toxins such as toxic heavy metals, pesticides, herbicides, fungicides, and petrochemicals causing thickened, dehydrated blood. Often triggered by years of a high-fat/high-protein diet and low-grade viral infection.

- **Fresh celery juice:** work up to 32 ounces daily
- **5-MTHF:** 1 capsule daily
- **Aloe vera:** 2 or more inches of fresh gel (skin removed) daily

- **Barley grass juice powder:** 2 teaspoons or 6 capsules daily
- **Burdock root:** 1 cup of tea or 1 root freshly juiced daily
- **Curcumin:** 2 capsules twice a day
- **EPA and DHA (fish-free):** 2 capsules daily (taken with dinner)
- **Glutathione:** 1 capsule daily
- **Lemon balm:** 2 dropperfuls twice a day
- **L-lysine:** 2 500-milligram capsules twice a day
- **Magnesium glycinate:** 2 capsules daily
- **Milk thistle:** 1 dropperful daily
- **MSM:** 1 capsule twice a day
- **Nettle leaf:** 2 dropperfuls twice a day
- **Selenium:** 1 capsule daily
- **Spirulina:** 2 teaspoons or 6 capsules daily
- **Vitamin B$_{12}$ (as adenosylcobalamin with methylcobalamin):** 2 dropperfuls twice a day
- **Vitamin C (as Micro-C):** 4 capsules twice a day
- **Wild blueberry powder:** 2 teaspoons daily
- **Zinc (as liquid zinc sulfate):** 1 dropperful twice a day

Dry Eye Syndrome

True cause: Low-grade chronic dehydration in combination with chronic deficiency of trace mineral salts and, in some cases, overactive or underactive, weakened adrenals.

- **Fresh celery juice:** work up to at least 16 ounces daily
- **Celeryforce:** 1 capsule twice a day
- **Aloe vera:** 2 or more inches of fresh gel (skin removed) daily
- **Ashwagandha:** 3 dropperfuls twice a day
- **Barley grass juice powder:** 2 teaspoons or 6 capsules daily

- **Ginger:** 1 cup of tea or freshly grated or juiced to taste daily
- **Lemon balm:** 4 dropperfuls twice a day
- **Licorice root:** 1 dropperful twice a day (two weeks on, two weeks off)
- **Magnesium glycinate:** 1 capsule twice a day
- **Nettle leaf:** 2 dropperfuls twice a day
- **Spirulina:** 2 teaspoons or 6 capsules daily
- **Vitamin B$_{12}$ (as adenosylcobalamin with methylcobalamin):** 1 dropperful twice a day
- **Vitamin C (as Micro-C):** 2 capsules twice a day
- **Zinc (as liquid zinc sulfate):** 1 dropperful daily

Ear Infections

True cause: Middle ear infections (sometimes called *otitis media*) are caused by one or more strains from the over 50 groups of *Streptococcus* bacteria.

Inner ear infections are mostly strep-caused too, although there can also be a co-infection of one of the over 60 varieties of Epstein-Barr virus or one of the over 30 varieties of shingles virus. Sometimes a viral infection on its own is the cause of inner ear infections, leading to chronic balance issues, pain, and mucus production.

As usual, the supplements that follow are listed in adult dosages.

- **Fresh celery juice:** work up to 32 ounces daily
- **Barley grass juice powder:** 2 teaspoons or 6 capsules daily
- **Cat's claw:** 3 dropperfuls twice a day
- **Curcumin:** 2 capsules twice a day
- **Eyebright:** 4 dropperfuls twice a day
- **Goldenseal:** 4 dropperfuls three times a day (two weeks on, two weeks off until ear infection subsides)

- **Lemon balm:** 3 dropperfuls three times a day
- **Licorice root:** 2 dropperfuls twice a day (two weeks on, two weeks off)
- **L-lysine:** 5 500-milligram capsules twice a day
- **Lomatium root:** 3 dropperfuls three times a day
- **Monolaurin:** 1 capsule twice a day
- **Mullein leaf:** 3 dropperfuls three times a day
- **Nascent iodine:** 3 small drops (not dropperfuls) daily until ear infection subsides
- **Olive leaf:** 2 dropperfuls twice a day
- **Oregano oil:** 2 capsules twice a day
- **Oregon grape root:** 2 dropperfuls three times a day until infection subsides
- **Raw honey:** 1 tablespoon a day
- **Spirulina:** 2 teaspoons or 6 capsules daily
- **Thyme:** 2 sprigs of fresh thyme in hot water as tea or 4 sprigs in room temperature water twice a day
- **Vitamin B$_{12}$ (as adenosylcobalamin with methylcobalamin):** 1 dropperful twice a day
- **Vitamin C (as Micro-C):** 6 capsules twice a day
- **Zinc (as liquid zinc sulfate):** 2 dropperfuls twice a day (try to let it sit in the mouth and throat for 30 seconds)

Eczema and Psoriasis (including Rosacea, Lupus-Style Rashes, Age Spots, Lichen Sclerosus, Scleroderma, Vitiligo, Seborrheic Dermatitis, Classic Dermatitis, Actinic Keratosis, and Cellulitis)

True cause: One of the over 60 varieties of Epstein-Barr virus living inside the liver, feeding on an abundance of the toxic heavy metal copper there, releasing a copper-infused dermatoxin that circulates through the body and can't detoxify properly due to a high-fat/high-protein diet and other food choices that are unproductive to the condition. When these dermatoxins float to the surface of the skin, they cause the sores and rashing of eczema and psoriasis. With vitiligo, it's an aluminum-based dermatoxin. Different pathogen-toxin brews are behind different variations of these skin conditions—for details on each specific cause, see *Liver Rescue*.

- **Fresh celery juice:** work up to 32 ounces daily
- **Celeryforce:** 2 capsules twice a day
- **5-MTHF:** 1 capsule daily
- **Aloe vera:** 2 or more inches of fresh gel (skin removed) daily
- **Barley grass juice powder:** 2 teaspoons or 6 capsules daily
- **Cat's claw:** 1 dropperful twice a day
- **Chaga mushroom:** 1 teaspoon or 3 capsules daily
- **Curcumin:** 1 capsule twice a day
- **EPA and DHA (fish-free):** 2 capsules daily (taken with dinner)
- **Lemon balm:** 2 dropperfuls twice a day or 1 cup of tea twice a day
- **Licorice root:** 1 dropperful daily (two weeks on, two weeks off)
- **L-lysine:** 4 500-milligram capsules twice a day
- **Mullein leaf:** 1 dropperful twice a day
- **Nettle leaf:** 1 dropperful or 1 cup of tea twice a day
- **Selenium:** 1 capsule daily
- **Spirulina:** 2 teaspoons or 6 capsules daily
- **Vitamin B$_{12}$ (as adenosylcobalamin with methylcobalamin):** 1 dropperful twice a day
- **Vitamin C (as Micro-C):** 6 capsules twice a day
- **Zinc (as liquid zinc sulfate):** up to 1 dropperful twice a day

Edema and Swelling

True cause: If a heart condition, kidney disease, or other obvious illness cannot directly explain this symptom, then a stagnant, sluggish liver that's filled with various toxins while battling a low-grade viral infection is the source, accelerated by a high-fat/high-protein diet. A sluggish, viral liver can also occur simultaneous to an obvious heart or kidney condition.

- **Fresh celery juice:** work up to 32 ounces daily
- **Celeryforce:** 2 capsules daily
- **5-MTHF:** 1 capsule daily
- **Ashwagandha:** 1 dropperful daily
- **Barley grass juice powder:** 2 teaspoons or 6 capsules daily
- **Cat's claw:** 1 dropperful daily
- **Curcumin:** 2 capsules twice a day
- **Glutathione:** 1 capsule daily
- **Lemon balm:** 2 dropperfuls twice a day
- **L-lysine:** 2 500-milligram capsules twice a day
- **Magnesium glycinate:** 1 capsule daily
- **Nettle leaf:** 4 dropperfuls twice a day
- **Peppermint:** 1 cup of tea twice a day
- **Raspberry leaf:** 1 cup of tea twice a day
- **Spirulina:** 1 teaspoon or 3 capsules daily
- **Vitamin B$_{12}$ (as adenosylcobalamin with methylcobalamin):** 1 dropperful twice a day
- **Vitamin C (as Micro-C):** 3 capsules twice a day
- **Wild blueberry powder:** 2 teaspoons daily
- **Zinc (as liquid zinc sulfate):** 1 dropperful daily

Endometriosis

True cause: Viruses and bacteria feeding on sources that include foreign hormones from animal products and synthetic, manufactured sources to which we're commonly exposed.

The byproduct that these pathogens produce in and around the female reproductive system activates and prompts abnormal tissue growth in order to trap and encase this toxic byproduct so it doesn't injure the uterus and other critical parts of the reproductive system. This tissue has the tendency to spread faster when on a high-fat/high-protein diet that includes foods such as eggs, milk, cheese, and butter because these are troublemaker foods that feed the pathogens, leading to increased production of viral and bacterial byproduct. Toxic heavy metal exposure can also exacerbate endometriosis.

- **Fresh celery juice:** work up to 32 ounces daily
- **Amla berry:** 1 teaspoon daily
- **Ashwagandha:** 1 dropperful twice a day
- **Barley grass juice powder:** 2 teaspoons or 6 capsules daily
- **Cat's claw:** 1 dropperful twice a day
- **Chaga mushroom:** 2 teaspoons or 6 capsules daily
- **Curcumin:** 1 capsule twice a day
- **D-mannose:** 1 tablespoon daily in water
- **Lemon balm:** 3 dropperfuls twice a day
- **L-lysine:** 2 500-milligram capsules twice a day
- **Nascent iodine:** 3 small drops (not dropperfuls) daily
- **Nettle leaf:** 5 dropperfuls twice a day
- **Raspberry leaf:** 1 cup of tea with 2 bags twice a day
- **Schisandra berry:** 1 cup of tea twice a day
- **Spirulina:** 2 teaspoons or 6 capsules daily
- **Vitamin B$_{12}$ (as adenosylcobalamin with methylcobalamin):** 1 dropperful daily
- **Vitamin C (as Micro-C):** 5 capsules twice a day
- **Wild blueberry powder:** 2 teaspoons daily
- **Zinc (as liquid zinc sulfate):** 1 dropperful daily

Energy Issues and Fatigue

True cause: Often diagnosed as adrenal fatigue when that's only one factor that contributes to chronic low energy and fatigue. The deeper cause is a stagnant, sluggish liver overburdened with toxins such as toxic heavy metals as well as viruses (such as strains of the over 60 varieties of Epstein-Barr or strains of the over 30 varieties of shingles) and their toxic viral byproduct. That waste matter usually comes in the form of viral neurotoxins that are released from the liver and create a mild to severe energy draw upon the central nervous system that elevates inflammation throughout the body and weakens the adrenal glands. This is an intermittent version of what I call *neurological fatigue*.

- **Fresh celery juice:** work up to 32 ounces daily
- **Celeryforce:** 3 capsules twice a day
- **5-MTHF:** 1 capsule daily
- **Ashwagandha:** 1 dropperful daily
- **Barley grass juice powder:** 2 teaspoons or 6 capsules daily
- **Chaga mushroom:** 2 teaspoons or 6 capsules daily
- **Ginger:** 1 cup of tea or freshly grated or juiced to taste daily
- **Lemon balm:** 2 dropperfuls daily
- **Licorice root:** 1 dropperful daily (two weeks on, two weeks off)
- **Mullein leaf:** 2 dropperfuls daily
- **Nascent iodine:** 6 small drops (not dropperfuls) daily
- **Oregon grape root:** 1 dropperful daily (two weeks on, two weeks off)
- **Raw honey:** 1 tablespoon daily
- **Spirulina:** 2 teaspoons or 6 capsules daily
- **Turmeric:** 2 capsules daily
- **Vitamin B$_{12}$ (as adenosylcobalamin with methylcobalamin):** 1 dropperful twice a day
- **Vitamin C (as Micro-C):** 4 capsules daily
- **Zinc (as liquid zinc sulfate):** up to 1 dropperful daily

Eye Floaters

True cause: When obvious, diagnosable injury is ruled out, eye floaters are the result of neurotoxins produced by one or more of the over 60 varieties of Epstein-Barr virus, along with toxic heavy metals such as mercury and aluminum that enter and saturate eye tissue.

- **Fresh celery juice:** work up to 32 ounces daily
- **Celeryforce:** 2 capsules twice a day
- **5-MTHF:** 1 capsule daily
- **Barley grass juice powder:** 2 teaspoons or 6 capsules daily
- **B-complex:** 1 capsule daily
- **Cat's claw:** 2 dropperfuls twice a day
- **Curcumin:** 2 capsules twice a day
- **Glutathione:** 1 capsule daily
- **Lemon balm:** 3 dropperfuls twice a day
- **Licorice root:** 1 dropperful daily (two weeks on, two weeks off)
- **L-lysine:** 4 500-milligram capsules twice a day
- **Lomatium root:** 1 dropperful twice a day
- **Monolaurin:** 2 capsules daily
- **Mullein leaf:** 3 dropperfuls twice a day
- **Nascent iodine:** 3 small drops (not dropperfuls) daily
- **Nettle leaf:** 2 dropperfuls daily
- **Olive leaf:** 2 dropperfuls daily
- **Spirulina:** 2 teaspoons or 6 capsules daily
- **Vitamin B$_{12}$ (as adenosylcobalamin with methylcobalamin):** 2 dropperfuls twice a day
- **Vitamin C (as Micro-C):** 4 capsules twice a day
- **Wild blueberry powder:** 2 teaspoons daily
- **Zinc (as liquid zinc sulfate):** 2 dropperfuls daily

Fatty Liver, Pre-Fatty Liver, and Sluggish Liver

True cause: A diet too high in fat/protein for too long, coupled with a liver overburdened by toxins such as pesticides and herbicides; toxic heavy metals such as mercury, aluminum, and copper; plastics and other petrochemical byproducts; old pharmaceuticals; chronic, low-grade viral and bacterial infections; and cologne, perfume, air fresheners, and scented candles. Troublemaker foods worsen these liver conditions.

- **Fresh celery juice:** work up to 32 ounces twice a day if possible; if not, work up to 32 ounces every morning
- **Aloe vera:** 2 or more inches of fresh gel (skin removed) daily
- **Amla berry:** 2 teaspoons daily
- **Barley grass juice powder:** 2 teaspoons or 6 capsules daily
- **Burdock root:** 1 cup of tea or 1 root freshly juiced daily
- **Cardamom:** sprinkle on food to taste daily
- **Chicory root:** 1 cup of tea daily
- **Dandelion root:** 1 cup of tea daily
- **Ginger:** 1 cup of tea or freshly grated or juiced to taste daily
- **Milk thistle:** 1 dropperful daily
- **Spirulina:** 1 tablespoon or 9 capsules daily
- **Yellow dock:** 1 cup of tea daily
- **Wild blueberry powder:** 1 tablespoon daily

Fibroids

True cause: One or more of the over 60 varieties of Epstein-Barr virus, or one or more strains from the over 50 groups of *Streptococcus* bacteria, feeding on both toxic hormones that enter the body from outside sources as well as toxic heavy metals. As a result, healthy cells become poisoned and injured, and these mutated, injured living cells fight to stay alive by forming groups that eventually solidify into fibroids. Blood vessels stem out of the fibroids and absorb nutrients from eggs, milk, cheese, and butter for these cells to feed on. The condition is greatly worsened by a high-fat/high-protein diet.

- **Fresh celery juice:** work up to 32 ounces daily
- **5-MTHF:** 1 capsule daily
- **ALA (alpha lipoic acid):** 1 capsule twice a week
- **Aloe vera:** 2 or more inches of fresh gel (skin removed) daily
- **Ashwagandha:** 1 dropperful twice a day
- **Barley grass juice powder:** 2 teaspoons or 6 capsules daily
- **Cat's claw:** 1 dropperful twice a day
- **Chaga mushroom:** 2 teaspoons or 6 capsules daily
- **Curcumin:** 2 capsules twice a day
- **D-mannose:** 1 tablespoon daily in water
- **Goldenseal:** 1 dropperful daily (two weeks on, two weeks off)
- **Hibiscus:** 1 cup of tea daily
- **Lemon balm:** 3 dropperfuls twice a day
- **L-lysine:** 3 500-milligram capsules twice a day
- **Nascent iodine:** 3 small drops (not dropperfuls) daily
- **Nettle leaf:** 5 dropperfuls twice a day
- **Oregano oil:** 1 capsule daily
- **Raspberry leaf:** 1 cup of tea with 2 bags twice a day
- **Raw honey:** 2 teaspoons daily
- **Spirulina:** 2 teaspoons or 6 capsules daily
- **Turmeric:** 2 capsules twice a day
- **Vitamin B$_{12}$ (as adenosylcobalamin with methylcobalamin):** 1 dropperful twice a day
- **Vitamin C (as Micro-C):** 4 capsules twice a day

- Wild blueberry powder: 2 teaspoons daily
- Zinc (as liquid zinc sulfate): 1 dropperful daily

Fibromyalgia

True cause: One or more of the over 60 varieties of Epstein-Barr virus inflaming the nervous system, with or without toxic heavy metals such as mercury present at the same time. A high-fat/high-protein diet tends to worsen the condition.

- Fresh celery juice: work up to 32 ounces daily
- Celeryforce: 2 capsules twice a day
- 5-MTHF: 1 capsule daily
- Ashwagandha: 1 dropperful daily
- Barley grass juice powder: 2 teaspoons or 6 capsules daily
- Cat's claw: 1 dropperful twice a day
- Curcumin: 2 capsules twice a day
- EPA and DHA (fish-free): 1 capsule daily (taken with dinner)
- Lemon balm: 4 dropperfuls twice a day
- Licorice root: 1 dropperful daily (two weeks on, two weeks off)
- L-lysine: 3 500-milligram capsules twice a day
- Magnesium glycinate: 1 capsule twice a day
- Monolaurin: 1 capsule daily
- MSM: 1 capsule daily
- Nettle leaf: 3 dropperfuls twice a day
- Spirulina: 2 teaspoons or 6 capsules daily
- Vitamin B$_{12}$ (as adenosylcobalamin with methylcobalamin): 2 dropperfuls twice a day
- Vitamin C (as Micro-C): 3 capsules twice a day
- Vitamin D$_3$: 1,000 IU daily
- Wild blueberry powder: 1 tablespoon daily
- Zinc (as liquid zinc sulfate): 1 dropperful twice a day

Gallbladder Infections

True cause: Acute or chronic, long-term bacterial infection inside the gallbladder, usually from one or more strains from the over 50 groups of *Streptococcus* bacteria or food-borne bacteria from contaminated foods or food poisoning. Worsened when consuming a high-fat/high-protein diet.

- Fresh celery juice: work up to 32 ounces twice a day, if possible; if not, work up to 32 ounces every morning
- Barley grass juice powder: 1 teaspoon or 3 capsules daily
- Cat's claw: 2 dropperfuls twice a day
- Ginger: 1 cup of tea twice a day or freshly grated or juiced to taste daily
- Goldenseal: 3 dropperfuls twice a day (two weeks on, two weeks off)
- Lemon balm: 3 dropperfuls or 1 cup of tea with 2 bags twice a day
- Licorice root: 1 dropperful twice a day (two weeks on, two weeks off)
- Mullein leaf: 2 dropperfuls twice a day
- Oregon grape root: 1 dropperful twice a day (two weeks on, two weeks off)
- Peppermint: 1 cup of tea with 2 bags twice a day
- Vitamin C (as Micro-C): 5 capsules twice a day
- Zinc (as liquid zinc sulfate): up to 1 dropperful twice a day

Gallstones

True cause: Sludge that has built up over the years from toxins, pathogens, and pathogenic byproduct inside the liver, eventually forming into stones inside the gallbladder.

- Fresh celery juice: work up to 32 ounces daily

- **Barley grass juice powder:** 2 teaspoons or 6 capsules daily
- **Cardamom:** sprinkled on food to taste daily
- **Chicory root:** 1 cup of tea daily
- **Dandelion root:** 1 cup of tea daily
- **Ginger:** 1 cup of tea or freshly grated or juiced to taste daily
- **Hibiscus:** 1 cup of tea daily
- **Nettle leaf:** 1 cup of tea or 2 dropperfuls daily
- **Peppermint:** 1 cup of tea daily
- **Raw honey:** 1 tablespoon daily
- **Rose hips:** 1 cup of tea daily
- **Spirulina:** 2 teaspoons or 6 capsules daily
- **Vitamin C (as Micro-C):** 2 capsules twice a day
- **Wild blueberry powder:** 1 tablespoon daily

- **Curcumin:** 2 capsules twice a day
- **Eyebright:** 1 dropperful twice a day
- **Lemon balm:** 2 dropperfuls twice a day
- **L-lysine:** 4 500-milligram capsules twice a day
- **Monolaurin:** 2 capsules twice a day
- **Mullein leaf:** 2 dropperfuls twice a day
- **Nascent iodine:** 4 small drops (not dropperfuls) daily
- **Nettle leaf:** 2 dropperfuls daily
- **Rose hips:** 1 cup of tea daily
- **Spirulina:** 2 teaspoons or 6 capsules daily
- **Vitamin B$_{12}$ (as adenosylcobalamin with methylcobalamin):** 2 dropperfuls twice a day
- **Vitamin C (as Micro-C):** 6 capsules twice a day
- **Wild blueberry powder:** 1 tablespoon daily
- **Zinc (as liquid zinc sulfate):** 2 dropperfuls daily

Glaucoma

True cause: One of the over 60 varieties of Epstein-Barr virus invading the eye and causing inflammation that spurs fluid development, in turn creating elevated pressure.

- **Fresh celery juice:** work up to 32 ounces daily
- **5-MTHF:** 1 capsule daily
- **ALA (alpha lipoic acid):** 1 capsule twice a week
- **Aloe vera:** 2 or more inches of fresh gel (skin removed) daily
- **Amla berry:** 2 teaspoons daily
- **Barley grass juice powder:** 2 teaspoons or 6 capsules daily
- **B-complex:** 1 capsule daily
- **Cat's claw:** 2 dropperfuls twice a day
- **Chaga mushroom:** 2 teaspoons or 6 capsules daily
- **CoQ10:** 1 capsule daily

Gout

True cause: A sluggish, stagnant liver over-burdened from any of a variety of toxins, normally coupled with a high-fat/high-protein diet.

- **Fresh celery juice:** work up to 32 ounces daily
- **Amla berry:** 2 teaspoons daily
- **Barley grass juice powder:** 2 teaspoons or 6 capsules daily
- **Cat's claw:** 1 dropperful twice a day
- **Chaga mushroom:** 2 teaspoons or 6 capsules daily
- **Curcumin:** 2 capsules twice a day
- **EPA and DHA (fish-free):** 1 capsule daily (taken with dinner)
- **Lemon balm:** 2 dropperfuls or 1 cup of tea with 2 bags twice a day
- **L-lysine:** 3 500-milligram capsules twice a day

- MSM: 2 capsules twice a day
- Nettle leaf: 2 dropperfuls or 1 cup of tea with 2 bags twice day
- Rose hips: 1 cup of tea daily
- Spirulina: 2 teaspoons or 6 capsules daily
- Turmeric: 2 capsules twice a day
- Vitamin B$_{12}$ (as adenosylcobalamin with methylcobalamin): 1 dropperful twice a day
- Vitamin C (as Micro-C): 4 capsules twice a day
- Wild blueberry powder: 2 tablespoons daily
- Zinc (as liquid zinc sulfate): up to 1 dropperful twice a day

Guilt and Sadness

True cause: Emotional struggles and difficult circumstances that have either happened in the past or are occurring in the present can potentially lower our immune system and deplete us of critically needed nutrients.

- Fresh celery juice: work up to 16 ounces daily
- Celeryforce: 2 capsules three times a day
- 5-MTHF: 1 capsule twice a day
- Ashwagandha: 1 dropperful twice a daily
- Barley grass juice powder: 2 teaspoons or 6 capsules daily
- B-complex: 1 capsule daily
- CoQ10: 1 capsule daily
- Curcumin: 2 capsules daily
- EPA and DHA (fish-free): 1 capsule daily (taken with dinner)
- Hibiscus: 3 cups of tea daily
- Lemon balm: 3 dropperfuls three times a day
- Licorice root: 1 dropperful daily (two weeks on, two weeks off)
- Magnesium glycinate: 2 capsules daily

- Melatonin: 5 milligrams at bedtime daily
- Nascent iodine: 3 small drops (not dropperfuls) daily
- Rose hips: 1 cup of tea daily
- Spirulina: 2 teaspoons or 6 capsules daily
- Vitamin B$_{12}$ (as adenosylcobalamin with methylcobalamin): 2 dropperfuls twice a day
- Zinc (as liquid zinc sulfate): 1 dropperful daily

Hair Thinning and Loss

True cause: A stagnant, sluggish liver containing toxic heavy metals and/or pathogens combined with deficiencies in the critical hormone produced by the adrenal glands that keeps hair follicles alive and stimulates hair growth.

- Fresh celery juice: work up to 32 ounces daily
- 5-MTHF: 1 capsule daily
- Ashwagandha: 3 dropperfuls twice a day
- Barley grass juice powder: 1 tablespoon or 9 capsules daily
- Burdock root: 1 cup of tea or 1 root freshly juiced daily
- Chaga mushroom: 1 tablespoon or 9 capsules daily
- CoQ10: 1 capsule daily
- Curcumin: 2 capsules twice a day
- EPA and DHA (fish-free): 1 capsule daily (taken with dinner)
- Lemon balm: 2 dropperfuls twice a day
- L-glutamine: 2 capsules twice a day
- Licorice root: 1 dropperful daily (two weeks on, two weeks off)
- Magnesium glycinate: 2 capsules twice a day
- MSM: 1 capsule daily
- Nascent iodine: 2 small drops (not dropperfuls) daily

- **Nettle leaf:** 4 dropperfuls daily
- **Raspberry leaf:** 1 cup of tea with 2 bags twice a day
- **Spirulina:** 2 teaspoons or 6 capsules daily
- **Vitamin B$_{12}$ (as adenosylcobalamin with methylcobalamin):** 2 dropperfuls twice a day
- **Vitamin C (as Micro-C):** 4 capsules twice a day
- **Vitamin D$_3$:** 1,000 IU every other day
- **Wild blueberry powder:** 1 tablespoon daily
- **Zinc (as liquid zinc sulfate):** 1 dropperful twice a day

Headaches and Migraines

True cause: When physical injury is not a factor, commonly caused by one of the over 30 varieties of shingles virus creating inflammation of the trigeminal, phrenic, or vagus nerves *or* one of the over 60 varieties of Epstein-Barr virus producing neurotoxins that saturate and inflame neurons inside the brain or inflame the phrenic or vagus nerves. Various triggers can contribute, including chronic dehydration from a sluggish, stagnant liver and a high-fat/high-protein diet that depletes organs such as the brain of oxygen; excessive adrenaline from stress, emotional turmoil, or struggle; and toxic heavy metals such as mercury, aluminum, and copper residing inside the brain and saturating neurons. Migraines and headaches can also be triggered by perfumes, colognes, scented candles, and air fresheners.

- **Fresh celery juice:** work up to 32 ounces daily
- **Celeryforce:** 3 capsules three times a day
- **Ashwagandha:** 1 dropperful twice a day
- **Barley grass juice powder:** 2 teaspoons or 6 capsules daily
- **Cat's claw:** 2 dropperfuls twice a day

- **CoQ10:** 1 capsule daily
- **Curcumin:** 3 capsules twice a day
- **Elderflower:** 1 cup of tea daily
- **Feverfew:** 2 dropperfuls or 2 capsules daily
- **Goldenseal:** 1 dropperful twice a day (two weeks on, two weeks off)
- **Kava kava:** 2 dropperfuls or 2 capsules daily
- **Lemon balm:** 4 dropperfuls twice a day
- **L-lysine:** 4 500-milligram capsules twice a day
- **Magnesium glycinate:** 2 capsules twice a day
- **Nettle leaf:** 4 dropperfuls twice a day
- **Oregano oil:** 2 capsules daily
- **Skullcap:** 2 dropperfuls or 2 capsules twice a day
- **Spirulina:** 2 teaspoons or 6 capsules daily
- **Turmeric:** 2 capsules twice a day
- **Vitamin B$_{12}$ (as adenosylcobalamin with methylcobalamin):** 2 dropperfuls twice a day
- **Vitamin C (as Micro-C):** 4 capsules twice a day
- **White willow bark:** 2 dropperfuls or 2 capsules daily
- **Wild blueberry powder:** 1 tablespoon daily

Heart Palpitations

True cause: When heart palpitations and fibrillations occur for no reason that a doctor can identify, what's usually going on is a low-grade viral infection (from one of the over 60 varieties of Epstein-Barr virus) sitting inside a stagnant, sluggish liver, creating byproduct and viral sludge (such as neurotoxins and viral cell casings) that leave the liver and accumulate in the heart valves. This jelly-like residue buildup can create inconsistencies in heart rhythm as the heart valves sometimes stick slightly. Also, viral neurotoxins can enter the brain and contaminate neurons that are associated with nerves that travel directly to the heart. This can provide an electrical inconsistency, prompting the heart to palpitate. Both of these causes are unknown to medical research and science.

- **Fresh celery juice:** work up to 32 ounces daily
- **Celeryforce:** 2 capsules twice a day
- **5-MTHF:** 1 capsule daily
- **Barley grass juice powder:** 2 teaspoons or 6 capsules daily
- **Cat's claw:** 2 dropperfuls daily
- **Chaga mushroom:** 2 teaspoons or 6 capsules daily
- **CoQ10:** 2 capsules daily
- **Curcumin:** 2 capsules daily
- **Lemon balm:** 3 dropperfuls daily
- **Magnesium glycinate:** 3 capsules daily
- **Nascent iodine:** 4 small drops (not dropperfuls) daily
- **Nettle leaf:** 2 dropperfuls daily
- **Raspberry leaf:** 1 cup of tea with 2 bags daily
- **Spirulina:** 2 teaspoons or 6 capsules daily
- **Vitamin B$_{12}$ (as adenosylcobalamin with methylcobalamin):** 2 dropperfuls daily
- **Vitamin C (as Micro-C):** 4 capsules daily
- **Wild blueberry powder:** 1 tablespoon daily
- **Zinc (as liquid zinc sulfate):** up to 1 dropperful daily

Hepatitis

True cause: An acute or chronic, low-grade viral infection in the liver, most commonly one of the over 60 varieties of Epstein-Barr virus. For further explanation, see *Liver Rescue*.

- **Fresh celery juice:** try to work up to 32 ounces twice a day
- **Barley grass juice powder:** 2 teaspoons or 6 capsules daily
- **Cat's claw:** 1 dropperful twice a day
- **Chaga mushroom:** 2 teaspoons or 6 capsules daily
- **Curcumin:** 3 capsules twice a day
- **Eyebright:** 1 dropperful twice a day
- **Goldenseal:** 2 dropperfuls twice a day (two weeks on, two weeks off)
- **Lemon balm:** 1 cup of tea with 2 bags or 2 dropperfuls twice a day
- **Licorice root:** 1 dropperful twice a day (two weeks on, two weeks off)
- **Mullein leaf:** 2 dropperfuls twice a day
- **Raw honey:** 1 tablespoon daily
- **Spirulina:** 2 teaspoons or 6 capsules daily
- **Vitamin C (as Micro-C):** 4 capsules twice a day
- **Wild blueberry powder:** 3 tablespoons daily
- **Zinc (as liquid zinc sulfate):** up to 2 dropperfuls twice a day

Herpes Simplex

True cause: There are many strains and mutations of herpes simplex 1 (HSV 1) and herpes simplex 2 (HSV 2). Symptoms that can arise from these viruses include fatigue, jaw pain, ear pain, pain in the lower neck, pain in the upper neck, pain in the back of the head, pain in the genital area, bladder pain and inflammation, sore throat, mild fever, mouth sores, and sores on the genitals or adjacent areas. In many cases, someone is actually dealing with shingles, and it's misdiagnosed as herpes simplex 1 or 2.

- **Fresh celery juice:** work up to 32 ounces daily

- **Aloe vera:** 2 or more inches of fresh gel (skin removed) daily; also apply fresh gel to herpes sores
- **Barley grass juice powder:** 2 teaspoons or 6 capsules daily
- **Cat's claw:** 2 dropperfuls twice a day
- **Curcumin:** 2 capsules twice a day
- **Lemon balm:** 5 dropperfuls twice a day
- **Licorice root:** 2 dropperfuls twice a day (two weeks on, two weeks off)
- **L- lysine:** 8 capsules twice a day
- **Lomatium root:** 2 dropperfuls twice a day
- **Mullein leaf:** 4 dropperfuls twice a day
- **Nascent iodine:** 3 small drops (not dropperfuls) twice a day
- **Nettle leaf:** 4 dropperfuls twice a day
- **Oregon grape root:** 2 dropperfuls twice a day (two weeks on, two weeks off)
- **Propolis:** 5 dropperfuls twice a day; also dab on herpes sores
- **Raw honey:** 1 tablespoon daily
- **Spirulina:** 6 capsules or 2 teaspoons daily
- **Thyme:** 2 sprigs of fresh thyme in hot water as tea or 4 sprigs in room temperature water twice a day
- **Vitamin B$_{12}$ (as adenosylcobalamin with methylcobalamin):** 2 dropperfuls twice a day
- **Vitamin C (as Micro-C):** 8 capsules twice a day
- **Zinc (as liquid zinc sulfate):** 2 dropperfuls twice a day

High Blood Pressure

True cause: If a heart problem is not discovered to explain it, what's usually behind mystery hypertension is a stagnant, sluggish, toxic, pre-fatty, or fatty liver filled with a combination of toxins and pathogens, along with a high-fat/high-protein diet and chronic dehydration.

- **Fresh celery juice:** work up to 32 ounces daily
- **Celeryforce:** 2 capsules twice a day
- **5-MTHF:** 1 capsule daily
- **Ashwagandha:** 1 dropperful daily
- **Barley grass juice powder:** 2 teaspoons or 6 capsules daily
- **B-complex:** 1 capsule daily
- **CoQ10:** 2 capsules daily
- **Curcumin:** 2 capsules twice a day
- **EPA and DHA (fish-free):** 1 capsule daily (taken with dinner)
- **Lemon balm:** 2 dropperfuls daily
- **Milk thistle:** 1 dropperful daily
- **Magnesium glycinate:** 4 capsules daily
- **Spirulina:** 2 teaspoons or 6 capsules daily
- **Turmeric:** 2 capsules daily
- **Vitamin B$_{12}$ (as adenosylcobalamin with methylcobalamin):** 1 dropperful daily
- **Vitamin C (as Micro-C):** 6 capsules daily
- **Zinc (as liquid zinc sulfate):** up to 1 dropperful daily

High Cholesterol

True cause: A liver that has become stagnant and sluggish from multiple toxins and pathogens and a long-term high-fat/high-protein diet, causing the organ to lose its ability to create good cholesterol and store bad cholesterol.

- **Fresh celery juice:** work up to 32 ounces daily
- **Aloe vera:** 2 or more inches of fresh gel (skin removed) daily
- **Amla berry:** 2 teaspoons daily
- **Barley grass juice powder:** 2 teaspoons or 6 capsules daily
- **CoQ10:** 2 capsules daily
- **Curcumin:** 2 capsules twice a day
- **EPA and DHA (fish-free):** 1 capsule daily (taken with dinner)

- **Ginger:** 1 cup of tea with 2 bags or freshly grated or juiced to taste daily
- **Milk thistle:** 1 dropperful daily
- **Peppermint:** 1 cup of tea daily
- **Spirulina:** 2 teaspoons or 6 capsules daily
- **Vitamin B$_{12}$ (as adenosylcobalamin with methylcobalamin):** 1 dropperful daily
- **Vitamin C (as Micro-C):** 4 capsules daily
- **Wild blueberry powder:** 2 tablespoons daily
- **Zinc (as liquid zinc sulfate):** up to 1 dropperful daily

Hormonal Problems

True cause: A low-grade viral infection, most commonly from one or more of the over 60 varieties of Epstein-Barr virus, combined with a stagnant, sluggish liver filled with toxins such as toxic heavy metals, pesticides, herbicides, plastics and other petrochemical byproducts, old pharmaceuticals, perfumes, colognes, scented candles, air fresheners, and troublemaker foods such as eggs.

- **Fresh celery juice:** work up to 32 ounces daily
- **Celeryforce:** 2 capsules twice a day
- **Ashwagandha:** 1 dropperful daily
- **Barley grass juice powder:** 2 teaspoons or 6 capsules daily
- **Hibiscus:** 1 cup of tea with 2 bags daily
- **Lemon balm:** 2 dropperfuls daily
- **Milk thistle:** 1 dropperful daily
- **Nascent iodine:** 6 small drops (not dropperfuls) daily
- **Nettle leaf:** 4 dropperfuls daily
- **Raspberry leaf:** 1 cup of tea with 3 bags twice a day
- **Schisandra berry:** 1 cup of tea daily
- **Spirulina:** 2 teaspoons or 6 capsules daily

- **Vitamin B$_{12}$ (as adenosylcobalamin with methylcobalamin):** 2 dropperfuls daily
- **Vitamin C (as Micro-C):** 2 capsules daily
- **Wild blueberry powder:** 2 tablespoons daily

Hot Flashes, Chills, Night Sweats, Running Hot, and Body Temperature Fluctuations

True cause: A sluggish, stagnant liver filled with a variety of toxins, including toxic hormones from years of fight or flight, toxic heavy metals (such as mercury, aluminum, and copper), poisonous viral byproduct and other waste matter (from any of the over 60 varieties of Epstein-Barr virus, over 30 varieties of shingles virus, or many varieties of HHV-6, herpes simplex 1 and 2, or cytomegalovirus), plus old pharmaceuticals, pesticides, herbicides, fungicides, air fresheners, scented candles, perfumes, colognes, and a long-term high-fat/high-protein diet.

- **Fresh celery juice:** work up to 32 ounces daily
- **Amla berry:** 2 teaspoons daily
- **Ashwagandha:** 1 dropperful daily
- **Barley grass juice powder:** 2 teaspoons or 6 capsules daily
- **Cat's claw:** 1 dropperful twice a day
- **Celeryforce:** 2 capsules twice a day
- **Chaga mushroom:** 2 teaspoons or 6 capsules daily
- **CoQ10:** 1 capsule daily
- **Curcumin:** 2 capsules daily
- **Lemon balm:** 2 dropperfuls or 1 cup of tea with 2 bags daily
- **Licorice root:** 1 dropperful daily (two weeks on, two weeks off)
- **L-lysine:** 2 500-milligram capsules daily
- **Monolaurin:** 1 capsule daily

- **Nascent iodine:** 4 small drops (not dropperfuls) daily
- **Nettle leaf:** 2 dropperfuls or 1 cup of tea with 2 bags daily
- **Raspberry leaf:** 1 cup of tea with 2 bags daily
- **Schisandra berry:** 2 dropperfuls daily
- **Spirulina:** 2 teaspoons or 6 capsules daily
- **Vitamin B$_{12}$ (as adenosylcobalamin with methylcobalamin):** 1 dropperful daily
- **Vitamin C (as Micro-C):** 4 capsules daily
- **Wild blueberry powder:** 2 teaspoons daily
- **Zinc (as liquid zinc sulfate):** up to 1 dropperful daily

Human Papillomavirus (HPV)

True cause: A virus, highly fueled by various troublemaker foods such as eggs in the diet, that takes advantage of an immune system already lowered by low-grade infections in the body, such as from one of the over 60 varieties of Epstein-Barr virus or one or more strains from the over 50 groups of *Streptococcus* bacteria, which in turn allows HPV to proliferate. The problems with HPV do not stem from HPV itself. HPV is a docile virus that causes little to no harm *unless* there are multiple systemic, chronic, low-grade infections occurring in the body at the same time, going undiagnosed and unhealed long term.

- **Fresh celery juice:** work up to 16 ounces daily
- **5-MTHF:** 1 capsule daily
- **Aloe vera:** 2 or more inches of fresh gel (skin removed) daily
- **Ashwagandha:** 1 dropperful daily
- **Barley grass juice powder:** 2 teaspoons or 6 capsules daily
- **B-complex:** 1 capsule daily
- **Cat's claw:** 2 dropperfuls twice a day

- **Chaga mushroom:** 2 teaspoons or 6 capsules daily
- **Curcumin:** 2 capsules twice a day
- **Eyebright:** 1 dropperful daily (two weeks on, two weeks off)
- **Lemon balm:** 4 dropperfuls twice a day
- **Licorice root:** 1 dropperful daily (two weeks on, two weeks off)
- **L-lysine:** 3 500-milligram capsules twice a day
- **Lomatium root:** 2 dropperfuls daily (two weeks on, two weeks off)
- **Monolaurin:** 1 capsule twice a day
- **Nascent iodine:** 3 small drops (not dropperfuls) daily
- **Nettle leaf:** 4 dropperfuls twice a day
- **Spirulina:** 2 teaspoons or 6 capsules daily
- **Turmeric:** 2 capsules daily
- **Vitamin B$_{12}$ (as adenosylcobalamin with methylcobalamin):** 1 dropperful twice a day
- **Vitamin C (as Micro-C):** 6 capsules twice a day
- **Vitamin D$_3$:** 1,000 IU daily
- **Wild blueberry powder:** 1 tablespoon daily
- **Zinc (as liquid zinc sulfate):** 1 dropperful twice a day

Infertility

True cause: Individuals with infertility issues experience them for varied reasons. It could be one of the over 60 varieties of Epstein-Barr virus affecting the reproductive system and causing mystery female infertility. It could be toxic heavy metals and pesticides causing mystery male infertility. Or it could be a little of both, or radiation, or "low reproductive battery," or it could be all of these and more at once. The most common causes are toxic heavy metals, viral activity, radiation, and DDT and its pesticide cousins, although every person will experience these at different levels. A high-fat/high-protein diet worsens mystery infertility. For a much more detailed look at this topic, see "Fertility and Our Future" in my book *Life-Changing Foods*.

Supplements for Female Infertility

- **Fresh celery juice:** work up to 32 ounces daily
- **5-MTHF:** 1 capsule twice a day
- **Ashwagandha:** 1 dropperful daily
- **Barley grass juice powder:** 1 tablespoon or 9 capsules daily
- **B-complex:** 1 capsule daily
- **Curcumin:** 2 capsules twice a day
- **Elderflower:** 1 cup of tea daily
- **EPA and DHA (fish-free):** 1 capsule daily (taken with dinner)
- **Hibiscus:** 1 cup of tea daily
- **Lemon balm:** 2 dropperfuls twice a day
- **Licorice root:** 1 dropperful daily (two weeks on, two weeks off)
- **L-lysine:** 3 500-milligram capsules twice a day
- **Nascent iodine:** 3 small drops (not dropperfuls) daily
- **Nettle leaf:** 4 dropperfuls twice a day
- **Raspberry leaf:** 1 cup of tea with 2 bags three times a day
- **Raw honey:** 1 tablespoon daily
- **Rose hips:** 1 cup of tea daily
- **Selenium:** 1 capsule daily
- **Spirulina:** 2 teaspoons or 6 capsules daily
- **Vitamin B$_{12}$ (as adenosylcobalamin with methylcobalamin):** 1 dropperful twice a day
- **Vitamin C (as Micro-C):** 4 capsules twice a day
- **Vitamin D$_3$:** 1,000 IU daily
- **Wild blueberry powder:** 2 tablespoons daily

- **Zinc (as liquid zinc sulfate):** 1 dropperful daily

Supplements for Male Infertility

- **Fresh celery juice:** work up to 16 ounces daily
- **Celeryforce:** 3 capsules twice a day
- **Ashwagandha:** 2 dropperfuls twice a day
- **Barley grass juice powder:** 1 tablespoon or 9 capsules daily
- **B-complex:** 1 capsule daily
- **Chaga mushroom:** 4 teaspoons or 12 capsules daily
- **CoQ10:** 1 capsule twice a day
- **Curcumin:** 3 capsules twice a day
- **EPA and DHA (fish-free):** 1 capsule daily (taken with dinner)
- **Lemon balm:** 4 dropperfuls twice a day
- **L-glutamine:** 2 capsules twice a day
- **Licorice root:** 1 dropperful twice a day (two weeks on, two weeks off)
- **L-lysine:** 2 500-milligram capsules twice a day
- **Magnesium glycinate:** 1 capsule twice a day
- **Melatonin:** 5 milligrams at bedtime daily
- **Nettle leaf:** 2 dropperfuls twice a day
- **Olive leaf:** 2 dropperfuls twice a day
- **Selenium:** 1 capsule daily
- **Spirulina:** 1 tablespoon or 9 capsules daily
- **Turmeric:** 2 capsules twice a day
- **Vitamin B$_{12}$ (as adenosylcobalamin with methylcobalamin):** 1 dropperful twice a day
- **Vitamin C (as Micro-C):** 4 capsules twice a day
- **Wild blueberry powder:** 2 tablespoons daily
- **Yellow dock:** 1 cup of tea daily
- **Zinc (as liquid zinc sulfate):** 2 dropperfuls twice a day

Inflammation

True cause: When inflammation is mysterious and not the result of a physical injury, the hidden cause is a pathogen such as a virus feeding on both toxic heavy metals (such as mercury, aluminum, and copper) and troublemaker foods (such as eggs, gluten, and dairy products) and as a result, producing chemical compounds called neurotoxins and dermatoxins that raise inflammation levels throughout the body. A high-fat/high-protein diet interferes with healing inflammation.

- **Fresh celery juice:** work up to 32 ounces daily
- **Celeryforce:** 2 capsules twice a day
- **5-MTHF:** 1 capsule daily
- **Aloe vera:** 2 or more inches of fresh gel (skin removed) daily
- **Barley grass juice powder:** 2 teaspoons or 6 capsules daily
- **Cat's claw:** 2 dropperfuls daily
- **Chaga mushroom:** 2 teaspoons or 6 capsules daily
- **Curcumin:** 3 capsules twice a day
- **Lemon balm:** 3 dropperfuls twice a day
- **Licorice root:** 1 dropperful daily (two weeks on, two weeks off)
- **L-lysine:** 4 500-milligram capsules twice a day
- **Magnesium glycinate:** 2 capsules daily
- **MSM:** 2 capsules daily
- **Mullein leaf:** 2 dropperfuls daily
- **Nascent iodine:** 4 small drops (not dropperfuls) daily
- **Nettle leaf:** 2 dropperfuls daily
- **Olive leaf:** 1 dropperful daily
- **Spirulina:** 2 teaspoons or 6 capsules daily
- **Turmeric:** 2 capsules daily

- **Vitamin B₁₂ (as adenosylcobalamin with methylcobalamin):** 2 dropperfuls twice a day
- **Vitamin C (as Micro-C):** 6 capsules twice a day
- **Wild blueberry powder:** 1 tablespoon daily
- **Zinc (as liquid zinc sulfate):** up to 2 dropperfuls twice a day

Insomnia

True cause: Causes can include emotional disturbance (anything from heartbreak to loss to an unresolved matter in life); excess stress and overactive or underactive adrenals; a sluggish, stagnant liver causing mild liver spasms that lead to restlessness in the night; a low-grade chronic viral infection (such as one of the over 60 varieties of Epstein-Barr virus or one of the over 30 varieties of shingles) that leads to restless leg syndrome; or weakened or dehydrated neurotransmitters due to toxic heavy metals such as mercury or neurotoxins produced by viruses such as EBV. You'll find much more about insomnia and sleep disturbances in *Thyroid Healing*'s "Secrets of Sleep."

- **Fresh celery juice:** work up to 32 ounces daily
- **Celeryforce:** 3 capsules three times a day
- **5-MTHF:** 1 capsule daily
- **Aloe vera:** 2 or more inches of fresh gel (skin removed) daily
- **Ashwagandha:** 2 dropperfuls twice a day
- **Barley grass juice powder:** 2 teaspoons or 6 capsules daily
- **Cat's claw:** 1 dropperful twice a day
- **Curcumin** 2 capsules twice a day
- **D-mannose:** 1 tablespoon in water daily
- **GABA:** 1 250-milligram capsule three times a day

- **Ginger:** 2 cups of tea or freshly grated or juiced to taste daily
- **Hibiscus:** 1 cup of tea with 2 bags (combined with the lemon balm tea) at bedtime daily
- **Lemon balm:** 4 dropperfuls three times a day *plus* 1 cup of lemon balm tea (combined with the hibiscus tea) at bedtime daily
- **Licorice root:** 1 dropperful daily (two weeks on, two weeks off)
- **Magnesium glycinate:** 2 capsules twice a day
- **Melatonin:** 5 to 20 milligrams at bedtime daily
- **Raw honey:** 1 tablespoon daily, preferably at night (for example, in tea)
- **Spirulina:** 2 teaspoons or 6 capsules daily
- **Vitamin B$_{12}$ (as adenosylcobalamin with methylcobalamin):** 2 dropperfuls twice a day
- **Vitamin C (as Micro-C):** 4 capsules twice a day
- **Wild blueberry powder:** 2 teaspoons daily
- **Zinc (as liquid zinc sulfate):** 1 dropperful daily

Irritable Bowel Syndrome (IBS)

True cause: Low production of hydrochloric acid and bile allowing bacteria such as strains from the over 50 groups of *Streptococcus* bacteria to proliferate inside the intestinal tract. Often the intestinal tract will also harbor toxic heavy metals such as mercury and the liver will be stagnant and sluggish due to an overload of toxins. A high-fat/high-protein diet accelerates the condition.

- **Fresh celery juice:** work up to 32 ounces daily
- **Celeryforce:** 1 capsule twice a day
- **Aloe vera:** 2 or more inches of fresh gel (skin removed) daily

- **Barley grass juice powder:** 1 teaspoon or 3 capsules daily
- **Burdock root:** 1 cup of tea or 1 root freshly juiced daily
- **Cat's claw:** 1 dropperful twice a day
- **Dandelion root:** 1 cup of tea daily
- **Ginger:** 1 cup of tea or freshly grated or juiced to taste daily
- **Hibiscus:** 1 cup of tea daily
- **Lemon balm:** 1 dropperful or 1 cup of tea daily
- **Licorice root:** 1 dropperful or 1 cup of tea with 2 bags daily (two weeks on, two weeks off)
- **Nettle leaf:** 1 dropperful or 1 cup of tea daily
- **Spirulina:** 1 teaspoon or 3 capsules daily
- **Vitamin B$_{12}$ (as adenosylcobalamin with methylcobalamin):** 1 dropperful twice a day

Jaundice

True cause: A liver condition from pathogens and toxic heavy metals creating bouts of acute inflammation or long-term chronic liver diseases, tumors, or cysts. Please note that while jaundice is common in babies, these are adult dosages.

- **Fresh celery juice:** work up to 32 ounces twice a day
- **Amla berry:** 1 teaspoon twice a day
- **Barley grass juice powder:** 2 teaspoons or 6 capsules daily
- **Hibiscus:** 1 cup of tea twice a day
- **Lemon balm:** 1 dropperful twice a day
- **Nettle leaf:** 1 dropperful or 1 cup of tea twice a day
- **Peppermint:** 1 cup of tea twice a day
- **Red clover:** 1 cup of tea or 1 dropperful twice a day
- **Vitamin C (as Micro-C):** 2 capsules twice a day

Joint Pain

True cause: An overabundance of acids and various toxins throughout the body due to a stagnant, sluggish, overburdened liver. Alternatively, low-grade viral infection from one of the over 60 varieties of Epstein-Barr virus feeding on mercury, aluminum, and/or copper in the body, releasing neurotoxins that cause the joints to ache. Together, these causes can contribute to joint pain at the same time, or someone may be suffering from only a stagnant liver or viral infection. Sometimes, rather than EBV, one of the over 30 varieties of shingles is the cause, creating viral inflammation around joint areas. Both viruses can create excess fluid and swelling, leading to a myriad of joint pain–related diagnoses. Joint pain can worsen on a high-fat/high-protein diet.

At times, joint pain is clearly the result of injury. When someone continues to experience sustained pain after the injury should have healed, it's often the result of a low-grade viral infection.

- **Fresh celery juice:** work up to 32 ounces daily
- **5-MTHF:** 1 capsule daily
- **Aloe vera:** 2 or more inches of fresh gel (skin removed) daily
- **Barley grass juice powder:** 2 teaspoons or 6 capsules daily
- **B-complex:** 1 capsule daily
- **Cat's claw:** 1 dropperful daily
- **CoQ10:** 1 capsule daily
- **Curcumin:** 3 capsules twice a day
- **Glutathione:** 1 capsule daily
- **Lemon balm:** 3 dropperfuls twice a day
- **Licorice root:** 1 dropperful twice a day (two weeks on, two weeks off)
- **L-lysine:** 4 500-milligram capsules twice a day
- **Magnesium glycinate:** 2 capsules twice a day

- **Milk thistle:** 1 dropperful daily
- **Monolaurin:** 1 capsule daily
- **MSM:** 2 capsules daily
- **Nettle leaf:** 4 dropperfuls twice a day
- **Spirulina:** 2 teaspoons or 6 capsules daily
- **Turmeric:** 4 capsules daily
- **Vitamin B$_{12}$ (as adenosylcobalamin with methylcobalamin):** 2 dropperfuls twice a day
- **Vitamin C (as Micro-C):** 4 capsules twice a day
- **Vitamin D$_3$:** 1,000 IU daily
- **Wild blueberry powder:** 1 tablespoon daily
- **Zinc (as liquid zinc sulfate):** 1 dropperful twice a day

Kidney Disease

True cause: Pathogenic injury (from bacterial or viral infection), toxic injury (from pharmaceuticals, recreational drugs, or toxic heavy metals), or diet injury (from a high-fat/high-protein diet). Someone can experience one of these causes on its own or more than one in combination.

- **Fresh celery juice:** work up to 16 ounces daily
- **Aloe vera:** 2 or more inches of fresh gel (skin removed) daily
- **Ashwagandha:** 6 small drops (not dropperfuls) daily
- **Barley grass juice powder:** 2 teaspoons or 6 capsules daily
- **Burdock root:** 1 cup of tea or 1 root freshly juiced daily
- **Curcumin:** 1 capsule daily
- **D-mannose:** 1 tablespoon twice a day in water
- **Elderberry:** 1 dropperful or capsule daily
- **Elderflower:** 1 cup of tea daily
- **L-lysine:** 1 500-milligram capsule twice a day

- **Lemon balm:** 2 dropperfuls twice a day
- **Magnesium glycinate:** 1 capsule twice a day
- **Rose hips:** 1 cup of tea daily
- **Spirulina:** 1 teaspoon or 3 capsules daily
- **Vitamin B$_{12}$ (as adenosylcobalamin with methylcobalamin):** 1 dropperful twice a day
- **Vitamin C (as Micro-C):** 2 capsules twice a day
- **Zinc (as liquid zinc sulfate):** 1 dropperful daily

Kidney Stones

True cause: A stagnant, sluggish, toxic liver coupled with a high-fat/high-protein diet. Learn more in *Liver Rescue*.

- **Fresh celery juice:** work up to 32 ounces daily
- **Barley grass juice powder:** 1 tablespoon or 9 capsules daily
- **Burdock root:** 2 cups of tea or 2 roots freshly juiced daily
- **Chaga mushroom:** 2 teaspoons or 6 capsules daily
- **Curcumin:** 2 capsules twice a day
- **Dandelion root:** 1 cup of tea daily
- **D-mannose:** 1 tablespoon twice a day in water
- **Lemon balm:** 2 dropperfuls twice a day
- **Magnesium glycinate:** 1 capsule twice a day
- **Milk thistle:** 1 dropperful twice a day
- **Red clover:** 1 dropperful or 1 cup of tea twice a day
- **Turmeric:** 2 capsules twice a day
- **Vitamin C (as Micro-C):** 4 capsules twice a day
- **Wild blueberry powder:** 1 tablespoon daily

Loss of Libido (Female)

True cause: When a woman's sex drive disappears mysteriously, the cause is weakened adrenal glands. Sometimes, one adrenal is weakened more than the other.

- **Fresh celery juice:** work up to at least 16 ounces daily
- **Celeryforce:** 2 capsules twice a day
- **Aloe vera:** 2 or more inches of fresh gel (skin removed) daily
- **Ashwagandha:** 2 dropperfuls twice a day
- **Barley grass juice powder:** 2 teaspoons or 6 capsules daily
- **Chaga mushroom:** 2 teaspoons or 6 capsules daily
- **Ginger:** 2 cups of tea or 1 tablespoon freshly grated into hot water as tea daily
- **Hibiscus:** 1 cup of tea daily
- **Lemon balm:** 2 dropperfuls twice a day
- **Licorice root:** 2 dropperfuls twice a day (two weeks on, two weeks off)
- **Magnesium glycinate:** 1 capsule twice a day
- **Nascent iodine:** 4 small drops (not dropperfuls) daily
- **Raspberry leaf:** 1 cup of tea with 2 bags three times a day
- **Schisandra berry:** 1 cup of tea three times a day
- **Spirulina:** 2 teaspoons or 6 capsules daily
- **Vitamin B$_{12}$ (as adenosylcobalamin with methylcobalamin):** 2 dropperfuls twice a day
- **Vitamin C (as Micro-C):** 4 capsules twice a day
- **Wild blueberry powder:** 1 tablespoon daily
- **Zinc (as liquid zinc sulfate):** 1 dropperful twice a day

Loss of Libido (Male) and Erectile Dysfunction

True cause: When a man's libido disappears mysteriously, the cause is a stagnant, sluggish liver that's overrun with fat to the point that the liver's fat "storage bin" is overfilled. In other words, it's fatty liver—or pre-fatty liver, in the case of men who haven't been diagnosed with fatty liver yet. This doesn't mean excess weight is necessarily visible on the body; you can have a pre-fatty or fatty liver without excess fat showing itself on the outside. A high-fat/high-protein diet can worsen this condition.

Erectile dysfunction is caused by toxic heavy metals such as mercury and aluminum oxidizing around neurons in the brain, in turn causing dysfunction of electrical impulses and neurotransmitters.

- **Fresh celery juice:** work up to at least 16 ounces daily
- **Celeryforce:** 4 capsules twice a day
- **Ashwagandha:** 1 dropperful twice a day
- **Barley grass juice powder:** 1 tablespoon or 9 capsules daily
- **Burdock root:** 3 cups of tea or 3 roots freshly juiced daily
- **Cat's claw:** 1 dropperful twice a day
- **Chaga mushroom:** 1 tablespoon or 9 capsules daily
- **Curcumin:** 3 capsules twice a day
- **GABA:** 1 250-milligram capsule daily
- **Lemon balm:** 4 dropperfuls three times a day
- **Licorice root:** 2 dropperfuls twice a day (two weeks on, two weeks off)
- **L-lysine:** 4 500-milligram capsules twice a day
- **Magnesium glycinate:** 2 capsules twice a day
- **Melatonin:** 10 milligrams at bedtime daily
- **Milk thistle:** 1 dropperful twice a day
- **Spirulina:** 1 tablespoon or 9 capsules daily
- **Vitamin B$_{12}$ (as adenosylcobalamin with methylcobalamin):** 3 dropperfuls twice a day
- **Vitamin C (as Micro-C):** 6 capsules twice a day

Low Vision

True cause: Mysterious low vision where the cause can't be diagnosed is a result of weakening nerve cells due to a chronic, low-grade viral infection, coupled with toxic heavy metals such as mercury and aluminum and other toxins such as pesticides, herbicides, fungicides, and petrochemicals.

- **Fresh celery juice:** work up to at least 16 ounces daily
- **Celeryforce:** 3 capsules twice a day
- **5-MTHF:** 1 capsule daily
- **ALA (alpha lipoic acid):** 1 capsule every other day
- **Amla berry:** 1 teaspoon daily
- **Barley grass juice powder:** 2 teaspoons or 6 capsules daily
- **Cat's claw:** 2 dropperfuls twice a day
- **Curcumin:** 3 capsules twice a day
- **EPA and DHA (fish-free):** 1 capsule daily (taken with dinner)
- **Glutathione:** 1 capsule daily
- **Lemon balm:** 3 dropperfuls twice a day
- **Licorice root:** 1 dropperful daily (two weeks on, two weeks off)
- **L-lysine:** 4 500-milligram capsules twice a day
- **Magnesium glycinate:** 2 capsules twice a day
- **Monolaurin:** 1 capsule daily
- **Mullein leaf:** 2 dropperfuls twice a day
- **Olive leaf:** 2 dropperfuls twice a day
- **Rose hips:** 1 cup of tea daily

- **Spirulina:** 2 teaspoons or 6 capsules daily
- **Vitamin B$_{12}$ (as adenosylcobalamin with methylcobalamin):** 2 dropperfuls twice a day
- **Vitamin C (as Micro-C):** 6 capsules twice a day
- **Vitamin D$_3$:** 1,000 IU daily
- **Wild blueberry powder:** 1 tablespoon daily
- **Zinc (as liquid zinc sulfate):** 1 dropperful daily

Lyme Disease

True cause: The true cause of Lyme disease is viral, not bacterial. If this is surprising to you, please know that the medical industry has started to move Lyme disease out of the bacterial category and place it instead in the autoimmune category. What this autoimmune designation means is that medical research and science have lost their belief that Lyme is bacterial, even though the system has been set up for decades to make us believe the disease is caused by bacteria. Lyme disease bloodwork labs still test for and indicate that the disease is bacterial, although this process will eventually shift with time.

Calling Lyme autoimmune is the medical industry saying, "We don't know the cause of Lyme." The reason for this recent development—the reason that medical research and science now doubt that Lyme disease is bacterial—is because of the Medical Medium book series. With the release of the first book, *Medical Medium*, which provided the truth of what causes Lyme disease, millions of people worldwide, including doctors and other health professionals, started to shift their perspective. Now there are doctors helping their patients heal by realizing that viruses such as Epstein-Barr, shingles, HHV-6, HHV-7, herpes simplex 1, herpes simplex 2, and cytomegalovirus are causing their Lyme symptoms. Keep in mind that there are over 60 varieties of EBV, over 30 varieties of shingles, and multiple varieties of these other herpetic viruses.

Bacteria cannot cause neurological symptoms, which is what Lyme disease patients suffer from. Aches and pains, tingles and numbness, dizziness, floaters in the eyes, weak limbs, heart palpitations, burning skin, jaw pain, neck pain, twitches, tics, and spasms are some of these neurological symptoms, and viruses create them, not bacteria. Viruses such as the over 60 varieties of EBV, over 30 varieties of shingles, and multiple varieties of HHV-6, HHV-7, herpes simplex, and CMV release neurotoxins—and it's neurotoxins that are responsible for these neurological symptoms. Bacteria cannot release neurotoxins; bacteria cannot create the neurological symptoms associated with Lyme disease.

Borrelia, *Bartonella*, *Babesia*, and other bacteria assumed to cause Lyme are not superbugs. They don't have the antibiotic resistance that, for example, MRSA does, and bacteria that aren't antibiotic-resistant are no match for antibiotics. The reason we've faced decades of people not recovering from Lyme disease despite taking multiple courses of antibiotics is that what they were battling this whole time were viruses.

This is why Lyme disease patients first started showing improvements when natural therapies were introduced in addition to antibiotic treatments. Some of those natural therapies, which were guessing games, happened to reduce patients' viral load, with nobody realizing that was what prompted symptom relief. Cat's claw is one natural herb that became popular for helping Lyme patients, and it didn't start as a guessing game. That therapy began as Medical Medium information more than three and a half decades ago, and over the years, it has helped tens of thousands of individuals with Lyme disease, including some of the original people who were first diagnosed with it. Cat's claw has shifted the medical system, both alternative and conventional, to accept it as a very helpful therapy for Lyme disease.

Originally, in the 1970s, when medical doctors were noticing an increase of symptoms in both children and adults with no explanation of what was happening, they theorized correctly that Lyme disease was viral. Because there were no medications to offer for viruses at the time, though, antibiotics became the treatment method, in part because they offered monetary gain for Big Pharma. For decades now, billions have been sold on antibiotics for Lyme disease. Even though doctors believed Lyme was viral to begin with, they had to shift the explanation and call it bacterial in order to support the treatment.

Viruses such as EBV and shingles feed on toxic heavy metals such as mercury, aluminum, and copper, and people with Lyme symptoms are higher in mercury than other metals. The neurotoxins released from a virus that has consumed mercury are far more aggressive than others, creating the neurological symptoms that Lyme sufferers know all too well. Again, bacteria don't create neurotoxins. The condition is worsened by troublemaker foods such as eggs, milk, cheese, butter, and gluten as well as a high-fat/high-protein diet.

There's a wake of people injured—not because of Lyme itself, but because of Lyme treatments they've gone through over the decades. It's time you know the truth, so you can protect yourself and anyone else you know. For information on how Lyme is not caused by tick bites—and can only be *triggered* by a tick bite—as well as answers to your other Lyme questions, see *Medical Medium*, the first book in this series.

If you'd like more supplement options in addition to the below, you are welcome to add supplements from the "Autoimmune Disorders and Diseases" list earlier in this chapter.

- **Fresh celery juice:** work up to 32 ounces twice a day if possible; if not, work up to 32 ounces every morning
- **Celeryforce:** 4 capsules twice a day
- **5-MTHF:** 1 capsule twice a day
- **Barley grass juice powder:** 2 teaspoons or 6 capsules twice a day
- **Cat's claw:** 3 dropperfuls twice a day
- **Curcumin:** 3 capsules twice a day
- **Glutathione:** 1 capsule daily
- **Lemon balm:** 4 dropperfuls twice a day
- **Licorice root:** 1 dropperful twice a day (two weeks on, two weeks off)
- **L-lysine:** 5 500-milligram capsules twice a day
- **Mullein leaf:** 4 dropperfuls twice a day
- **Nascent iodine:** 3 small drops (not dropperfuls) twice a day
- **Nettle leaf:** 3 dropperfuls twice a day
- **Raw honey:** 1 to 3 teaspoons daily
- **Spirulina:** 2 teaspoons or 6 capsules daily
- **Vitamin B$_{12}$ (as adenosylcobalamin with methylcobalamin):** 3 dropperfuls twice a day
- **Vitamin C (as Micro-C):** 8 capsules twice a day
- **Zinc (as liquid zinc sulfate):** up to 2 dropperfuls twice a day

Macular Degeneration

True cause: Toxic heavy metals such as mercury and aluminum, along with viral activity from one of the over 60 varieties of Epstein-Barr virus.

- **Fresh celery juice:** work up to at least 16 ounces daily
- **Celeryforce:** 1 capsule twice a day

- **5-MTHF:** 1 capsule daily
- **Barley grass juice powder:** 2 teaspoons or 6 capsules daily
- **B-complex:** 1 capsule daily
- **CoQ10:** 1 capsule daily
- **Curcumin:** 2 capsules twice a day
- **EPA and DHA (fish-free):** 1 capsule daily (taken with dinner)
- **Hibiscus:** 1 cup of tea daily
- **Lemon balm:** 2 dropperfuls twice a day
- **L-lysine:** 2 500-milligram capsules twice a day **Magnesium glycinate:** 2 capsules twice a day
- **Nettle leaf:** 4 dropperfuls daily
- **Spirulina:** 2 teaspoons or 6 capsules daily
- **Vitamin B$_{12}$ (as adenosylcobalamin with methylcobalamin):** 1 dropperful twice a day
- **Vitamin C (as Micro-C):** 4 capsules twice a day
- **Wild blueberry powder:** 2 tablespoons daily
- **Zinc (as liquid zinc sulfate):** 1 dropperful daily

Menopause Symptoms

True cause: Symptoms of menopause are not caused by aging. Rather, the source is a stagnant, sluggish liver filled with decades of viral and bacterial toxins (from pathogens such as the over 60 varieties of Epstein-Barr virus, the over 30 varieties of shingles virus, other herpetic viruses, and bacterial strains from the over 50 groups of *Streptococcus*), along with a liver "storage bin" overfilled with toxic heavy metals, herbicides, pesticides, perfumes, colognes, air fresheners, and residues from scented candles accumulated over the decades. These different factors contribute at different levels for each individual, leading to the variety of symptoms that for the past 70 years have been blamed on hormones and menopause. A high-fat/high-protein diet worsens these symptoms.

- **Fresh celery juice:** work up to 32 ounces daily
- **Celeryforce:** 2 capsules twice a day
- **5-MTHF:** 1 capsule daily
- **Ashwagandha:** 2 dropperfuls twice a day
- **Barley grass juice powder:** 1 tablespoon or 9 capsules daily
- **B-complex:** 1 capsule daily
- **Burdock root:** 1 cup of tea or 1 root freshly juiced daily
- **Cat's claw:** 2 dropperfuls twice a day
- **Chaga mushroom:** 1 tablespoon or 9 capsules daily
- **Curcumin:** 2 capsules twice a day
- **Dandelion root:** 1 cup of tea daily
- **EPA and DHA (fish-free):** 1 capsule daily (taken with dinner)
- **Ginger:** 2 cups of tea or freshly grated to taste daily
- **Glutathione:** 1 capsule daily
- **Goldenseal:** 1 dropperful daily (two weeks on, two weeks off)
- **Lemon balm:** 4 dropperfuls twice a day
- **L-lysine:** 4 500-milligram capsules twice a day
- **Magnesium glycinate:** 2 capsules twice a day
- **Melatonin:** 5 milligrams at bedtime daily
- **Milk thistle:** 1 dropperful twice a day
- **MSM:** 1 capsule daily
- **Nascent iodine:** 3 small drops (not dropperfuls) daily
- **Nettle leaf:** 4 dropperfuls twice a day
- **Raspberry leaf:** 1 cup of tea with 2 bags daily
- **Spirulina:** 2 teaspoons or 6 capsules daily
- **Vitamin B$_{12}$ (as adenosylcobalamin with methylcobalamin):** 2 dropperfuls twice a day

- **Vitamin C (as Micro-C):** 4 capsules twice a day
- **Wild blueberry powder:** 1 tablespoon daily
- **Zinc (as liquid zinc sulfate):** 1 dropperful twice a day

Methylation Problems

True cause: A liver unable to convert or create vitamins, minerals, and other nutrients due to a chronic, low-grade infection, most commonly from one or more of the over 60 varieties of Epstein-Barr virus. This also leads to a detoxification problem, where the liver is overrun with viral toxins, toxic heavy metals, and other poisons and toxins to the point that it can't filter properly, which slows down the nutrient conversion function for which the liver is responsible. (The liver is meant to take in nutrients and convert them into usable forms for specific areas of the body.) Too many poisons and toxins floating in the bloodstream also prevent the lymphatic system from filtering properly. These liver and lymphatic detox problems lead to elevated inflammation, which can trigger any number of tests, including the MTHFR gene mutation test, to indicate a problem. The MTHFR gene mutation test is merely another glorified inflammation test, not too different from the ANA or C-reactive protein tests as far as what it detects. Contrary to what it seems, the MTHFR test does not actually pinpoint a mutated gene. See more on this in *Liver Rescue*.

- **Fresh celery juice:** work up to 32 ounces daily
- **Celeryforce:** 2 capsules twice a day
- **5-MTHF:** 1 capsule twice a day
- **Barley grass juice powder:** 2 teaspoons or 6 capsules daily
- **B-complex:** 1 capsule twice a day

- **Cat's claw:** 2 dropperfuls twice a day
- **Glutathione:** 1 capsule twice a day
- **L-lysine:** 4 500-milligram capsules twice a day
- **NAC:** 1 capsule daily
- **Selenium:** 1 capsule daily
- **Spirulina:** 2 teaspoons or 6 capsules daily
- **Vitamin B$_{12}$ (as adenosylcobalamin with methylcobalamin):** 2 dropperfuls twice a day
- **Vitamin C (as Micro-C):** 4 capsules twice a day
- **Wild blueberry powder:** 1 tablespoon daily
- **Zinc (as liquid zinc sulfate):** 1 dropperful twice a day

Mononucleosis (Mono, an early stage of Epstein-Barr virus, EBV)

True cause: Mononucleosis is caused by any of the over 60 varieties of Epstein-Barr virus. Once the virus is contracted, mono is the beginning of EBV's second stage. The virus is transferred most commonly through bodily fluids—often in relationships or when sharing utensils, glasses, plates, and food. The virus's first stage begins when EBV exposure first happens, and during this Stage One it lies dormant in the body, waiting for stressful events, hardships, losses, fight or flight, deficiencies, or toxic exposure to weaken the immune system enough to take advantage. When EBV enters Stage Two, that's mononucleosis, an active viral infection. Mono often goes undiagnosed, unless it's a severe episode and a physician properly analyzes the person's white count. Otherwise, mono usually occurs in a mild form, where someone dismisses their scratchy throat or fatigue and thinks they're just run down, burnt out, or dealing with a cold or flu.

- **Fresh celery juice:** work up to 32 ounces daily

- **Cat's claw:** 3 dropperfuls twice a day
- **Eyebright:** 3 dropperfuls twice a day
- **Ginger:** 1 cup of tea or freshly grated or juiced to taste four times a day
- **Goldenseal:** 4 dropperfuls twice a day (two weeks on, two weeks off)
- **Lemon balm:** 4 dropperfuls twice a day
- **Licorice root:** 1 dropperful twice a day (two weeks on, two weeks off)
- **L-lysine:** 6 500-milligram capsules twice a day
- **Lomatium root:** 3 dropperfuls twice a day
- **Monolaurin:** 2 capsules twice a day
- **Mullein leaf:** 4 dropperfuls twice a day
- **Oregon grape root:** 2 dropperfuls twice a day (two weeks on, two weeks off)
- **Osha:** 3 dropperfuls twice a day
- **Thyme:** 2 sprigs fresh thyme in hot water as tea or 4 sprigs in room temperature water daily
- **Vitamin C (as Micro-C):** after optional Medical Medium Vitamin C Shock Therapy, 10 capsules twice a day
- **Zinc (as liquid zinc sulfate):** after optional Medical Medium Zinc Shock Therapy for two days, 3 dropperfuls twice a day

Mood Swings, Irritability, Mood Struggles, and Emotional Liver

True cause: A stagnant, sluggish liver overburdened with low-grade bacterial and/or viral infections combined with toxic heavy metals; residues from scented candles, air fresheners, perfumes, colognes, plastics, petrochemicals, household cleaners, and fabric softeners; and other toxins inside both the liver and the intestinal tract.

- **Fresh celery juice:** work up to 32 ounces daily
- **Celeryforce:** 2 capsules twice a day

- **Aloe vera:** 2 or more inches of fresh gel (skin removed) daily
- **Barley grass juice powder:** 2 teaspoons or 6 capsules daily
- **GABA:** 1 250-milligram capsule daily
- **Hibiscus:** 1 cup of tea twice a day
- **Lemon balm:** 4 dropperfuls twice a day
- **Magnesium glycinate:** 2 capsules twice a day
- **Nascent iodine:** 3 small drops (not dropperfuls) daily
- **Nettle leaf:** 1 dropperful or 1 cup of tea twice a day
- **Spirulina:** 2 teaspoons or 6 capsules daily
- **Vitamin B$_{12}$ (as adenosylcobalamin with methylcobalamin):** 1 dropperful twice a day
- **Vitamin C (as Micro-C):** 2 capsules twice a day
- **Vitamin D$_3$:** 1,000 IU daily
- **Wild blueberry powder:** 1 tablespoon daily
- **Zinc (as liquid zinc sulfate):** up to 1 dropperful daily

Multiple Sclerosis (MS)

True cause: Viral neurotoxins from one or more strains of Epstein-Barr virus floating through the body and inflaming the central nervous system. Elevated mercury is usually present too. The condition worsens with a high-fat/high-protein diet. Only a few out of the over 60 varieties of EBV can cause MS; particularly aggressive strains can directly damage the nerves as well as produce these inflammatory neurotoxins. Lesions found in the brain with MRIs are caused by mercury-aluminum deposits that are oxidizing and in turn staining the brain tissue. Sometimes the more aggressive Epstein-Barr viral strains can enter the brain and feed on this oxidized toxic heavy metal, causing additional symptoms.

- **Fresh celery juice:** work up to 32 ounces daily, then work up to 64 ounces if possible
- **Celeryforce:** 2 capsules three times a day
- **5-MTHF:** 2 capsules twice a day
- **ALA (alpha lipoic acid):** 1 capsule daily
- **Barley grass juice powder:** 2 to 4 teaspoons or 6 to 12 capsules daily
- **B-complex:** 1 capsule daily
- **Cat's claw:** 3 dropperfuls twice a day
- **CoQ10:** 1 capsule daily
- **Curcumin:** 3 capsules twice a day
- **EPA and DHA (fish-free):** 1 capsule daily (taken with dinner)
- **GABA:** 1 250-milligram capsule daily
- **Glutathione:** 1 capsule daily
- **Lemon balm:** 4 dropperfuls twice a day
- **L-glutamine:** 1 capsule twice a day
- **Licorice root:** 1 dropperful twice a day (two weeks on, two weeks off)
- **L-lysine:** 4 500-milligram capsules twice a day
- **Magnesium glycinate:** 2 capsules twice a day
- **Monolaurin:** 1 capsule twice a day
- **MSM:** 1 capsule twice a day
- **Mullein leaf:** 2 dropperfuls twice a day
- **Nettle leaf:** 4 dropperfuls twice a day
- **Spirulina:** 1 tablespoon or 9 capsules daily
- **Vitamin B$_{12}$ (as adenosylcobalamin with methylcobalamin):** 2 dropperfuls twice a day
- **Vitamin C (as Micro-C):** 6 capsules twice a day
- **Zinc (as liquid zinc sulfate):** 2 dropperfuls twice a day

Myalgic Encephalomyelitis/Chronic Fatigue Syndrome (ME/CFS), Chronic Fatigue Immune Dysfunction Syndrome (CFIDS), Systemic Exertion Intolerance Disease (SEID)

True cause: Any of the over 60 varieties of Epstein-Barr virus, accompanied by toxic heavy metals such as mercury and aluminum, can create this condition that I call *neurological fatigue*, which is far more pronounced and limiting than simply being tired. A high-fat/high-protein diet accelerates the condition.

- **Fresh celery juice:** work up to 32 ounces daily, then work up to 64 ounces daily if possible
- **Celeryforce:** 2 capsules three times a day
- **5-MTHF:** 1 capsule twice a day
- **Ashwagandha:** 1 dropperful daily
- **Barley grass juice powder:** 4 teaspoons or 12 capsules daily
- **Cat's claw:** 2 dropperfuls twice a day
- **Chaga mushroom:** 2 teaspoons or 6 capsules daily
- **Curcumin:** 2 capsules twice a day
- **EPA and DHA (fish-free):** 1 capsule daily (taken with dinner)
- **Eyebright:** 1 dropperful daily
- **Glutathione:** 1 capsule daily
- **Goldenseal:** 2 dropperfuls twice a day (two weeks on, two weeks off)
- **Lemon balm:** 3 dropperfuls twice a day
- **Licorice root:** 1 dropperful twice day (two weeks on, two weeks off)
- **L-lysine:** 4 500-milligram capsules twice a day
- **Magnesium glycinate:** 1 capsule twice a day
- **Monolaurin:** 2 capsules twice a day
- **Mullein:** 2 dropperfuls twice a day

- **Oregon grape root:** 1 dropperful daily (two weeks on, two weeks off)
- **Spirulina:** 1 tablespoon or 9 capsules daily
- **Vitamin B$_{12}$ (as adenosylcobalamin with methylcobalamin):** 2 dropperfuls twice a day
- **Vitamin C (as Micro-C):** 3 capsules twice a day
- **Zinc (as liquid zinc sulfate):** 2 dropperfuls twice a day

Nail Fungus

True cause: An overburdened, toxic liver unable to convert vitamins and minerals into more usable nutrients, leading in particular to a zinc deficiency. Often triggered by a weakened immune system.

- **Fresh celery juice:** work up to 32 ounces daily
- **5-MTHF:** 1 capsule daily
- **Amla berry:** 1 teaspoon daily
- **Barley grass juice powder:** 2 teaspoons or 6 capsules daily
- **B-complex:** 1 capsule daily
- **Burdock root:** 1 cup of tea or 1 root freshly juiced daily
- **Cat's claw:** 1 dropperful daily
- **Chaga mushroom:** 2 teaspoons or 6 capsules daily
- **Curcumin:** 2 capsules daily
- **Glutathione:** 1 capsule daily
- **Goldenseal:** 2 dropperfuls twice a day (two weeks on, two weeks off)
- **Hibiscus:** 1 cup of tea daily
- **Lemon balm:** 2 dropperfuls twice a day
- **L-lysine:** 2 500-milligram capsules twice a day
- **Mullein leaf:** 2 dropperfuls twice a day
- **Olive leaf:** 2 dropperfuls daily
- **Oregano oil:** 2 capsules daily

- **Spirulina:** 2 teaspoons or 6 capsules daily
- **Vitamin B$_{12}$ (as adenosylcobalamin with methylcobalamin):** 1 dropperful twice a day
- **Vitamin C (as Micro-C):** 5 capsules twice a day
- **Wild blueberry powder:** 2 teaspoons daily
- **Zinc (as liquid zinc sulfate):** 2 dropperfuls twice a day

Neurological Symptoms (Tightness in the Chest, Trembling Hands, Twitches and Spasms, Muscle Weakness, Tingles and Numbness, Restless Legs, Restlessness, Weakness of the Limbs, Muscle Spasms, Aches and Pains)

True cause: If physical injury has not occurred, neurological symptoms are caused by one or more of the over 60 varieties of Epstein-Barr virus, one or more of the over 30 varieties of shingles virus, or any of the multiple strains of herpes simplex 1 or herpes simplex 2. These viruses feed on mercury and other toxins that reside inside the body, and they release neurotoxins to which the nervous system is very sensitive, leading to inflammation of the brain that appears mysterious to medical research and science. Oftentimes, these viruses take advantage of previous injuries, where the nerves were weakened, allowing the viruses and the neurotoxins they produce to create bodily inflammation and discomfort. Troublemaker foods such as eggs, milk, cheese, butter, and gluten worsen these symptoms, as do colognes, perfumes, air fresheners, and scented candles, all of which can feed the viruses accelerating neurological issues. A high-fat/high-protein diet interferes with glucose that nerve cells need critically for rejuvenation.

- **Fresh celery juice:** work up to 32 ounces daily, then work up to 64 ounces daily if possible
- **Celeryforce:** 3 capsules twice a day
- **5-MTHF:** 1 capsule twice a day
- **Aloe vera:** 2 or more inches of fresh gel (skin removed) daily
- **Barley grass juice powder:** 2 teaspoons or 6 capsules daily
- **B-complex:** 1 capsule daily
- **Cat's claw:** 2 dropperfuls twice a day
- **Chaga mushroom:** 2 teaspoons or 6 capsules daily
- **Curcumin:** 3 capsules twice a day
- **EPA and DHA (fish-free):** 1 capsule daily (taken with dinner)
- **GABA:** 1 250-milligram capsule daily
- **Goldenseal:** 1 dropperful twice a day (two weeks on/two weeks off)
- **Lemon balm:** 4 dropperfuls twice a day
- **Licorice root:** 1 dropperful twice a day (two weeks on, two weeks off)
- **L-lysine:** 5 500-milligram capsules twice a day
- **Lomatium root:** 1 dropperful twice a day
- **Magnesium glycinate:** 1 capsule twice a day
- **Mullein leaf:** 3 dropperfuls twice a day
- **Nettle leaf:** 4 dropperfuls twice a day
- **Oregano oil:** 1 capsule daily
- **Spirulina:** 2 teaspoons or 6 capsules daily
- **Vitamin B$_{12}$ (as adenosylcobalamin with methylcobalamin):** 2 dropperfuls twice a day
- **Vitamin C (as Micro-C):** 5 capsules twice a day
- **Vitamin D$_3$:** 1,000 IU twice a week
- **Wild blueberry powder:** 1 tablespoon daily
- **Zinc (as liquid zinc sulfate):** 1 dropperful twice a day

Obsessive-Compulsive Disorder (OCD)

True cause: Either emotional injury or toxic heavy metals such as mercury, aluminum, and copper, or many times, both causes creating the symptoms of OCD in combination with each other. In some extreme cases of OCD, electrical impulses that travel down neurons in certain specific areas of the brain where there are mercury and aluminum deposits then collide with those deposits. Each time, this can cause a tiny "explosion" that temporarily sends a signal back the other way.

- **Fresh celery juice:** work up to 32 ounces daily
- **Celeryforce:** 3 capsules twice a day
- **Barley grass juice powder:** 2 teaspoons or 6 capsules daily
- **B-complex:** 1 capsule daily
- **Cat's claw:** 1 dropperful daily
- **CoQ10:** 1 capsule daily
- **Curcumin:** 1 capsule twice a day
- **Elderflower:** 1 cup of tea daily
- **EPA and DHA (fish-free):** 1 capsule daily (taken with dinner)
- **Lemon balm:** 3 dropperfuls twice a day
- **L-glutamine:** 1 capsule twice a day
- **Magnesium glycinate:** 1 capsule twice a day
- **Melatonin:** 5 milligrams at bedtime daily
- **Spirulina:** 2 teaspoons or 6 capsules daily
- **Vitamin B$_{12}$ (as adenosylcobalamin with methylcobalamin):** 1 dropperful twice a day
- **Vitamin C (as Micro-C):** 2 capsules twice a day
- **Wild blueberry powder:** 1 tablespoon daily

Optic Nerve Atrophy

True cause: Optic nerve cells weakening due to one of the over 60 varieties of Epstein-Barr virus feeding on toxic heavy metals such as mercury and other toxins such as pesticides and herbicides, creating neurotoxins that saturate the optic nerve. Occasionally, EBV can attach itself to the optic nerve, causing cell damage. Optic nerve atrophy can result from either cause—neurotoxins or direct damage—or both at once.

- **Fresh celery juice:** work up to 32 ounces daily
- **Celeryforce:** 2 capsules twice a day
- **5-MTHF:** 1 capsule daily
- **Aloe vera:** 2 or more inches of fresh gel (skin removed) daily
- **Amla berry:** 1 teaspoon daily
- **Barley grass juice powder:** 1 tablespoon or 9 capsules daily
- **Burdock root:** 1 cup of tea or 1 root freshly juiced daily
- **Cat's claw:** 3 dropperfuls twice a day
- **Chaga mushroom:** 2 teaspoons or 6 capsules daily
- **Curcumin:** 3 capsules twice a day
- **EPA and DHA (fish-free):** 1 capsule daily (taken with dinner)
- **Glutathione:** 1 capsule daily
- **Lemon balm:** 4 dropperfuls twice a day
- **Licorice root:** 1 dropperful twice a day (two weeks on, two weeks off)
- **L-lysine:** 6 500-milligram capsules twice a day
- **Lomatium root:** 2 dropperfuls twice a day
- **Monolaurin:** 2 capsules daily
- **MSM:** 1 capsule daily
- **Mullein leaf:** 3 dropperfuls twice a day
- **Olive leaf:** 2 dropperfuls twice a day
- **Oregano oil:** 2 capsules daily
- **Rose hips:** 1 cup of tea daily
- **Spirulina:** 2 teaspoons or 6 capsules daily
- **Vitamin B$_{12}$ (as adenosylcobalamin with methylcobalamin):** 2 dropperfuls twice a day
- **Vitamin C (as Micro-C):** 6 capsules twice a day
- **Wild blueberry powder:** 1 tablespoon daily
- **Zinc (as liquid zinc sulfate):** 1 dropperful twice a day

Overactive Bladder (OAB)

True cause: Chronic inflammation of the bladder is due to a low-grade infection, either in years past or present, from one or more strains of the over 50 groups of *Streptococcus* bacteria and/or a virus such as one or more of the over 60 varieties of Epstein-Barr. Normally both a virus and bacteria are present in combination, working with each other in the same environment: neurotoxins that the virus releases can irritate the lining of the bladder while bacteria nestle themselves into the bladder lining, both causing inflammation at once.

- **Fresh celery juice:** work up to 32 ounces daily
- **Aloe vera:** 2 or more inches of fresh gel (skin removed) daily
- **Barley grass juice powder:** 1 teaspoon or 3 capsules daily
- **Cat's claw:** 2 dropperfuls twice a day
- **Curcumin:** 2 capsules twice a day
- **D-mannose:** 1 tablespoon three times a day in water
- **GABA:** 1 250-milligram capsule daily
- **Lemon balm:** 2 dropperfuls three times a day
- **Licorice root:** 1 dropperful twice a day (two weeks on, two weeks off)
- **L-lysine:** 2 500-milligram capsules twice a day
- **Magnesium glycinate:** 1 capsule daily

- **Melatonin:** 5 milligrams at bedtime daily
- **Monolaurin:** 2 capsules daily
- **Mullein leaf:** 1 dropperful twice a day
- **Nascent iodine:** 3 small drops (not dropperfuls) daily
- **Nettle leaf:** 2 dropperfuls twice a day
- **Oregano oil:** 1 capsule daily
- **Oregon grape root:** 1 dropperful daily (two weeks on, two weeks off)
- **Raspberry leaf:** 1 cup of tea with 2 bags daily
- **Raw honey:** 2 teaspoons daily
- **Schisandra berry:** 1 cup of tea daily
- **Spirulina:** 1 teaspoon or 3 capsules daily
- **Vitamin B$_{12}$ (as adenosylcobalamin with methylcobalamin):** 1 dropperful twice a day
- **Vitamin C (as Micro-C):** 3 capsules twice a day
- **Zinc (as liquid zinc sulfate):** 1 dropperful daily

PANDAS (Pediatric Autoimmune Neuropsychiatric Disorders Associated with Streptococcal Infections)

True cause: A co-infection of one or more strains from the over 50 groups of *Streptococcus* bacteria plus a virus (most commonly HHV-6, or sometimes EBV or even a variety of shingles) that is feeding on toxic heavy metals (most commonly mercury) and releasing viral neurotoxins. This is an instance where dosages are geared to children.

- **Fresh celery juice:** refer to table on page 480 for children's amounts
- **Cat's claw:** 4 small drops (not dropperfuls) twice a day
- **Eyebright:** 4 small drops (not dropperfuls) twice a day

- **Goldenseal:** 10 small drops (not dropperfuls) twice a day (two weeks on, two weeks off)
- **Lemon balm:** 10 small drops (not dropperfuls) twice a day
- **Licorice root:** 10 small drops (not dropperfuls) twice a day (two weeks on, two weeks off)
- **Mullein leaf:** 10 small drops (not dropperfuls) twice day
- **Olive leaf:** 10 small drops (not dropperfuls) twice a day
- **Spirulina:** ½ teaspoon daily
- **Vitamin B$_{12}$ (as adenosylcobalamin with methylcobalamin):** 10 small drops (not dropperfuls) daily
- **Vitamin C (as Micro-C):** 2 capsules twice a day (if needed, open capsule and mix contents into juice, smoothie, or water)
- **Wild blueberry powder:** 1 teaspoon daily
- **Zinc (as liquid zinc sulfate):** up to 6 small drops (not dropperfuls) in juice, water, or directly in mouth twice a day

Parkinson's Disease

True cause: Neurons injured by toxic heavy metals (such as mercury, aluminum, and copper) oxidizing and creating discharge that spreads in the brain. The toxic heavy metals defuse electrical impulses and starve neurotransmitters of the electricity and fuel they need in order to stay healthy and active, and this starvation usually leads to a severe neurotransmitter deficiency. Often accelerated by a high-fat/high-protein diet.

- **Fresh celery juice:** work up to 32 ounces daily, then work up to 64 ounces if possible
- **Celeryforce:** 3 capsules three times a day
- **5-MTHF:** 1 capsule daily
- **Amla berry:** 2 teaspoons daily
- **Ashwagandha:** 1 dropperful daily

- **Barley grass juice powder:** 1 tablespoon or 9 capsules daily
- **California poppy:** 4 capsules or 4 dropperfuls daily
- **CoQ10:** 1 capsule daily
- **Curcumin:** 3 capsules twice a day
- **EPA and DHA (fish-free):** 1 capsule daily (taken with dinner)
- **GABA:** 1 250-milligram capsule twice a day
- **Kava kava:** 1 capsule or 1 dropperful twice a day
- **Lemon balm:** 4 dropperfuls twice a day
- **L-glutamine:** 2 capsules twice a day
- **Magnesium glycinate:** 2 capsules twice a day
- **Melatonin:** 5 milligrams twice a day
- **MSM:** 1 capsule daily
- **Nettle leaf:** 2 dropperfuls twice a day
- **Raw honey:** 1 tablespoon daily
- **Selenium:** 1 capsule daily
- **Spirulina:** 1 tablespoon or 9 capsules daily
- **Turmeric:** 4 capsules daily
- **Vitamin B$_{12}$ (as adenosylcobalamin with methylcobalamin):** 3 dropperfuls twice a day
- **Vitamin C (as Micro-C):** 4 capsules twice a day
- **Wild blueberry powder:** 1 tablespoon daily
- **Zinc (as liquid zinc sulfate):** 1 dropperful daily

Pelvic Inflammatory Disease (PID) and Prostatitis

True cause: Bacterial infection of one or more strains from the over 50 groups of *Streptococcus*. There are different levels of PID. Some are very mild, and some are severe, with more systemic, long-term, chronic pain. You don't need to be diagnosed with PID to have it. The mildest forms of PID are overactive bladder with occasional UTIs and pelvic discomfort that may be difficult to distinguish from gastric or intestinal bloating or discomfort. Often women with PID also struggle with recurrences of UTIs, vaginal discharge, bacterial vaginosis, or chronic yeast infections because they are all strep-caused as well.

The parallel experience for men is prostatitis, which is also caused by low-grade, chronic strep infection or an acute strep infection.

When someone has prostatitis or PID, they usually have strep in their lower colon too, leading to irritable bowel syndrome at the same time, because IBS is also a result of low-grade, chronic strep.

- **Fresh celery juice:** work up to 32 ounces daily
- **Aloe vera:** 2 or more inches of fresh gel (skin removed) daily
- **Barley grass juice powder:** 2 teaspoons or 6 capsules daily
- **Cat's claw:** 2 dropperfuls twice a day
- **Curcumin:** 2 capsules twice a day
- **D-mannose:** 1 tablespoon twice a day
- **Eyebright:** 1 dropperful twice a day
- **Goldenseal:** 3 dropperfuls three times a day (two weeks on, two weeks off)
- **Lemon balm:** 4 dropperfuls twice a day
- **Licorice root:** 1 dropperful daily (two weeks on, two weeks off)
- **L-lysine:** 2 500-milligram capsules twice a day
- **Lomatium root:** 2 dropperfuls twice a day
- **Mullein leaf:** 3 dropperfuls twice a day
- **Nascent iodine:** 2 small drops (not dropperfuls) daily
- **Nettle leaf:** 4 dropperfuls twice a day
- **Olive leaf:** 2 dropperfuls twice a day
- **Oregano oil:** 2 capsules daily
- **Oregon grape root:** 1 dropperful daily (two weeks on, two weeks off)

- **Raspberry leaf:** 1 cup of tea with 2 bags twice a day
- **Raw honey:** 2 teaspoons daily
- **Spirulina:** 2 teaspoons or 6 capsules daily
- **Thyme:** 2 sprigs of fresh thyme in hot water as tea or 4 sprigs in room temperature water daily
- **Vitamin B$_{12}$ (as adenosylcobalamin with methylcobalamin):** 1 dropperful twice a day
- **Vitamin C (as Micro-C):** 5 capsules twice a day
- **Zinc (as liquid zinc sulfate):** 1 dropperful twice a day

Polycystic Ovarian Syndrome (PCOS)

True cause: Fluid-filled cysts often caused by one or more of the over 60 varieties of Epstein-Barr virus, frequently creating injuries to cells in the ovaries and sometimes weakening the ovaries overall. Troublemaker foods such as eggs rapidly worsen the condition, and a high-fat/high-protein diet impedes the healing process of PCOS. For more on cysts, see "Reproductive Cysts" on pages 540–541.

- **Fresh celery juice:** work up to 32 ounces daily
- **5-MTHF:** 1 capsule daily
- **Ashwagandha:** 1 dropperful daily
- **Barley grass juice powder:** 2 teaspoons or 6 capsules daily
- **Cat's claw:** 2 dropperfuls twice a day
- **Curcumin:** 2 capsules twice a day
- **Glutathione:** 1 capsule daily
- **Lemon balm:** 4 dropperfuls twice a day
- **L-lysine:** 4 500-milligram capsules twice a day
- **Monolaurin:** 1 capsule twice a day
- **Mullein leaf:** 3 dropperfuls twice a day
- **Nascent iodine:** 2 small drops (not dropperfuls) daily

- **Nettle leaf:** 4 dropperfuls twice a day
- **Olive leaf:** 1 dropperful daily
- **Raspberry leaf:** 1 cup of tea with 2 bags three times a day
- **Spirulina:** 2 teaspoons or 6 capsules daily
- **Turmeric:** 2 capsules daily
- **Vitamin B$_{12}$ (as adenosylcobalamin with methylcobalamin):** 1 dropperful twice a day
- **Vitamin C (as Micro-C):** 5 capsules twice a day
- **Wild blueberry powder:** 1 tablespoon daily
- **Zinc (as liquid zinc sulfate):** 1 dropperful twice a day

Posttraumatic Stress Symptoms (PTSS, also known as Posttraumatic Stress Disorder, or PTSD)

True cause: Toxic heavy metal exposure (from sources such as mercury, aluminum, and copper) either on its own or combined with other compromises and exposures, such as from radiation, pesticides, herbicides, fungicides, petrochemicals, and even colognes, perfumes, air fresheners, and scented candles. Emotional injury from traumatic or compromising experiences can also be the sole cause of PTSS. Many times, toxic troublemaker exposure and emotional exposure in combination create PTSS.

- **Fresh celery juice:** work up to 32 ounces daily
- **Celeryforce:** 3 capsules three times a day
- **5-MTHF:** 1 capsule daily
- **Aloe vera:** 2 or more inches of fresh gel (skin removed) daily
- **Ashwagandha:** 2 dropperfuls twice a day
- **Barley grass juice powder:** 1 tablespoon or 9 capsules daily
- **B-complex:** 1 capsule daily

- **California poppy:** 3 capsules or 3 dropperfuls daily at bedtime
- **Cat's claw:** 1 dropperful daily
- **CoQ10:** 1 capsule daily
- **Curcumin:** 2 capsules twice a day
- **D-mannose:** 1 tablespoon daily in water
- **Elderflower:** 1 cup of tea daily
- **EPA and DHA (fish-free):** 1 capsule daily (taken with dinner)
- **GABA:** 1 250-milligram capsule daily
- **Lemon balm:** 5 dropperfuls three times a day
- **Licorice root:** 1 dropperful daily (two weeks on, two weeks off)
- **Magnesium glycinate:** 2 capsules twice a day
- **Melatonin:** 5 milligrams at bedtime daily
- **NAC:** 1 capsule daily
- **Nascent iodine:** 4 small drops (not dropperfuls) daily
- **Nettle leaf:** 3 dropperfuls twice a day
- **Peppermint:** 1 cup of tea twice a day
- **Spirulina:** 1 tablespoon or 9 capsules daily
- **Vitamin B$_{12}$ (as adenosylcobalamin with methylcobalamin):** 3 dropperfuls twice a day
- **Vitamin C (as Micro-C):** 2 capsules twice a day
- **Wild blueberry powder:** 1 tablespoon daily

Psoriatic Arthritis

True cause: One or more of the over 60 varieties of Epstein-Barr virus residing inside the liver, feeding on copper and mercury there and releasing both neurotoxins and dermatoxins into the bloodstream that mostly settle in the joint regions. Most cases of psoriatic arthritis come with either mild or more severe fatigue, because neurotoxins can predominate over dermatoxins. A high-fat/high-protein diet interferes with the detoxification of heavy metals.

- **Fresh celery juice:** work up to 32 ounces daily
- **Celeryforce:** 1 capsule twice a day
- **5-MTHF:** 1 capsule daily
- **Aloe vera:** 2 or more inches of fresh gel (skin removed) daily
- **Barley grass juice powder:** 2 teaspoons or 6 capsules daily
- **B-complex:** 1 capsule daily
- **Cat's claw:** 1 dropperful twice a day
- **Curcumin:** 2 capsules twice a day
- **EPA and DHA (fish-free):** 1 capsule daily (taken with dinner)
- **Lemon balm:** 4 dropperfuls twice a day
- **Licorice root:** 1 dropperful daily (two weeks on, two weeks off)
- **L-lysine:** 4 500-milligram capsules twice a day
- **Magnesium glycinate:** 1 capsule twice a day
- **MSM:** 1 capsule daily
- **Mullein leaf:** 1 dropperful twice a day
- **Nettle leaf:** 2 dropperfuls twice a day
- **Spirulina:** 2 teaspoons or 6 capsules daily
- **Vitamin B$_{12}$ (as adenosylcobalamin with methylcobalamin):** 2 dropperfuls twice a day
- **Vitamin C (as Micro-C):** 4 capsules twice a day
- **Wild blueberry powder:** 2 teaspoons daily
- **Zinc (as liquid zinc sulfate):** 1 dropperful twice a day

Raynaud's Syndrome

True cause: A chronic, long-term, low-grade viral infection (most commonly one of the over 60 varieties of Epstein-Barr virus, sometimes in combination with one of the over 30 varieties of shingles virus) plus a stagnant, sluggish liver in which the virus or viruses have resided for quite some time, potentially years. This leads to viral neurotoxins, dermatoxins, and other viral waste matter floating through the bloodstream and, because the liver is too hindered to detoxify properly, causing the symptoms of Raynaud's. These toxins, in combination with a high-fat/high-protein diet, cause the blood to thicken, which reduces circulation and in turn leads toxins, sludge, and debris to start to settle in the extremities and cause heightened discoloration in the hands and feet.

- **Fresh celery juice:** work up to 32 ounces daily
- **Celeryforce:** 2 capsules twice a day
- **5-MTHF:** 1 capsule daily
- **Amla berry:** 2 teaspoons daily
- **Ashwagandha:** 1 dropperful daily
- **Barley grass juice powder:** 2 teaspoons or 6 capsules daily
- **Cat's claw:** 1 dropperful twice a day
- **Chaga mushroom:** 2 teaspoons or 6 capsules daily
- **Curcumin:** 1 capsule daily
- **Lemon balm:** 2 dropperfuls twice a day
- **Licorice root:** 1 dropperful daily (two weeks on, two weeks off)
- **L-lysine:** 6 500-milligram capsules daily
- **Nettle leaf:** 2 dropperfuls daily
- **Olive leaf:** 2 dropperfuls daily
- **Spirulina:** 2 teaspoons or 6 capsules daily
- **Thyme:** 2 sprigs of fresh thyme in hot water as tea or 4 sprigs in room temperature water daily
- **Vitamin B$_{12}$ (as adenosylcobalamin with methylcobalamin):** 1 dropperful twice a day
- **Vitamin C (as Micro-C):** 6 capsules daily
- **Wild blueberry powder:** 1 tablespoon daily
- **Zinc (as liquid zinc sulfate):** up to 2 dropperfuls daily

Reproductive Cysts (including Uterine Cysts, Ovarian Cysts, Vaginal Cysts, and Cervical Cysts)

True cause: One or more of the over 60 varieties of Epstein-Barr virus, combined with a variety of toxins and poisons. Viruses and toxins are in relationship: a virus in the body consumes toxins there, and then releases more destructive chemical compounds that denature and injure healthy cells. As this pattern repeats itself, injured cells form into living scar tissue, with the virus trapped inside. The cyst formation process is how a healthy body protects itself, making sure this activity happens within the cyst and not outside of it, in other places in the body. While trapped, the virus works to survive. Blood vessels develop out of the cyst in order to draw nutrients and fuel back inside to feed these injured, unhealthy cells and viruses and keep them alive. The fuel that the cyst draws in makes the difference in whether it continues to grow or starts to reduce. A high-fat/high-protein diet, especially one that includes eggs, milk, cheese, and butter, worsens reproductive cysts. Eggs are a leading fuel that can make cysts grow larger over time, because eggs feed viruses, which means that more unhealthy cells grow and develop inside the cysts.

- **Fresh celery juice:** work up to 32 ounces daily
- **ALA (alpha lipoic acid):** 1 capsule every other day
- **Aloe vera:** 2 or more inches of fresh gel (skin removed) daily
- **Amla berry:** 1 teaspoon daily
- **Barley grass juice powder:** 1 tablespoon or 9 capsules daily
- **Cat's claw:** 3 dropperfuls twice a day
- **Chaga mushroom:** 1 tablespoon or 9 capsules daily
- **Chrysanthemum:** 1 cup of tea daily

- **Curcumin:** 3 capsules twice a day
- **D-mannose:** 1 tablespoon daily in water
- **Glutathione:** 1 capsule daily
- **Lemon balm:** 4 dropperfuls twice a day
- **Melatonin:** 5 milligrams at bedtime daily
- **Milk thistle:** 1 dropperful daily
- **Monolaurin:** 1 capsule daily
- **Nascent iodine:** 8 small drops (not dropperfuls) daily
- **Nettle leaf:** 5 dropperfuls twice a day
- **Raspberry leaf:** 2 cups of tea with 2 bags daily
- **Spirulina:** 2 teaspoons or 6 capsules daily
- **Vitamin B$_{12}$ (as adenosylcobalamin with methylcobalamin):** 1 dropperful daily
- **Vitamin C (as Micro-C):** 6 capsules twice a day
- **Wild blueberry powder:** 1 tablespoon daily

Retinopathy (including Diabetic Retinopathy)

True cause: A weakened, stagnant, sluggish liver leading to diminished nutrient storage in the organ as toxins dominate, in turn leading to severe nutrient deficiencies throughout the body. This can lead to an eye compromise. A high-fat/high-protein diet can accelerate the condition. Diabetic retinopathy is not due to diabetes; there are just as many people who have retinopathy without diabetes.

- **Fresh celery juice:** work up to 32 ounces daily
- **5-MTHF:** 1 capsule daily
- **ALA (alpha lipoic acid):** 1 capsule twice a week
- **Amla berry:** 1 teaspoon daily
- **Barley grass juice powder:** 2 teaspoons or 6 capsules daily
- **B-complex:** 1 capsule daily
- **Cat's claw:** 1 dropperful daily

- **CoQ10:** 1 capsule daily
- **Curcumin:** 2 capsules twice a day
- **EPA and DHA (fish-free):** 1 capsule daily (taken with dinner)
- **Lemon balm:** 2 dropperfuls twice a day
- **Magnesium glycinate:** 1 capsule daily
- **MSM:** 1 capsule daily
- **Nascent iodine:** 4 small drops (not dropperfuls) daily
- **Nettle leaf:** 4 dropperfuls daily
- **Rose hips:** 1 cup of tea daily
- **Selenium:** 1 capsule daily
- **Spirulina:** 2 teaspoons or 6 capsules daily
- **Vitamin B$_{12}$ (as adenosylcobalamin with methylcobalamin):** 2 dropperfuls daily
- **Vitamin C (as Micro-C):** 4 capsules twice a day
- **Vitamin D$_3$:** 1,000 IU daily
- **Wild blueberry powder:** 1 tablespoon daily
- **Zinc (as liquid zinc sulfate):** 1 dropperful daily

Scar Tissue

True cause: When mysterious scar tissue appears—for example, in the liver—it's caused by pathogens feeding on toxic heavy metals and troublemaker foods in the diet (such as eggs, dairy products, and gluten) and then burrowing themselves into healthy cells, causing damage. The bacterial strains within the over 50 groups of *Streptococcus* are common instigators of scar tissue. Strep is the cause of acne scarring as well as the scar tissue left behind in the sinus cavities by chronic sinusitis, scar tissue in the bladder, and scar tissue in the intestinal tract, both large and small. Mild levels of scar tissue can also be caused by other common pathogens, such as Epstein-Barr virus, herpes simplex 1 and 2, and shingles. EBV, for example, causes sarcoidosis, which is scar tissue of the lymphatic system.

This protocol is also helpful for scar tissue caused by surgical procedures, wounds, and injury; the antioxidants it provides help heal scars of any kind.

- **Fresh celery juice:** work up to 32 ounces daily
- **5-MTHF:** 1 capsule daily
- **ALA (alpha lipoic acid):** 1 capsule daily
- **Aloe vera:** 2 or more inches of fresh gel (skin removed) daily
- **Barley grass juice powder:** 2 teaspoons or 6 capsules daily
- **B-complex:** 1 capsule daily
- **Cat's claw:** 2 dropperfuls daily
- **Chaga mushroom:** 2 teaspoons or 6 capsules daily
- **Curcumin:** 3 capsules daily
- **L-lysine:** 4 500-milligram capsules daily
- **Milk thistle:** 1 dropperful daily
- **MSM:** 2 capsules daily
- **NAC:** 1 capsule daily
- **Nettle leaf:** 2 dropperfuls daily
- **Silica:** 1 teaspoon daily
- **Spirulina:** 2 teaspoons or 6 capsules daily
- **Turmeric:** 2 capsules daily
- **Vitamin B$_{12}$ (as adenosylcobalamin with methylcobalamin):** 2 dropperfuls twice a day
- **Vitamin C (as Micro-C):** 6 capsules twice a day
- **Wild blueberry powder:** 2 tablespoons daily
- **Zinc (as liquid zinc sulfate):** up to 1 dropperful twice a day

Seasonal Affective Disorder (SAD)

True cause: Toxic heavy metals (such as mercury, aluminum, and copper) in both the liver and brain in combination with viruses or bacteria in the liver (such as strains of the over 60 varieties of Epstein-Barr virus or over 50 groups of *Streptococcus* bacteria) plus a long-term, high-fat/ high-protein diet. Blood sugar imbalances, which can cause mood shifts, can also contribute. SAD can be seasonal because we tend to eat higher-fat foods in the colder months; these burden our liver and aggravate underlying health conditions at the same time we're eating fewer productive foods such as leafy greens, fruits, and vegetables. A low-grade viral infection can land somebody a SAD diagnosis at first that eventually leads to a more advanced diagnosis such as fibromyalgia, ME/CFS, fatigue, RA, anxiety, or depression. For much more on SAD, see the chapter on this topic in *Liver Rescue*.

- **Fresh celery juice:** work up to 32 ounces daily
- **Celeryforce:** 3 capsules three times a day
- **5-MTHF:** 1 capsule daily
- **Ashwagandha:** 1 dropperful daily
- **Barley grass juice powder:** 2 teaspoons or 6 capsules daily
- **B-complex:** 1 capsule daily
- **Curcumin:** 2 capsules twice a day
- **EPA and DHA (fish-free):** 1 capsule daily (taken with dinner)
- **Lemon balm:** 2 dropperfuls daily
- **Lemon balm:** 4 dropperfuls twice a day
- **Melatonin:** 5 milligrams at bedtime daily
- **Nascent iodine:** 6 small drops (not dropperfuls) daily
- **Raw honey:** 1 tablespoon daily
- **Red clover:** 1 cup of tea daily
- **Spirulina:** 1 tablespoon or 9 capsules daily
- **Turmeric:** 2 capsules daily
- **Vitamin B$_{12}$ (as adenosylcobalamin with methylcobalamin):** 2 dropperfuls twice a day
- **Vitamin C (as Micro-C):** 6 capsules daily
- **Vitamin D$_3$:** 2,000 IU daily
- **Wild blueberry powder:** 1 tablespoon daily
- **Zinc (as liquid zinc sulfate):** up to 2 dropperfuls daily

Sensitivity to Cold, Heat, Sun, or Humidity; Cold Hands and Feet

True cause: A sensitive central nervous system caused by an elevated low-grade viral load inside the liver and throughout the body. Viruses that create these symptoms are varieties that release neurotoxins, which circulate throughout the bloodstream and attach to nerves, causing mild to more extreme inflammation. This can cause nerves throughout the body to become more sensitive, so that when cold air or cold water hits the skin, it creates discomfort that can lead to a misdiagnosis of poor circulation. Physical injury can also create the nerve damage that leads to these symptoms, although in many cases viruses are still present, taking advantage of the damaged nerves and elevating inflammation.

- **Fresh celery juice:** work up to 32 ounces daily
- **Celeryforce:** 2 capsules twice a day
- **5-MTHF:** 1 capsule daily
- **Aloe vera:** 2 or more inches of fresh gel (skin removed) daily
- **Barley grass juice powder:** 2 teaspoons or 6 capsules daily
- **Cat's claw:** 1 dropperful twice a day
- **Chaga mushroom:** 1 teaspoon or 6 capsules daily
- **Curcumin:** 3 capsules twice a day
- **Ginger:** 1 cup of tea or freshly grated or juiced to taste daily
- **Glutathione:** 1 capsule daily
- **Lemon balm:** 2 dropperfuls three times a day
- **L-lysine:** 2 500-milligram capsules twice a day
- **Magnesium glycinate:** 2 capsules twice a day
- **MSM:** 1 capsule daily
- **Mullein leaf:** 1 dropperful twice a day

- **Spirulina:** 2 teaspoons or 6 capsules daily
- **Vitamin B$_{12}$ (as adenosylcobalamin with methylcobalamin):** 2 dropperfuls twice a day
- **Vitamin C (as Micro-C):** 4 capsules twice a day
- **Vitamin D$_3$:** 1,000 IU daily
- **Wild blueberry powder:** 2 teaspoons daily
- **Zinc (as liquid zinc sulfate):** 1 dropperful twice a day

Shingles

True cause: The shingles virus is the true cause of trigeminal neuralgia, frozen shoulder, ulcerative colitis, and many cases of neck pain, jaw pain, gum and tooth pain, tongue pain, burning sensations inside the mouth, burning sensations on the skin, pain in the back of the head, some migraine-related pain, mystery sciatica, mystery lower back pain, neuropathy, and a stagnant, sluggish liver. There are shingles infections without rashes and with rashes, and there are over 30 varieties of shingles, all but one undiscovered. See the shingles chapter in *Medical Medium* for more.

- **Fresh celery juice:** work up to 32 ounces daily
- **Aloe vera:** 2 or more inches of fresh gel (skin removed) daily; also apply fresh gel to shingles rash
- **California poppy:** 3 capsules or 3 dropperfuls twice a day
- **Cat's claw:** 2 dropperfuls twice a day
- **Curcumin:** 3 capsules three times a day
- **Lemon balm:** 4 dropperfuls three times a day
- **Licorice root:** 2 dropperfuls twice a day (two weeks on, two weeks off)
- **L-lysine:** 6 capsules twice a day
- **Mullein leaf:** 4 dropperfuls twice a day
- **Nettle leaf:** 4 dropperfuls twice a day

- **Propolis:** 3 dropperfuls three times a day
- **Spirulina:** 1 teaspoon or 3 capsules daily
- **Vitamin B$_{12}$ (as adenosylcobalamin with methylcobalamin):** 3 dropperfuls twice a day
- **Vitamin C (as Micro-C):** 8 capsules twice a day
- **Zinc (as liquid zinc sulfate):** 2 dropperfuls twice a day

SIBO (Small Intestinal Bacterial Overgrowth)

True cause: One or more strains from the over 50 groups of *Streptococcus* bacteria residing in the small intestinal tract and colon, feeding on putrefying, decayed proteins and rancid fats that have lined the walls of the gut. Troublemaker foods such as eggs, milk, cheese, butter, and gluten can feed the strep bacteria, allowing it to proliferate. SIBO often accompanies a liver and lymphatic system that have become weakened, sluggish, and stagnant due to toxin overload and a high-fat/high-protein diet. Someone with SIBO has a very good chance of having a history of acne, sinus infections, UTIs, yeast infections, bladder infections, strep throat, bloating, or acid reflux—any of which might have been treated with antibiotics that allowed the strep that survived the antibiotics to strengthen over time and make a home in the gut and throughout the body. *Streptococcus* can contribute to low hydrochloric acid and low bile production. Within our relationships, we often pass around different strains of strep from different groups of the bacteria.

- **Fresh celery juice:** work up to 32 ounces daily
- **Aloe vera:** 2 or more inches of fresh gel (skin removed) twice a day
- **Barley grass juice powder:** 2 teaspoons or 6 capsules daily

- **Burdock root:** 1 cup of tea or 1 root freshly juiced daily
- **Cat's claw:** 3 dropperfuls twice a day
- **Chaga mushroom:** 2 teaspoons or 6 capsules daily
- **Curcumin:** 1 capsule twice a day
- **Ginger:** 1 cup of tea twice a day or freshly grated or juiced to taste daily
- **Goldenseal:** 4 dropperfuls twice a day (two weeks on, two weeks off)
- **Lemon balm:** 4 dropperfuls twice a day
- **Licorice root:** 1 dropperful twice a day (two weeks on, two weeks off)
- **Mullein leaf:** 4 dropperfuls twice a day
- **Olive leaf:** 3 dropperfuls twice a day
- **Oregano oil:** 1 capsule twice a day
- **Oregon grape root:** 2 dropperfuls twice a day (two weeks on, two weeks off)
- **Spirulina:** 2 teaspoons or 6 capsules daily
- **Turmeric:** 2 capsules daily
- **Vitamin B$_{12}$ (as adenosylcobalamin with methylcobalamin):** 1 dropperful twice a day
- **Vitamin C (as Micro-C):** 4 capsules twice a day
- **Zinc (as liquid zinc sulfate):** up to 1 dropperful twice a day

Sinusitis, Sinus Infections, and Lung Infections

True cause: One or more strains from the over 50 groups of *Streptococcus* bacteria nestling in the sinus cavities, creating long-term, chronic sinus issues from mild to severe, resulting in scar tissue or even polyps. Normally misconstrued as chronic allergies or environmental or air quality sensitivities without an understanding that strep is creating the underlying sinus problem. Sinus inflammation and infections are instigated by feeding strep bacteria their favorite foods such as eggs, dairy, and gluten. Irritants to these conditions are air fresheners, scented candles, perfumes, and colognes, which often lower the immune system, allowing flare-ups to occur.

- **Fresh celery juice:** work up to 32 ounces daily
- **Amla berry:** 2 teaspoons twice a day
- **Barley grass juice powder:** 2 teaspoons or 6 capsules daily
- **Cat's claw:** 2 dropperfuls twice a day
- **CoQ10:** 1 capsule daily
- **Ginger:** 2 cups of tea twice a day or freshly grated or juiced to taste daily
- **Goldenseal:** 4 dropperfuls twice a day (two weeks on, two weeks off)
- **Hibiscus:** 2 cups of tea daily
- **Lemon balm:** 4 dropperfuls twice a day
- **L-lysine:** 4 500-milligram capsules twice a day
- **Mullein leaf:** 4 dropperfuls twice a day
- **NAC:** 1 capsule twice a day
- **Olive leaf:** 3 dropperfuls twice a day
- **Oregon grape root:** 2 dropperfuls twice a day (two weeks on, two weeks off)
- **Peppermint:** 1 cup of tea with 2 bags twice a day
- **Rose hips:** 2 cups of tea daily
- **Spirulina:** 2 teaspoons or 6 capsules daily
- **Thyme:** 2 sprigs of fresh thyme in hot water as tea or 4 sprigs in room temperature water daily
- **Turmeric:** 3 capsules twice a day
- **Vitamin C (as Micro-C):** after optional Medical Medium Vitamin C Shock Therapy, 6 capsules twice a day
- **Vitamin D$_3$:** 1,000 IU daily
- **Zinc (as liquid zinc sulfate):** after optional Medical Medium Zinc Shock Therapy for two days, up to 3 dropperfuls twice a day

Strep Throat, Viral Sore Throat, Mystery Sore Throat, and Sties

True cause: A strain of the over 50 groups of *Streptococcus* bacteria residing inside the lymphatic system and tonsils, often surfacing to the top of the throat and made visible by white spots, or not directly visible and experienced as inflammation, redness, and pain. Some of the time, discovered with a swab of the throat at your doctor's office, although many times undetectable.

One or more of the over 60 varieties of Epstein-Barr virus can also cause chronic, on-off, mystery sore throats. Someone in this case will often exhibit a little patch of redness on each side of the throat, occasionally accompanied by a sharp pain when swallowing. This type of sore throat is impossible to diagnose at the doctor's office because a throat culture won't show strep, nor will it usually be diagnosed as mono, since EBV can live out of reach of current medical testing. Nevertheless, a chronic, low-grade viral infection that comes and goes periodically when someone becomes run down from a high-fat/high-protein diet and little sleep is a common cause of sore throats.

- **Fresh celery juice:** work up to 32 ounces daily
- **Cat's claw:** 3 dropperfuls twice a day
- **Eyebright:** 2 dropperfuls twice a day
- **Ginger:** 2 cups of tea twice a day or freshly grated or juiced to taste daily
- **Goldenseal:** 5 dropperfuls twice a day (two weeks on, two weeks off)
- **Lemon balm:** 4 dropperfuls twice a day
- **Licorice root:** 1 dropperful twice a day (two weeks on, two weeks off)
- **L-lysine:** 6 500-milligram capsules twice a day
- **Mullein leaf:** 3 dropperfuls twice a day

- **Olive leaf:** 3 dropperfuls twice a day
- **Rose hips:** 2 cups of tea twice a day
- **Thyme:** 2 sprigs of fresh thyme in hot water as tea or 4 sprigs in room temperature water daily
- **Vitamin C (as Micro-C):** after optional Medical Medium Vitamin C Shock Therapy, 8 capsules twice a day
- **Zinc (as liquid zinc sulfate):** after optional Medical Medium Zinc Shock Therapy for two days, up to 3 dropperfuls twice a day

Thyroid Conditions

True cause: One or more of the over 60 varieties of Epstein-Barr virus entering and inhabiting the thyroid gland, causing cell injury there as it burrows into thyroid tissue and slowly produces byproduct and other toxic waste matter. Fuels for the EBV behind thyroid issues can range from mercury to unproductive hormones to residue from troublemaker foods such as eggs. In other words, thyroid conditions are low-grade viral infections. A more aggressive, acute infection can take someone out of the realm of mild thyroid inflammation and hypothyroidism that are unseen on medical tests and into Hashimoto's thyroiditis, a much more advanced inflammation that can be detected by a physician both by touch and medical testing. Two varieties of EBV can subsist in the thyroid together, having two different effects, which is how someone can find themselves with hypothyroidism and hyperthyroidism seemingly at the same time. Or one variety of EBV may be creating nodules while another variety causes a tumor in a different area of the thyroid. EBV causes most goiters of this day and age because iodine deficiency is becoming rarer than ever before. For more information on thyroid disease, check out the Medical Medium book *Thyroid Healing*.

Supplements for Hypothyroidism; Hashimoto's Thyroiditis; Goiters; Thyroid Nodules, Cysts, and Tumors

- **Fresh celery juice:** work up to 32 ounces daily, then work up to 64 ounces daily if possible
- **Celeryforce:** 1 capsule twice a day
- **5-MTHF:** 1 capsule daily
- **Barley grass juice powder:** 2 teaspoons or 6 capsules daily
- **B-complex:** 1 capsule daily
- **Cat's claw:** 2 dropperfuls twice a day
- **Chaga mushroom:** 2 teaspoons or 6 capsules daily
- **Curcumin:** 2 capsules twice a day
- **EPA and DHA (fish-free):** 1 capsule daily (taken with dinner)
- **Lemon balm:** 4 dropperfuls twice a day
- **Licorice root:** 1 dropperful twice a day (two weeks on, two weeks off)
- **L-lysine:** 5 500-milligram capsules twice a day
- **Lomatium root:** 1 dropperful twice a day
- **Magnesium glycinate:** 1 capsule twice a day
- **Melatonin:** 5 milligrams at bedtime daily
- **Monolaurin:** 1 capsule twice a day
- **Mullein leaf:** 2 dropperfuls twice a day
- **Nascent iodine:** 2 small drops (not dropperfuls) daily (or 1 capsule of bladderwrack daily)
- **Nettle leaf:** 2 dropperfuls twice a day
- **Spirulina:** 2 teaspoons or 6 capsules daily
- **Thyme:** 2 sprigs of fresh thyme in hot water as tea or 4 sprigs in room temperature water daily
- **Vitamin B$_{12}$ (as adenosylcobalamin with methylcobalamin):** 1 dropperful twice a day

- Vitamin C (as Micro-C): 6 capsules twice a day
- Vitamin D$_3$: 1,000 IU daily
- Wild blueberry powder: 2 tablespoons daily
- Zinc (as liquid zinc sulfate): 1 dropperful twice a day

Supplements for Hyperthyroidism and Graves' Disease

- Fresh celery juice: work up to 32 ounces daily
- Celeryforce: 1 capsule twice a day
- 5-MTHF: 1 capsule daily
- Amla berry: 2 teaspoons daily
- Ashwagandha: 1 dropperful daily
- Barley grass juice powder: 2 teaspoons or 6 capsules daily
- B-complex: 1 capsule daily
- Bladderwrack: 1 capsule daily
- Cat's claw: 1 dropperful twice a day
- Chaga mushroom: 2 teaspoons or 6 capsules daily
- Curcumin: 2 capsules twice a day
- Elderberry: 1 teaspoon daily
- EPA and DHA (fish-free): 1 capsule daily (taken with dinner)
- Glutathione: 1 capsule daily
- L-lysine: 4 500-milligram capsules twice a day
- Lemon balm: 3 dropperfuls twice a day
- Licorice root: 1 dropperful daily (two weeks on, two weeks off)
- Lomatium root: 1 dropperful daily
- Monolaurin: 1 capsule daily
- MSM: 1 capsule daily
- Nettle leaf: 2 dropperfuls twice a day
- Olive leaf: 1 dropperful daily
- Selenium: 1 capsule daily
- Spirulina: 2 teaspoons or 6 capsules daily

- Thyme: 2 sprigs of fresh thyme in hot water as tea or 4 sprigs in room temperature water daily
- Vitamin B$_{12}$ (as adenosylcobalamin with methylcobalamin): 1 dropperful twice a day
- Vitamin C (as Micro-C): 4 capsules twice a day
- Wild blueberry powder: 1 tablespoon daily
- Zinc (as liquid zinc sulfate): 1 dropperful twice a day

Tinnitus (Ringing, Vibrating, or Buzzing in the Ears) and Unexplained Hearing Loss

True cause: When decibel damage or injury to the ear have been ruled out, the cause here is one of the over 60 varieties of Epstein-Barr virus burrowing itself into the labyrinth of the inner ear, causing inflammation that's undetectable by current medical testing. The labyrinth swells, causing pitch to change when sounds enter the ear. When nerves are swollen inside the labyrinth, they can also vibrate and emit sounds such as ringing, buzzing, popping, and even fluttering.

- Celery juice: work up to 32 ounces daily, then work up to 64 ounces daily if possible
- Celeryforce: 1 capsule twice a day
- 5-MTHF: 1 capsule daily
- ALA (alpha lipoic acid): 1 capsule twice a week
- Barley grass juice powder: 2 teaspoons or 6 capsules daily
- Cat's claw: 2 dropperfuls twice a day
- Chaga mushroom: 2 teaspoons or 6 capsules daily
- Curcumin: 3 capsules twice a day
- Lemon balm: 4 dropperfuls twice a day

- **Licorice root:** 1 dropperful twice a day (two weeks on, two weeks off)
- **L-lysine:** 6 500-milligram capsules twice a day
- **Lomatium root:** 2 dropperfuls twice a day
- **Magnesium glycinate:** 1 capsule twice a day
- **Monolaurin:** 1 capsule daily
- **Mullein leaf:** 3 dropperfuls twice a day
- **Nettle leaf:** 3 dropperfuls twice a day
- **Olive leaf:** 1 dropperful twice a day
- **Oregano oil:** 1 capsule twice a day
- **Spirulina:** 2 teaspoons or 6 capsules daily
- **Vitamin B$_{12}$ (as adenosylcobalamin with methylcobalamin):** 3 dropperfuls twice a day
- **Vitamin C (as Micro-C):** 6 capsules twice a day
- **Wild blueberry powder:** 1 tablespoon daily
- **Zinc (as liquid zinc sulfate):** 2 dropperfuls twice a day

Tumors and Cysts (Benign—for cancerous varieties, see "Cancer")

True cause: Non-cancerous strains of viruses in the herpes family (including Epstein-Barr virus and HHV-6) feeding on toxic heavy metals and other toxins such as pesticides, herbicides, fungicides, plastics, other petrochemical byproducts, air fresheners, scented candles, perfumes, and colognes. When these particular viral strains feed on these aggressive toxins, they release toxic material through elimination that is very sticky and jelly-like. The waste byproduct clings to and suffocates adjacent living cells, keeping the cells from the critical life support provided by oxygen and nutrients, which causes them to denature, weaken, and die—all while the sticky byproduct blocks the dead cells from entering the bloodstream so the body can detoxify them.

Eventually, scar tissue forms around the damaged and dead cells, and that's the beginning of a benign cyst or tumor. The virus will stay alive inside of the cyst or tumor, and blood vessels will even form out of the growth to bring in more oxygen, nutrients, and other fuel to feed the virus in its core. This allows the virus to continue its cycle of producing more toxic materials, which allows the cyst or tumor to grow until the virus is addressed. A high-fat/high-protein diet can accelerate the growth of cysts and tumors. Also be cautious of troublemaker foods such as eggs, as tumors and cysts feed on eggs, which allows tumors and cysts to grow.

- **Fresh celery juice:** work up to 32 ounces daily, then work up to 64 ounces daily if possible
- **ALA (alpha lipoic acid):** 1 capsule daily
- **Amla berry:** 2 teaspoons daily
- **Ashwagandha:** 2 dropperfuls daily
- **Barley grass juice powder:** 1 tablespoon or 9 capsules daily
- **Burdock root:** 1 cup of tea or 1 root freshly juiced daily
- **Cat's claw:** 3 dropperfuls twice a day
- **Chaga mushroom:** 1 tablespoon or 9 capsules daily
- **CoQ10:** 2 capsules daily
- **Curcumin:** 2 capsules daily
- **EPA and DHA (fish-free):** 1 capsule daily (taken with dinner)
- **Glutathione:** 1 capsule daily
- **Hibiscus:** 1 cup of tea with 2 bags daily
- **Lemon balm:** 4 dropperfuls daily
- **Melatonin:** work up to 20 milligrams at bedtime daily
- **Nascent iodine:** 6 small drops (not dropperfuls) daily
- **Nettle leaf:** 2 dropperfuls daily
- **Raspberry leaf:** 1 cup of tea with 2 bags twice a day

- **Raw honey:** 2 teaspoons daily
- **Schisandra berry:** 1 cup of tea with 2 bags twice a day
- **Spirulina:** 2 teaspoons or 6 capsules daily
- **Vitamin B$_{12}$ (as adenosylcobalamin with methylcobalamin):** 1 dropperful daily
- **Vitamin C (as Micro-C):** 6 capsules twice a day
- **Vitamin D$_3$:** 2,000 IU daily
- **Wild blueberry powder:** 2 tablespoons daily
- **Zinc (as liquid zinc sulfate):** up to 2 dropperfuls daily

UTIs (Urinary Tract Infections), Bladder Infections, Yeast Infections, and Bacterial Vaginosis (BV)

True cause: One or more strains from the over 50 groups of *Streptococcus* bacteria either causing an acute infection for the first time or hiding inside the liver long term, creating one or more of these problems chronically. Strep often causes symptoms near menstruation, as your overall immune system lowers by roughly 80 percent—because that 80 percent goes toward protecting your uterus and ovaries. This is a natural, built-in phenomenon to ensure life here on earth continues safely. Often when the uterus sheds its lining, it's trying to eliminate pathogens and other toxins that your immune system needs to be present for to help protect you. And at ovulation, your reproductive immune system strengthens to protect your ovaries, which means that your overall immune system lowers by about 40 percent, leaving the rest of your body more vulnerable to conditions and infections. So near menstruation and ovulation, when your body's overall immune system is lower, strep tends to reveal itself as a bladder infection or other UTI. While yeast may be present in yeast infections, the discomfort is caused by strep bacteria, and

this is most often missed at the doctor's office. Hormones are not the cause of acne near menstruation. Instead, it's this lowering of the overall immune system that allows the strep bacteria that cause acne to take advantage. Try to avoid troublemaker foods such as eggs. Also be aware that a high-fat/high-protein diet can worsen any of these conditions.

- **Fresh celery juice:** work up to 32 ounces daily
- **Aloe vera:** 2 or more inches of fresh gel (skin removed) daily
- **Amla berry:** 2 teaspoons twice a day
- **Barley grass juice powder:** 2 teaspoons or 6 capsules daily
- **Cat's claw:** 3 dropperfuls twice a day
- **Chaga mushroom:** 2 teaspoons or 6 capsules daily
- **D-mannose:** 1 tablespoon powder in water four times a day
- **Goldenseal:** 4 dropperfuls twice a day (two weeks on, two weeks off)
- **Hibiscus:** 2 cups of tea daily
- **Lemon balm:** 4 dropperfuls twice a day
- **Lomatium root:** 2 dropperfuls twice a day
- **Mullein leaf:** 3 dropperfuls twice a day
- **Olive leaf:** 2 dropperfuls twice a day
- **Oregon grape root:** 1 dropperful twice a day (two weeks on, two weeks off)
- **Raw honey:** 1 tablespoon daily
- **Rose hips:** 2 cups of tea daily
- **Thyme:** 2 sprigs of fresh thyme in hot water as tea or 4 sprigs in room temperature water twice a day
- **Vitamin C (as Micro-C):** after optional Medical Medium Vitamin C Shock Therapy, 6 capsules twice a day
- **Zinc (as liquid zinc sulfate):** after optional Medical Medium Zinc Shock Therapy for two days, up to 2 dropperfuls twice a day

Varicose and Spider Veins

True cause: A sluggish, stagnant liver toxic from a variety of poisons including toxic heavy metals, solvents, everyday conventional household cleaners, scented candles, air fresheners, colognes, perfumes, plastics and other petrochemical byproducts, and old pharmaceuticals. Varicose and spider veins are often accompanied by breast density (in both women and men), weight gain, and eventually blood sugar, cholesterol, and blood sugar issues, as a sluggish, stagnant liver is also behind these symptoms and conditions. High-fat/high-protein diets accelerate growth of varicose and spider veins.

- **Fresh celery juice:** work up to 32 ounces daily
- **ALA (alpha lipoic acid):** 1 capsule daily
- **Barley grass juice powder:** 2 teaspoons or 6 capsules daily
- **Burdock root:** 1 cup of tea or 1 root freshly juiced daily
- **Curcumin:** 2 capsules twice a day
- **Dandelion root:** 1 cup of tea daily
- **EPA and DHA (fish-free):** 1 capsule daily (taken with dinner)
- **Lemon balm:** 2 dropperfuls daily
- **Milk thistle:** 1 dropperful daily
- **MSM:** 2 capsules daily
- **Nettle leaf:** 2 dropperfuls daily
- **Red clover:** 1 cup of tea daily
- **Schisandra berry:** 1 cup of tea daily
- **Spirulina:** 2 teaspoons or 6 capsules daily
- **Vitamin B$_{12}$ (as adenosylcobalamin with methylcobalamin):** 1 dropperful daily
- **Vitamin C (as Micro-C):** 4 capsules daily
- **Wild blueberry powder:** 1 tablespoon daily

Vertigo & Ménière's Disease

True cause: Vertigo is caused by one or more of the over 60 varieties of Epstein-Barr virus releasing neurotoxins that adhere to the vagus nerve, inflaming and irritating it. This causes a range of symptoms, including dizziness or the feeling that you're on a moving boat, since the vagus nerve is mainly responsible for equilibrium.

With Ménière's, the theoretical belief that calcium crystals and stones cause this disease is inaccurate. In truth, Ménière's is neurological, caused by a low-grade viral infection affecting the vagus nerves and nerves inside the inner ear.

- **Fresh celery juice:** work up to 32 ounces daily
- **Celeryforce:** 2 capsules twice a day
- **Barley grass juice powder:** 2 teaspoons or 6 capsules daily
- **B-complex:** 1 capsule daily
- **Cat's claw:** 2 dropperfuls twice a day
- **Chaga mushroom:** 2 teaspoons or 6 capsules daily
- **Curcumin:** 2 capsules twice a day
- **EPA and DHA (fish-free):** 1 capsule daily (taken with dinner)
- **Eyebright:** 1 dropperful daily
- **Lemon balm:** 3 dropperfuls three times a day
- **L-glutamine:** 1 capsule daily
- **Licorice root:** 1 dropperful daily (two weeks on, two weeks off)
- **L-lysine:** 5 500-milligram capsules twice a day
- **Lomatium root:** 2 dropperfuls twice a day
- **Magnesium glycinate:** 1 capsule daily
- **Monolaurin:** 1 capsule daily
- **Mullein leaf:** 3 dropperfuls twice a day
- **Olive leaf:** 1 dropperful twice a day
- **Spirulina:** 2 teaspoons or 6 capsules daily
- **Vitamin B$_{12}$ (as adenosylcobalamin with methylcobalamin):** 2 dropperfuls twice a day

- **Vitamin C (as Micro-C):** 4 capsules twice a day
- **Wild blueberry powder:** 2 teaspoons daily
- **Zinc (as liquid zinc sulfate):** 2 dropperfuls twice a day

- **Vitamin C (as Micro-C):** 6 capsules daily
- **Wild blueberry powder:** 2 tablespoons daily
- **Zinc (as liquid zinc sulfate):** up to 1 dropperful daily

Weight Gain

True cause: Often mistaken for the theory of slow metabolism, the true cause of mystery weight gain is usually a sluggish, stagnant liver overburdened from a diet too high in fat/protein combined with toxins such as toxic heavy metals, pesticides, herbicides, plastics and other petro-chemical byproducts, solvents, old pharmaceuticals, air fresheners, scented candles, colognes, and perfumes. Low-grade viral and bacterial infections inside the liver can also be a factor, causing someone to over-exercise to constantly battle pounds adding up on the scale. For more, refer to the weight section in Chapter 20, "Your Body's Healing Power."

- **Fresh celery juice:** work up to 32 ounces daily
- **5-MTHF:** 1 capsule daily
- **Aloe vera:** 2 or more inches of fresh gel (skin removed) daily
- **Ashwagandha:** 1 dropperful daily
- **Barley grass juice powder:** 2 teaspoons or 6 capsules daily
- **Chaga mushroom:** 2 teaspoons or 6 capsules daily
- **Lemon balm:** 2 dropperfuls daily
- **Milk thistle:** 1 dropperful daily
- **Nascent iodine:** 3 small drops (not dropperfuls) daily
- **Nettle leaf:** 2 dropperfuls daily
- **Raspberry leaf:** 1 cup of tea with 2 bags daily
- **Schisandra berry:** 1 cup of tea daily
- **Spirulina:** 2 teaspoons or 6 capsules daily
- **Vitamin B$_{12}$ (as adenosylcobalamin with methylcobalamin):** 1 dropperful daily

Worms and Parasites

True cause: Consuming raw fish, shellfish, meat, poultry, or pork; food or dishware accidentally contaminated by their raw juices; other contaminated food that hasn't been heated enough; or a contaminated water-based beverage.

- **Fresh celery juice:** work up to 32 ounces twice a day
- **Barley grass juice powder:** 2 teaspoons or 6 capsules daily
- **Black walnut:** 1 dropperful twice a day
- **Burdock root:** 1 cup of tea or 1 root freshly juiced twice a day
- **Cat's claw:** 4 dropperfuls twice a day
- **Chaga mushroom:** 2 teaspoons or 6 capsules twice a day
- **Dandelion root:** 1 cup of tea twice a day
- **Eyebright:** 2 dropperfuls twice a day
- **Ginger:** 1 tablespoon freshly grated into room temperature or hot water daily
- **Lemon balm:** 5 dropperfuls twice a day
- **Olive leaf:** 4 dropperfuls twice a day
- **Oregano oil:** 3 capsules twice a day
- **Oregon grape root:** 3 dropperfuls twice a day (two weeks on/two weeks off)
- **Rosemary:** 2 sprigs fresh rosemary in hot water as tea or 4 sprigs in room temperature water daily
- **Spirulina:** 2 teaspoons or 6 capsules daily
- **Thyme:** 2 sprigs of fresh thyme in hot water as tea or 4 sprigs in room temperature water twice a day
- **Wild blueberry powder:** 2 tablespoons daily
- **Yellow dock:** 1 cup of tea twice a day

INDEX

Note: Page numbers in *italics* indicate recipes;
page numbers in **bold** indicate the true cause of conditions and symptoms with
dosages to heal. Parentheses around page numbers indicate intermittent references.

ACKNOWLEDGMENTS

Thank you to Patty Gift, Anne Barthel, Reid Tracy, Margarete Nielsen, Diane Hill, everyone at Hay House Radio, and the rest of the Hay House team for your faith and commitment to getting Spirit of Compassion's wisdom out into the world so it can continue to change lives.

Hilary Swank and Philip Schneider, your dedication to the healing truth and wisdom is remarkable, and I am deeply honored. Your support is immensely powerful.

Helen Lasichanh and Pharrell Williams, you are extraordinarily kind-hearted seers.

Sylvester Stallone, Jennifer Flavin Stallone, and family, your support has been legendarily game-changing.

Kate Hudson, Danny Fujikawa, Erinn and Oliver Hudson, and Elisabeth Stassen, having you guys on my side with your love and support is a blessing.

Miranda Kerr and Evan Spiegel, it's so amazing to have your hands of light and compassion behind the healing movement.

Laura Dern, thank you for spreading your light and changing the world for the better.

Novak and Jelena Djokovic, you are pioneers in advancing health and teaching the world how to thrive.

Gwyneth Paltrow, Elise Loehnen, and your devoted GOOP crew, your caring and generosity are a profound inspiration.

Sage and Tony Robbins, it's an honor to be part of your world that's helping so many.

Martin, Jean, Elizabeth, and Jacqueline Shafiroff, thank you for always being there, believing in me, and helping to spread the message so that others can heal.

Dr. Alejandro Junger, life would not be the same without you, brother.

Dr. Ilana Zablozki-Amir, your willingness to support the Medical Medium cause is epic.

Dr. Christiane Northrup, your inexhaustible devotion to the health of womankind has become its own star in the universe.

Dr. Prudence Hall, your selfless work to enlighten patients who need answers renews the true, heroic meaning of the word *doctor*.

Craig Kallman, thank you for your support, advocacy, and friendship on this journey.

Caroline Fleming, you're truly a blessing because you have the gift to always care about everyone around you as you share your light.

Chelsea Field and Scott, Wil, and Owen Bakula, how did I get so blessed to have you in my life? You are true crusaders for the Medical Medium cause.

Kimberly and James Van Der Beek, there's a special place in my heart for you and your family. I'm truly thankful to have crossed paths with you in this lifetime.

Kerri Walsh Jennings, you truly amaze me with your hopeful nature and endless positive energy.

John Donovan, it's an honor to be on the planet with such a peace-seeking soul.

Nanci Chambers and David James, Stephanie, and Wyatt Elliott, I can't thank you enough for your dear friendship and everlasting encouragement.

Suze Orman and KT, your determination and commitment are exceptional.

Lisa Gregorisch-Dempsey, your acts of kindness have been deeply meaningful.

Grace Hightower De Niro, Robert De Niro, and family, you are precious, gracious beings.

Liv Tyler, it's such a great honor to be a part of your world.

Jenna Dewan, your fighting spirit is an inspiration to behold.

Debra Messing, you are bettering people's lives with your vision for a healthy planet.

Alexis Bledel, your strength in this world is extraordinarily heartening.

Lisa Rinna, thank you for tirelessly using your influence to spread the message.

Jennifer Aniston, your kindness, caring, and support are on another level.

Taylor Schilling, what a joy to know you and have your support.

Marcela Valladolid, knowing you is a gift in my life.

Kelly Noonan and Alec Gores, thank you for always looking out for me. It means so much.

Jennifer Meyer, I'm beyond grateful for your friendship and how you're always spreading the word.

Calvin Harris, you've changed the world with a powerful rhythm.

Courteney Cox, thank you for having such a pure, loving heart.

Hunter Mahan and Kandi Harris, I'm proud of you for always being game to take on a challenge.

Kidada Jones and Rashida Jones, the deep care and compassion you bring to life mean more than you know. Your mother was a treasure who lives on in you.

Andrew Kusatsu: love you, brother, for persevering past the pain and fighting for health freedom.

To the following special souls whose loyalty I treasure, my thanks go out: Naomi Campbell; Eva Longoria; Lewis Howes; Carla Gugino; Mario Lopez; Renee Bargh; Tanika Ray; Maria Menounos; Michael Bernard Beckwith; Jay Shetty; Alex Kushneir; LeAnn Rimes Cibrian; Hana Hollinger; Sharon Levin; Nena, Robert, and Uma Thurman; Jenny Mollen; Jessica Seinfeld; Kelly Osbourne; Demi Moore; Kyle Richards; India.Arie; Kristen Bower; Rozonda Thomas; Peggy Rometo; Debbie Gibson; Carol, Scott, and Christiana Ritchie; Jamie-Lynn Sigler; Amanda de Cadenet; Marianne Williamson; Erin Johnson; Gabrielle Bernstein; Sophia Bush; Maha Dakhil; Bhavani Lev and Bharat Mitra; Woody Fraser, Milena Monrroy, Midge Hussey, and everyone at Hallmark's Home & Family; Morgan Fairchild; Patti Stanger; Catherine, Sophia, and Laura Bach; Annabeth Gish; Robert Wisdom; Danielle LaPorte; Nick and Brenna Ortner; Jessica Ortner; Mike Dooley; Kris Carr; Kate Northrup; Ann Louise Gittleman; Jan and Panache Desai; Ami Beach and Mark Shadle; Brian Wilson; John Holland; Jill Black Zalben; Alexandra Cohen; Christine Hill; Carol Donahue; Caroline Leavitt; Michael Sandler and Jessica Lee; Koya Webb; Jenny Hutt; Adam Cushman; Sonia Choquette; Colette Baron-Reid; Denise Linn; and Carmel Joy Baird. I deeply value you all.

To the compassionate doctors and other healers of the world who have changed the lives of so many: I have tremendous respect for you. Dr. Masha Kogan, Dr. Virginia Romano, Dr. Habib Sadeghi, Dr. Carol Lee, Dr. Richard Sollazzo, Dr. Jeff Feinman, Dr. Deanna Minich, Dr. Ron Steriti,

Dr. Nicole Galante, Dr. Diana Lopusny, Dr. Dick and Noel Shepard, Dr. Aleksandra Phillips, Dr. Chris Maloney, Drs. Tosca and Gregory Haag, Dr. Dave Klein, Dr. Deborah Kern, Dr. Darren and Suzanne Boles, and Dr. Robin Karlin—it's an honor to call you friends. Thank you for your endless dedication to the field of healing.

Thanks to David Schmerler, Kimberly S. Grimsley, and Susan G. Etheridge for being there for me.

A very warm, heartfelt thanks to Muneeza Ahmed; Kimberly Spair; Amber Stone; Lauren Henry; Tara Tom; Bella; Gretchen Manzer; Victoria and Michael Arnstein; Nina Leatherer; Michelle Sutton; Haily Cataldo; Kerry; Amy Bacheller; Michael McMenamin; Alexandra Laws; Ester Horn; Linda and Robert Coykendall; Setareh Khatibi; Heather Coleman; Glenn Klausner; Carolyn DeVito; Michael Monteleone; Bobbi and Leslie Hall; Katherine Belzowski; Matt and Vanessa Houston; David, Holly, and Ginnie Whitney; Melody Lee Pence; Terra Appelman; Eileen Crispell; Kristin Cassidy; Calvin Stebbins; Catherine Lawton; Taylor Call; Alana DiNardo; Min Lee; and Eden Epstein Hill.

Thank you to the countless people, including those in the Medical Medium communities, whom I've had the privilege and honor of seeing blossom, heal, and transform.

Sally Arnold, thank you for shining your light so brightly and lending your voice to the movement.

Ruby Scattergood, your masterful patience and countless hours of dedication have heroically formed the true spine of this book. The Medical Medium series would not be possible without your writing and editing. Thank you for your literary counsel.

Vibodha and Tila Clark, your creative genius has been astoundingly instrumental to the cause of helping others. Thank you for standing with us throughout the years.

Friar and Clare: *And God said, Let the earth bring forth grass, the herb yielding seed, and the fruit tree yielding fruit after his kind, whose seed is in itself, upon the earth: and it was so . . . And God said, Behold, I have given you every herb bearing seed, which is upon the face of all the earth, and every tree, in the which is the fruit of a tree yielding seed; to you it shall be for meat* (Gen. 1:11; 1:29).

Quincy: Thank you for your invaluable support and hard work.

Sepideh Kashanian and Ben, thank you for your warm, loving care.

Jeff Skeirik, thank you for the best pictures, man.

Jon Morelli and Noah, you two are all heart.

Robby Barbaro, your unwavering positivity lifts up everyone around you.

For your love and support, as always, I thank my family: my luminous wife; Dad and Mom; my brothers, nieces, nephews, aunts, and uncles; my champions Indigo, Ruby, and Great Blue; Hope; Marjorie and Robert; Laura; Rhia and Byron; Alayne Serle and Scott, Perri, Lissy, and Ari Cohn; David Somoroff; Joel, Liz, Kody, Jesse, Lauren, Joseph, and Thomas; Brian, Joyce, and Josh; Jarod; Brent; Kelly and Evy; Danielle, Johnny, and Declan; and all my loved ones who are on the other side.

Finally, thank you, Spirit of the Most High (a.k.a. Spirit of Compassion), for providing all of us with compassionate wisdom from the heavens that inspires us to keep our heads up and carry the sacred gifts you've been so kind to give us. Thank you for putting up with me over the years and reminding me to keep a light heart with your never-ending patience and willingness to answer my questions in search of the truth.

CONVERSION CHARTS

The recipes in this book use the standard United States method for measuring liquid and dry or solid ingredients (teaspoons, tablespoons, and cups). The following charts are provided to help cooks outside the U.S. successfully use these recipes. All equivalents are approximate.

Standard Cup	Fine Powder (e.g., flour)	Grain (e.g., rice)	Granular (e.g., sugar)	Liquid Solids (e.g., butter)	Liquid (e.g., milk)
1	140 g	150 g	190 g	200 g	240 ml
¾	105 g	113 g	143 g	150 g	180 ml
⅔	93 g	100 g	125 g	133 g	160 ml
½	70 g	75 g	95 g	100 g	120 ml
⅓	47 g	50 g	63 g	67 g	80 ml
¼	35 g	38 g	48 g	50 g	60 ml
⅛	18 g	19 g	24 g	25 g	30 ml

Useful Equivalents for Liquid Ingredients by Volume					
¼ tsp				1 ml	
½ tsp				2 ml	
1 tsp				5 ml	
3 tsp	1 tbsp		½ fl oz	15 ml	
	2 tbsp	⅛ cup	1 fl oz	30 ml	
	4 tbsp	¼ cup	2 fl oz	60 ml	
	5⅓ tbsp	⅓ cup	3 fl oz	80 ml	
	8 tbsp	½ cup	4 fl oz	120 ml	
	10⅔ tbsp	⅔ cup	5 fl oz	160 ml	
	12 tbsp	¾ cup	6 fl oz	180 ml	
	16 tbsp	1 cup	8 fl oz	240 ml	
	1 pt	2 cups	16 fl oz	480 ml	
	1 qt	4 cups	32 fl oz	960 ml	
			33 fl oz	1000 ml	1 l

Useful Equivalents for Dry Ingredients by Weight		
(TO CONVERT OUNCES TO GRAMS, MULTIPLY THE NUMBER OF OUNCES BY 30.)		
1 oz	1/16 lb	30 g
4 oz	1/4 lb	120 g
8 oz	1/2 lb	240 g
12 oz	3/4 lb	360 g
16 oz	1 lb	480 g

Useful Equivalents for Cooking/Oven Temperatures			
PROCESS	FAHRENHEIT	CELSIUS	GAS MARK
Freeze Water	32° F	0° C	
Room Temperature	68° F	20° C	
Boil Water	212° F	100° C	
Bake	325° F	160° C	3
	350° F	180° C	4
	375° F	190° C	5
	400° F	200° C	6
	425° F	220° C	7
	450° F	230° C	8
Broil			Grill

Useful Equivalents for Length				
(TO CONVERT INCHES TO CENTIMETERS, MULTIPLY THE NUMBER OF INCHES BY 2.5.)				
1 in			2.5 cm	
6 in	1/2 ft		15 cm	
12 in	1 ft		30 cm	
36 in	3 ft	1 yd	90 cm	
40 in			100 cm	1 m

ABOUT THE AUTHOR

Anthony William, the originator of the global celery juice movement and #1 *New York Times* best-selling author of *Medical Medium Celery Juice: The Most Powerful Medicine of Our Time Healing Millions Worldwide*; *Medical Medium Liver Rescue: Answers to Eczema, Psoriasis, Diabetes, Strep, Acne, Gout, Bloating, Gallstones, Adrenal Stress, Fatigue, Fatty Liver, Weight Issues, SIBO & Autoimmune Disease*; *Medical Medium Thyroid Healing: The Truth behind Hashimoto's, Graves', Insomnia, Hypothyroidism, Thyroid Nodules & Epstein-Barr*; *Medical Medium Life-Changing Foods: Save Yourself and the Ones You Love with the Hidden Healing Powers of Fruits & Vegetables*; and *Medical Medium: Secrets Behind Chronic and Mystery Illness and How to Finally Heal*, was born with the unique ability to converse with the Spirit of Compassion, who provides him with extraordinarily advanced healing medical information that's far ahead of its time. Since age four, Anthony has been using his gift to "read" people's conditions and tell them how to recover their health. His unprecedented accuracy and success rate as the Medical Medium have earned him the trust and love of millions worldwide, among them movie stars, rock stars, billionaires, professional athletes, and countless other people from all walks of life who couldn't find a way to heal until he provided them with insights from above. Over the decades, Anthony has also been an invaluable resource to doctors who need help solving their most difficult cases.

Learn more at www.medicalmedium.com